Monoclonal Antibodies and Their Functional Fragments in Research, Diagnosis and Therapy

Monoclonal Antibodies and Their Functional Fragments in Research, Diagnosis and Therapy

Editor

Menotti Ruvo

MDPI • Basel • Beijing • Wuhan • Barcelona • Belgrade • Manchester • Tokyo • Cluj • Tianjin

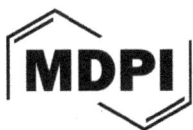

Editor
Menotti Ruvo
Institute of Biostructure and
Bioimaging
National Research Council
Napoli
Italy

Editorial Office
MDPI
St. Alban-Anlage 66
4052 Basel, Switzerland

This is a reprint of articles from the Special Issue published online in the open access journal *International Journal of Molecular Sciences* (ISSN 1422-0067) (available at: www.mdpi.com/journal/ijms/special_issues/mabs).

For citation purposes, cite each article independently as indicated on the article page online and as indicated below:

LastName, A.A.; LastName, B.B.; LastName, C.C. Article Title. *Journal Name* **Year**, *Volume Number*, Page Range.

ISBN 978-3-0365-3167-0 (Hbk)
ISBN 978-3-0365-3166-3 (PDF)

© 2022 by the authors. Articles in this book are Open Access and distributed under the Creative Commons Attribution (CC BY) license, which allows users to download, copy and build upon published articles, as long as the author and publisher are properly credited, which ensures maximum dissemination and a wider impact of our publications.

The book as a whole is distributed by MDPI under the terms and conditions of the Creative Commons license CC BY-NC-ND.

Contents

About the Editor vii

Preface to "Monoclonal Antibodies and Their Functional Fragments in Research, Diagnosis and Therapy" ix

André L. B. Bitencourt, Raquel M. Campos, Erika N. Cline, William L. Klein and Adriano Sebollela
Antibody Fragments as Tools for Elucidating Structure-Toxicity Relationships and for Diagnostic/Therapeutic Targeting of Neurotoxic Amyloid Oligomers
Reprinted from: *Int. J. Mol. Sci.* **2020**, *21*, 8920, doi:10.3390/ijms21238920 1

Manali S. Sawant, Craig N. Streu, Lina Wu and Peter M. Tessier
Toward Drug-Like Multispecific Antibodies by Design
Reprinted from: *Int. J. Mol. Sci.* **2020**, *21*, 7496, doi:10.3390/ijms21207496 19

Ashley R. Sutherland, Madeline N. Owens and C. Ronald Geyer
Modular Chimeric Antigen Receptor Systems for Universal CAR T Cell Retargeting
Reprinted from: *Int. J. Mol. Sci.* **2020**, *21*, 7222, doi:10.3390/ijms21197222 61

Julie Pelletier, Hervé Agonsanou, Fabiana Manica, Elise G. Lavoie, Mabrouka Salem and Patrick Luyindula et al.
A Simple and Efficient Genetic Immunization Protocol for the Production of Highly Specific Polyclonal and Monoclonal Antibodies against the Native Form of Mammalian Proteins
Reprinted from: *Int. J. Mol. Sci.* **2020**, *21*, 7074, doi:10.3390/ijms21197074 75

Zora Novakova, Nikola Belousova, Catherine A. Foss, Barbora Havlinova, Marketa Gresova and Gargi Das et al.
Engineered Fragments of the PSMA-Specific 5D3 Antibody and Their Functional Characterization
Reprinted from: *Int. J. Mol. Sci.* **2020**, *21*, 6672, doi:10.3390/ijms21186672 91

Kyungjae Kang, Kicheon Kim, Se-Ra Lee, Yoonji Kim, Joo Eon Lee and Yong Sun Lee et al.
Selection and Characterization of YKL-40-Targeting Monoclonal Antibodies from Human Synthetic Fab Phage Display Libraries
Reprinted from: *Int. J. Mol. Sci.* **2020**, *21*, 6354, doi:10.3390/ijms21176354 113

Annamaria Sandomenico, Jwala P. Sivaccumar and Menotti Ruvo
Evolution of *Escherichia coli* Expression System in Producing Antibody Recombinant Fragments
Reprinted from: *Int. J. Mol. Sci.* **2020**, *21*, 6324, doi:10.3390/ijms21176324 131

Sara Ponziani, Giulia Di Vittorio, Giuseppina Pitari, Anna Maria Cimini, Matteo Ardini and Roberta Gentile et al.
Antibody-Drug Conjugates: The New Frontier of Chemotherapy
Reprinted from: *Int. J. Mol. Sci.* **2020**, *21*, 5510, doi:10.3390/ijms21155510 171

Hanley N. Abramson
B-Cell Maturation Antigen (BCMA) as a Target for New Drug Development in Relapsed and/or Refractory Multiple Myeloma
Reprinted from: *Int. J. Mol. Sci.* **2020**, *21*, 5192, doi:10.3390/ijms21155192 197

Dario Roccatello, Roberta Fenoglio, Savino Sciascia, Carla Naretto, Daniela Rossi and Michela Ferro et al.
CD38 and Anti-CD38 Monoclonal Antibodies in AL Amyloidosis: Targeting Plasma Cells and beyond
Reprinted from: *Int. J. Mol. Sci.* **2020**, *21*, 4129, doi:10.3390/ijms21114129 . . . . **223**

Sebastian W. Meister, Linnea C. Hjelm, Melanie Dannemeyer, Hanna Tegel, Hanna Lindberg and Stefan Ståhl et al.
An Affibody Molecule Is Actively Transported into the Cerebrospinal Fluid via Binding to the Transferrin Receptor
Reprinted from: *Int. J. Mol. Sci.* **2020**, *21*, 2999, doi:10.3390/ijms21082999 . . . . **235**

Jiayu Fu, Rui Chen, Jingfei Hu, Huan Qu, Yujia Zhao and Sanjie Cao et al.
Identification of a Novel Linear B-Cell Epitope on the Nucleocapsid Protein of Porcine Deltacoronavirus
Reprinted from: *Int. J. Mol. Sci.* **2020**, *21*, 648, doi:10.3390/ijms21020648 . . . . **249**

About the Editor

Menotti Ruvo

Dr. Ruvo graduated in Chemistry at the University of Naples in 1991. During the first 10 years of his career, he worked in industry, as a researcher in charge of the protein and peptide laboratory and contributing to the development of several bioactive molecules. In 2002, he joined the Institute of Biostructure and Bioimaging of the National Research Council (IBB-CNR) in Naples, Italy, leading several projects focused on the development of novel bioactive peptides and monoclonal antibodies against therapeutically relevant targets. Among others, he has developed peptides modulating the activity of PlGF, Cripto and Gadd45beta and monoclonal antibodies against Nodal, HCV E2 protein, Cripto, Ape1 and PRAME. He was one of the founders of Kesios Therapeutics Ltd (London) and Anbition (Naples). He is the author of about 170 papers and inventor of >30 patents.

Preface to "Monoclonal Antibodies and Their Functional Fragments in Research, Diagnosis and Therapy"

Monoclonal antibodies ($mAbs$) are among the most specialized molecules for the recognition and capture of specific analytes. Hundreds of thousands of $mAbs$ have been generated, targeting a large number of different antigens with ever-increasing affinity and specificity, and are available for diverse purposes. Many of them have been validated as irreplaceable agents for diagnosis and therapy or as unique reagents for research. Others are being developed using a plethora of emerging technologies that provide new molecular tools to overcome the need for animal immunization. This Special Issue has strived to collect prospective visions and to survey new strategic assets adopted by the main research groups engaged in this field, focusing in particular on the generation of new monoclonal or surrogate antibodies, such as Fab, Fab2, ScFv and nanobodies, which have an increasing impact in biomedicine as therapeutic or diagnostic assets in various diseases.

Menotti Ruvo
Editor

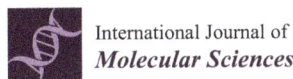

Review

Antibody Fragments as Tools for Elucidating Structure-Toxicity Relationships and for Diagnostic/Therapeutic Targeting of Neurotoxic Amyloid Oligomers

André L. B. Bitencourt [1,†], Raquel M. Campos [1,†], Erika N. Cline [2], William L. Klein [2] and Adriano Sebollela [1,*]

1. Department of Biochemistry and Immunology, Ribeirao Preto Medical School, University of São Paulo, Ribeirão Preto, SP 14049-900, Brazil; brandaobqi@hotmail.com (A.L.B.B.); raquelmariacampos@usp.br (R.M.C.)
2. Department of Neurobiology, Northwestern University, Evanston, IL 60208-3520, USA; erika.cline@northwestern.edu (E.N.C.); wklein@northwestern.edu (W.L.K.)
* Correspondence: sebollela@fmrp.usp.br; Tel.: +55-16-3315-3109
† These authors contributed equally to this work.

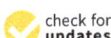

Received: 9 September 2020; Accepted: 1 October 2020; Published: 24 November 2020

Abstract: The accumulation of amyloid protein aggregates in tissues is the basis for the onset of diseases known as amyloidoses. Intriguingly, many amyloidoses impact the central nervous system (CNS) and usually are devastating diseases. It is increasingly apparent that neurotoxic soluble oligomers formed by amyloidogenic proteins are the primary molecular drivers of these diseases, making them lucrative diagnostic and therapeutic targets. One promising diagnostic/therapeutic strategy has been the development of antibody fragments against amyloid oligomers. Antibody fragments, such as fragment antigen-binding (Fab), scFv (single chain variable fragments), and VHH (heavy chain variable domain or single-domain antibodies) are an alternative to full-length IgGs as diagnostics and therapeutics for a variety of diseases, mainly because of their increased tissue penetration (lower MW compared to IgG), decreased inflammatory potential (lack of Fc domain), and facile production (low structural complexity). Furthermore, through the use of in vitro-based ligand selection, it has been possible to identify antibody fragments presenting marked conformational selectivity. In this review, we summarize significant reports on antibody fragments selective for oligomers associated with prevalent CNS amyloidoses. We discuss promising results obtained using antibody fragments as both diagnostic and therapeutic agents against these diseases. In addition, the use of antibody fragments, particularly scFv and VHH, in the isolation of unique oligomeric assemblies is discussed as a strategy to unravel conformational moieties responsible for neurotoxicity. We envision that advances in this field may lead to the development of novel oligomer-selective antibody fragments with superior selectivity and, hopefully, good clinical outcomes.

Keywords: antibody fragments; single chain; amyloid; oligomer; neurotoxicity; NUsc1

1. Toxic Protein Oligomers in Central Nervous System Diseases

In living systems, proteins must assume and maintain a three-dimensional conformation, which dictates their biological functions. Under certain conditions, however, monomeric protein units may self-associate to form oligomeric structures that display both loss of biological, and gain of toxic, function [1]. Ultimately, these oligomers have the potential to aggregate into insoluble amyloid fibrils, highly stable non-branched insoluble structures rich in β-sheet content [2–4]. Although this property is inherent to all proteins [5–7], a number of amyloidogenic proteins accumulate in tissues, causing diseases known as amyloidoses, which can be systemic but commonly impact the central nervous system (CNS) [1,8–11].

It is now evident that soluble oligomers are the most toxic form of amyloidogenic proteins, more so than their monomeric or fibrillar forms, disrupting, e.g., synaptic function, membrane permeability, calcium homeostasis, gene transcription, mitochondrial activity, autophagy, and/or endosomal transport in an array of disease models [12–15]. The first reports on the brain accumulation of toxic soluble oligomers were in Alzheimer's disease (AD); the associated oligomers mainly composed of the 4.5 kDa amyloid β (Aβ) peptide [16–18]. Since then, toxic soluble oligomers of other proteins have been implicated in the onset and progression of several debilitating CNS diseases, e.g., tau, α-synuclein, the prion protein (PrP^c), and huntingtin protein (htt) in Alzheimer's, Parkinson's, prion, and Huntington's diseases, respectively [19–24]. In fact, many of these protein oligomers are found together in multiple diseases [25,26].

Amyloidogenic oligomers have been frequently implicated as promising diagnostic and therapeutic targets for CNS amyloidoses [12,14,27–33]. Despite their disease relevance, the structural hallmarks of such soluble oligomers remain elusive due to their metastability and heterogeneity, hampering our ability to target them therapeutically and diagnostically [12,34–36]. One promising strategy in the structural analysis of amyloidogenic oligomers is the utilization of antibody fragments, which can achieve high conformational selectivity, enabling the isolation and stabilization of different oligomeric species. Furthermore, the structural properties of the antibody fragments themselves make them promising diagnostic/therapeutic tools. In this review, we discuss their application as tools for structural research and diagnostic/therapeutic targeting of oligomers acting in brain amyloidoses.

2. Antibody Fragments

Monoclonal antibodies (mAbs) are currently the largest, and most rapidly growing, class of biopharmaceuticals on the market to treat a variety of diseases [37,38]. However, only four mAbs have been approved to treat a neurodegenerative disease (multiple sclerosis), and these antibodies are thought to work primarily in the periphery [37]. There are a number of challenges in utilizing monoclonal antibodies for the diagnosis or treatment of brain diseases. For one, their large molecular mass hinders their ability to cross the blood–brain barrier [38,39]. Moreover, the crystallizable fraction (Fc) of mAbs can mediate deleterious inflammatory responses resulting in, e.g., meningoencephalitis, vasogenic edema, cerebral microhemorragies, and even death [40–47]. Regarding diagnostics, poor contrast of mAbs in imaging applications due to a long serum half-life has been reported as a drawback [48].

During the past 20 years, antibody fragments have been developed as an alternative to full-length IgGs for the diagnosis and treatment of a variety of diseases, including brain disorders [13,38,39,47,49–52]. These molecules are simple protein motifs of large diversity that include the IgG antigen-binding domain(s) but lack the inflammatory Fc domain, retaining the total (fragment antigen-binding: Fab and single-chain variable fragment: scFv) or partial (VH) antigen specificity of intact IgGs [38,39,52].

Compared to full-length IgGs, antibody fragments have advantages and disadvantages as therapeutics. An important advantage is their smaller size (12–50 kDa), thought to potentiate the blood–brain barrier crossing and tissue penetration and enable access to challenging, cryptic epitopes [38,39,52]. Furthermore, their fast blood clearance makes them ideal imaging agents [39]. On the other hand, their smaller size leads to a shorter half-life in vivo, in part due to rapid kidney clearance, which limits the chance of target engagement without the addition of half-life extension moieties (e.g., PEG and albumin-binding fragments) [38,44]. Another advantage of antibody fragments, is their lack of the inflammatory Fc domain (see discussion above). On the other hand, it is noteworthy that the lack of Fc-dependent activation of immune cells may reduce the efficiency of an immunotherapy when a robust inflammatory response is required [53,54], as in cancer immunotherapy, which requires T cell recruiting [55].

Another advantage of antibody fragments, is their excellent manufacturability and low cost of production [38,39]. They can be efficiently selected from in vitro display libraries (phage or yeast) and cloned and expressed in heterologous expression systems (e.g., bacteria); this facilitates the production of large quantities in an easy and affordable way. Importantly, the in vitro approach eliminates animal immunization, which may be key when the conformation of the immunogen plays a role in antibody specificity [46,56]. Finally, engineered antibody fragments yielding multimers (diabodies, triabodies, and tetrabodies) have been shown to present higher avidity and lower blood clearance than their monomeric counterparts without compromising tissue penetration abilities [38,48,54].

The main types of antibody fragments under development are Fab, scFv (single chain variable fragments), and heavy chain variable domain VH/VHH (single-domain antibodies) fragments [38,39,49,52,57]. The potential of isolated light chain variable domain (VL) chains has not been significantly investigated due to their low stability [56]. An overview of the structures of these molecules is presented in Figure 1. The first artificial antibody fragments reported in the literature were initially obtained by removing the Fc domain through proteolysis [44]. Later advances have enabled the further reduction of antibody structure to scFv and VH/VHH (also called minibodies or nanobodies) [38,39,52–54,57]. These fragment types are described in more detail below.

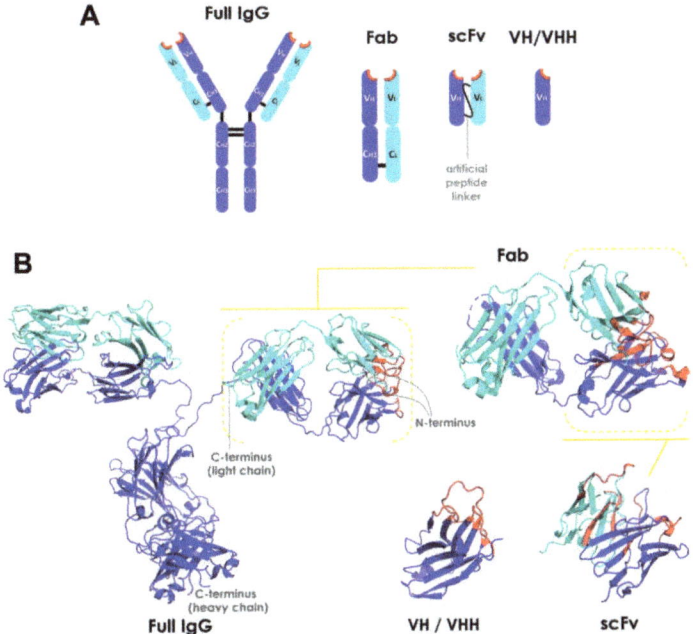

Figure 1. Overview of the structure of antibody fragments. (**A**) General schematic of domain framework and (**B**) ribbon diagrams of full-length IgG and fragment molecules. Structures were obtained from the Protein Data Bank (http://www.rcsb.org/pdb/). CH, CL, VH, and VL stand for constant heavy, constant light, variable heavy, and variable light domains, respectively. Heavy or light chains are depicted in dark blue or cyan, respectively. Complementarity-determining region (CDR) segments are highlighted in red. PDB codes: 1IGT (full length IgG), 5VH3 (Fab), 4NKO (scFv), and 3R0M (VHH) [58]. Fab: fragment antigen-binding; scFv: single chain variable fragments; VH/VHH: heavy chain variable domain fragment.

Fab fragments are independent structural units of ~50 kDa containing two antigen-binding sites, with the heavy chain variable domain (VH) linked to the heavy constant domain 1 (CH1) and the light chain variable domain (VL) linked to the light constant domain (CL) [44]. These domains interact through a large interface between the chains (VH/VL and CH1/CL) and a small one between the variable and the constant domains (VH/CH1 and VL/CL) of each chain [59]. The packing between the variable domains creates the antigen binding site [56]. The CH1 and CL domains are also covalently connected by a disulfide bond between Cys residues at their carboxyl terminal region [60,61]. Each Ig domain presents two layers of β-sheet structures, with three to five β-sheets per layer. The variable Ig domains (cyan; Figure 1B) are slightly longer than the constant domains (dark blue; Figure 1B), as they contain two more β-sheets per layer. The β-sheets are connected through loops, and the β-sheet layers of constant domains are attached through a disulfide bond. All amino terminal variable domain loops pack together in a β-sheet motif arranged as an antiparallel barrel-like structure, forming the complete complementarity-determining region (CDR), which is ultimately responsible for the antibody specificity (highlighted in red in Figure 1B) [44,59]. Each Ig domain contains three amino terminal loops encoding different CDR segments. Since the sequence variation associated with the specificity of immunoglobulins is found in CDRs, these regions are also referred to as hypervariable regions [59]. The hypervariable regions assemble into the antigen binding site and interact directly with the epitope. The framework regions, those comprising the variable domain sequences besides CDRs, fold into β-sheet motif structures and provide the scaffold for antibody-antigen interactions [62].

Single-chain variable fragments (scFvs), the smallest antibody fragments containing a complete antigen binding site, are recombinant molecules of ~30 kDa in which the variable domains of both VL and VH chains are engineered into a single polypeptide chain connected by a flexible peptide linker and/or a disulfide bond [20,43,45,46]. Their hypervariable segments (amino terminal loops) are approximately 10 amino acid residues long and, as in full length IgGs, form the antigen binding site [59]. The length and amino acid composition of the linker are crucial in maintaining the correct fold of these proteins [54]. The linker is typically about 3.5 nm in length and must contain small, hydrophilic residues (typically Gly and Ser) for enhanced solubility and flexibility [44,54].

VH/VHH fragments (~15–20 kDa) are N-terminal Ig domains derived only from the heavy chain, thus retaining antigen binding specificity within a single polypeptide domain [53,59,63]. Similar to VH fragments (Figure 1), VHHs (high affinity variable domains naturally found in camelids) contain three CDRs forming the antigen binding site [59,62]. Human VH domains and camelid VHH framework regions show a high sequence homology [61]. VHH fragments are naturally occurring [38,39,49,52] and especially stable.

3. Antibody Fragments Assisting the Study, and Diagnostic/Therapeutic Targeting, of Neurotoxic Amyloid Oligomers in CNS Amyloidoses

In the last two decades, several studies using antibody fragments to study the role of protein oligomers in CNS amyloidoses have been published (Table 1). Considering the discussion in the first two sections above, a major motivation for the use of antibody fragments as research and diagnostic/therapeutic tools for this disease class is the augmented chance of obtaining high affinity, conformation-sensitive antibodies over the typical animal immunization approach. Antibody fragments that display high selectivity for toxic oligomeric conformations are likely to be capable of neutralizing these neurotoxic aggregates without interfering with the physiological function of their monomeric counterparts, therefore presenting as preferred candidates for immunotherapies to treat amyloidogenic diseases. In the following sections, we review studies describing conformational antibody fragments capable of recognizing soluble oligomeric species formed by distinct proteins linked to prevalent CNS amyloidosis that currently lack a cure. We also highlight reports that, in our view, should provide guidance for the development of improved antibody fragments targeting neurotoxic oligomers.

Table 1. Conformation-sensitive antibody fragments directed to oligomeric species of proteins implicated in central nervous system (CNS) amyloidoses.

Antibody	Fragment Type	CNS Amyloidosis	Target High Affinity *	Target Low Affinity	Ref.
NUsc1	scFv	AD	Aβ42 Oligomers (>50 kDa) ¶	not reported	[64,65]
MO6	scFv	AD	Aβ42 Oligomers and Immature fibrils (18–37 kDa #)	not reported	[66]
AS	scFv	AD	Aβ42 Oligomers and Immature Protofibrils (25–55 kDa #)	not reported	[67]
HT6	scFv	AD	Aβ42 Oligomers (18–45 kDa #)	not reported	[68]
11A5	scFv	AD	Aβ42 Oligomers (34 kDa #)	not reported	[69]
A4	scFv	AD	Aβ42 Oligomers	Aβ42 Monomers and Fibrils	[70]
E1	scFv	AD	Aβ42 Oligomers	not reported	[71]
scFv59	scFv	AD	Aβ42 Oligomers and Plaques	not reported	[72]
scFv235	scFv	AD	phosphoTau Oligomers (50–70 kDa) #	Tau monomers	[73]
F9T, D11C, H2A	scFv	AD	Tau Oligomers (Trimers) ¶	not reported	[74]
RN2N	scFv	AD	Tau Oligomers	not reported	[75]
D5	scFv	PD	α-Synuclein Oligomers	not reported	[76]
10H	scFv	PD	α-Synuclein Oligomers (Trimers and Hexamers) ¶	α-Synuclein Monomers	[77]
VH14, NbSyn87	VH	PD	α-Synuclein Oligomers	not reported	[78]
D5-apoB	scFv	PD	α-Synuclein Oligomers (28–80 kDa) #	not reported	[79]
W20	scFv	Various diseases	Oligomers of Aβ40 and Aβ42, PrP^C, α-Syn, amylin, insulin, lysozyme	not reported	[80]

* MW/size of targeted oligomers is presented when available. It is also indicated whether MW/size have been determined under non-denaturing ¶ or denaturing # conditions. AD: Alzheimer's Disease; PD: Parkinson's Disease; PrP^c: cellular prion protein.

3.1. Alzheimer's Disease

3.1.1. Amyloid β

The increasing collection of antibody fragments against toxic aggregates associated with Alzheimer's Disease (AD) has enabled the elucidation of important information related to the biochemical nature of these toxic aggregates and their contribution to AD pathogenesis. As discussed above, a major challenge for all amyloidogenic proteins, but perhaps especially for the AD toxins Aβ oligomers (AβOs), has been to identify the most toxic aggregated species. This difficulty in characterization is due to the heterogeneous distribution of metastable species (including non-toxic or differentially toxic species) formed during the aggregation process [81]. Although robust evidence suggests that soluble AβOs and protofibrils play a prominent role in AD progression [12,82], the precise structural features of these soluble aggregates that contribute to AD pathogenesis remain elusive [1,12,81]. However, recent advances in this area have been made possible with the use of conformation-selective fragment antibodies [64–72,82,83]. One of those is the scFv antibody NUsc1, selected from a phage-display library by our group [64,65]. NUsc1 presents a marked selectivity for soluble AβOs compared to monomers or fibrils (Figure 2A) and, importantly, provides neuroprotection against AβO toxicity in cell cultures, blocking AβO binding and reducing AβO-induced oxidative stress and Tau hyperphosphorylation [64,65]. NUsc1 is of particular interest since it recognizes a unique conformational epitope displayed on oligomers of Aβ but not those formed by other proteins (such as Tau or Lysozyme); other anti-AβO scFvs have been shown to recognize a common epitope present on oligomers formed by different proteins [73,81,84]. Moreover, NUsc1 exhibits a marked oligomer size-dependent selectivity, preferentially targeting neurotoxic AβO species larger than 50 kDa, as analyzed under non-denaturing conditions by size-exclusion chromatography (Figure 2B).

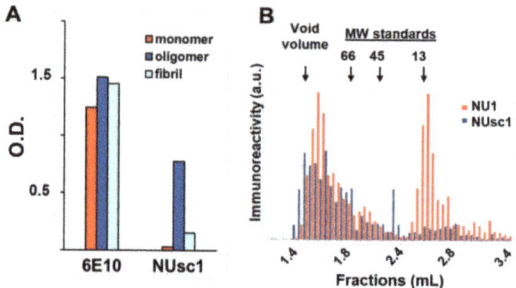

Figure 2. The scFv antibody NUsc1 is highly selective to high molecular weight Aβ oligomers (AβO). (**A**) NUsc1 shows high selectivity for Aβ oligomers over monomers and fibrils as determined via ELISA. The anti-pan Aβ IgG 6E10 is shown for comparison. Adapted with permission from (Velasco et al., ACS Chem. Neurosci. 2012 [64]). Copyright (2020) American Chemical Society. (**B**) Within a synthetic AβO population, NUsc1 selectively targets a high molecular weight subset, showing little binding to a lower molecular weight subset that is readily bound by the anti-AβO IgG NU1. Reactivity of both antibodies to AβO fractions separated by size-exclusion chromatography under non-denaturing conditions was determined by dot immunoblotting. Reprinted with permission from (Sebollela et al., Journal of Neurochem. 2017 [65]). Copyright (2020) John Wiley and Sons.

Other anti-AβO scFvs have been reported that are promising tools for the study of AβO structure–toxicity relationships as well as their diagnostic and therapeutic targeting. The scFv MO6 was found to target AβO species (18–37 kDa) that are on-pathway to fibril formation and toxic to SH-SY5Y cells [66]. Important to its diagnostic/therapeutic potential, MO6 was demonstrated to cross the blood–brain barrier (BBB) in an in vitro BBB model with a delivery efficiency of 66% 60 min post-administration. Another study reported the scFv b4.4, which recognized an epitope in the central region of Aβ42 (comprising residues H^{13}, K^{16} V^{18}, F^{19}) and was able to neutralize the toxicity of either AβOs or fibrillar Aβ to SH-SY5Y cells [83]. The scFv AS was found to recognize cytotoxic medium-sized AβO species (25–55 kDa) and protofibrils [67]. While scFvs are commonly identified via phage display, AS was identified from a library constructed from the immune repertoire of AD patients. The scFv HT6 also was found to bind efficiently to an N-terminal epitope present in cytotoxic medium-sized AβOs (mainly 18–45 kDa) in vitro [68]. Significantly, the anti-AβO scFv 11A5, selected by phage display and found to target a 34 kDa assembly, has been reported to ameliorate cognitive decline in rats induced by injection of AβOs [69]. It is important to consider that in all of these studies, AβO size has been evaluated by denaturing SDS-PAGE/Western immunoblotting, and therefore may not accurately reflect the AβO size in the physiological milieu. Additionally, an interesting approach has been developed wherein atomic force microscopy is utilized to biopan for conformation-selective antibodies by phage display. Following this approach, two scFvs were identified, named A4 and E1, that targeted distinct oligomeric species presenting either high [70] or low [71] cytotoxicity potentials. Further studies with these conformer-selective scFvs, and others like them, promise to shed additional light on the AβO structural properties contributing to AD pathogenesis.

The scFvs highlighted above were all identified by their unique selectivities from antibody libraries. One promising strategy for the rational engineering of scFvs with even further improved selectivity for oligomeric species of interest, is complementarity-determining region (CDR) mapping (i.e., determination of the complementarity-determining region (CDR) amino acid sequences, the regions responsible for antibody specificity) of existing scFvs. So far, CDR mapping has only been reported for non-conformational anti-Aβ scFvs. In one of these reports, Tiller and colleagues (2017) used a series of mutations in the CDR sequences of scFvs to identify the contribution of arginine residues to the affinity and selectivity for Aβ monomers [85]. Other recent studies have contributed to the identification and importance of particular amino acids within CDRs, e.g., tyrosine, glycine, serine, and especially arginine, in the binding to different Aβ aggregated species [86,87]. If similar studies are conducted with anti-AβO scFvs in the future, comparison to these data obtained with non-conformational anti-Aβ scFvs may indicate the key interactions underlying conformational preference for oligomeric over monomeric and fibrillar species. From a therapeutic perspective, the ectopic expression of neurotoxic-selective fragment antibodies by using brain-optimized viral vectors is emerging as an exciting path to be exploited. For instance, recent data in AD-mouse models indicate a cognitive benefit provided by the brain expression of the scFv NUsc1, which was discussed above (unpublished data [88]).

3.1.2. Tau

Another AD-relevant amyloidogenic protein is the microtubule-associated protein Tau. Upon abnormal hyperphosphorylation or co-factor binding, this protein forms oligomers and larger aggregates that contribute to neuronal dysfunction and death in AD and other tauopathies (reviewed in [89,90]). Since Tau oligomers have been linked to neurodegeneration, structural studies aimed to unravel the conformation of soluble Tau aggregates have been the focus of recent investigations [91]. As with AβOs, antibody fragments are emerging as promising tools for these studies [74,75,92]. For instance, Tian et al. (2015) reported the selection of three conformation-selective anti-Tau scFvs (F9T, D11C, H2A) capable of binding trimeric but not monomeric or fibrillar Tau [74]. These scFvs distinguished AD from cognitively normal post-mortem human brains and are capable of detecting oligomeric Tau at earlier ages, compared to typical ages in which neurofibrillary tangles can be detected. In terms of therapy, these oligomer-selective scFv antibodies represent an advantage over non-conformational antibodies as they do not block the physiological functions carried out by monomeric Tau.

3.2. Parkinson's Disease

Parkinson's disease (PD) is a neurodegenerative disorder associated with the abnormal aggregation of the neuronal membrane protein alpha synuclein (α-syn) (reviewed in Shulz-Schaeffer [93]). It has been shown that, besides the formation of insoluble aggregates that deposit inside neurons as inclusion bodies, termed Lewy bodies, α-syn also forms neurotoxic soluble oligomers/protofibrils [94,95]. As with Aβ and Tau, antibody fragments are beginning to emerge in the literature with selectivity for oligomeric over monomeric or fibrillar forms of α-syn. Emadi and colleagues have identified two scFv antibodies of particular use in elucidating α-syn oligomer structure–function relationships. The scFv D5 was found to be selective for oligomers more abundant in initial stages of α-syn aggregation and to block further aggregation of these oligomers and their toxicity in SH-SY5Y cells [76]. D5 was also seen to interact with oligomers formed by the Huntington's disease-associated protein htt51Q [96], in line with the notion that many antibodies raised against amyloid oligomers cross-react with structurally similar oligomers formed by non-related proteins [97]. In contrast, 10H, an scFv that targets oligomers more abundant in later stages of α-syn aggregation, appears to be selective for oligomers of α-syn [77]. Both scFvs D5 and 10H provided neuroprotection in an α-syn overexpressing transgenic mouse model when fused to penetratin (a cell-penetrating peptide), raising a potential immunotherapeutic benefit of these scFvs in PD [98]. Although in principle antibodies targeting pan-amyloid aggregates such as scFv D5 may represent a promising therapeutic strategy, it is also important to consider that cross-reactivity may be harmful in some cases. For instance, Kvam et al. (2009) showed that the anti-fibrillar α-syn scFv-6E, which also binds mutant huntingtin and ataxin-3, increased the aggregation of these polyglutamine-rich proteins in striatal cells, aggravating intracellular dysfunction and cell death [99].

Although few antibody fragments selective for oligomeric α-syn conformations have been reported in the literature, studies utilizing antibody fragments selective for linear α-syn sequences (i.e., non-conformational antibodies) have increased our understanding of α-syn aggregation and toxicity. Zhou et al. (2004) reported the scFv antibody D10, which presented nanomolar affinity for α-syn monomers and inhibited aggregation to oligomeric and protofibrillar forms. The authors localized the D10 epitope within the C-terminus of α-syn, suggesting that perturbation in this region interferes with the aggregation process. In the same study, it was also shown that co-expression of D10 in HEK293 cells engineered to overexpresses α-syn reduced the formation of high-molecular weight α-syn aggregates, thus suggesting a positive action of D10 as an intrabody [100] (i.e., a fragment antibody engineered to accumulate within its producing cell). The VHH single domain antibodies NbSyn2 and NbSyn87 have been used to identify the role of different C-terminal regions of α-syn in fibril formation [101–103]. NbSyn2, which recognizes an epitope between residues 136–140, did not affect fibril formation [78,102,103]. In contrast, NbSyn87, which recognizes an epitope comprised by residues 118–128, induced conformational changes on both secondary and tertiary structures of α-syn, consequentially reducing the half-time of fibril formation [78,101].

scFvs targeting the α-syn nonamyloid component (NAC) have also shown therapeutic promise in pre-clinical studies. The NAC presents a high tendency to adopt β-pleated sheet structures and is known to play a key role in the aggregation and toxicity of α-syn in vitro and in vivo [104]. In 2008, Lynch and colleagues showed a novel NAC-selective scFv named NAC32 capable of reducing the aggregation and neurotoxicity of α-syn aggregates [105]. Other single domain antibodies targeting the NAC, NAC1 and VH14, acted similarly to NAC32 in preventing a-syn aggregation [106].

Although considerable advances towards the understanding of α-syn aggregation and toxicity have been attained by the use of fragment antibodies, few reports have been published so far evaluating the consequences of the in vivo expression/administration of these antibody fragments. Although few, these reports do demonstrate therapeutic promise. In one of these studies, the single-domain antibodies VH14 and NbSyn87 were expressed in fusion with the proteasome-targeting PEST motif, resulting in increased cytoplasmic solubility and enhanced degradation of α-syn in neuronal cell lines [78]. In another interesting piece of work, Spencer et al. (2014) induced the expression of a scFv directed to α-syn oligomers in fusion with the low-density lipoprotein receptor-binding domain from apolipoprotein B (LDL ApoB) in vivo [79]. This construction increased the penetration of the scFv into the brain via the endosomal sorting complex required for transport (ESCRT) pathway, consequently leading to lysosomal degradation of α-syn aggregates [79]. These exciting reports suggest the feasibility of in vivo expression of engineered anti-oligomeric scFvs as a therapeutic alternative for PD.

3.3. Huntington's Disease

Huntingtin (HTT) is a ubiquitously expressed large protein (3144 amino acids) involved in the pathogenesis of Huntington's disease (HD) [107]. Although the diverse physiological roles of HTT are not yet fully understood, it is well known that its aggregation and neurotoxicity are dependent on the presence of an aberrant polyglutamine (polyQ) stretch encoded in exon 1 of the htt gene (corresponding to the N-terminus in the protein) [108–110]. In mutant-disease-associated HTT, this polyQ stretch is longer than in wild type HTT, reaching 40 or more glutamine residues (as opposed to normally 20 on average) [110]. Interestingly, this increment is enough to impact the stability of the whole molecule, driving its aggregation into both soluble oligomers and insoluble aggregates [111].

Since HTT aggregates are exclusively intraneuronal, intrabodies have been the antibody fragment type preferentially applied to their structure-function study and their therapeutic targeting. One of the first scFv-type intrabodies directed to huntingtin was reported by Lecerf et al. (2001). Named C4, this scFv binds to residues 1–17 of HTT, a sequence N-terminal to the polyQ repeat in HTT exon 1, stabilizing an alpha helix-rich oligomeric complex and preventing amyloid formation [112,113]. When co-expressed with HTT exon 1 in non-neuronal cells, C4 was capable of reducing the amount of HTT aggregates and redirecting the subcellular localization of HTT exon 1. Moreover, C4 efficiently reduced cell death in malonate-treated brain slice cultures expressing mutant HTT [114]. Additionally of importance, expression of C4 in the HD disease mouse model B6.HDR6/1, via AAV2/1 vector, led to delayed HTT aggregation in both early and late disease stages [115]. The authors also generated scFv-C4 in fusion with the PEST domain to increase proteasomal degradation of the antigen–antibody complex [115].

A piece of pioneering work by Khoshnan et al. (2002) reported three scFvs (MW1, MW2, and MW7) produced by cloning the antigen-binding domains of monoclonal IgGs targeting either polyQ or an adjacent domain in HTT exon 1 rich in proline residues (named PRD) into scFv scaffolds [116]. The scFv MW7, selective for PRD, inhibited cell death induced by mutant HTT in co-transfected HEK293 cells [116]. Surprisingly MW1 and MW2, both selective for polyQ, accelerated aggregation and cell death in the same culture model. Possible explanations for this unexpected result are that MW1 and MW2 either stabilized a toxic aggregated conformation of HTT or interfered with the binding of HTT to other molecules mediating HTT toxicity [116]. These findings highlight the complexity and importance of identifying fragment antibodies that indeed target toxic oligomeric species, which are expected to show promise as therapeutics and/or diagnostics.

In another piece of work, multiple intrabodies targeting HTT PRD domains (scFv MW7; VL Happ1; VL Happ3) or the HTT N-terminus (VL 12.3) were used to investigate the role of these domains in HTT aggregation and toxicity [117]. VL 12.3 had been previously shown to reduce toxicity in a neuronal culture model of HD [118]. All of these intrabodies reduced mutant HTT exon 1 aggregation and toxicity in both cell culture and brain slice models of HD, although the mechanisms of protection were different. While the N-terminus-targeting intrabody altered HTT subcellular localization, the PRD-targeting intrabodies were seen to increase the turnover rate of HTT [119]. These results reinforce the notion of a strong correlation between the structural domains targeted by each intrabody and their mechanism of neuroprotection. Fragment antibodies VL 12.3 and Haap1 were also employed to investigate the contribution of N-terminus and PRD domains to HD pathology in vivo using five different HD mouse models. While VL 12.3 showed no significant effects on one model, and increased mortality in another, Haap1 alleviated HD neuropathology in all the five animal models tested, including prolonged lifespan in one model [120].

Finally, the scFv-EM48, which targets the C-terminus of human mutant HTT exon 1, also showed promising results in an HD mouse model, as decreased formation of neuropil aggregates and cognitive HD-like symptoms [114]. In conjunction with data obtained with antibody fragments targeting the N-terminus, the polyQ domain, and the PRD domain, these data indicate that all domains within HTT exon 1 play a role in mutant HTT aggregation and toxicity. When used as an intrabody, scFv-EM48 also suppressed the toxicity of mutant HTT in HEK293 cells. The ability of this antibody fragment to increase the ubiquitination and consequent degradation of cytoplasmatic HTT suggests that scFv-EM48 acts by promoting the cytoplasmic clearance of mutant HTT thereby preventing its accumulation.

3.4. Prion Diseases

Prion diseases are characterized by the brain accumulation of aggregated and neurotoxic forms of the prion protein (PrP). Under physiological conditions, PrP presents as a ~24 kDa transmembrane protein that exerts a number of functions, such as metal ion hemostasis and cell adhesion [121]. On the other hand, in diseased brains, it converts into a beta-sheet-rich confirmation named PrP^{sc} (i.e., the scrapie isoform), which forms both soluble oligomers and amyloid fibrils [122–124]. Importantly, PrP^{sc} is known to catalyze the conversion of harmless PrP molecules into the aggregation-prone conformation PrP^{sc}, thus conferring to Prion diseases their unique infectious nature [123]. Finding molecules capable of inhibiting either the formation or the toxicity of PrP^{sc} aggregates, including soluble oligomers, has been a major goal in the prion diseases field, as a way to provide a disease-modifying therapy for patients. In this regard, some fragment antibodies have been selected that display promising inhibitory activity on PrP^{sc} oligomerization and fibrillization both in vitro and in cellular models [125,126].

In 2001, Peretz et al. reported the Fab antibody fragment D18, which binds to an epitope within residues 132–156 in helix 1 of the Prion protein in its native conformation, a region thought to contribute to PrP^{sc} assembly and prion elongation. Although the aggregation states targeted by D18 have not yet been identified experimentally, D18 was found to inhibit prion elongation in cultured mouse neuroblastoma cells infected with PrP^{sc} [126]. Subsequently, Campana et al. (2009) engineered scFv-D18 from Fab-D18 and used in silico tools to create a structural model of scFv-D18 bound to PrP. In that model, PrP residue Arg151 was seen to be key in the interaction with the antibody fragment, by anchoring PrP to the cavity formed on antigen binding site of the scFv [127].

More recently, Fujita et al. (2011) cloned the variable region of mAb 3S9—previously shown to inhibit PrP^{sc} accumulation in cell lines infected with mouse-adapted scrapie strains [128,129]—into the scaffold of a scFv antibody. The resulting antibody, named scFv-3S9, recognized an epitope containing Tyr154 in the helix 1 of PrP. When injected into mice brains, Prion-infected cells expressing scFv-3S9 presented less Prion pathology than infected cells not expressing this scFv [128].

Lastly, Sonati and coworkers (2013) used a panel composed of full-length antibodies and antibody fragments (Fab and scFv) directed to either the globular domain or the flexible tail on PrP, to investigate the role of these regions in oligomerization and neurotoxicity. Results generated on cerebellar organotypic cultured slices showed that both domains are required for toxicity, as the flexible tail acquires oxidative stress-mediated toxicity upon undergoing a conformational change originated from the globular domain [130]. This comprehensive work reinforced the notion that antibody-based therapeutic developments against Prion diseases must include a detailed analysis of the targeted structural epitope of each antibody candidate as well as the molecular and clinical outcomes of targeting these epitopes.

4. Concluding Remarks

Increased knowledge about the aggregation pathways and conformations of the toxic aggregate species relevant to CNS amyloidoses has been obtained with the use of fragment antibodies, in particular Fab, scFv, and VHH (Table 1). As technologies for engineering fragment antibodies are constantly improving, the perspective for the generation of novel fragment antibodies with high selectivity for toxic oligomeric conformations as diagnostic and/or therapeutic candidates for CNS amyloidoses, is also rising.

Methodologies for rational Aβ-targeting antibody design have been reviewed (e.g., Plotkin and Cashman, 2020 [131]). For example, just as our group has successfully generated full-length IgGs with selectivity for AβOs over monomers and fibrils [132], rational immunization with specific toxic AβO species can be employed, followed by conversion of the resulting anti-AβO IgG to an antibody fragment. Alternatively, specific toxic AβO species can be utilized in rational bio-panning of antibody fragment libraries. These specific AβO species can be generated by size-based separation methods (reviewed in [12]) or by utilizing specific Aβ monomeric proteoforms ([133,134]) and can be stabilized by various methods. For example, chemical crosslinking via DFDNB (1,5-difluoro-2,4-dinitrobenzene) has been shown to stabilize high molecular weight AβOs that exhibit toxicity in cell cultures and in vivo [135]. Alternatively, computational prediction of regions present on the surface of toxic oligomeric species is emerging as an additional strategy for rational identification of target species [136].

We envision that the use of fragment antibodies in structural studies aimed to unravel the molecular mechanisms of protein aggregation and related toxicity has a strong potential to make unique contributions to the field. In conjunction with CDR mapping and the detailed analysis of the assembly selectivity of each fragment antibody described, this approach may significantly improve our knowledge regarding key atomic contacts between antibodies and toxic oligomers, and as a consequence, the structural moieties that confer toxicity to amyloid oligomers. These advances could enhance the field's capability of engineering antibody fragments able to selectively target neurotoxic aggregates amongst a multitude of oligomeric assemblies co-existing in diseased human tissue. Even in a likely case in which different oligomeric species contribute to neurotoxicity, and thus a single, highly specific antibody would not able to fully neutralize the pathogenic cascade, a therapeutic strategy based on the combination of multiple oligomer-selective antibody fragments directed against different species could be employed to circumvent this issue.

The cognitive benefit and lowering of multiple AD markers reported in AD patients treated with the antibody aducanumab (Biogen)—a monoclonal IgG that preferentially targets aggregated Aβ [137,138]—has brought hope, reinforcing the notion that selectively targeting neurotoxic aggregates would guide the field toward disease-modifying treatments against brain amyloidosis. Indeed, the FDA has recently granted aducanumab priority review [139]. However, there is still room for improvement in the field as the therapeutic benefits of aducanumab were only apparent following a re-analysis of the phase three trials that were initially halted due to a lack of efficacy [138]. In our view, this improvement will stem from the development of antibodies even more selective to neurotoxic oligomeric assemblies. In this context, detailed structural information on these toxic oligomers will be invaluable to the targeted design of new oligomer-selective fragment antibodies with improved specificity and clinical outcomes.

Author Contributions: All authors have read and agree to the published version of the manuscript. Conceptualization, A.L.B.B., R.M.C. and A.S.; data curation, A.L.B.B., R.M.C. and E.N.C.; writing—original draft preparation, A.L.B.B., R.M.C. and A.S.; writing—review and editing, E.N.C., W.L.K. and A.S.; supervision, A.S. All authors have read and agreed to the published version of the manuscript.

Funding: This research was funded by FAPESP (Grant 2014/25681-3 to AS), CNPq (Pre-Doctoral fellowship to ALBB), CAPES (Pre-Doctoral fellowship to RMC) and the NIH (1RF1AG063903 to WLK).

Conflicts of Interest: The authors declare no conflict of interest. The funders had no role in the design of the study; in the collection, analyses, or interpretation of data; in the writing of the manuscript, or in the decision to publish the results.

Abbreviations

AD	Alzheimer's Disease
Aβ	Amyloid-β
AβOs	Amyloid-β Peptide Oligomers
CDR	Complementary-determining Region
CNS	Central Nervous System
Fab	Fragment Antigen-Binding
Fc	Fragment Crystallizable
HD	Huntington's Disease
HTT	Huntingtin Protein
IgG	Immunoglobulin G
mAbs	Monoclonal Antibodies
NAC	Nonamyloid Component
PD	Parkinson's Disease
PrP^c	Cellular Prion Protein
PrP^{sc}	Scrapie Prion Protein
scFv	Single-chain Variable Fragment

References

1. Chiti, F.; Dobson, C.M. Protein Misfolding, Amyloid Formation, and Human Disease: A Summary of Progress Over the Last Decade. *Annu. Rev. Biochem.* **2017**, *86*, 27–68. [CrossRef]
2. Bleiholder, C.; Dupuis, N.F.; Wyttenbach, T.; Bowers, M.T. Ion mobilityg-mass spectrometry reveals a conformational conversion from random assembly to β-sheet in amyloid fibril formation. *Nat. Chem.* **2011**, *3*, 172–177. [CrossRef]
3. Lomont, J.P.; Rich, K.L.; Maj, M.; Ho, J.-J.; Ostrander, J.S.; Zanni, M.T. Spectroscopic Signature for Stable β-Amyloid Fibrils versus β-Sheet-Rich Oligomers. *J. Phys. Chem. B* **2018**, *122*, 144–153. [CrossRef]
4. Lu, J.-X.; Qiang, W.; Yau, W.-M.; Schwieters, C.D.; Meredith, S.C.; Tycko, R. Molecular structure of β-amyloid fibrils in Alzheimer's disease brain tissue. *Cell* **2013**, *154*, 1257–1268. [CrossRef]
5. Kayed, R.; Head, E.; Thompson, J.L.; McIntire, T.M.; Milton, S.C.; Cotman, C.W.; Glabel, C.G. Common structure of soluble amyloid oligomers implies common mechanism of pathogenesis. *Science* **2003**, *300*, 486–489. [CrossRef]
6. Chiti, F.; Webster, P.; Taddei, N.; Clark, A.; Stefani, M.; Ramponi, G.; Dobson, C.M. Designing conditions for in vitro formation of amyloid protofilaments and fibrils. *Proc. Natl. Acad. Sci. USA* **1999**, *96*, 3590–3594. [CrossRef]
7. Bucciantini, M.; Giannoni, E.; Chiti, F.; Baroni, F.; Taddei, N.; Ramponi, G.; Dobson, C.M.; Stefani, M. Inherent toxicity of aggregates implies a common mechanism for protein misfolding diseases. *Nature* **2002**, *416*, 507–511. [CrossRef]
8. Dobson, C.M. The structural basis of protein folding and its links with human disease. *Proc. Philos. Trans. R. Soc. B Biol. Sci.* **2001**, *356*, 133–145. [CrossRef]
9. Kelly, J.W. The alternative conformations of amyloidogenic proteins and their multi-step assembly pathways. *Curr. Opin. Struct. Biol.* **1998**, *8*, 101–106. [CrossRef]
10. Hardy, J.A.; Higgins, G.A. Alzheimer's disease: The amyloid cascade hypothesis. *Science* **1992**, *256*, 184–185. [CrossRef]
11. Vieira, M.N.N.; Forny-Germano, L.; Saraiva, L.M.; Sebollela, A.; Martinez, A.M.B.; Houzel, J.C.; De Felice, F.G.; Ferreira, S.T. Soluble oligomers from a non-disease related protein mimic Aβ-induced tau hyperphosphorylation and neurodegeneration. *J. Neurochem.* **2007**, *103*, 736–748. [CrossRef]
12. Cline, E.N.; Bicca, M.A.; Viola, K.L.; Klein, W.L. The Amyloid-β Oligomer Hypothesis: Beginning of the Third Decade. *J. Alzheimer's Dis.* **2018**, *64*, S567–S610. [CrossRef]
13. Valera, E.; Spencer, B.; Masliah, E. Immunotherapeutic Approaches Targeting Amyloid-β, α-Synuclein, and Tau for the Treatment of Neurodegenerative Disorders. *Neurotherapeutics* **2016**, *13*, 179–189. [CrossRef]
14. Bittar, A.; Bhatt, N.; Kayed, R. Advances and considerations in AD tau-targeted immunotherapy. *Neurobiol. Dis.* **2020**, *134*, 104707. [CrossRef]
15. Choi, M.L.; Gandhi, S. Crucial role of protein oligomerization in the pathogenesis of Alzheimer's and Parkinson's diseases. *FEBS J.* **2018**, *285*, 3631–3644. [CrossRef]
16. Gong, Y.; Chang, L.; Viola, K.L.; Lacor, P.N.; Lambert, M.P.; Finch, C.E.; Krafft, G.A.; Klein, W.L. Alzheimer's disease-affected brain: Presence of oligomeric A ligands (ADDLs) suggests a molecular basis for reversible memory loss. *Proc. Natl. Acad. Sci. USA* **2003**, *100*, 10417–10422. [CrossRef]
17. Shankar, G.M.; Li, S.; Mehta, T.H.; Garcia-Munoz, A.; Shepardson, N.E.; Smith, I.; Brett, F.M.; Farrell, M.A.; Rowan, M.J.; Lemere, C.A.; et al. Amyloid-β protein dimers isolated directly from Alzheimer's brains impair synaptic plasticity and memory. *Nat. Med.* **2008**, *14*, 837–842. [CrossRef]
18. Lambert, M.P.; Barlow, A.K.; Chromy, B.A.; Edwards, C.; Freed, R.; Liosatos, M.; Morgan, T.E.; Rozovsky, I.; Trommer, B.; Viola, K.L.; et al. Diffusible, nonfibrillar ligands derived from A 1-42 are potent central nervous system neurotoxins. *Proc. Natl. Acad. Sci. USA* **1998**, *95*, 6448–6453. [CrossRef]
19. Theillet, F.X.; Binolfi, A.; Bekei, B.; Martorana, A.; Rose, H.M.; Stuiver, M.; Verzini, S.; Lorenz, D.; Van Rossum, M.; Goldfarb, D.; et al. Structural disorder of monomeric α-synuclein persists in mammalian cells. *Nature* **2016**. [CrossRef]
20. Spillantini, M.G.; Schmidt, M.L.; Lee, V.M.Y.; Trojanowski, J.Q.; Jakes, R.; Goedert, M. Alpha-synuclein in Lewy bodies. *Nature* **1997**, *388*, 839–840. [CrossRef]
21. Hatters, D.M. Protein misfolding inside cells: The case of Huntingtin and Huntington's disease. *IUBMB Life* **2008**, *60*, 724–728. [CrossRef]

22. Imarisio, S.; Carmichael, J.; Korolchuk, V.; Chen, C.W.; Saiki, S.; Rose, C.; Krishna, G.; Davies, J.E.; Ttofi, E.; Underwood, B.R.; et al. Huntington's disease: From pathology and genetics to potential therapies. *Biochem. J.* **2008**, *412*, 191–209. [CrossRef]
23. Grassmann, A.; Wolf, H.; Hofmann, J.; Graham, J.; Vorberg, I. Cellular aspects of prion replication in vitro. *Viruses* **2012**, *5*, 374–405. [CrossRef]
24. Soto, C.; Satani, N. The intricate mechanisms of neurodegeneration in prion diseases. *Trends Mol. Med.* **2011**, *17*, 14–24. [CrossRef]
25. Rabinovici, G.D.; Carrillo, M.C.; Forman, M.; DeSanti, S.; Miller, D.S.; Kozauer, N.; Petersen, R.C.; Randolph, C.; Knopman, D.S.; Smith, E.E.; et al. Multiple comorbid neuropathologies in the setting of Alzheimer's disease neuropathology and implications for drug development. *Alzheimer's Dement. Transl. Res. Clin. Interv.* **2017**, *3*, 83–91. [CrossRef]
26. Visanji, N.P.; Lang, A.E.; Kovacs, G.G. Beyond the synucleinopathies: Alpha synuclein as a driving force in neurodegenerative comorbidities. *Transl. Neurodegener.* **2019**, *8*, 28. [CrossRef]
27. Goure, W.F.; Krafft, G.A.; Jerecic, J.; Hefti, F. Targeting the proper amyloid-beta neuronal toxins: A path forward for Alzheimer's disease immunotherapeutics. *Alzheimer's Res. Ther.* **2014**, *6*, 42. [CrossRef]
28. Sengupta, U.; Nilson, A.N.; Kayed, R. The Role of Amyloid-β Oligomers in Toxicity, Propagation, and Immunotherapy. *EBioMedicine* **2016**, *6*, 42–49. [CrossRef]
29. Oertel, W.H. Recent advances in treating Parkinson's disease. *F1000Research* **2017**, *6*, 260. [CrossRef]
30. Masnata, M.; Cicchetti, F. The evidence for the spread and seeding capacities of the mutant huntingtin protein in in vitro systems and their therapeutic implications. *Front. Neurosci.* **2017**, *11*, 647. [CrossRef]
31. Jankovic, J.; Rousseaux, M.W.C.; Shulman, J.M. Progress toward an integrated understanding of Parkinson's disease. *F1000Research* **2017**, *6*, 1121.
32. Velayudhan, L.; Ffytche, D.; Ballard, C.; Aarsland, D. New Therapeutic Strategies for Lewy Body Dementias. *Curr. Neurol. Neurosci. Rep.* **2017**, *17*, 68. [CrossRef]
33. Zella, S.M.A.; Metzdorf, J.; Ciftci, E.; Ostendorf, F.; Muhlack, S.; Gold, R.; Tönges, L. Emerging Immunotherapies for Parkinson Disease. *Neurol. Ther.* **2019**, *8*, 29–44. [CrossRef]
34. De Genst, E.; Messer, A.; Dobson, C.M. Antibodies and protein misfolding: From structural research tools to therapeutic strategies. *Biochim. Biophys. Acta* **2014**, *8*, 29–44. [CrossRef]
35. Villar-Piqué, A.; Lopes da Fonseca, T.; Outeiro, T.F. Structure, function and toxicity of alpha-synuclein: the Bermuda triangle in synucleinopathies. *J. Neurochem.* **2016**, *139*, 240–255. [CrossRef]
36. Hoffner, G.; Djian, P. Polyglutamine Aggregation in Huntington Disease: Does Structure Determine Toxicity? *Mol. Neurobiol.* **2015**, *52*, 1297–1314. [CrossRef]
37. Carter, L.; Kim, S.J.; Schneidman-Duhovny, D.; Stöhr, J.; Poncet-Montange, G.; Weiss, T.M.; Tsuruta, H.; Prusiner, S.B.; Sali, A. Prion Protein—Antibody Complexes Characterized by Chromatography-Coupled Small-Angle X-Ray Scattering. *Biophys. J.* **2015**, *109*, 793–805. [CrossRef]
38. Bates, A.; Power, C.A. David vs. Goliath: The Structure, Function, and Clinical Prospects of Antibody Fragments. *Antibodies* **2019**, *8*, 28. [CrossRef]
39. Bélanger, K.; Iqbal, U.; Tanha, J.; MacKenzie, R.; Moreno, M.; Stanimirovic, D. Single-Domain Antibodies as Therapeutic and Imaging Agents for the Treatment of CNS Diseases. *Antibodies* **2019**, *8*, 27. [CrossRef]
40. Nicoll, J.A.; Wilkinson, D.; Holmes, C.; Steart, P.; Markham, H.; Weller, R.O. Neuropathology of human Alzheimer disease after immunization with amyloid-beta peptide: a case report. *Nat Med* **2003**, *9*, 448–452. [CrossRef]
41. Ferrer, I.; Rovira, M.B.; Guerra, M.L.S.; Rey, M.J.; Costa-Jussá, F. Neuropathology and Pathogenesis of Encephalitis following Amyloid β Immunization in Alzheimer's Disease. *Brain Pathol.* **2004**, *14*, 11–20. [CrossRef]
42. Gilman, S.; Koller, M.; Black, R.S.; Jenkins, L.; Griffith, S.G.; Fox, N.C.; Eisner, L.; Kirby, L.; Boada Rovira, M.; Forette, F.; et al. Clinical effects of Aβ immunization (AN1792) in patients with AD in an interrupted trial. *Neurology* **2005**, *64*, 1553–1562. [CrossRef]
43. Lee, M.; Bard, F.; Johnson-Wood, K.; Lee, C.; Hu, K.; Griffith, S.G.; Black, R.S.; Schenk, D.; Seubert, P. Aβ42 immunization in Alzheimer's disease generates Aβ N-terminal antibodies. *Ann. Neurol.* **2005**, *28*, 430–435. [CrossRef]
44. Strohl, W.R.; Strohl, L.M. *Therapeutic Antibody Engineering: Current and Future Advances Driving the Strongest Growth Area in the Pharmaceutical Industry*; Woodhead Publishing: Cambridge, UK, 2012; ISBN 9781907568374.

45. Meyer-Luehmann, M.; Spires-Jones, T.L.; Prada, C.; Garcia-Alloza, M.; De Calignon, A.; Rozkalne, A.; Koenigsknecht-Talboo, J.; Holtzman, D.M.; Bacskai, B.J.; Hyman, B.T. Rapid appearance and local toxicity of amyloid-β plaques in a mouse model of Alzheimer's disease. *Nature* **2008**, *451*, 720–724. [CrossRef]
46. Esquerda-Canals, G.; Martí-Clúa, J.; Villegas, S. Pharmacokinetic parameters and mechanism of action of an efficient anti-Aβ single chain antibody fragment. *PLoS One* **2019**, *14*, e0217793. [CrossRef]
47. Manoutcharian, K.; Perez-Garmendia, R.; Gevorkian, G. Recombinant Antibody Fragments for Neurodegenerative Diseases. *Curr. Neuropharmacol.* **2016**, *5*, 779–788. [CrossRef]
48. Holliger, P.; Hudson, P.J. Engineered antibody fragments and the rise of single domains. *Nat. Biotechnol.* **2005**, *23*, 1126–1136. [CrossRef]
49. Pain, C.; Dumont, J.; Dumoulin, M. Camelid single-domain antibody fragments: Uses and prospects to investigate protein misfolding and aggregation, and to treat diseases associated with these phenomena. *Biochimie* **2015**, *111*, 82–106. [CrossRef]
50. Chia, K.Y.; Ng, K.Y.; Koh, R.Y.; Chye, S.M. Single-chain Fv Antibodies for Targeting Neurodegenerative Diseases. *CNS Neurol. Disord.* **2018**, *17*, 671–679. [CrossRef]
51. Chatterjee, D.; Kordower, J.H. Immunotherapy in Parkinson's disease: Current status and future directions. *Neurobiol. Dis.* **2019**, *132*, 104587. [CrossRef]
52. Messer, A.; Butler, D.C. Optimizing intracellular antibodies (intrabodies/nanobodies) to treat neurodegenerative disorders. *Neurobiol. Dis.* **2020**, *134*, 104619. [CrossRef]
53. Nelson, A.L.; Reichert, J.M. Development trends for therapeutic antibody fragments. *Nat. Biotechnol.* **2009**, *27*, 331–337. [CrossRef]
54. Monnier, P.; Vigouroux, R.; Tassew, N. In Vivo Applications of Single Chain Fv (Variable Domain) (scFv) Fragments. *Antibodies* **2013**, *2*, 193–208. [CrossRef]
55. Alspach, E.; Lussier, D.M.; Miceli, A.P.; Kizhvatov, I.; DuPage, M.; Luoma, A.M.; Meng, W.; Lichti, C.F.; Esaulova, E.; Vomund, A.N.; et al. MHC-II neoantigens shape tumour immunity and response to immunotherapy. *Nature* **2019**, *574*, 696–701. [CrossRef]
56. Ewert, S.; Huber, T.; Honegger, A.; Plückthun, A. Biophysical properties of human antibody variable domains. *J. Mol. Biol.* **2003**, *325*, 531–553. [CrossRef]
57. Nelson, A.L. Antibody fragments: Hope and hype. *MAbs* **2010**, *2*, 77–83. [CrossRef]
58. Rose, A.S.; Hildebrand, P.W. NGL Viewer: A web application for molecular visualization. *Nucleic Acids Res.* **2015**, *43*, W576–W579. [CrossRef]
59. Abbas, A.K.; Lichtman, A.H. *Cellular and Molecular Immunology*; Saunders: Philadelphia, PA, USA, 2014; ISBN 9780323315937.
60. Wörn, A.; Plückthun, A. Stability engineering of antibody single-chain Fv fragments. *J. Mol. Biol.* **2001**, *305*, 989–1010. [CrossRef]
61. Harmsen, M.M.; De Haard, H.J. Properties, production, and applications of camelid single-domain antibody fragments. *Appl. Microbiol. Biotechnol.* **2007**, *77*, 13–22. [CrossRef]
62. Paul, W.E. *Fundamental Immunology*; LWW: Philadelphia, PA, USA, 2012; ISBN 9781451117837.
63. Mitchell, L.S.; Colwell, L.J. Comparative analysis of nanobody sequence and structure data. *Proteins Struct. Funct. Bioinforma.* **2018**, *86*, 697–706. [CrossRef]
64. Velasco, P.T.; Heffern, M.C.; Sebollela, A.; Popova, I.A.; Lacor, P.N.; Lee, K.B.; Sun, X.; Tiano, B.N.; Viola, K.L.; Eckermann, A.L.; et al. Synapse-binding subpopulations of Abeta oligomers sensitive to peptide assembly blockers and scFv antibodies. *ACS Chem Neurosci* **2012**, *3*, 972–981. [CrossRef]
65. Sebollela, A.; Cline, E.N.; Popova, I.; Luo, K.; Sun, X.; Ahn, J.; Barcelos, M.A.; Bezerra, V.N.; Lyra e Silva, N.M.; Patel, J.; et al. A human scFv antibody that targets and neutralizes high molecular weight pathogenic amyloid-β oligomers. *J. Neurochem.* **2017**, *142*, 934–947. [CrossRef]
66. Zhang, Y.; Chen, X.; Liu, J.; Zhang, Y. The protective effects and underlying mechanism of an anti-oligomeric Aβ42 single-chain variable fragment antibody. *Neuropharmacology* **2015**, *99*, 387–395. [CrossRef]
67. Zhang, Y.; Sun, Y.; Huai, Y.; Zhang, Y.J. Functional Characteristics and Molecular Mechanism of a New scFv Antibody Against Aβ42 Oligomers and Immature Protofibrils. *Mol. Neurobiol.* **2015**, *52*, 1269–1281. [CrossRef]
68. Zhang, X.; Huai, Y.; Cai, J.; Song, C.; Zhang, Y. Novel antibody against oligomeric amyloid-β: Insight into factors for effectively reducing the aggregation and cytotoxicity of amyloid-β aggregates. *Int. Immunopharmacol.* **2019**, *67*, 176–185. [CrossRef]

69. Wang, J.; Wang, J.; Li, N.; Ma, J.; Gu, Z.; Yu, L.; Fu, X.; Liu, X. Effects of an amyloid-beta 1-42 oligomers antibody screened from a phage display library in APP/PS1 transgenic mice. *Brain Res.* **2016**, *1635*, 169–179. [CrossRef]
70. Zameer, A.; Kasturirangan, S.; Emadi, S.; Nimmagadda, S. V.; Sierks, M.R. Anti-oligomeric Aβ Single-chain Variable Domain Antibody Blocks Aβ-induced Toxicity Against Human Neuroblastoma Cells. *J. Mol. Biol.* **2008**, *384*, 917–928. [CrossRef]
71. Kasturirangan, S.; Li, L.; Emadi, S.; Boddapati, S.; Schulz, P.; Sierks, M.R. Nanobody specific for oligomeric beta-amyloid stabilizes nontoxic form. *Neurobiol. Aging* **2012**, *33*, 1320–1328. [CrossRef]
72. Yang, J.; Pattanayak, A.; Song, M.; Kou, J.; Taguchi, H.; Paul, S.; Ponnazhagan, S.; Lalonde, R.; Fukuchi, K.I. Muscle-directed anti-Aβ Single-Chain Antibody Delivery Via AAV1 reduces cerebral Aβ load in an Alzheimer's disease mouse model. *J. Mol. Neurosci.* **2013**, *49*, 277–288. [CrossRef]
73. Krishnaswamy, S.; Lin, Y.; Rajamohamedsait, W.J.; Rajamohamedsait, H.B.; Krishnamurthy, P.; Sigurdsson, E.M. Antibody-derived in Vivo imaging of tau pathology. *J. Neurosci.* **2014**, *34*, 16835–16850. [CrossRef]
74. Tian, H.; Davidowitz, E.; Lopez, P.; He, P.; Schulz, P.; Moe, J.; Sierks, M.R. Isolation and characterization of antibody fragments selective for toxic oligomeric tau. *Neurobiol. Aging* **2015**, *36*, 1342–1355. [CrossRef]
75. Nisbet, R.M.; Van Der Jeugd, A.; Leinenga, G.; Evans, H.T.; Janowicz, P.W.; Götz, J. Combined effects of scanning ultrasound and a tau-specific single chain antibody in a tau transgenic mouse model. *Brain* **2017**, *140*, 1220–1230. [CrossRef]
76. Emadi, S.; Barkhordarian, H.; Wang, M.S.; Schulz, P.; Sierks, M.R. Isolation of a Human Single Chain Antibody Fragment Against Oligomeric α-Synuclein that Inhibits Aggregation and Prevents α-Synuclein-induced Toxicity. *J. Mol. Biol.* **2007**, *368*, 1132–1144. [CrossRef]
77. Emadi, S.; Kasturirangan, S.; Wang, M.S.; Schulz, P.; Sierks, M.R. Detecting morphologically distinct oligomeric forms of α-synuclein. *J. Biol. Chem.* **2009**, *284*, 11048–11058. [CrossRef]
78. Butler, D.C.; Joshi, S.N.; De Genst, E.; Baghel, A.S.; Dobson, C.M.; Messer, A. Bifunctional anti-non-amyloid component α-Synuclein nanobodies are protective in situ. *PLoS ONE* **2016**, *11*, e0165964. [CrossRef]
79. Spencer, B.; Emadi, S.; Desplats, P.; Eleuteri, S.; Michael, S.; Kosberg, K.; Shen, J.; Rockenstein, E.; Patrick, C.; Adame, A.; et al. ESCRT-mediated uptake and degradation of brain-targeted α-synuclein single chain antibody attenuates neuronal degeneration in vivo. *Mol. Ther.* **2014**, *22*, 1753–1767. [CrossRef]
80. Zhang, X.; Sun, X.X.; Xue, D.; Liu, D.G.; Hu, X.Y.; Zhao, M.; Yang, S.G.; Yang, Y.; Xia, Y.J.; Wang, Y.; et al. Conformation-dependent scFv antibodies specifically recognize the oligomers assembled from various amyloids and show colocalization of amyloid fibrils with oligomers in patients with amyloidoses. *Biochim. Biophys. Acta* **2011**, *1814*, 1703–1712. [CrossRef]
81. Benilova, I.; Karran, E.; De Strooper, B. The toxic Aβ oligomer and Alzheimer's disease: An emperor in need of clothes. *Nat. Neurosci.* **2012**, *15*, 349–357. [CrossRef]
82. Haass, C.; Selkoe, D.J. Soluble protein oligomers in neurodegeneration: Lessons from the Alzheimer's amyloid β-peptide. *Nat. Rev. Mol. Cell Biol.* **2007**, *8*, 101–112. [CrossRef]
83. Solórzano-Vargas, R.S.; Vasilevko, V.; Acero, G.; Ugen, K.E.; Martinez, R.; Govezensky, T.; Vazquez-Ramirez, R.; Kubli-Garfias, C.; Cribbs, D.H.; Manoutcharian, K.; et al. Epitope mapping and neuroprotective properties of a human single chain FV antibody that binds an internal epitope of amyloid-beta 1-42. *Mol. Immunol.* **2008**. [CrossRef]
84. Williams, S.M.; Schulz, P.; Sierks, M.R. Oligomeric α-synuclein and β-amyloid variants as potential biomarkers for Parkinson's and Alzheimer's diseases. *Eur. J. Neurosci.* **2016**. [CrossRef]
85. Tiller, K.E.; Li, L.; Kumar, S.; Julian, M.C.; Garde, S.; Tessier, P.M. Arginine mutations in antibody complementarity-determining regions display context-dependent affinity/specificity trade-offs. *J. Biol. Chem.* **2017**, *45*, 881–886. [CrossRef]
86. Das, U.; Hariprasad, G.; Ethayathulla, A.S.; Manral, P.; Das, T.K.; Pasha, S.; Mann, A.; Ganguli, M.; Verma, A.K.; Bhat, R.; et al. Inhibition of protein aggregation: Supramolecular assemblies of Arginine hold the key. *PLoS ONE* **2007**, *2*, e1176. [CrossRef]
87. Kawasaki, T.; Onodera, K.; Kamijo, S. Selection of peptide inhibitors of soluble Aβ1-42 oligomer formation by phage display. *Biosci. Biotechnol. Biochem.* **2010**, *74*, 2214–2219. [CrossRef]
88. Sellés, M.C.; Fortuna, J.; Cercato, M.; Bitencourt, A.; Souza, A.; Prado, V.; Prado, M.; Sebollela, A.; Arancio, O.; Klein, W.; et al. Neuronal expression of NUsc1, a single-chain variable fragment antibody against Aβ oligomers, protects synapses and rescues memory in Alzheimer's disease models. *IBRO Rep.* **2019**, *6*, S497. [CrossRef]

89. Castellani, R.J.; Perry, G.; Tabaton, M. Tau biology, tauopathy, traumatic brain injury, and diagnostic challenges. *J. Alzheimer's Dis.* **2019**, *67*, 447–467. [CrossRef]
90. Buée, L.; Bussière, T.; Buée-Scherrer, V.; Delacourte, A.; Hof, P.R. Tau protein isoforms, phosphorylation and role in neurodegenerative disorders. *Brain Res. Rev.* **2000**, *33*, 95–130. [CrossRef]
91. Kundel, F.; Hong, L.; Falcon, B.; McEwan, W.A.; Michaels, T.C.T.; Meisl, G.; Esteras, N.; Abramov, A.Y.; Knowles, T.J.P.; Goedert, M.; et al. Measurement of Tau Filament Fragmentation Provides Insights into Prion-like Spreading. *ACS Chem. Neurosci.* **2018**, *9*, 1276–1282. [CrossRef]
92. Ising, C.; Gallardo, G.; Leyns, C.E.G.; Wong, C.H.; Jiang, H.; Stewart, F.; Koscal, L.J.; Roh, J.; Robinson, G.O.; Serrano, J.R.; et al. AAV-mediated expression of anti-tau scFvs decreases tau accumulation in a mouse model of tauopathy. *J. Exp. Med.* **2017**, *214*, 1227–1238. [CrossRef]
93. Schulz-Schaeffer, W.J. The synaptic pathology of α-synuclein aggregation in dementia with Lewy bodies, Parkinson's disease and Parkinson's disease dementia. *Acta Neuropathol.* **2010**, *12*, 131–143. [CrossRef]
94. Langston, J.W.; Sastry, S.; Chan, P.; Forno, L.S.; Bolin, L.M.; Di Monte, D.A. Novel α-synuclein-immunoreactive proteins in brain samples from the Contursi kindred, Parkinson's, and Alzheimer's disease. *Exp. Neurol.* **1998**, *154*, 684–690. [CrossRef]
95. Conway, K.A.; Harper, J.D.; Lansbury, P.T. Fibrils formed in vitro from α-synuclein and two mutant forms linked to Parkinson's disease are typical amyloid. *Biochemistry* **2000**, *39*, 2552–2563. [CrossRef]
96. Nannenga, B.L.; Zameer, A.; Sierks, M.R. Anti-oligomeric single chain variable domain antibody differentially affects huntingtin and α-synuclein aggregates. *FEBS Lett.* **2008**, *582*, 517–522. [CrossRef]
97. Kayed, R.; Head, E.; Sarsoza, F.; Saing, T.; Cotman, C.W.; Necula, M.; Margol, L.; Wu, J.; Breydo, L.; Thompson, J.L.; et al. Fibril specific, conformation dependent antibodies recognize a generic epitope common to amyloid fibrils and fibrillar oligomers that is absent in prefibrillar oligomers. *Mol. Neurodegener.* **2007**, *2*, 18. [CrossRef]
98. Spencer, B.; Williams, S.; Rockenstein, E.; Valera, E.; Xin, W.; Mante, M.; Florio, J.; Adame, A.; Masliah, E.; Sierks, M.R. α-synuclein conformational antibodies fused to penetratin are effective in models of Lewy body disease. *Ann. Clin. Transl. Neurol.* **2016**, *3*, 588–606. [CrossRef]
99. Kvam, E.; Nannenga, B.L.; Wang, M.S.; Jia, Z.; Sierks, M.R.; Messer, A. Conformational targeting of fibrillar polyglutamine proteins in live cells escalates aggregation and cytotoxicity. *PLoS One* **2009**, *4*, e5727. [CrossRef]
100. Zhou, C.; Emadi, S.; Sierks, M.R.; Messer, A. A human single-chain Fv intrabody blocks aberrant cellular effects of overexpressed α-synuclein. *Mol. Ther.* **2004**, *10*, 1023–1031. [CrossRef]
101. De Genst, E.J.; Guilliams, T.; Wellens, J.; Day, E.M.; Waudby, C.A.; Meehan, S.; Dumoulin, M.; Hsu, S.T.D.; Cremades, N.; Verschueren, K.H.G.; et al. Structure and properties of a complex of α-synuclein and a single-domain camelid antibody. *J. Mol. Biol.* **2010**, *402*, 326–343. [CrossRef]
102. Vuchelen, A.; O'Day, E.; De Genst, E.; Pardon, E.; Wyns, L.; Dumoulin, M.; Dobson, C.M.; Christodoulou, J.; Hsu, S.T.D. 1H, 13C and 15N assignments of a camelid nanobody directed against human α-synuclein. *Biomol. NMR Assign.* **2009**, *3*, 231–233. [CrossRef]
103. El-Turk, F.; Newby, F.N.; De Genst, E.; Guilliams, T.; Sprules, T.; Mittermaier, A.; Dobson, C.M.; Vendruscolo, M. Structural Effects of Two Camelid Nanobodies Directed to Distinct C-Terminal Epitopes on α-Synuclein. *Biochemistry* **2016**, *55*, 3116–3122. [CrossRef]
104. Emamzadeh, F.N. Alpha-synuclein structure, functions, and interactions. *J. Res. Med. Sci.* **2016**, *9*, 21–29. [CrossRef]
105. Lynch, S.M.; Zhou, C.; Messer, A. An scFv Intrabody against the Nonamyloid Component of α-Synuclein Reduces Intracellular Aggregation and Toxicity. *J. Mol. Biol.* **2008**, *377*, 136–147. [CrossRef]
106. Guilliams, T.; El-Turk, F.; Buell, A.K.; O'Day, E.M.; Aprile, F.A.; Esbjörner, E.K.; Vendruscolo, M.; Cremades, N.; Pardon, E.; Wyns, L.; et al. Nanobodies raised against monomeric α-synuclein distinguish between fibrils at different maturation stages. *J. Mol. Biol.* **2013**, *425*, 2397–2411. [CrossRef]
107. Ross, C.A.; Tabrizi, S.J. Huntington's disease: From molecular pathogenesis to clinical treatment. *Lancet Neurol.* **2011**, *10*, 83–98. [CrossRef]
108. Davies, S.W.; Turmaine, M.; Cozens, B.A.; DiFiglia, M.; Sharp, A.H.; Ross, C.A.; Scherzinger, E.; Wanker, E.E.; Mangiarini, L.; Bates, G.P. Formation of neuronal intranuclear inclusions underlies the neurological dysfunction in mice transgenic for the HD mutation. *Cell* **1997**, *90*, 537–548. [CrossRef]
109. Lecerf, J.M.; Shirley, T.L.; Zhu, Q.; Kazantsev, A.; Amersdorfer, P.; Housman, D.E.; Messer, A.; Huston, J.S. Human single-chain Fv intrabodies counteract in situ huntingtin aggregation in cellular models of Huntington's disease. *Proc. Natl. Acad. Sci. USA* **2001**, *98*, 4764–4769. [CrossRef]

110. Saudou, F.; Humbert, S. The Biology of Huntingtin. *Neuron* **2016**, *89*, 910–926. [CrossRef]
111. Koyuncu, S.; Fatima, A.; Gutierrez-Garcia, R.; Vilchez, D. Proteostasis of huntingtin in health and disease. *Int. J. Mol. Sci.* **2017**, *18*, 1568. [CrossRef]
112. De Genst, E.; Chirgadze, D.Y.; Klein, F.A.C.; Butler, D.C.; Matak-Vinković, D.; Trottier, Y.; Huston, J.S.; Messer, A.; Dobson, C.M. Structure of a single-chain Fv bound to the 17 N-terminal residues of huntingtin provides insights into pathogenic amyloid formation and suppression. *J. Mol. Biol.* **2015**, *427*, 2166–2178. [CrossRef]
113. Murphy, R.C.; Messer, A. A single-chain Fv intrabody provides functional protection against the effects of mutant protein in an organotypic slice culture model of Huntington's disease. *Mol. Brain Res.* **2004**, *121*, 141–145. [CrossRef]
114. Butler, D.C.; Messer, A. Bifunctional anti-huntingtin proteasome-directed intrabodies mediate efficient degradation of mutant huntingtin exon 1 protein fragments. *PLoS One* **2011**, *6*, e29199. [CrossRef]
115. Snyder-Keller, A.; McLear, J.A.; Hathorn, T.; Messer, A. Early or late-stage anti-N-terminal huntingtin intrabody gene therapy reduces pathological features in B6.HDR6/1 mice. *J. Neuropathol. Exp. Neurol.* **2010**, *69*, 1078–1085. [CrossRef]
116. Khoshnan, A.; Ko, J.; Patterson, P.H. Effects of intracellular expression of anti-huntingtin antibodies of various specificities on mutant huntingtin aggregation and toxicity. *Proc. Natl. Acad. Sci. USA* **2002**, *99*, 1002–1007. [CrossRef]
117. Southwell, A.L.; Khoshnan, A.; Dunn, D.E.; Bugg, C.W.; Lo, D.C.; Patterson, P.H. Intrabodies binding the proline-rich domains of mutant Huntingtin increase its turnover and reduce neurotoxicity. *J. Neurosci.* **2008**, *28*, 9013–9020. [CrossRef]
118. Shimizu, Y.; Kaku-Ushiki, Y.; Iwamaru, Y.; Muramoto, T.; Kitamoto, T.; Yokoyama, T.; Mohri, S.; Tagawa, Y. A novel anti-prion protein monoclonal antibody and its single-chain fragment variable derivative with ability to inhibit abnormal prion protein accumulation in cultured cells. *Microbiol. Immunol.* **2010**, *54*, 112–121. [CrossRef]
119. Wang, C.E.; Zhou, H.; McGuire, J.R.; Cerullo, V.; Lee, B.; Li, S.H.; Li, X.J. Suppression of neuropil aggregates and neurological symptoms by an intracellular antibody implicates the cytoplasmic toxicity of mutant huntingtin. *J. Cell Biol.* **2008**, *181*, 803–816. [CrossRef]
120. Southwell, A.L.; Ko, J.; Patterson, P.H. Intrabody gene therapy ameliorates motor, cognitive, and neuropathological symptoms in multiple mouse models of Huntington's disease. *J. Neurosci.* **2009**, *29*, 13589–13602. [CrossRef]
121. Biasini, E.; Turnbaugh, J.A.; Unterberger, U.; Harris, D.A. Prion protein at the crossroads of physiology and disease. *Trends Neurosci.* **2012**, *35*, 92–103. [CrossRef]
122. Martins, S.M.; Frosoni, D.J.; Martinez, A.M.B.; De Felice, F.G.; Ferreira, S.T. Formation of soluble oligomers and amyloid fibrils with physical properties of the scrapie isoform of the prion protein from the C-terminal domain of recombinant murine prion protein mPrP-(121-231). *J. Biol. Chem.* **2006**, *281*, 26121–26128. [CrossRef]
123. Aguzzi, A.; Lakkaraju, A.K.K. Cell Biology of Prions and Prionoids: A Status Report. *Trends Cell Biol.* **2016**, *26*, 40–51. [CrossRef]
124. Pan, K.M.; Baldwin, M.; Nguyen, J.; Gasset, M.; Serban, A.; Groth, D.; Mehlhorn, I.; Huang, Z.; Fletterick, R.J.; Cohen, F.E.; et al. Conversion of α-helices into β-sheets features in the formation of the scrapie prion proteins. *Proc. Natl. Acad. Sci. USA* **1993**. [CrossRef]
125. Donofrio, G.; Heppner, F.L.; Polymenidou, M.; Musahl, C.; Aguzzi, A. Paracrine Inhibition of Prion Propagation by Anti-PrP Single-Chain Fv Miniantibodies. *J. Virol.* **2005**. [CrossRef]
126. Peretz, D.; Williamson, R.A.; Kaneko, K.; Vergara, J.; Leclerc, E.; Schmitt-Ulms, G.; Mehlhorn, I.R.; Legname, G.; Wormald, M.R.; Rudd, P.M.; et al. Antibodies inhibit prion propagation and clear cell cultures of prion infectivity. *Nature* **2001**, *412*, 739–743. [CrossRef]
127. Campana, V.; Zentilin, L.; Mirabile, I.; Kranjc, A.; Casanova, P.; Giacca, M.; Prusiner, S.B.; Legname, G.; Zurzolo, C. Development of antibody fragments for immunotherapy of prion diseases. *Biochem. J.* **2009**, *418*, 507–515. [CrossRef]
128. Fujita, K.; Yamaguchi, Y.; Mori, T.; Muramatsu, N.; Miyamoto, T.; Yano, M.; Miyata, H.; Ootsuyama, A.; Sawada, M.; Matsuda, H.; et al. Effects of a brain-engraftable microglial cell line expressing anti-prion scFv antibodies on survival times of mice infected with scrapie prions. *Cell. Mol. Neurobiol.* **2011**, *31*, 999–1008. [CrossRef]
129. Miyamoto, K.; Nakamura, N.; Aosasa, M.; Nishida, N.; Yokoyama, T.; Horiuchi, H.; Furusawa, S.; Matsuda, H. Inhibition of prion propagation in scrapie-infected mouse neuroblastoma cell lines using mouse monoclonal antibodies against prion protein. *Biochem. Biophys. Res. Commun.* **2005**, *335*, 197–204. [CrossRef]

130. Sonati, T.; Reimann, R.R.; Falsig, J.; Baral, P.K.; O'Connor, T.; Hornemann, S.; Yaganoglu, S.; Li, B.; Herrmann, U.S.; Wieland, B.; et al. The toxicity of antiprion antibodies is mediated by the flexible tail of the prion protein. *Nature* **2013**, *501*, 102–106. [CrossRef]
131. Plotkin, S.S.; Cashman, N.R. Passive immunotherapies targeting Aβ and tau in Alzheimer's disease. *Neurobiol. Dis.* **2020**, *144*, 26. [CrossRef]
132. Lambert, M.P.; Velasco, P.T.; Chang, L.; Viola, K.L.; Fernandez, S.; Lacor, P.N.; Khuon, D.; Gong, Y.; Bigio, E.H.; Shaw, P.; et al. Monoclonal antibodies that target pathological assemblies of Aβ. *J. Neurochem.* **2007**, *100*, 23–35. [CrossRef]
133. Wildburger, N.C.; Esparza, T.J.; Leduc, R.D.; Fellers, R.T.; Thomas, P.M.; Cairns, N.J.; Kelleher, N.L.; Bateman, R.J.; Brody, D.L. Diversity of Amyloid-beta Proteoforms in the Alzheimer's Disease Brain. *Sci. Rep.* **2017**, *7*, 9520. [CrossRef]
134. Condello, C.; Stöehr, J. Aβ propagation and strains: Implications for the phenotypic diversity in Alzheimer's disease. *Neurobiol. Dis.* **2018**, *109*, 191–200. [CrossRef]
135. Cline, E.N.; Das, A.; Bicca, M.A.; Mohammad, S.N.; Schachner, L.F.; Kamel, J.M.; DiNunno, N.; Weng, A.; Paschall, J.D.; Bu, R. Lo; et al. A novel crosslinking protocol stabilizes amyloid β oligomers capable of inducing Alzheimer's-associated pathologies. *J. Neurochem.* **2019**, *148*, 822–836. [CrossRef]
136. Gibbs, E.; Silverman, J.M.; Zhao, B.; Peng, X.; Wang, J.; Wellington, C.L.; Mackenzie, I.R.; Plotkin, S.S.; Kaplan, J.M.; Cashman, N.R. A Rationally Designed Humanized Antibody Selective for Amyloid Beta Oligomers in Alzheimer's Disease. *Sci. Rep.* **2019**, *9*, 9870. [CrossRef]
137. Sevigny, J.; Chiao, P.; Bussière, T.; Weinreb, P.H.; Williams, L.; Maier, M.; Dunstan, R.; Salloway, S.; Chen, T.; Ling, Y.; et al. The antibody aducanumab reduces Aβ plaques in Alzheimer's disease. *Nature* **2016**, *537*, 50–56. [CrossRef]
138. Rogers, M.B. Exposure, Exposure, Exposure? At CTAD, Aducanumab Scientists Make a Case. Available online: https://www.alzforum.org/news/conference-coverage/exposure-exposure-exposure-ctad-aducanumab-scientists-make-case#comment-34176 (accessed on 29 September 2020).
139. Biogen. FDA Accepts Biogen's Aducanumab Biologics License Application for Alzheimer's Disease with Priority Review|Biogen. Available online: https://investors.biogen.com/news-releases/news-release-details/fda-accepts-biogens-aducanumab-biologics-license-application (accessed on 29 September 2020).

Publisher's Note: MDPI stays neutral with regard to jurisdictional claims in published maps and institutional affiliations.

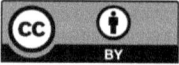

© 2020 by the authors. Licensee MDPI, Basel, Switzerland. This article is an open access article distributed under the terms and conditions of the Creative Commons Attribution (CC BY) license (http://creativecommons.org/licenses/by/4.0/).

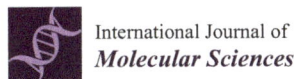

Review

Toward Drug-Like Multispecific Antibodies by Design

Manali S. Sawant [1,2,†], Craig N. Streu [1,2,3,†], Lina Wu [2,4] and Peter M. Tessier [1,2,4,5,*]

1. Department of Pharmaceutical Sciences, University of Michigan, Ann Arbor, MI 48109, USA; manalis@med.umich.edu (M.S.S.); cstreu@albion.edu (C.N.S.)
2. Biointerfaces Institute, University of Michigan, Ann Arbor, MI 48109, USA; linawu@umich.edu
3. Department of Chemistry, Albion College, Albion, MI 49224, USA
4. Department of Chemical Engineering, University of Michigan, Ann Arbor, MI 48109, USA
5. Department of Biomedical Engineering, University of Michigan, Ann Arbor, MI 48109, USA
* Correspondence: ptessier@umich.edu; Tel.: +1-734-763-1486
† These authors contributed equally to this work.

Received: 1 September 2020; Accepted: 2 October 2020; Published: 12 October 2020

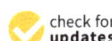

Abstract: The success of antibody therapeutics is strongly influenced by their multifunctional nature that couples antigen recognition mediated by their variable regions with effector functions and half-life extension mediated by a subset of their constant regions. Nevertheless, the monospecific IgG format is not optimal for many therapeutic applications, and this has led to the design of a vast number of unique multispecific antibody formats that enable targeting of multiple antigens or multiple epitopes on the same antigen. Despite the diversity of these formats, a common challenge in generating multispecific antibodies is that they display suboptimal physical and chemical properties relative to conventional IgGs and are more difficult to develop into therapeutics. Here we review advances in the design and engineering of multispecific antibodies with drug-like properties, including favorable stability, solubility, viscosity, specificity and pharmacokinetic properties. We also highlight emerging experimental and computational methods for improving the next generation of multispecific antibodies, as well as their constituent antibody fragments, with natural IgG-like properties. Finally, we identify several outstanding challenges that need to be addressed to increase the success of multispecific antibodies in the clinic.

Keywords: bispecific; polyspecificity; pharmacokinetics; solubility; aggregation; viscosity; developability; stability; affinity; specificity; protein engineering; self-association; non-specific binding; immunogenicity

1. Introduction

Antibodies are among the most well-established biologics and are widely employed as therapeutics. Their success as therapeutics is largely due to their unique combination of properties, including their favorable activities, safety profiles, and physical and chemical properties (also known as developability properties). The activity of antibodies is linked to their high binding affinities and specificities as well as their Fc-mediated interactions with receptors that enable extended half-lives and, in some cases, effector functions. The safety of antibodies is due to their low off-target binding, low immunogenicity (for human or humanized antibodies), and non-toxic breakdown products (amino acids). The desirable developability properties of antibodies are due to their high folding stabilities, high solubilities, low viscosities and high chemical stabilities. The combination of these key properties has led to >80 approved antibody drugs and hundreds more in clinical trials [1].

Nevertheless, most lead antibody (IgG) candidates do not have the required combination of activity, safety, and developability properties for therapeutic applications, and must be further engineered to achieve drug-like molecules. Overcoming these issues is even more challenging for multispecific antibodies, a class of engineered antibodies that seeks to engage either two or more targets or two or more epitopes on the same target. Generally, multispecifics are chimeric proteins composed of IgGs and smaller antibody fragments or multiple antibody fragments (Figure 1). Given their ability to bind more than one target, multispecific antibodies have functional advantages for applications in which it is necessary to bring together two targets in close proximity. This is a key feature of the two multispecific antibodies blinatumomab and emicizumab that have been approved for use in humans and are currently being marketed [2–6]. Although the full potential of multispecific antibodies is just beginning to be tapped [7], one particularly notable therapeutic application has been the recruitment of immune effector cells, such as T cells [8–11] or natural killer (NK) cells [12–15], to tumor cells using multispecific formats that recognize antigens on both cell types. Still other potential advantages of binding multiple targets include synergistic effects, improved specificity, and reduced incidence of drug-resistance.

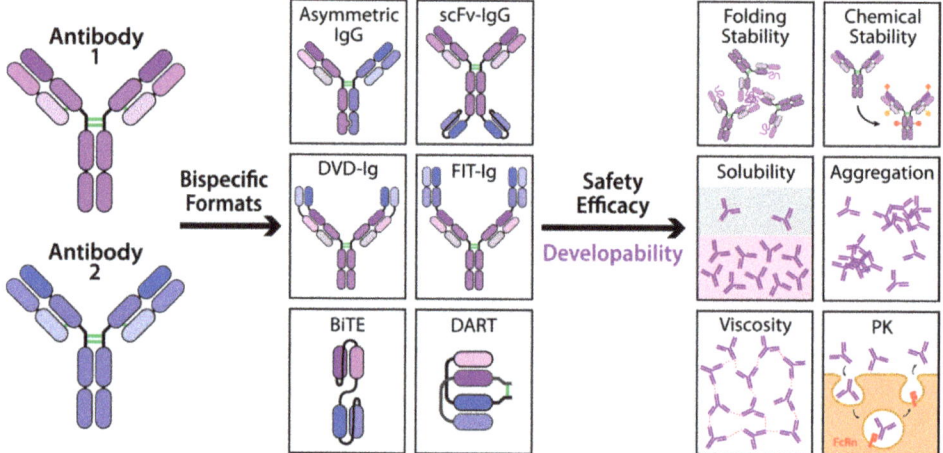

Figure 1. Antigen-binding regions of monospecific IgGs can be combined into various multispecific formats that have unique developability concerns, including those related to their stability, solubility, aggregation, viscosity, and pharmacokinetics. The abbreviations are scFv-IgG for single-chain variable fragment immunoglobulin, DVD-Ig for dual variable domain immunoglobulin, FIT-Ig for fabs-in-tandem immunoglobulin, BiTE for bispecific T-cell engager and DART for dual-affinity re-targeting antibody fragment.

Despite their impressive therapeutic potential, much less is known about the developability properties of multispecifics with respect to conventional antibodies (IgGs), which is a major limitation to their development and broad adoption as therapeutics. Further exacerbating the knowledge gap is the sheer number of multispecific antibody formats that have been developed, each with its own specific advantages and liabilities as therapeutics [16–18]. Recent advances in the ability to screen antibodies for developability parameters earlier in the discovery process are likely to streamline the development of antibody therapeutics but, to date, no such general approach exists for multispecific antibodies. Because many multispecific antibodies are composed of recombined antibody fragments, and stabilization of the individual fragments is a common component of multispecific design strategies, this review will focus on the latest methods for optimizing the drug-like properties of antibody fragments in addition to strategies for optimizing multispecific antibodies. Here we divide the critical antibody properties into three broad categories, namely: (i) physical and chemical stability, (ii) self-association and high concentration properties, and (iii) polyspecificity and in vivo properties. For each category, we highlight the latest advances in understanding how to design and engineer multispecific antibodies and their constituent antibody fragments with drug-like properties as well as outline the outstanding challenges.

2. Physical and Chemical Stability

2.1. Folding and Assembly

Many new multispecific formats are generated from constituent antibody fragments. Typically, the folding stability of these fragments is lower than that for full-length IgGs, which can be problematic following incorporation into multispecific formats. Much previous work has focused on the thermostabilization of antibody fragments and full-length antibodies [19–22], while comparatively less is known about the thermostability of diverse multispecific formats [23]. However, it is possible to improve the stability of multispecific antibodies by optimization of their component parts. Therefore, thermostabilization of antibody fragments is an important strategy for producing multispecific antibodies with improved overall stability.

One established method for improving the thermostability of antibody fragments is disulfide engineering. The addition of well-positioned disulfide bonds is known to improve the thermostability of antibodies and fragments thereof, and the number of engineered disulfide bond variants validated for stabilization, as well as the list of successful applications, continues to expand [24–27]. Disulfide engineering has been particularly successful in generating stabilized single-domain antibodies with one recent example generating an extremely stable nanobody with a melting temperature exceeding 90 °C [28–31]. The ability to generate such highly stable single-domain antibodies is likely to shift the developmental bottleneck for multispecifics that contain these fragments away from thermal stabilization of the constituent fragments toward optimization of other developability properties.

One such property is proper folding. Despite the success of disulfide engineering in protein stabilization, introducing additional non-canonical disulfide bonds to proteins, such as scFvs, comes at the risk of scrambled or mismatched disulfides. This scrambling can lead to incorrect folding or multimerization, resulting in lost production yield and purity [32]. Therefore, when considering disulfide engineering as an approach to antibody fragment thermostabilization, the potential stabilizing effects must be weighed against the potential for disulfide scrambling and misfolding. In multispecific formats that may contain increased numbers of disulfide bonds, the potential for mispairing may be magnified. Fortunately, novel approaches for improving the yield of proteins with engineered disulfide bonds have been investigated [33]. One particularly powerful method is the co-expression of four proteins that promote folding and disulfide bond formation in the periplasm of *E. coli* from a single helper plasmid [34]. These helper proteins include DsbA and DsbC, which are thiol-disulfide oxidoreductases that are responsible for the reduction and subsequent rearrangement of improperly formed disulfide bonds. In addition, the other two proteins include peptidyl-prolyl *cis/trans*-isomerases FkpA and SurA. These enzymes promote sampling both *cis* and *trans* isomeric forms of proline during protein refolding. Application of this technology to nanobodies containing a second stabilizing disulfide bond has been reported to increase expression yield by 2- to 10-fold, approaching and occasionally exceeding the expression yields for nanobodies containing a single canonical disulfide bond [35].

Given the added risk of disulfide scrambling and subsequently reduced yields associated with disulfide engineering, other approaches for antibody fragment thermostabilization are of broad interest. One strategy for generating antibody fragments with high stability is to graft portions of a known antibody or antibody fragment, especially the CDRs, onto a thermostable scaffold [22,36]. However, the affinity and stability of an antibody or antibody fragment is generally highly dependent upon the compatibility of the framework and CDR regions since CDRs make many contacts that can drastically alter these properties [37,38]. This means that grafted CDR regions or affinity-improving mutations cannot be incorporated into a thermostable framework without risk of compromising antibody stability. Although compensatory mutations can offset this loss of stability, iterative rounds of affinity and stability maturation are generally required [21,22,37,39]. A related strategy that involves thermostabilization of the framework has recently been demonstrated that involves V_L framework swapping [40]. The investigators identified a suboptimal lambda V_L domain in an anti-epidermal growth factor receptor (EGFR) scFv and replaced it with more stable kappa3 framework regions, generating a scFv variant with greater stability, improved expression in *E. coli*, and similar binding to the parental antibody fragment.

Yet another method for generating thermally stable antibodies is the use of high-throughput biophysical profiling. Among the most common strategies for selecting stabilized antibody fragments is the use of thermal challenge assays of libraries displayed on phage or yeast [41–45]. In these assays, libraries are heat shocked before selection for antigen binding. This strategy was recently used successfully to improve the stability of a bispecific tetravalent antibody by allowing the rapid optimization of its scFv subunits [46]. Of course, this type of assay relies on the viability of the display system following heat shock, which has led to the development of a new thermostable yeast strain for use in such heat shock screens [47]. Although this fragment-based approach has proven effective, recent advances in screening intact bispecific antibodies suggests that the final format of an antibody can have unexpected consequences for potency, and may therefore identify variants with optimal properties that may be missed by the fragment-based approaches [48].

Despite the success of these and other approaches [47,49–52], stabilizing mutations in the CDRs or frameworks would be highly valuable. Fortunately, computational approaches for the design of antibodies with high affinity and thermostability have made significant recent advances [53–58]. One notable method also approaches the problem by computationally recombining antibody variable domains to generate variants with improved biophysical properties [53]. Specifically, stabilized antibodies against multiple antigens were designed by a computational algorithm known as AbDesign [53,59]. The AbDesign algorithm optimizes both binding and stability by first generating recombinations of known F_V backbone fragments, which are docked against a desired target. Next, affinity and stability are simultaneously optimized by sampling different natural conformations of the F_V backbone fragments and optimizing their sequences using Rosetta. The corresponding scFvs could then be further affinity matured into nanomolar binders experimentally using error-prone PCR and in vitro library sorting methods. After five rounds of design, the resulting antibody fragments contained more than 30 backbone mutations with respect to the mammalian germline sequence and achieved respectable folding stabilities, as measured in terms of their melting temperatures (57–79 °C relative to 70 °C for similar wild-type constructs). To achieve this level of affinity and stability, the authors conclude that it is critical to both maintain residues required for proper F_V backbone configurations, such as buried polar networks, and segment the F_V backbone fragments during the design process in a manner that keeps the CDRs and their closest framework contacts on the same fragment. Using those constraints, the authors suggest that their fragmentation strategy is a generally applicable approach to computational design of stabilized antibodies, which will be important to further evaluate in future studies.

Another streamlined computational approach to antibody fragment affinity maturation and stabilization focuses on optimization of the V_H-V_L interface (Figure 2) [60]. This strategy was inspired by deep mutational analysis data for anti-lysozyme antibody D44.1 suggesting that, in addition to the CDRs, many affinity-enhancing mutations occur at the V_H-V_L interface. From this mutational data, Rosetta was used to generate optimized multipoint mutants from combinations of the affinity-enhancing mutations at eight interface positions. This method yielded an antibody with nearly ten-fold greater affinity than wild type with substantially improved thermal stability (melting temperature increase of 9 °C relative to wild type) and aggregation resistance (aggregation temperature increase of 7 °C relative to wild type). Comparison of the X-ray structures of the wild type and designed Fabs showed a high degree of structural similarity in the lysozyme binding site. Furthermore, the designed antibody had a 25-fold slower off rate than the parental antibody. Taken together, these results suggest that the improvements in affinity are likely a result of improved stabilization of the binding conformation, as well as improved packing, solvation and/or rigidity in the resulting framework backbone. Therefore, optimization of the V_H-V_L interface has the potential to improve binding and developability properties in a number of ways. This method was then automated into a freely available web-based platform known as AbLIFT, which was validated on two additional antibodies, both of which showed substantial improvements in affinity, thermal stability, and aggregation resistance [60]. Recently, a related strategy was employed for scFv and single-chain antibody (scAb) formats, placing special emphasis not necessarily on domain interfaces, but on local regions that are particularly susceptible to unfolding [57]. Once again, the application of Rosetta to determine multipoint mutants with enhanced properties within a defined region yielded significant enhancements in thermal stability, suggesting that these approaches are not necessarily format specific and therefore hold potential for engineering multispecific antibodies.

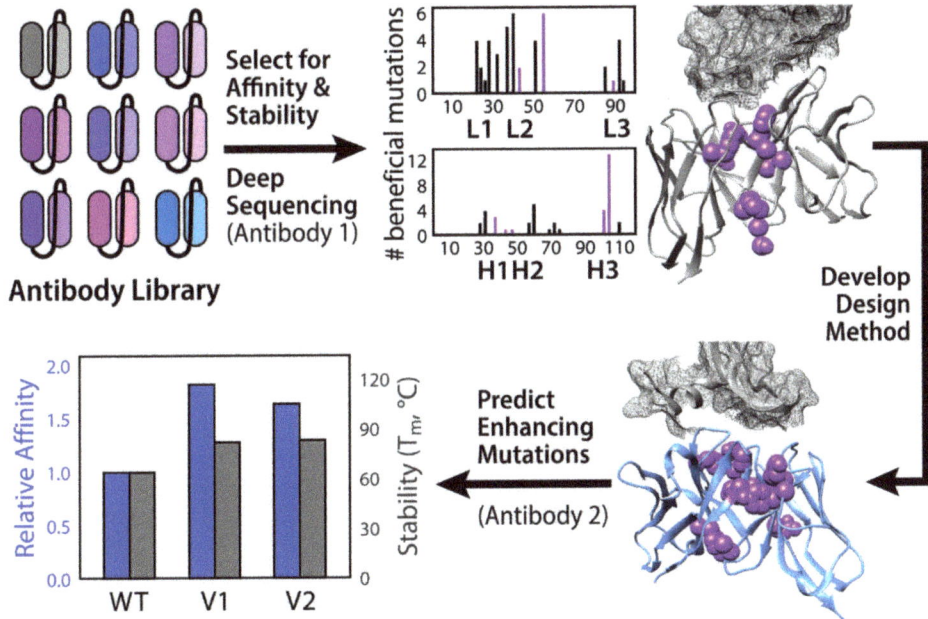

Figure 2. Evaluation and prediction of mutations in the V_H/V_L interface that enhance the stability and affinity of single-chain antibodies. Deep mutational analysis of a scFv library (top left) identified eight interface residues tolerant of mutations (purple, top right). Combinations of affinity-maintaining mutations at these sites were analyzed with Rosetta to predict those that also improve thermal stability. After development using the anti-lysozyme antibody D44.1, the automated design method (AbLift) was validated on two additional antibodies, including the anti-VEGF antibody G6 (bottom right). AbLift designed G6 variants 1 (V1) and 2 (V2) displayed both improved affinity and thermal stability (bottom left). The figure is adapted from a previous publication [60].

Although multispecific antibodies face their own challenges associated with thermal stability, their proper and efficient assembly into relatively large and complex molecular formats is one of the greatest barriers to their successful development into viable therapeutics. In traditional antibody-like formats, this includes proper heavy chain pairing as well as heavy-light chain pairing. These assembly issues have generally impaired high-throughput study of multispecific properties, slowing their development.

Multiple approaches for the efficient production of multispecific antibodies have recently been reported, including those that range from improved purification procedures [61] to novel strategies for reducing mispairing [62–66]. These later strategies can broadly be divided into two categories:

novel multispecific formats that are less prone to mispairing and new strategies for assembling multispecifics. For example, common light chain approaches have been developed to address the light chain pairing problem while generating different F_v antigen-binding sites using divergent heavy chains [67–69]. Given that the light chains for each binding site are the same, this eliminates the possibility of heavy chain-light chain mispairing. However, identifying a promiscuous light chain that enables binding of two different antigens can be a significant undertaking. Still others have engineered the heavy chain-light chain interface to promote selective association of the correct heavy chain-light chain pairs, or perhaps just as importantly, disfavor incorrect chain pairing [70–73]. This type of engineering has the potential to allow direct expression and production of heterodimeric antibodies, which are antibodies composed of half of two different antibodies dimerized into a full IgG through heterotypic Fc pairing [74,75]. Given that the engineered sites are buried at antibody domain interfaces, these frameworks are anticipated to exhibit minimal immunogenicity, which is an important consideration for their viability as potential therapeutics [67].

Assembly issues notwithstanding, multispecific antibody formats have the potential to show highly favorable drug-like properties. For example, the Bispecific T-Cell Engager (BiTE) format, which is composed of two scFvs linked in sequence, was the first bispecific drug format to earn FDA approval [76]. By making use of the propensity of scFvs to atypically heterodimerize through intermolecular disulfide formation, another related bispecific antibody fragment (Dual-Affinity Re-Targeting, DART) has been produced [77]. These bispecific antibody fragments, which are composed of sets of heterodimerized scFvs that are stabilized by interstrand disulfide bonds, have shown even greater bioactivity and stability than the equivalent BiTE format [78,79]. Other recent additions to the growing list of multispecific formats include bivalent tandem Fabs [80], as well as the related tetravalent bispecific IgG1-Fabs [80] and Fabs-in-tandem (FIT-Ig) [81]. Unlike BiTEs that are single-chain antibodies, or DARTs that are composed of two chains, all three of these formats are expressed as three chains. IgG1-Fabs contain a Fab recombinantly fused to a parent antibody V_H through the Fab C_H1 with a linker. On the other hand, Fabs-in-tandem are composed of two Fabs linked from the V_H of one Fab to the C_L of another (instead of to C_H1 for IgG1-Fabs), leading to a "crisscross" Fab orientation. Bivalent Fabs-in-tandem composed of anti-EGFR and anti-CD3 Fabs showed excellent antigen binding and superior thermostability, aggregation propensity and expression compared to the corresponding tandem scFv, demonstrating its potential as a multispecific scaffold [81]. Similar improvements in stability, aggregation, and expression were observed for the IgG1-Fab constructed from the Fab of pertuzumab fused to the IgG1 of trastuzumab relative to the corresponding IgG1-scFv [80]. It is worth noting that both formats demonstrated excellent bioactivity and that the IgG1-Fab also showed improved bioactivity with respect to the combination of parental antibodies, further highlighting the unique therapeutic potential of multispecific formats. Such bispecific antibodies composed of the anti-IL-17 Fab of ixekizumab fused to the anti-IL-20 antibody 15D2 showed little mispairing during assembly except for a small quantity of light chain dimerization [81]. Like the other recent Fab-based multispecific formats [80,82], these Fabs-in-tandem displayed excellent biophysical properties [81].

While these new antibody formats have significant advantages, each new antibody format brings with it uncertainties about drug-like properties and developability. Therefore, multispecific antibodies with native IgG frameworks are still considered most desirable. Recently, intein-based protein splicing methods have proven highly effective for generating multispecific antibodies from antibody fragments [83,84] as well as native IgG frameworks [85,86]. Although the full impact of this technology has yet to be realized, the ability to make multispecifics with fully native IgG Fc regions will undoubtedly have significant implications for multispecific antibody production for a variety of reasons. For example, this intein approach will enable generation of complex multispecific antibodies in a much higher throughput fashion than is currently possible. Such methods will be necessary for generating early-stage developability data to assess the biophysical properties of multispecifics, which is one area where multispecifics lag far behind traditional monospecific antibody formats. Fortunately, the unique advantages of intein splicing have already been applied in a generalizable high-throughput screen for bispecific antibodies, demonstrating the applicability of the technology for screening applications [87].

2.2. Aggregation

Aggregation is a particularly important liability for biotherapeutic drug development because it can impact all stages of production and, therefore, strategies for reducing aggregation are an important part of antibody design efforts. For example, high levels of aggregate formation during protein expression and cell culture can cause low purification yields of the antibody of interest [32]. Even more important, aggregates can also form during formulation and storage, and dimers, trimers, and higher order multimers can lead to undesirable immunogenic responses [88,89].

Although aggregation is commonly associated with reduced folding stability, leading to unfolding or misfolding, these properties are not always linked. For example, we and others have shown that antibody fragments can display large differences in their aggregation propensities despite having similar folding stabilities [90–93]. Additionally, it is difficult to identify a single attribute that can be used to predict protein aggregation due to the complexities of the locations of aggregation-prone regions in antibodies and other proteins, as some are solvent-exposed in the folded state and others become solvent exposed upon unfolding [94,95]. Moreover, the propensity of antibody fragments to aggregate may be amplified by avidity effects when reformatted as multispecifics or in conditions that may be encountered during bioprocessing, such as freeze-thaw cycles, pH changes or mechanical stresses such as shaking and stirring [94,96,97].

Several powerful methods have been developed recently to experimentally and computationally identify antibody variants that are resistant to aggregation [98,99]. One general strategy is to modify the charge of antibodies or antibody fragments. Applications that address the aggregation of antibody fragments are important because a significant challenge in developing multispecific antibodies as drugs is that the constituent antibody fragments used in common multispecific antibody formats are generally more prone to aggregation than conventional IgGs. The most common approach to suppress antibody aggregation is to replace hydrophobic residues with charged residues, which generates aggregation-resistant variants by reducing hydrophobic association between species [92,100]. For example, phage display has been used for mutational screening of CDR1 and CDR2 in human variable domains to determine the contribution of individual residues to aggregation [92]. This analysis revealed a set of seven positions localized in or near CDR1 of V_H and six positions localized in or near CDR2 of V_L that were responsible for the greatest contributions to the aggregation of human antibody variable domains. Mutational analysis was also used to show that inclusion of aspartate or, less favorably, glutamate residues at these positions resulted in substantially reduced aggregation behavior. Interestingly, the results suggested that the contribution of each position were generally independent and qualitatively additive, such that multiple mutations led to the highest levels of aggregation resistance. Not only did these substitutions improve aggregation behavior, they also resulted in generally improved biophysical properties. Surprisingly, an earlier study of the same aggregation-prone V_H domain identified a novel negatively-charged mutation near the edge of heavy chain CDR1 (F29D) that was as effective at preventing aggregation as multiple negatively-charged mutations in the middle of the same CDR [90]. It was also demonstrated that residues near the edges of CDR3 in human single-domain antibodies contribute disproportionately to aggregation and that the most effective mutations for reducing aggregation vary with respect to the overall charge of the antibody fragment [93]. A similar mutational strategy was used to improve the solubility and aggregation profile of a F(ab')$_2$ [100]. Interestingly, the sites that were found to be critical for these improvements were located along the perimeter of the paratope. This finding, which is similar to those for other types of protein-protein interactions [101–103], may explain the results of the mutational analysis and influence future design strategies.

While these mutational strategies have proven highly effective at improving the aggregation behavior of antibodies and antibody fragments, it would ideally be possible to select for aggregation-resistant variants earlier in the development process and with higher accuracy. Important progress has been made in recent years to accomplish this ambitious goal by combining these mutational strategies with computational predictive methods. For example, using previously identified sites in antibody variable regions that mediate aggregation [92], an in silico library of 393 single, double, and triple aspartate mutants were generated and screened using Rosetta to identify those that retain thermodynamic stability [104]. Those mutants predicted to retain high thermodynamic stability were produced and tested for various developability attributes. Of the 26 variants produced, half showed reduced aggregation, while nearly all (25 of 26) demonstrated reduced non-specific binding. Interestingly, the judiciously identified mutations had a negligible impact on antigen-binding affinity, demonstrating the tremendous potential of this approach for streamlining antibody development.

One potential consequence of mutational design strategies that alter antibody charge is that added surface charge may increase transient local unfolding, which could lead to an increase in aggregate nucleation [105]. To investigate this, the electrostatic potential of a model scFv was systematically modified by insertion of three different sets of five charged residues (Glu, Lys or Arg residues) into a hydrophobic patch in such a way as to introduce new salt bridges [106]. In all cases, replacing arginine with lysine was shown to reduce aggregation, leading to the conclusion that lysine has an increased ability, relative to arginine, to reduce interactions between partially folded states, which may become more prominent after electrostatic engineering. More recently, the biophysical basis of this finding was shown to be a result of the propensity of arginine to form favorable interactions with the unfolded states of proteins, possibly through interactions with exposed aromatic residues [107]. Furthermore, the unique geometric structure afforded by the guanidinium group in arginine permits multiple types of intermolecular interactions and thus can promote aggregation [108]. As such, the authors conclude that the arginine:lysine ratio may be a useful parameter for predicting antibody aggregation propensities and for designing antibody variants with reduced aggregation behavior [107].

Several additional notable studies in predicting aggregation behavior have focused on single-chain (scFv) antibodies, which are one of the most aggregation-prone antibody fragments. This is due in large part to the relatively weak interactions between V_H and V_L domains in the absence of the stabilizing constant (C_H1 and C_L) domains, which results in a dynamic equilibrium between open and closed forms of the fragment. This process facilitates the formation of intermolecular domain swapping and high levels of aggregation. Rational design and high-throughput mutagenesis methods have both been used successfully to reduce aggregation by improving the stability of the V_H/V_L interface and promoting the closed state of the scFv [40,109–113].

Although interface stabilization strategies have proven effective, a broadly generalizable approach for aggregation reduction across many different types of scFv frameworks would be highly desirable. Interestingly, intramolecular chain cyclization of scFvs has been shown to be effective at reducing the propensity of scFvs to dissociate and subsequently aggregate [114]. Specifically, sortase-cyclized scFvs demonstrated an increased fraction of closed states as well as reduced separation between V_H and V_L domains in the open states. In addition, these improvements came at little cost to the overall thermostability and antigen binding. This strategy was also demonstrated to be generalizable to other scFvs. However, cyclic scFv fragments cannot be incorporated into traditional multispecific frameworks such as IgG-scFv formats in the same ways as the conventional (acyclic) versions, necessitating the development of novel strategies for linking cyclic scFvs into multivalent therapeutics.

As advances in assays for aggregation have improved, so too have high-throughput methods for analyzing aggregation propensity early in development [92,115]. Two particularly notable studies have sought correlations between early-stage analyses of biophysical parameters and late-stage developability [116,117]. In the first study, the results of twelve different biophysical assays for 137 antibodies that had advanced to at least phase II clinical studies were analyzed [116]. This information was used to correlate biophysical assay results, many of which can be performed in a high-throughput fashion early in the discovery process, to drug-like properties and to establish thresholds for each of these properties. Interestingly, the results from multiple assays could be correlated with each other, such as strong correlations between different types of non-specific and self-interaction assays. However, accelerated stability (aggregation) results could not be quantitatively correlated with the results from other assays, highlighting the distinctive nature of antibody aggregation and the difficulty in assessing aggregation behavior using early-stage screens [116].

In the second related study, the results of a largely different set of early-stage biophysical assays for 152 human or humanized monoclonal antibodies were evaluated for correlations between early-stage screening results and downstream developmental parameters [117]. The authors observed a significant number of correlations between early-stage high-throughput assays and later stage analytical methods that often require much more sample. For example, aggregation is generally evaluated using size-exclusion chromatography. However, this type of analysis is relatively low throughput and requires quantities of protein beyond what would be desirable for early-stage screening. Fortunately, measurements of the melting temperature (T_m) and aggregation temperature (T_{agg}), obtained from intrinsic differential scanning fluorimetry (T_m) and near-UV light scattering (T_{agg}), correlated well with measurements of aggregation during expression, accelerated stability, and particle formation, as well as with various purification properties. Furthermore, high melting and aggregation temperatures were correlated with the best colloidal properties. Using a strategy based largely around early-stage optimization of aggregation behavior, an antibody with a substantially improved developability profile was produced, suggesting that measurements of melting and aggregation temperatures are indeed useful early surrogates for predicting and optimizing some late-stage developability parameters of antibodies [117]. While these findings may have important implications for multispecific antibodies, it is not known if the same correlations apply to such non-traditional formats.

Another powerful way to screen for antibody fragments with favorable developability properties is to use rodents engineered to express human V_H repertoires [118]. To realize this goal, transgenic rats containing chimeric heavy chain only antibodies with fully human V_H domains have been generated. These transgenic animals are engineered to express a wide range of human sequences that are available from V(D)J recombination and develop large numbers of stable and high-affinity heavy chain antibodies in response to immunization. Such antigen-specific heavy chain antibodies demonstrate favorable stability and aggregation profiles despite the absence of stabilizing V_L domains. These uniquely stable V_H domains were attributed to specific frameworks and CDRs found in traditional IgGs. The ability to generate highly stable, fully human single-domain antibodies by immunization has tremendous potential for generating antibody fragments with favorable developability profiles for incorporation into multispecific antibodies.

Computation has also been a valuable resource for evaluating the physical processes that lead to aggregation and semi-rational design of aggregation-resistant proteins. The ultimate goal in this area of research is to fully predict antibody aggregation profiles based solely on their primary sequences. One early major step in the computational prediction of antibody properties, including aggregation propensities, was the Developability Index (DI) [119], which is based upon the spatial aggregation propensity (SAP) [96]. This algorithm, which was originally developed using the long-term stability data of a panel of twelve antibodies, correlated antibody hydrophobicity and electrostatic properties, as well as 3D structural information, to aggregation propensity. This enabled the prediction of lead antibodies as well as mutated variants with high stability with respect to aggregation [108,119].

As expected, the generation of more extensive experimental data sets that correlate antibody sequence with aggregation behavior has led to improved computational predictions of antibodies with aggregation-resistant properties. For example, computational methods have been developed for predicting antibody aggregation based upon experimental aggregation data generated from size-exclusion chromatography and an oligomer detection assay [120]. These computational methods, which do not require detailed structural models, were generated using statistical modeling of antibody properties in combination with machine learning. Importantly, these methods were validated by selecting anti-interferon γ (IFN-γ) antibodies that are less aggregation prone and have overall better developability profiles. Although the sequence-based method and the Developability Index method both performed well in terms of predicting antibodies with high aggregation propensity, the former method outperformed the latter one in terms of correctly identifying antibodies with low aggregation propensities, which is important for early-stage antibody screening efforts.

One of the challenges in early-stage screening for aggregation behavior has been the poor correlation between global protein folding stability (as measured by the melting temperature) or fraction of unfolded protein and aggregation at native conditions. This disconnect is attributed to the fact that the dominant aggregation pathway for proteins at native conditions is likely due to local structural perturbations or partial unfolding rather than global protein unfolding. At near-native conditions, local flexible or unfolded protein regions may form intermolecular interactions, leading to protein aggregation without global unfolding. To test this hypothesis, potential aggregation-prone regions that mediate aggregate formation were first identified in the A33 Fab by molecular dynamic simulations and analysis of relevant crystal structure B-factors, which are related to thermal motions of each residue [121]. Rosetta was then used to predict stabilizing and destabilizing mutants, which were tested for their ability to mediate differences in folding cooperativity. As expected, none of the selected single point mutations produced significant changes in the global stability of the Fab, but half of these mutants increased unfolding cooperativity. This cooperativity could be correlated with reductions in conformational flexibility, making it possible to evaluate the role of conformational flexibility in aggregation processes, independent of changes in global stability. The results of this study suggest that aggregation behavior at near-native conditions can indeed be related to short flexible regions of protein structure and that aggregation behavior can be improved by simple mutations that reduce conformational flexibility in these regions.

Although the previous study specifically avoided mutations in the CDRs of the Fab regions in order to preserve the paratope, CDRs are often predicted to be aggregation-prone regions (APRs) [122,123]. These predictions are consistent with findings that show CDRs are often the chief determinants of antibody aggregation behavior [90–93,119,124–126]. Solubis, a computational tool for predicting aggregation propensity of mutants, was used to identify critical APRs in antibodies [94]. This method first uses computational tools to distinguish between structural APRs that are typically buried, and those that are critical for aggregation, by determining their overall contribution to the stability of the antibody as well as their ability to form conformers likely to aggregate without significant unfolding. Once the critical APRs are identified, mutants can be generated that are predicted to both reduce aggregation and maintain the local and global stability of the protein. Interestingly, several of the mutations predicted in this study maintained antigen binding along with their predicted reduction in aggregation behavior. Gratifyingly, the reduction in aggregation propensity also corresponded to an improved expression profile [94].

Despite the significant advances in predicting aggregation propensities of antibodies and antibody fragments, much is unknown about the applicability of these models to multispecific antibodies. For example, most models rely on structural homology modeling or large sets of aggregation data taken from traditional antibody frameworks. In fact, one recent study suggests that the aggregation properties of a multispecific antibody can be more complicated than the sum of its parts [32]. In this study, the levels of aggregation for a Fab attached to a disulfide linked Fv (Fab-ds-Fv) and a Fab attached to a disulfide linked scFv (Fab-ds-scFv) were compared. Note that the first construct involves an Fv fragment stabilized by an additional disulfide bond, while the second construct involves a single-chain (scFv) fragment also stabilized by an additional disulfide bond. These two formats were chosen as simple representations of bispecific formats containing attached Fv or scFv domains. Interestingly, the ranking of the fragments in terms of the % monomer levels of the free ds-Fv and ds-scFv fragments did not correlate with the ranking of the % monomer levels for the corresponding bispecific Fab-ds-Fv and Fab-ds-scFv fragments. This finding implies the distinct nature of "free" versus "tethered" intermolecular association properties and suggests that aggregation screening of multispecifics, at least in some cases, must be conducted in the context of the final antibody format. Fortunately, with advances in multispecific expression and assembly technologies (Section 2.1), it is increasingly possible to produce multispecific constructs en masse. This development, and the high-throughput accumulation of data on multispecific formats, will facilitate the transition from tools that require detailed structural models to those that can make predictions with sequence information alone.

As it is not always possible to engineer multispecific antibodies that do not aggregate, advances in manufacturing have provided an important alternative. For example, flocculation-based pretreatments of mammalian cell cultures have recently been demonstrated as an alternate strategy to reduce aggregates [127]. While the majority of known flocculants adequately remove host cell impurities, one particular flocculant, partially benzylated poly(allylamine) (PAAm-Bn), shows promise in reducing aggregates, in addition to host cell impurities. One study tested the treatment of this flocculant in cell cultures of multiple monospecific and bispecific antibodies, and showed a variable yet PAAm-Bn concentration-dependent removal of aggregates. Multispecific antibodies tend to have higher aggregate levels compared to monospecific antibodies, and therefore require higher concentrations of PAAm-Bn. It is clear that a combination of improved screening, design, analysis and manufacturing procedures will all play important roles in the development of multispecific antibodies with improved aggregation profiles.

2.3. Chemical Stability

Although much progress has been made in the efficient assembly of multispecific antibodies with desirable drug-like properties, a somewhat less appreciated barrier to their development as therapeutics is the ability to control and monitor their chemical stability throughout the development process. Chemical stability is of course an essential property for the developability of any therapeutic. In general, the major issues that antibody fragments or multispecific antibodies face (e.g., oxidation, deamidation and isomerization) are also found in traditional IgGs.

Although the issues are the same, their study may be complicated by the increased complexity of multispecifics. For example, in order to understand the impact of post-translational modifications on bioactivity, it may be necessary to generate symmetrically or asymmetrically modified antibodies. Even bispecifics based on a traditional IgG scaffold, but comprising of two different variable regions, are likely to contain differences not only in the variable regions but also in the constant regions, which are often mutated to direct heavy or light chain pairing. To address this issue, a strategy based upon the DuoBody platform [63,64] has been developed for generating symmetrically or asymmetrically modified IgG bispecific antibodies (Figure 3). To understand how chemical instabilities impact bispecific antibodies, the DuoBody platform was used to recombine two parental antibodies into a bispecific antibody with high fidelity, such that the parental antibodies could first be modified by chemical degradation (e.g., oxidation or deamidation) [128]. Next, the antibodies were recombined to give four possible variants for analysis (symmetric modified, symmetric unmodified, and both asymmetrically modified bispecific antibodies). Methionine oxidized and asparagine deamidated versions were then used to analyze the effects of such chemical modifications on Protein A, FcRn and FcγRIIIa binding. Interestingly, this study confirmed the proposed stoichiometric binding between antibody Fc and FcγRIIIa receptor, which has implications for predicting the impacts of chemical degradation on multispecific antibody biological activity. Such methods will be critical for evaluating critical quality attributes in IgG-based bispecific antibodies.

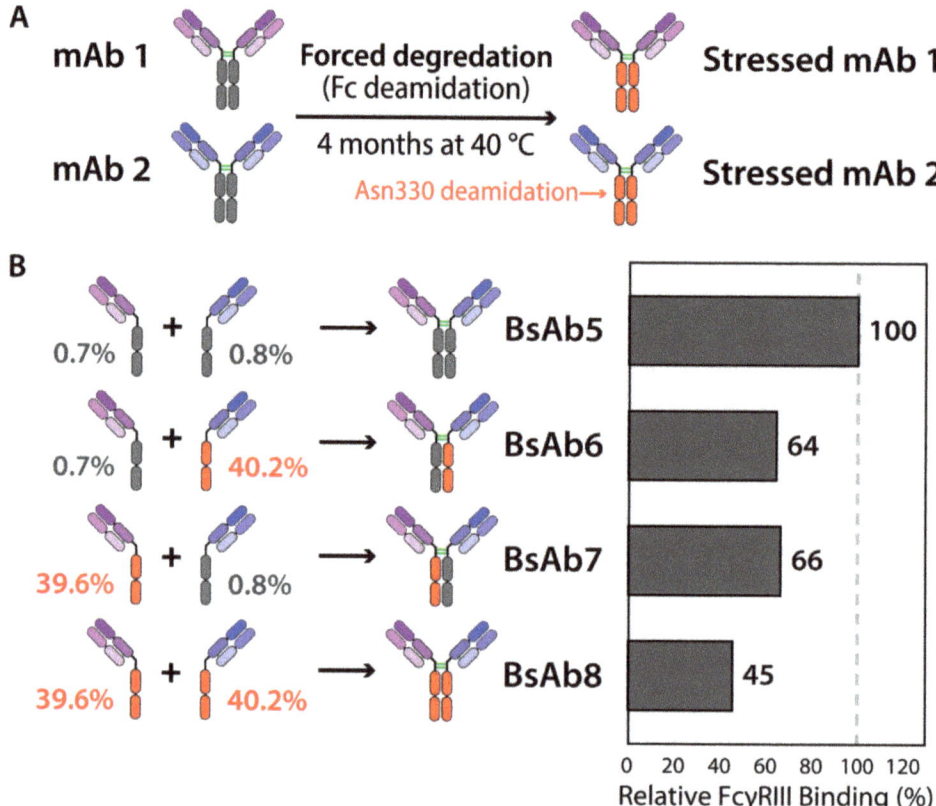

Figure 3. Evaluation of the role of chemical modifications (deamidation) on Fc-mediated receptor binding for bispecific antibodies. Bispecific mAbs were generated with asymmetric levels of deamidation and evaluated for their binding to FcγRIII. (**A**) mAbs 1 and 2 were heat stressed for 4 months to force deamidation in the Fc region (Asn 330). (**B**) Bispecific mAbs with various levels of symmetric (BsAb5, BsAb 8) or asymmetric (BsAb6, BsAb7) deamidation were produced through Fab-arm exchange of pooled native and stressed mAbs. The resulting bispecific antibodies display reduced levels of FcγRIII binding relative to BsAb5 in a manner consistent with total levels of deamidation. The figure is adapted from a previous publication [128].

Given that the primary analysis technique for most antibody chemical modifications is mass spectrometry, the additional complexity of evaluating chemical modifications in multispecific antibodies is not insurmountable but does complicate the analysis. Fortunately, a combined top-down fragmentation and cation-exchange chromatography method coupled with mass spectrometry has been developed for the site-specific identification of chemical variants that result in charge differences, specifically methionine oxidation. Furthermore, this technology was applied to the analysis of a bispecific antibody [129]. One notable advantage of the top-down methodology is the reduced need for peptide mapping, which is a major drawback of previous strategies. This approach is expected to be useful for future analysis of the impacts of chemical modifications on multispecific antibodies properties.

In addition to the added complexities associated with multispecific analysis, disulfide bond scrambling is another major area where antibody fragments and/or multispecifics present unique challenges. These challenges are especially prominent in multispecifics, particularly those composed of scFvs, because they can also contain additional (engineered) intrachain disulfide bonds that promote domain pairing [130–137]. Mispairing of disulfide bonds can result in complex mixtures and aggregates with reduced activity and/or potential immunogenicity. While many engineering strategies exist to overcome these challenges, a basic understanding of the chemical processes that contribute to mispairing is necessary. Although some of the challenges of intermolecular disulfide scrambling between scFvs were highlighted above, the possible chemical modification of these cysteines through disulfide formation with free cysteine or glutathione can have significant implications for clinical applications and these small modifications can be difficult to detect [138]. Even if the desired intramolecular disulfide bonds are formed during protein expression, reductases found in the harvest cell culture media may promote scrambling by reducing properly formed disulfide bonds [139–142]. The reduced disulfides can then become mispaired by reoxidation in downstream manufacturing processes [143]. Fortunately, it has recently been demonstrated that high-resolution size exclusion chromatography can, in fact, be used to monitor the levels of undesired species during production [138], which is significant considering the relative similarity of the cysteine or glutathione modified variants to the parental antibodies. This method can be used to accurately monitor these impurities in the production of bispecific IgG-scFvs. However, similar approaches must be extended from traditional IgG-based bispecifics to take full advantage of the diverse array of multispecific formats that have been developed.

3. Self-Association and High Concentration Properties

3.1. Self-Association and Solubility

The increasing trend toward subcutaneous administration of antibodies requires large quantities of antibodies to be delivered in small volumes [144]. While concentrated antibody formulations provide the benefits of reduced dosing frequency and compatibility with devices used to self-administer antibody-based therapeutics, high concentration formulations also produce crowded environments for antibody molecules. The decreased intermolecular distances and increased molecular collisions in these formulations promotes reversible self-association. Self-association not only contributes to undesirable solubility and viscosity properties but also has the potential to adversely affect shelf-life, pharmacokinetic properties, efficacy, safety and immunogenicity.

The majority of knowledge on antibody self-association is derived from studies of IgGs and efforts to reduce IgG self-association using rational approaches supported by computational insights or predictions. For example, a structural approach was developed to identify sites in antibody variable regions that caused uncontrolled self-association of an anti-nerve growth factor antibody and formation of dimers and higher order oligomers [144]. The researchers mapped the self-association interface to nine amino acids in the V_H domain and used computational methods (SAP) [96] to identify solvent-exposed hydrophobic patches. Combining hydrogen-deuterium exchange mass spectrometry data with predictions of aggregation hot spots allowed for the design of a triple mutant with improved solubility [144]. Further analysis of the wild-type and triple mutant antibodies confirmed that the triple mutant primarily existed as a monomeric antibody in solution while the wild-type antibody assembled into oligomeric structures. Furthermore, the triple mutant demonstrated a two-fold improvement in the half-life and decreased nonspecific binding while maintaining high binding affinity.

A separate study on an IgG1 antibody also employed hydrogen-deuterium exchange mass spectrometry in conjunction with structural modelling to identify two regions prone to self-interaction and associated viscous behavior [145]. The investigators identified sites in these regions to mutate to reduce hydrophobicity, including those initially solvent exposed (W50 in V_H and Y49 and L54 in V_L) and solvent shielded (H35 in V_H). In contrast to the intuitive contributions of solvent-exposed hydrophobic residues to self-association, the effect of buried residues on self-association is more complex. In this case, the buried residue (H35) is positioned within a hydrophobic cavity between V_H and V_L, modifying the local structure and reducing the surface hydrophobicity. While electrostatic interactions typically drive reversible self-association in monoclonal antibodies, this study presents an example in which reversible self-association is predominantly induced by short-range hydrophobic interactions rather than long-range electrostatic interactions. A similar finding was observed for a different monoclonal antibody, containing mutations in the V_H and V_L regions of the Fab that had a larger contribution to self-association behavior than those mutations in Fc due to their limited surface exposure [108]. These discoveries hold potential for guiding rational design and systematic protein engineering approaches to control self-association behavior in multispecific antibody formats.

One specific result of increased self-association on formulation stability and manufacturing processes is thermodynamically driven liquid-liquid phase separation (LLPS) [146]. The formation of a protein-rich bottom layer and protein-depleted top layer, characteristic of LLPS, typically occurs for highly concentrated solutions at low temperatures (2–8 °C), such as refrigerated formulations [147]. It can also occur during large-scale purification in which intermediates are kept either at room temperature or 2–8 °C for extended periods of time. Low pH elution during Protein A chromatography can also cause LLPS when antibodies elute at high concentration. Although addition of excipients such as sucrose and arginine can prevent LLPS [148], high concentrations of some of these excipients can lead to adverse manufacturing outcomes, such as decreased chromatography performance. Therefore, it would be desirable to minimize LLPS with early-stage property engineering. Recent work has used protein engineering to investigate the mechanistic foundations of antibody site-specific contributions to LLPS behavior [147]. One study found that strong self-association between the light chains of a mAb contributed to electrostatic interactions resulting in LLPS. Homology modeling of the antibody revealed five charged, surface-exposed residues, and AC-SINS and DLS measurements of rationally engineered variants allowed for the identification of key residues responsible for self-association. Disrupting the charge patches or inserting charged residues to increase repulsive interactions substantially decreased LLPS behavior, suggesting that this may be a generalizable engineering strategy.

As the low solubility of antibody fragments often restricts the overall solubility of multispecifics, approaches for studying isolated fragments are advantageous. A majority of preclinical and clinical ocular therapies utilize antibody fragments rather than full-length antibody formats, as their smaller size enables the fragments to cross the cornea in topical applications, which is the preferred route of administration with minimal systemic side effects [149]. Additionally, due to the small acceptable volumes required for both topical and intravitreal administration of antibody-based therapies for ocular targets, such as age-related macular degeneration, the final drug products need to be formulated at high protein concentrations [150]. While antibody fragments are generally less soluble than full-length antibodies, Fab fragments have the potential to be very soluble. One ocular therapeutic against Factor D initially showed limited solubility at low ionic strength, possibly due to weak intermolecular electrostatic interactions that induce assembly of higher-order structures. Although solubility enhancements can be achieved with higher ionic strength formulations that prevent electrostatic association, these formulations can cause adverse reactions, such as detachment and retinal edema [151], which motivates the use of protein engineering strategies to improve solubility. While CDRs are known to play a dominant role in antibody stability and affinity, they may also be large contributors to solubility [90,91,93,99,125,152–154]. As such, CDR engineering is a major focus in the development of antibodies with favorable solubility in concentrated formulations. Researchers increased the solubility of anti-Factor D by light chain CDR1 engineering, resulting in a variant that can be formulated at high concentrations (>250 mg/mL) and low viscosities (<17 cP) for intravitreal injection [150]. Importantly, the mutations that improved solubility and stability also retained antigen-binding capacity and favorable PK properties.

Rational design of antibody fragments has been successfully used to enhance stability and reduce reversible self-association in a multispecific IgG-scFv (Figure 4). Specifically, an anti-IL17A scFv was grafted onto an anti-BAFF IgG4 heavy chain C-terminus via a glycine-rich flexible linker to create a tetravalent bispecific IgG-scFv [155]. The original IgG-scFv displayed poor biophysical properties, including aggregation and concentration-, pH-, and salt-dependent self-association, which was not observed for the parental antibodies. While the scFv purified at 0.55 mg/mL consisted primarily of monomers, concentration to 15 mg/mL created oligomeric species that dissociated upon dilution, indicating reversible association. Given the high melting temperature of the parental scFv, this reversible self-association suggests that dynamic domain exchange between the V_H and V_L at high concentrations can cause oligomeric species to form between scFvs in the open configuration. Furthermore, chemical degradation of the scFv attached to the IgG was also observed, including clipping of the anti-IL17A scFv tether, heavy chain oxidation, and light chain deamidation. As these issues were not apparent in the parental anti-IL17A antibody, the poor biophysical properties were linked to the scFv. The scFv was therefore rationally engineered by replacing labile CDR residues with stability-enhancing and affinity-maintaining mutations, balancing the CDR charge distribution to disrupt charged patches, and inserting a H44-L100 disulfide bond at the scFv interface to halt the dynamic domain exchange between the V_H and V_L. This strategy proved highly effective, as the disulfide-stabilized scFv showed no apparent self-association up to 71 mg/mL. Once formulated into the final IgG-scFv, the engineered antibody showed improved physical and chemical stability, as well as decreased aggregation propensity, which could be explained by the lower measured hydrophobicity using ANS fluorescence measurements.

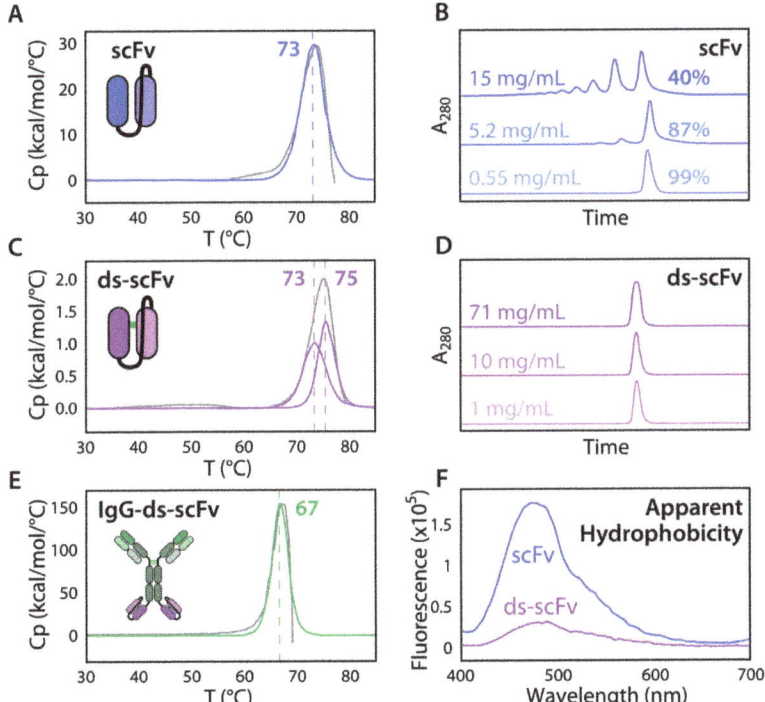

Figure 4. Impact of an additional intramolecular disulfide bond in single-chain antibody fragments, either in isolation or as IgG-scFv bispecific antibodies, on their biophysical properties. Comparison of an anti-IL17 scFv with and without an additional intramolecular (H44-L100) disulfide bond as isolated scFvs or IgG-scFv fusions. (**A**) Differential scanning calorimetry (DSC) thermogram and (**B**) analytical SEC chromatograms for the wild-type scFv. (**C**) DSC thermogram and (**D**) analytical SEC chromatograms for the disulfide-stabilized scFv. (**E**) DSC thermogram of the disulfide-stabilized bispecific antibody. (**F**) ANS fluorescence emission (300 μM ANS) of the wild-type (blue) and disulfide-stabilized (purple) scFvs. In (**A**,**C**,**E**), the raw data are shown in grey, and the fitted data are shown in color (blue, purple or green). The figure is adapted from a previous publication [155].

While systematic protein engineering studies are important for understanding the determinants of protein self-association and solubility, there is great need for experimental screening methods that identify highly soluble antibodies early in discovery to reduce the need for protein engineering and formulation development at later stages. To this end, there has been significant effort in developing high-throughput, early-stage experimental methods to identify highly soluble antibodies. To be of maximal utility, these early-stage assays must accurately predict solubility behavior using low protein quantities available at the discovery stage. Assays that measure self-association using small amounts of protein, such as AC-SINS [156–158], can be used in the early stages of antibody development to eliminate antibody candidates with high self-association that may display poor solubility. The AC-SINS assay has also been used to characterize unpurified, ultra-dilute mAbs directly in cell culture media, eliminating the need for antibody purification in order to measure self-association [159]. This study tested the self-association propensities of 87 unpurified antibodies and found that extremely dilute solution measurements of self-association (~0.001 mg/mL), as identified from the assay, correlated with high solubility at three to five orders of magnitude higher concentrations (>100 mg/mL). This finding underscores the potential of the AC-SINS assay for measuring antibody self-association in the presence of cell culture contaminants at extremely low antibody concentrations.

More recently, a tour de force study was reported that used a large panel of clinical-stage antibodies and a panel of early-stage assays to evaluate antibody biophysical properties, including self-association, which may be important in the success of antibody therapeutics [116]. Two self-interaction assays, clone self-interaction by biolayer interferometry and AC-SINS, ranked in the top five biophysical assays for identifying drug-like antibodies, second to assays that measured non-specific interactions. A separate, equally impressive study utilized sequence-based data analysis and Pearson and Spearman correlations on early-stage assay measurements of IgG1 and IgG4 antibodies to predict antibody developability [117]. The discovery-stage assays were prioritized into two categories, with a higher priority assigned to assays that determine unacceptable properties. In general, IgG4 antibodies were found to have a greater tendency to self-associate in comparison to IgG1 antibodies. This finding is in agreement with an even more recent study [160], the fact that IgG4 antibodies tend to have lower isoelectric points compared to IgG1 antibodies, and that antibodies with higher isoelectric points generally have improved biophysical properties. Multiple case studies were conducted with the goals of improving aggregation propensity and self-association behavior. For example, an attempted reparation of a heavy chain CDR3 tryptophan oxidation site in a humanized IgG1 kappa antibody (termed wild type) led to the evaluation of ten variants, each with a different mutation at position W104 in heavy chain CDR3 [117]. The W104X variants exhibited comparable measurements to wild type for a majority of biophysical properties except AC-SINS and dynamic light scattering. The W104X variants that showed increased self-association using AC-SINS were also confirmed to display unusually large hydrodynamic radii by light scattering. Only one of these variants (W104F) retained antigen binding, but displayed unacceptably high self-association, preventing its therapeutic development.

Another early-stage screening approach for identifying antibodies that are likely to be well behaved at high concentrations is the addition of crowding reagents such as polyethylene glycol (PEG) or ammonium sulfate to antibody solutions [161–163]. These crowding reagents lower the intrinsic maximum protein solubility, which can be evaluated in moderate throughput by quantifying the apparent solubility using a fraction of the amount of protein in comparison to traditional solubility measurements (e.g., concentration by ultrafiltration). A combination of two assays (a vapor diffusion technique and PEG-induced precipitation) carried out in a high-throughput, automated manner has been used to rank order monoclonal antibodies based on their relative solubilities [164]. However, it is unclear whether methods such as PEG-induced precipitation can be used to probe solubility of a wide variety of multispecific formats. For example, in one study, PEG-induced precipitation accurately predicted solubilities of Fc-fusion proteins and mAbs, but was not able to predict solubility of single-domain antibodies [165]. Because methods that use crowding reagents rely on excluded volume effects, it is unclear how useful they will be for evaluating multispecific antibodies.

Given the difficulty associated with measuring reversible self-association, computational methods that can accurately predict this property are highly desirable. However, as reversible self-association can be induced by a sophisticated interplay of hydrophobic and electrostatic interactions, creating prediction algorithms that identify interaction hot-spots is challenging [108]. One key approach for computationally predicting self-association is through quantitative structure-property relationship (QSPR) predictions, a technique that uses scoring functions derived from antibody primary sequence and/or structural descriptors [166–168]. However, the accuracy of this method is limited by the composition of the antibodies in the training set, and for novel antibody formats such as those employed in multispecific antibody design, there is no optimal training set currently available.

For these reasons, there is strong interest in improving the current standard of physics-based simulations, which are not limited on training data. Physics-based simulations, however, can be restricted by available computational resources, especially at increasing levels of detail (e.g., fully atomistic). To overcome these constraints, coarse-grain simulations may prove to be a suitable solution. Coarse-grain molecular simulations at the one bead-per-amino-acid degree of coarse-graining have been used to evaluate protein-protein interactions computationally, as this amount of detail was found to best balance trade-offs between accuracy and computational load [169]. The results from these models have been correlated with light scattering data across a range of formulation conditions (pH 5, 6.5, and 8, and ionic strengths varying between 5 to 300 mM) [170]. These models were used to effectively predict the B_{22} values of three monoclonal antibodies that exhibit a range of colloidal behaviors, demonstrating the utility of the potential generality of the approach. Further research on solubility predictions using computational methods should address current limitations, such as finite computational resources, and supplement the predictions with accelerated antibody design and experimental assessment of solubility and reversible self-association at the preliminary stages of candidate screening. Models that rely on Lennard-Jones potentials are less effective when evaluating self-association at low concentrations [166]. To overcome this limitation, longer range van der Waals potentials can be employed [171]. A different coarse-grain model that also accounts for electrostatic and hydrophobic interactions was applied to two model mAbs, and while the original model was able to predict the equilibrium self-associated structure, it overpredicted self-diffusivity and underpredicted viscosity. An improvement was observed when the protein clusters in the simulations were rigidified. Future developments in computational modelling should focus on better quantifying the dynamics of closely interacting entities to yield more accurate predictions of self-association.

3.2. Viscosity

Viscosity is another property of unique concern for concentrated antibody solutions that affects almost every stage of development, including protein purification, formulation, and delivery. High viscosity is caused by an amalgam of intermolecular interactions, including electrostatic, hydrophobic, dipole-dipole, hydrogen bonding, and van der Waals interactions. The viscosity threshold for subcutaneous injection formulations is less than ~15–30 centipoise [138]. High concentration formulations with increased viscosity above this threshold can make injection either extremely difficult or painful for the patient [149]. Thus, significant efforts are devoted to develop high concentration formulations required for dosing with acceptable viscosity.

To better understand the molecular origins of viscous antibody formulations and particularly for bispecific antibodies, a previous theoretical study used covalently-linked hard spheres with different attractive interactions to model antibodies as Y-shaped molecules [172]. Interestingly, such models show that bispecific antibodies with two different binding arms tend to be less viscous than monospecific IgG, as linkages through a single Fab arm form dimers instead of the higher-order networks formed by bivalent monospecific antibodies with similar Fab arms. However, when three sites are involved, such as in the case of an antibody in which the Fc regions also mediates attractive interactions, the formation of branched clusters generates high viscosities [173,174].

Antibody fragments, in general, do not exhibit viscosity-related issues, because most fragments cannot be concentrated to sufficient levels for abnormally high viscosity and their monovalent formats are less likely to lead to network-like structures often found in highly viscous solutions. In contrast, multispecifics have the potential to demonstrate high viscosity. It has previously been determined that asymmetric distributions of positive and negative charge [175] in antibodies can create dipole-like electrostatic attraction [175,176], increasing reversible self-association and the formation of transient antibody networks associated with viscosity [177].

To further study the impact of asymmetric charge distributions on reversible self-association, researchers evaluated the effects of charge neutralization on mAb solubility and viscosity. Specifically, a mAb known to display electrostatically-driven viscosity was mutated within and near charge patches in the CDRs. The mutations included both charge neutralization (E59Y) and charge reversal (E59K/R) variants [178]. This site (light chain E59) was in one of the largest negatively-charged patches in the variable regions and was located at the outskirts of the antigen-binding site. Interestingly, charge neutralization was able to decrease viscosity while charge reversal increased self-association. This finding is significant as multispecific antibodies may consist of a large number of charged patches, and further investigation on how such patches interact with each other can provide insights into viscosity-reducing strategies for multispecifics. Furthermore, the large variability in multispecific formats may demand unique strategies for controlling viscosity. Nevertheless, some multispecific antibodies do not contain Fc regions, such as bispecific antibody fragments (e.g., BiTES and DARTs), and are expected to display unique viscosity profiles. Another finding from this study was that certain mutations can affect the structure of antibody subunits distant from the mutational site. Such interdomain contacts and allosteric influences may be even more pronounced in multispecific antibodies that consist of a greater number of adjoined fragments. A double mutant (V44K/E59Y) in V_L was generated with the E59Y charge neutralization mutation and a second mutation (V44K) that disrupted a solvent-exposed hydrophobic patch [179]. The double mutant exhibited higher apparent solubilities in comparison to the single mutations. Another promising double mutant (V44K/E59S) in V_L showed improved properties such as enhanced solubility, decreased viscosity, increased stability, and greater activity. The synergistic effects of the mutations at positions 44 and 59 revealed that hydrophobic and electrostatic interactions work in concert to increase viscosity. For viscous effects that arise from a combination of long-range electrostatic interactions and short-range hydrophobic interactions, understanding the relative contribution of these interactions is important, because a strategy that addresses both issues is often required.

Although electrostatic contributions to viscosity are significant, recent studies have examined the role of other molecular determinants of viscosity, as multispecific antibodies can display complex viscosity behavior that deserves further consideration [174,180,181]. In comparison to monoclonal antibodies, multispecifics can be larger molecules and typically display asymmetrical shape, charge distribution, and hydrophobicity [180]. A study of Dual Variable Domain Immunoglobulin (DVD-Ig) bispecific antibodies was conducted to examine the effect of molecular size, excluded volume, charge patches, and protein-protein interactions on viscosity. The DVD-Ig was considerably more viscous than the mAbs and the effect was pronounced at very low ionic strength (water). In comparison to globular proteins, the Y-shape of monoclonal antibodies leads to higher intrinsic viscosities. The DVD-Ig format consists of additional variable domains that account for a significant increase in the intrinsic viscosity. Excluded volume calculations highlight the significant impact of molecular size on viscosity for high concentration formulations (>100 mg/mL). Multispecific antibodies at pH values near their pIs can also display high viscosity due to attractive electrostatic interactions between oppositely charged patches on their surfaces.

In the process of studying the viscosities of multispecific antibodies, the contributions of additional intermolecular forces, apart from electrostatics and hydrophobic interactions, have been elucidated. For instance, the anti-IL13/IL17 bispecific IgG4 antibody displayed a significant increase in viscosity compared to the parent monospecific antibodies (Figure 5) [174]. Interestingly, a 1:1

mixture of the two parental antibodies (anti-IL13 IgG4 and anti-IL17 IgG1) also exhibited increased viscosity. A further investigation showed that bivalency is required for network formation and high viscosity solutions. To determine the contribution of different intermolecular interactions to reversible self-association, viscosity was measured under different solution conditions. Arginine-HCl and guanidine-HCl excipients were more effective than NaCl at decreasing viscosity by reducing intermolecular interactions, revealing the significant contributions of cation-π and π-π interactions relative to electrostatic interactions. This is in agreement with previous computational studies that suggest cation-π interactions are stronger than analogous salt bridges in aqueous solutions [182]. Molecular dynamics simulations confirmed that arginine significantly interacts with solvent-exposed aromatic residues and mutation of such CDR residues led to the discovery of two anti-IL13 variants with reduced viscosities that were similar to those of the parental antibodies [174]. This case study corroborates the current theory that interactions between different Fab regions can form networks of bivalent molecules, leading to increased viscosity. Moreover, this study highlights the potential importance of cation-π and π-π interactions in mediating viscous solution behavior.

The use of antibody mixtures to predict the viscoelastic behavior of bispecific antibodies has also been reported in another study [181]. The investigators compared viscosities of equimolar mixtures of two sets of parental mAb pairs and their bispecific counterparts, and compared these measurements to predictions of viscosities of mixtures using the Arrhenius mixture model. This study consisted of a slightly viscous antibody (mAb A), a highly viscous antibody (mAb C), and its bispecific counterpart (BsAb A/C). The viscosity of the bispecific variant was similar to the 1:1 mixture of each mAb, as the two parental mAbs participate in similar protein-protein cross interactions. A similar experiment was carried out with a separate set of antibodies that displayed similar viscosity profiles and significantly different isoelectric points (pI 6.3 for mAb A and 9.3 for mAb B). Because mAb A and mAb B have dissimilar intermolecular interactions, the mixture and bispecific antibody displayed much higher viscosities than the individual mAbs and deviated significantly from the Arrhenius mixing prediction. Interestingly, Rayleigh scattering experiments indicated a large contribution of short-ranged, non-electrostatic attractive interactions to the observed viscoelastic behavior in addition to the expected contribution of attractive electrostatic interactions.

As demonstrated in diverse previous studies, predictions of diverse antibody biophysical properties rely on trends that are gathered from experimental data [116,117]. A recent study on engineering antibodies with reduced viscosities extensively sampled Fv and CDR charge mutations and measured the viscosity of 40 unique variants [183]. The viscosity of the parental antibody was 40 cP (measured) at ~100 mg/mL and 250–300 cP (extrapolated) at 150 mg/mL. In order to be suitable for subcutaneous injections, the viscosity needed to be lowered to below 20 cP for a 150 mg/mL antibody formulation. Two rounds of structure-based design allowed for the identification of a variant that met these criteria while maintaining binding affinity. The most promising mutations were located in a negative charge patch in the middle of light chain CDR2. Furthermore, because charge asymmetry is influenced by individual residues, computational models that only use domain-level charges were not able to discriminate the differences in viscosity of the antibody variants in this study. It is also important to note that the rational design process benefited from the accessibility of an X-ray crystal structure, as this structural information greatly reduced the total mutational space that needed to be scanned.

Given the challenges in experimental viscosity analysis due to unrealistic requirements for large (mg) amounts of antibody, computational methods for predicting antibody variants with low viscosity are particularly valuable. One proposed computational method is referred to as the spatial charge map (SCM) method, which uses antibody sequences and corresponding homology models to detect highly viscous antibodies at the initial stages of the development process [184]. Analysis is only performed on the Fv region, which contains the majority of the variability between antibodies. The SCM tool uses hydrophobicity (hydrophobicity index), net charge, and charge asymmetry properties to generate an SCM score. This method has been validated using multiple panels of IgG1 antibodies, and the model is able to accurately identify highly viscous antibodies. It should be noted that solution conditions, such as buffer components and temperature, are not accounted for in the analysis. Therefore, the ability of the SCM score to predict high viscosities can vary and is expected to be more successful when comparing antibodies of the same isotype at similar formulation and temperature conditions. Future work is needed to not only account for different formulation conditions but also for applications to multispecific antibodies.

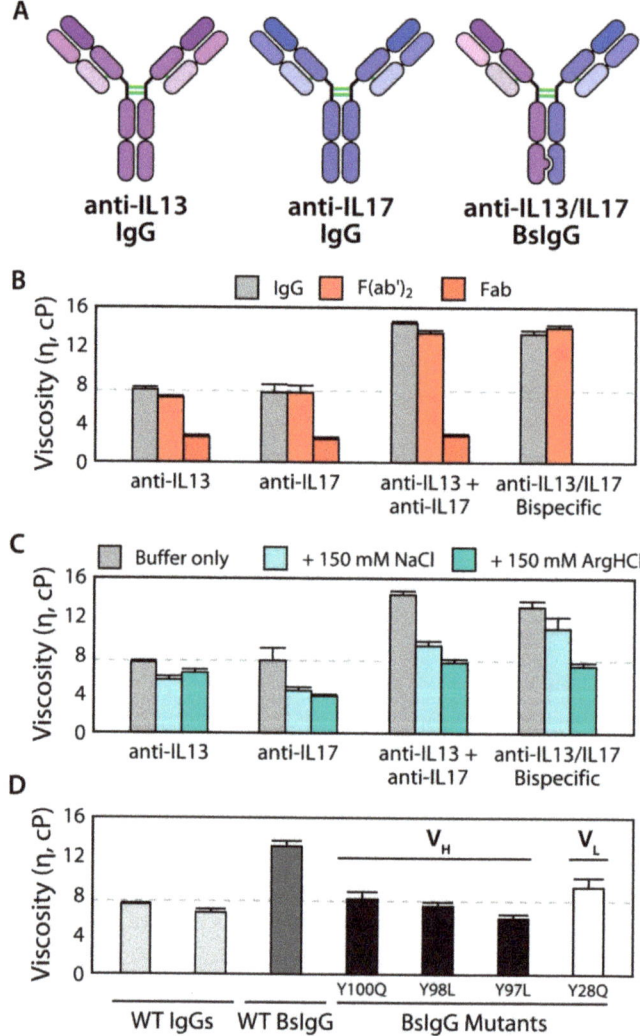

Figure 5. Evaluation of the viscoelastic properties of bispecific antibodies and approaches for reducing their viscosities using formulation and mutational strategies. (**A**) Structures of anti-IL13/IL17 mono- and bi-specific antibodies, the latter of which were generated using knob-in-hole heavy chain pairing methods. (**B–D**) Measured viscosities at 150 mg/mL in standard formulation conditions (20 mM His-HCl, pH 6.0) for (**B**) various antibody formats, (**C**) IgGs at different formulation conditions, and (**D**) IgGs with various point mutations in the anti-IL13 variable domains. The viscosity of one of the parental IgGs is shown with a grey dotted line. The figure is adapted from a previous publication [174].

Similar to solubility predictions, coarse-grain models can also be used to predict viscosity [166]. A recently developed, novel coarse-grained simulation method analyzes molecular dynamics simulations of highly concentrated full-length antibodies at the microsecond time-scale. This new method differs from previous coarse-grain simulation methods in that the model accounts for the high-order electrostatic multipole moments, charge asymmetry, and hydrophobic character of full-length antibodies, all of which are factors that contribute to self-association. High-order electrostatic interactions, which are generally negligible in dilute conditions, are significant at high concentration, and the notably different electrostatic potentials between mAbs can lead to differences in viscosity. However, the importance of accounting for hydrophobicity in the viscosity predictions should not be underestimated, as evidenced by antibodies that show minimal differences in their electrostatic fields and multipole moments but large differences in their hydrophobicities. Accurate values for both the hydrophobicity and electrostatic components are also necessary when accounting for the impacts of changes in ionic strength on the viscosity of mAbs in different formulations, as the viscosity of concentrated antibody solutions is generally mitigated by the addition of salt and excipients [185–188].

As molecular crowding also influences the diffusion of antibodies in solution, diffusivity measurements can be used to assess intermolecular interaction strength that is often inversely correlated with viscosity. This novel coarse-grain model was applied to a set of fifteen antibodies, and the results highlight the influence of intermolecular interactions on the diffusion coefficients of antibodies in crowded environments [166]. Interestingly, an inaccurate prediction of a highly viscous antibody led to further investigation on the causes behind the inconsistency. The calculated modest hydrophobicity and comparatively large net charge anticipated repulsive intermolecular interactions and therefore low viscosity. The discrepancy is speculated to arise from errors in homology modeling, particularly those related to heavy chain CDR3 loop, as the crowded environment in viscous, high-concentration formulations may destabilize the antibody structure and alter the antibody conformation.

Coarse-grain simulations have also been used to further understand the molecular basis for antibody network formation and discern whether the number or frequency of domain-domain interactions are linked to greater antibody self-association [177]. Unlike previous simulations, the use of an asymmetric mAb in which one Fab arm is located much closer to the Fc fragment compared to the other Fab arm showed that the asymmetry significantly impacts the prevalence of intermolecular interactions. Inspiration for the modeling of an asymmetric mAb was derived from the preferred conformation of an HIV-1 neutralizing IgG1 antibody in solution, in which the non-flexible asymmetric shape is a property inherent to the antibody [189]. As many multispecific antibodies are asymmetric by design, this model can potentially be extended to such entities as well. Researchers have used this model to quantify features of mAb network formation for high and low viscous mAbs at different concentrations [177]. In general, viscous antibodies with more negatively charged Fv regions tend to have more nodes, defined as mAbs that are in contact with three or more mAbs (closer than the 35 Å cut-off), and the number of nodes increases with concentration. These models indicate that a larger network density (correlated with high viscosity) allows for a greater stress-bearing capacity and increased structure that withstands deformation under shear stress. Complementary charges between mAb domains increase viscosity by slowing molecular mobility, which is reflected in smaller diffusion coefficients for the highly viscous antibodies. In fact, domain-domain interactions play a greater role in comparison to contact frequency in highly viscous mAbs at the same concentration. Although the coarse-grain model can be improved by incorporating the effect of solvent on network formation (a feature that was omitted due to computational resource constraints), the study corroborates the use of coarse-grained simulations to predict viscosity. This newfound understanding of the molecular determinants of viscosity may hold promise for the prediction and design of multispecific antibodies with favorable viscoelastic properties.

4. Polyspecificty and In Vivo Properties

4.1. Polyspecificity and Pharmacokinetics

Since pharmacokinetic (PK) properties such as systemic clearance, volume of distribution, and half-life can influence efficacy and toxicity, accurate measurement of these properties is critical. Due to the low-throughput nature of many PK profiling strategies, PK properties are typically evaluated in the late stages of antibody development, presenting a considerable bottleneck to the development process. Although the full PK profile of an antibody is the result of a complex set of processes including non-specific binding, immunogenicity, and FcRn recycling, polyspecificity is a key contributor to poor antibody PK behavior because non-specific binding can lead to a number of unfavorable PK properties, including short half-lives and increased toxicity. Most of the available antibody polyspecificity data is for IgGs. Interestingly, a recent study of IgGs revealed that approved antibody therapeutics are generally more specific and display lower levels of non-specific binding than those in clinical trials, suggesting that high specificity may be a critical attribute of drug-like antibodies [116].

Current in vitro methods for measuring antibody polyspecificity, as reviewed elsewhere [190], involve evaluation of antibody interactions with polyclonal antibodies (cross-interaction chromatography) [191], baculovirus particles (BVP assay) [192], a combination of protein and non-protein antigens (DNA, lipids, proteins, and polysaccharides; ELISA) [193] or soluble membrane and cytosolic proteins (polyspecificity reagent, PSR assay) [116,194]. These types of non-specific reagents, such as PSR, are even being employed during the antibody discovery stage using in vitro high-throughput methods, such as yeast surface display, to select antibody candidates with low polyspecificity [194–198]. Removing nonspecific binders in the library-screening stage of antibody discovery prevents the arduous process of rectifying abnormal PK properties due to off-target binding for late-stage antibody candidates. The PSR reagent can be prepared using soluble membrane and cytosolic proteins obtained from either CHO or HEK cells [194]. This reagent is biotinylated and subsequently incubated with antibody-presenting yeast. Antibody binding to PSR can be probed via flow cytometry in a high-throughput manner (10^8 cells/h). Importantly, the PSR assay has been shown to correlate with antibody clearance rates in mice [195]. However, one drawback of using PSR to probe polyspecificity is that, due to the ill-defined nature of the reagent, lot-to-lot variability of the complex cell extract can lead to different assay results. The need for well-characterized, defined reagents has led to the use of Hsp90 and insulin as single-component specificity reagents that also correlate to antibody clearance rates in mice [196,199]. Previous specificity assays, employing microarray technologies or microtiter plate assays, afford much lower throughput (tens to hundreds) relative to FACS-based approaches that can process millions of variants [200].

Increased antibody non-specific binding in general, and in particular to FcRn, is generally linked to increased risk of fast antibody clearance [192,199,201–205]. Therefore, it is necessary to both obtain accurate PK measurements in a high-throughput manner at earlier stages of development and establish in vitro/in vivo correlations (IVIVC). In a recent study, researchers formulated a combinatorial triage approach to differentiate antibodies with favorable and unfavorable PK profiles [199]. This strategy involved a set of five in vitro assays that could be grouped into three categories—nonspecific binding assays (DNA- and insulin binding ELISAs), a self-association assay (affinity-capture self-interaction nanoparticle spectroscopy, AC-SINS), and two assays to measure interactions with matrix-immobilized human FcRn (surface plasmon resonance and column chromatography). Results showed a group of antibodies with low clearance and assay scores, enabling the demarcation of a clearance threshold at ≥7.7 mL/day/kg. Human clearance values were estimated by allometrically projecting clearance values measured in Tg32 mice. A threshold value for each in vitro assay was defined by applying this clearance threshold to each mAb set, and antibodies that scored below the threshold in all three categories were deemed to have favorable PK and those that scored above the threshold in all three categories were rejected due to unfavorable PK. The PK properties of antibodies with above-threshold scores in one or two assay categories were further investigated in mice. Notably, the correlations of these in vitro assays to allometrically projected human clearance based on mice clearance values were statistically significant. In another study, a novel assay was developed for PK analysis of a fully human anti-EGFRvIII/anti-CD3 bispecific T-cell engager (BiTE) using microflow liquid chromatography coupled to high resolution parallel reaction monitoring mass spectrometry [206]. Using this method it is possible to quantify the bispecific antibody levels in mice plasma and whole blood.

However, even early stage high-throughput screens for non-specific binding, which is only one property linked to antibody PK, can be time and resource intensive. The significant costs incurred from realizing unfavorable PK properties in late-stage antibody candidates incentivizes the use of predictive methods at even earlier stages of development, such as at the stage of in vitro antibody discovery. Advances in this area by several research teams have paved the way for generalized predictions of problematic amino acid motifs and nonspecific antibodies in general. While it has long been known that over enrichment in positive charge and hydrophobicity can lead to nonspecificity [144,197,207–210], one study used molecular modelling to determine residue substitutions in the CDRs that disrupt positively charged patches [211]. They were able to reduce the net positive charge of the Fv region without affecting the overall antibody pI, although the effect was more significant for IgG4s in comparison to IgG1s. In a separate study, panning nonimmune yeast display libraries elucidated the dominant role of a constrained β-sheet structure in heavy chain CDR2 of V_H6 antibodies in driving nonspecificity [198]. Furthermore, homology modeling showed that an Arg50 residue at the base of this CDR stabilizes the β-sheet and rigidifies the structure of this loop, allowing it to protrude farther than other heavy chain CDR2 loops. The exposure of other residues in the same loop could also account for the increased polyspecificity. This finding can be used to exclude V_H6-1 variants during future library generation. Other studies employing synthetic yeast libraries have identified motifs containing Trp, Val, and Arg in the center four positions of heavy chain CDR3 of nonspecific antibodies [197]. In order to further develop our understanding of nonspecificity motifs, approaches that combine next generation sequencing, homology modeling, and machine learning will be required in the future.

Computational models provide an alternate method to investigate sequence determinants of specificity. Analysis of published non-specific interaction data for clinical-stage antibodies revealed a strong positive correlation between non-specific binding and increasing numbers of arginine and lysine residues in antibody CDRs [212]. Conversely, the investigators found a strong negative correlation between non-specific binding and increasing numbers of aspartic acid and glutamic acid residues. These results further showed that arginine, in comparison to lysine, plays a greater role in mediating nonspecific interactions, and aspartic acid, in comparison to glutamic acid, plays a larger role in mediating highly specific interactions. In an effort to identify highly specific antibody candidates based primarily on antibody sequences, chemical rules based on physicochemical properties of different regions in antibody variable fragments have also been recently established [213]. Combinations of these chemical rules could be used to effectively identify antibodies with improved specificity during early-stage discovery and protein engineering.

Monoclonal antibodies typically exhibit slow systemic clearance and low volume of distribution (Vd) as their size and polarity confines their distribution to the vascular and interstitial spaces [199,214]. These two factors, combined with FcRn-mediated recycling, result in the prolonged half-life of mAbs. PK properties of mAb-based therapeutics can vary based on their nature (humanized vs. human), type (IgG1, 2, 3, or 4) and mode of binding (monospecific vs. multispecific) [215]. Systematically administered mAbs generally show biphasic PK profiles, characterized by a fast distribution phase followed by a slower elimination phase [214]. The general consensus for the threshold value that constitutes fast antibody clearance varies between >7.7 mL/day/kg to >20 mL/day/kg [192,195,199]. These clearance threshold values are determined from a variety of factors, including analysis of receiver operating characteristic (ROC) curves and allometric scaling of clearance thresholds values previously reported in cynomolgus monkeys. Clearance pathways for antibody therapeutics that are larger than ~55 kDa (the glomerular filtration threshold) are typically through pinocytosis and proteolysis (nonspecific), target-mediated specific clearance, and ADA-mediated clearance [214]. Multispecific antibodies have a higher risk for displaying anomalous PK properties, such as shorter half-lives and increased clearance rates compared to monoclonal antibodies [216–219].

One notable study evaluated the PK properties of a bispecific fusion protein in which a biologically active protein domain (termed extracellular domain or ECD) was attached to an IgG4 antibody via a flexible linker (Figure 6). This study evaluated the effect of the location of the fusion protein relative to the IgG (e.g., N-terminus of heavy chain) on its biophysical, biochemical, and PK properties [219]. The protein domain was attached to the N- and C- termini of the heavy and light chains of an IgG4 monoclonal antibody. The C-terminal light chain fusion construct was excluded from further studies due to poor expression. Notably, attachment of the protein domain to the N-terminus of the heavy chain (N-HC) lead to a variant with similar hydrophobicity as the wild type, while the other fusions [C-terminus of heavy chain (C-HC) and N-terminus of light chain (N-LC)] displayed higher hydrophobicity. Moreover, PK analysis of these constructs using cynomolgus monkeys and CD-1 mice revealed the least hydrophobic fusion protein (N-HC) displayed PK properties that were closest to the wild type, while the more hydrophobic variants displayed significantly worse PK properties. Given that the bispecific constructs were composed of the same IgG and fusion protein, the differences in hydrophobicity and PK properties demonstrate the importance of molecular architecture on the pharmacokinetic properties of bispecific antibodies.

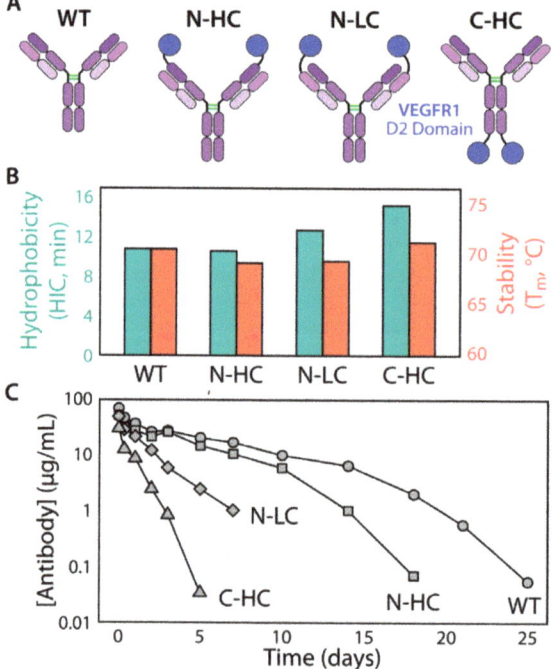

Figure 6. Effect of molecular architecture of IgG fusion proteins on their hydrophobicities, stabilities, and pharmacokinetic properties. (**A**) Representations of various IgG-extracellular domains (ECDs) with the D2 domain of VEGFR1 fused to different regions of the wild-type IgG. (**B**) Hydrophobicity measured by hydrophobic interaction chromatography (HIC; blue) and stability (first thermal unfolding transition, red) of the wild-type (WT) IgG and IgG-ECDs. (**C**) Pharmacokinetic profiles of the WT IgG and IgG-ECDs in cynomolgus monkeys (single 2 mg/kg iv dose) reveal increased clearance rates for more hydrophobic formats. The figure is adapted from a previous publication [219].

Multispecific formats can also be constructed to promote favorable PK properties, including longer half-lives [220]. For example, albumin-binding multispecific antibodies that extend systemic half-life have been reported [221–225]. Moreover, application of this concept to ocular therapies in an effort to reduce dosing frequency is particularly advantageous, as each intravitreal injection can expose the patient to a variety of complications, including vitreous hemorrhage, endophthalmitis, and uveitis [226]. In one study, researchers attached a 97-amino acid, hyaluronan-binding peptide to therapeutic antibodies and proteins [220]. Hyaluronan was chosen as the target over other vitreous components, such as collagen type II and albumin, based on three main criteria: (1) sufficient concentration and exposure of binding sites of a vitreous component to effectively bind a clinically relevant dosage of drug; (2) low concentration of vitreous target in non-ocular tissues and blood to minimize systemic retention; and (3) low turnover in the eye to reduce target-mediated drug clearance. Fusion proteins consisting of the hyaluronan-binding peptide and anti-VEGF therapeutics [ranibizumab, bevacizumab, aflibercept, NVS0 (Fab), and brolucizumab (scFv)] were injected into the vitreous of rabbits and cynomolgus monkeys. Fusion of the hyaluronan-binding peptide did not hamper the ability of anti-VEGF therapeutics to neutralize VEGF in vivo. In fact, a key finding was that reduced doses of these fusion proteins (as much as 50-fold lower) can demonstrate either commensurate or superior activity in comparison to the parental anti-VEGF antibody while exhibiting the desired half-life extension that enables reduced dosing frequency. The potential generality of using this type of approach in diverse multispecific antibody formats holds great therapeutic promise.

4.2. Immunogenicity

Another key challenge in developing antibody therapeutics is their potential immunogenicity [227,228]. This immunogenicity may be mediated by T cells, which recognize short peptide sequences displayed by MHC class II proteins on antigen-presenting cells, or B cells, which produce anti-drug antibodies capable of recognizing conformational epitopes on therapeutic proteins [229–231]. A variety of methods exist for determining the potential immunogenicity of protein therapeutics, although the measurement of anti-drug antibodies (ADAs) is the most common [228,231–234].

ADAs can impact the function of a drug in multiple ways [235]. One of the chief concerns with ADAs is the potential for neutralization of the activity of therapeutic antibodies by interfering with antigen binding. However, even ADAs that do not neutralize antigen binding may otherwise impact the pharmacodynamic or pharmacokinetic behavior of the drug. In addition, ADAs can elicit a potentially dangerous hypersensitive immune response. Therefore, immunogenicity is a primary concern for the development of safe and effective biologics. To this end, a number of strategies have been developed for reducing unwanted immunogenic activity of biologics [236,237], and the FDA has recently released guidance for developing and validating assays to assess immunogenicity of therapeutic proteins [234].

Multispecific antibodies may be particularly susceptible to immunogenic liabilities [238,239]. This is because divergence from the natural human antibody repertoire generally increases the potential for immunogenicity and multispecific antibodies are likely to include multiple unnatural features. For example, multispecific antibodies may contain sequences of non-human origin through the incorporation of antibody fragments such as scFvs or nanobodies. Although such fragments are generally considered to be of low risk for immunogenicity, both could theoretically represent risk factors for immunogenicity due to their linkers and, in the case of nanobodies, non-human origin [240,241]. Even in cases where scaffolds contain fully human sequences, changes in format, such as single-domain antibodies or scFvs derived from mAbs, can lead to exposure of epitopes that are normally buried in the parental mAb and which result in an immunogenic response. Additionally, upon antigen binding, a novel surface, known as a neoantigen, is created at the new binding interface that may be recognized by ADAs. In some cases, immunogenic response to one portion of a multi-domain drug can lead to a phenomenon known as epitope spreading where an immune response to a highly immunogenic subunit results in further responses to otherwise non-immunoreactive portions of a therapeutic. Given the multi-domain nature of many multispecific antibodies, this phenomenon may be of particular concern. The challenges associated with assembly and purification of multispecific antibodies may also result in an increased risk of immunogenicity. Moreover, critical quality attributes like aggregation, particle size, and polyspecificity are also thought to increase the likelihood of immunogenicity [88,89,239,242–244]. Given the unique immunogenic liabilities of multispecific antibodies and their increasing numbers in clinical trials, new tools for the analysis and reduction of immunogenic liabilities will be of increasing importance.

Typically, immunogenicity is measured late in the development process using immunosorbent assays to detect ADAs. Although there are some notable limits to these assays associated with interference or quantitation, which have been extensively reviewed elsewhere [233], they are particularly useful for qualitatively determining if ADAs are created in response to a therapeutic. It is also possible to determine the domain specificity of ADAs by evaluating antibody binding to individual domains of a therapeutic, a strategy that has been successfully adapted for use in determining ADA specificity in bispecific antibodies [245]. Interestingly, similar assays have been used to show that pre-existing ADAs for an IgG-scFv corresponded to the same domain as emergent ADAs for the same therapeutic, suggesting that the presence of pre-existing ADAs can be used to predict and even identify regions of immunogenic liability in multispecific antibodies [246]. Despite the utility of these assays, they require human testing, and are limited in their ability to quantify ADA interactions or precisely determine ADA epitopes [247].

To address these issues, a variety of approaches have been developed [228], including MHC-associated peptide proteomics (MAPPs) [248,249]. In this in vitro technique, human professional antigen-presenting cells are incubated with the biologic of interest, the biologic is then internalized, processed enzymatically, and presented at the surface by human leukocyte antigen (HLA) class II molecules. The antigen-presenting cells are then lysed and the HLA class II receptors are isolated by anti-HLA antibody coated beads. The antigenic peptides from the biologic of interest are then released from HLA by reducing the pH. The resulting antigen peptide sequences can be determined by LC-MS. Although these methods are highly validated for identifying immunogenic sequences, the assays require analysis of the blood from at least 20 donors to cover the processing and display variability that is often observed for antigen-presenting cells obtained from different individuals. Therefore, a full analysis can take up to eight weeks for approximately ten therapeutic candidates [249]. Although this method is valuable for determining antigenic liability of biologics without dosing human subjects, MAPPs assays are not practical for early-stage development decisions, as a consequence of the time-intensive and low-throughput nature of this approach.

Fortunately, for some biologics, such as camelid nanobody (V_HH) domains, it is possible to predict a higher-than-normal immunogenicity risk to humans without sophisticated analytical or computational methods. In such cases, a variety of approaches have been used to engineer out immunogenic properties in the late stages of antibody development, but one recent study described a strategy for engineering out immunogenic liabilities at the initial discovery stage. Specifically, the investigators sought to develop neutralizing single-domain human antibodies for the SARS-CoV-2 coronavirus [250]. Such single-domain antibodies have a variety of advantages over traditional antibodies such as ease of expression in bacterial cells and the ability to be administered to the lung by inhalation. However, single-domain human antibodies have not found wide application due to their poor biophysical properties in the absence of light chains [41]. Instead, nanobodies produced in camelid species make up the vast majority of reported single-domain antibodies. Because these species produce heavy chain only antibodies, their variable regions show superb stability and solubility when expressed in the absence of the conserved domains. Unfortunately, their camelid origin also increases their risk for inducing immunogenic responses in humans. To address this issue, investigators have screened human frameworks for stability, expression level, and Protein A binding [250]. Next, they created a library of human single-domain (heavy chain) antibodies by grafting human CDRs onto the preferred framework. This framework was then used to produce highly stable human single-domain antibodies for a variety of antigens, including the SARS-CoV-2 spike protein. Given the number of nanobody-based multispecific formats, this work is likely to have implications for multispecific antibody generation in the future.

Of course, not all immunogenic liabilities are as easily predictable as those for the camelid nanobodies. In these cases, new strategies to either predict or efficiently screen for protein sequences and structures with immunogenic liabilities would be highly desirable. In addition, once the liabilities can be efficiently identified, robust strategies for improving these liabilities early in screening or development are critical. For mAbs, there is a long history of successful humanization strategies [251–253]. For unconventional multispecific scaffolds, computational approaches may play a significant role in addressing both of these hurdles. For example, because immunogenicity arises from non-self-recognition, one major approach to predicting immunogenicity is to evaluate humanness of antibodies. Facilitated by the recent increase in next-generation sequencing data for B-cell repertoires, multiple approaches have recently been reported that demonstrate high fidelity predictions of antibody humanness [254,255]. Although it is now possible to clearly distinguish between therapeutic antibodies in terms of their degree of humanness, it is not clear how these methods will translate to multispecific antibodies.

Another way to evaluate the immunogenic liabilities of protein therapeutics is to predict the peptides that are likely to be displayed on MHC proteins and lead to immune responses. To this end, much effort has been directed toward developing algorithms to predict peptide presentation of MHC class I and MHC class II proteins [256]. These efforts began with peptide binding affinity measurements for MHC proteins, but have been improved by the inclusion of large mass spectrometry datasets from MAPPs-like experiments [257–259]. However, deconvolution of this data is difficult for many reasons, but particularly because the number of MHC alleles makes it is difficult to trace any given peptide to a specific MHC protein. Without that critical piece of information, it is difficult to develop a model for MHC peptide binding. To solve this problem, a variety of innovative approaches have been explored, the most recent of which is the development of artificial neural networks that can simultaneously analyze the mass spectrometry data while developing individual MHC binding models [257,260]. The authors report that this strategy results in an immunogenicity predictor that met or exceeded the predictive capacity of previous methods in their test system. Interestingly, this method also identified two regions with predicted immunogenicity in their test set that were not identified by MAPPs analysis, both of which ultimately showed immunogenicity in CD4 T-cell activation assays, suggesting that this method may be able to enhance or improve upon MAPPs analyses. In addition, because the MAPPs data can be generated for biologics in any format, these methods may hold the greatest potential for predicting multispecific antibody immunogenicity in the near term.

5. Conclusions and Future Directions

Multispecific antibodies present a number of advantages in terms of their biological activities and, therefore, it is likely that interest in using them in diverse therapeutic applications will increase in the coming years. To address the increased physical and chemical liabilities associated with such non-natural antibody formats, there are a number of challenges discussed in this review that must be met to advance their widespread application. In particular, it will be important to continue to improve expression and purification methods for simplifying the production of multispecific antibodies with high yields and minimal amounts of mispaired or incompletely assembled antibodies. This issue has greatly limited the development of multispecific antibodies and progress in the field in generating them in a rational and systematic manner. Given the vast number of possible multispecific antibody formats, it will also be critical to improve computational methods for predicting antibody variants with favorable biophysical properties to reduce the design and protein engineering space that needs to be explored to identify drug-like variants. This will require large experimental datasets to be generated for multispecific antibody biophysical properties, at least for a subset of the most promising formats, to train and optimize such predictive methods. The importance of such datasets, which are challenging and costly to generate, should not be underappreciated, as the field is unlikely to significantly advance without them due to the lack of systematic design and engineering strategies. It will also be critical to better define the immunogenicity risks of different multispecific antibody formats, which are inherently more likely to be recognized as foreign by the immune system, and improve the prediction of multispecific variants with low immunogenicity. Current methods are limited, even for analyzing immunogenicity risks for conventional IgGs, and significant advances are needed to reduce safety and efficacy risks associated with multispecific antibodies. Despite these challenges, it is likely that the rapid progress toward improving the prediction and identification of drug-like monospecific IgGs in the last decade will continue to inspire and guide related efforts to improve computational and high-throughput experimental developability analysis of multispecific antibodies with unprecedented therapeutic activities.

Author Contributions: M.S.S., C.N.S., and P.M.T. wrote the manuscript. L.W. prepared the figures and provided feedback on the manuscript. All authors have read and agreed to the published version of the manuscript.

Funding: This work was supported by the National Institutes of Health [R01GM104130, R01AG050598, RF1AG059723 and R35GM136300 to P.M.T., T32 fellowship to L.W. (T32-GM008353)], National Science Foundation [CBET 1813963, CBET 1605266 and CBET 1804313 to P.M.T.], and the Albert M. Mattocks Chair (to P.M.T.).

Acknowledgments: We thank Alec Desai, Jie Huang, Matthew Smith, and Edward Ionescu for their scientific input during the initial stages of this review.

Conflicts of Interest: The authors declare no conflict of interest.

References

1. Kaplon, H.; Muralidharan, M.; Schneider, Z.; Reichert, J.M. Antibodies to watch in 2020. *mAbs* **2020**, *12*, 1703531. [CrossRef]
2. Trabolsi, A.; Arumov, A.; Schatz, J.H. T Cell–Activating Bispecific Antibodies in Cancer Therapy. *J. Immunol.* **2019**, *203*, 585–592. [CrossRef]
3. Maher, J.; Adami, A.A. Antitumor Immunity: Easy as 1, 2, 3 with Monoclonal Bispecific Trifunctional Antibodies? *Cancer Res.* **2013**, *73*, 5613–5617. [CrossRef]
4. Linke, R.; Klein, A.; Seimetz, D. Catumaxomab: Clinical development and future directions. *mAbs* **2010**, *2*, 129–136. [CrossRef] [PubMed]
5. Lenting, P.J.; Denis, C.V.; Christophe, O.D. Emicizumab, a bispecific antibody recognizing coagulation factors IX and X: How does it actually compare to factor VIII? *Blood* **2017**, *130*, 2463–2468. [CrossRef] [PubMed]
6. Shima, M.; Hanabusa, H.; Taki, M.; Matsushita, T.; Sato, T.; Fukutake, K.; Fukazawa, N.; Yoneyama, K.; Yoshida, H.; Nogami, K. Factor VIII–Mimetic Function of Humanized Bispecific Antibody in Hemophilia A. *N. Engl. J. Med.* **2016**, *374*, 2044–2053. [CrossRef] [PubMed]
7. Deshaies, R.J. Multispecific drugs herald a new era of biopharmaceutical innovation. *Nature* **2020**, *580*, 329–338. [CrossRef] [PubMed]
8. Staerz, U.D.; Kanagawa, O.; Bevan, M.J. Hybrid antibodies can target sites for attack by T cells. *Nature* **1985**, *314*, 628–631. [CrossRef]
9. Bargou, R.; Leo, E.; Zugmaier, G.; Klinger, M.; Goebeler, M.; Knop, S.; Noppeney, R.; Viardot, A.; Hess, G.; Schuler, M.; et al. Tumor Regression in Cancer Patients by Very Low Doses of a T Cell-Engaging Antibody. *Science* **2008**, *321*, 974–977. [CrossRef] [PubMed]
10. Einsele, H.; Borghaei, H.; Orlowski, R.Z.; Subklewe, M.; Roboz, G.J.; Zugmaier, G.; Kufer, P.; Iskander, K.; Kantarjian, H. The BiTE (bispecific T-cell engager) platform: Development and future potential of a targeted immuno-oncology therapy across tumor types. *Cancer* **2020**, *126*, 3192–3201. [CrossRef]
11. Löffler, A.; Kufer, P.; Lutterbüse, R.; Zettl, F.; Daniel, P.T.; Schwenkenbecher, J.M.; Riethmüller, G.; Dörken, B.; Bargou, R.C. A recombinant bispecific single-chain antibody, CD19 x CD3, induces rapid and high lymphoma-directed cytotoxicity by unstimulated T lymphocytes. *Blood* **2000**, *95*, 2098–2103. [CrossRef]

12. Oberg, H.H.; Kellner, C.; Gonnermann, D.; Sebens, S.; Bauerschlag, D.; Gramatzki, M.; Kabelitz, D.; Peipp, M.; Wesch, D. Tribody [(HER2)2xCD16] Is More Effective Than Trastuzumab in Enhancing γδ T Cell and Natural Killer Cell Cytotoxicity Against HER2-Expressing Cancer Cells. *Front. Immunol.* **2018**, *9*, 814. [CrossRef] [PubMed]
13. Schmohl, J.U.; Felices, M.; Todhunter, D.; Taras, E.; Miller, J.S.; Vallera, D.A. Tetraspecific scFv construct provides NK cell mediated ADCC and self-sustaining stimuli via insertion of IL-15 as a cross-linker. *Oncotarget* **2016**, *7*, 73830–73844. [CrossRef] [PubMed]
14. Schmohl, J.U.; Gleason, M.K.; Dougherty, P.R.; Miller, J.S.; Vallera, D.A. Heterodimeric Bispecific Single Chain Variable Fragments (scFv) Killer Engagers (BiKEs) Enhance NK-cell Activity Against CD133+ Colorectal Cancer Cells. *Target. Oncol.* **2016**, *11*, 353–361. [CrossRef] [PubMed]
15. Gauthier, L.; Morel, A.; Anceriz, N.; Rossi, B.; Blanchard-Alvarez, A.; Grondin, G.; Trichard, S.; Cesari, C.; Sapet, M.; Bosco, F.; et al. Multifunctional Natural Killer Cell Engagers Targeting NKp46 Trigger Protective Tumor Immunity. *Cell* **2019**, *177*, 1701–1713.e16. [CrossRef]
16. Husain, B.; Ellerman, D. Expanding the Boundaries of Biotherapeutics with Bispecific Antibodies. *BioDrugs* **2018**, *32*, 441–464. [CrossRef] [PubMed]
17. Liu, H.; Saxena, A.; Sidhu, S.S.; Wu, D. Fc Engineering for Developing Therapeutic Bispecific Antibodies and Novel Scaffolds. *Front. Immunol.* **2017**, *8*, 38. [CrossRef]
18. Wang, Q.; Chen, Y.; Park, J.; Liu, X.; Hu, Y.; Wang, T.; McFarland, K.; Betenbaugh, M.J. Design and Production of Bispecific Antibodies. *Antibodies* **2019**, *8*, 43. [CrossRef]
19. Tiller, K.E.; Tessier, P.M. Advances in Antibody Design. *Annu. Rev. Biomed. Eng.* **2015**, *17*, 191–216. [CrossRef]
20. Rouet, R.; Lowe, D.; Christ, D. Stability engineering of the human antibody repertoire. *FEBS Lett.* **2014**, *588*, 269–277. [CrossRef]
21. McConnell, A.D.; Spasojevich, V.; Macomber, J.L.; Krapf, I.P.; Chen, A.; Sheffer, J.C.; Berkebile, A.; Horlick, R.A.; Neben, S.; King, D.J.; et al. An integrated approach to extreme thermostabilization and affinity maturation of an antibody. *Protein Eng. Des. Sel.* **2013**, *26*, 151–164. [CrossRef] [PubMed]
22. McConnell, A.D.; Zhang, X.; Macomber, J.L.; Chau, B.; Sheffer, J.C.; Rahmanian, S.; Hare, E.; Spasojevic, V.; Horlick, R.A.; King, D.J.; et al. A general approach to antibody thermostabilization. *mAbs* **2014**, *6*, 1274–1282. [CrossRef] [PubMed]
23. Gu, J.; Ghayur, T. Rationale and development of multispecific antibody drugs. *Expert Rev. Clin. Pharmacol.* **2010**, *3*, 491–508. [CrossRef] [PubMed]
24. Hagihara, Y.; Saerens, D. Engineering disulfide bonds within an antibody. *Biochim. Biophys. Acta* **2014**, *1844*, 2016–2023. [CrossRef] [PubMed]
25. Turner, K.; Liu, J.L.; Zabetakis, D.; Lee, A.B.; Anderson, G.P.; Goldman, E.R. Improving the biophysical properties of anti-ricin single-domain antibodies. *Biotechnol. Rep.* **2015**, *6*, 27–35. [CrossRef]
26. Anderson, G.P.; Liu, J.H.; Zabetakis, D.; Liu, J.L.; Goldman, E.R. Thermal stabilization of anti-α-cobratoxin single domain antibodies. *Toxicon* **2017**, *129*, 68–73. [CrossRef]
27. Kim, D.Y.; Kandalaft, H.; Hussack, G.; Raphael, S.; Ding, W.; Kelly, J.F.; Henry, K.A.; Tanha, J. Evaluation of a noncanonical Cys40-Cys55 disulfide linkage for stabilization of single-domain antibodies. *Protein Sci.* **2019**, *28*, 881–888. [CrossRef]
28. Kim, D.Y.; Kandalaft, H.; Ding, W.; Ryan, S.; Van Faassen, H.; Hirama, T.; Foote, S.J.; MacKenzie, C.R.; Tanha, J. Disulfide linkage engineering for improving biophysical properties of human VH domains. *Protein Eng. Des. Sel.* **2012**, *25*, 581–590. [CrossRef]
29. Hussack, G.; Hirama, T.; Ding, W.; MacKenzie, R.; Tanha, J. Engineered Single-Domain Antibodies with High Protease Resistance and Thermal Stability. *PLoS ONE* **2011**, *6*, e28218. [CrossRef]
30. Hagihara, Y.; Mine, S.; Uegaki, K. Stabilization of an Immunoglobulin Fold Domain by an Engineered Disulfide Bond at the Buried Hydrophobic Region. *J. Biol. Chem.* **2007**, *282*, 36489–36495. [CrossRef]
31. Zabetakis, D.; Olson, M.A.; Anderson, G.P.; Legler, P.M.; Goldman, E.R. Evaluation of Disulfide Bond Position to Enhance the Thermal Stability of a Highly Stable Single Domain Antibody. *PLoS ONE* **2014**, *9*, e115405. [CrossRef]
32. Bhatta, P.; Humphreys, D.T. Relative Contribution of Framework and CDR Regions in Antibody Variable Domains to Multimerisation of Fv- and scFv-Containing Bispecific Antibodies. *Antibodies* **2018**, *7*, 35. [CrossRef] [PubMed]

33. Liu, J.L.; Goldman, E.R.; Zabetakis, D.; Walper, S.A.; Turner, K.; Shriver-Lake, L.C.; Anderson, G.P. Enhanced production of a single domain antibody with an engineered stabilizing extra disulfide bond. *Microb. Cell Factories* **2015**, *14*, 158. [CrossRef] [PubMed]
34. Schlapschy, M.; Grimm, S.; Skerra, A. A system for concomitant overexpression of four periplasmic folding catalysts to improve secretory protein production in Escherichia coli. *Protein Eng. Des. Sel.* **2006**, *19*, 385–390. [CrossRef]
35. Shriver-Lake, L.C.; Goldman, E.R.; Zabetakis, D.; Anderson, G.P. Improved production of single domain antibodies with two disulfide bonds by co-expression of chaperone proteins in the Escherichia coli periplasm. *J. Immunol. Methods* **2017**, *443*, 64–67. [CrossRef] [PubMed]
36. Jung, S.; Plückthun, A. Improving in vivo folding and stability of a single-chain Fv antibody fragment by loop grafting. *Protein Eng.* **1997**, *10*, 959–966. [CrossRef] [PubMed]
37. Honegger, A.; Malebranche, A.D.; Röthlisberger, D.; Plückthun, A. The influence of the framework core residues on the biophysical properties of immunoglobulin heavy chain variable domains. *Protein Eng. Des. Sel.* **2009**, *22*, 121–134. [CrossRef] [PubMed]
38. Queen, C.; Schneider, W.P.; Selick, H.E.; Payne, P.W.; Landolfi, N.F.; Duncan, J.F.; Avdalovic, N.M.; Levitt, M.; Junghans, R.P.; Waldmann, T.A. A humanized antibody that binds to the interleukin 2 receptor. *Proc. Natl. Acad. Sci. USA* **1989**, *86*, 10029–10033. [CrossRef]
39. Julian, M.C.; Li, L.-J.; Garde, S.; Wilen, R.; Tessier, P.M. Efficient affinity maturation of antibody variable domains requires co-selection of compensatory mutations to maintain thermodynamic stability. *Sci. Rep.* **2017**, *7*, 45259. [CrossRef]
40. Lehmann, A.; Wixted, J.H.F.; Shapovalov, M.V.; Roder, H.; Dunbrack, R.L.; Robinson, M.K. Stability engineering of anti-EGFR scFv antibodies by rational design of a lambda-to-kappa swap of the VL framework using a structure-guided approach. *mAbs* **2015**, *7*, 1058–1071. [CrossRef]
41. Shusta, E.V.; Holler, P.D.; Kieke, M.C.; Kranz, D.M.; Wittrup, K. Directed evolution of a stable scaffold for T-cell receptor engineering. *Nat. Biotechnol.* **2000**, *18*, 754–759. [CrossRef]
42. Orr, B.; Carr, L.; Wittrup, K.; Roy, E.; Kranz, D.M. Rapid Method for Measuring ScFv Thermal Stability by Yeast Surface Display. *Biotechnol. Prog.* **2003**, *19*, 631–638. [CrossRef] [PubMed]
43. Franklin, E.; Cunningham, O.; Fennell, B. Parallel Evolution of Antibody Affinity and Thermal Stability for Optimal Biotherapeutic Development. *Adv. Struct. Safe. Stud.* **2018**, 457–477. [CrossRef]
44. Traxlmayr, M.W.; Obinger, C. Directed evolution of proteins for increased stability and expression using yeast display. *Arch. Biochem. Biophys.* **2012**, *526*, 174–180. [CrossRef] [PubMed]
45. Traxlmayr, M.W.; Shusta, E.V. Directed Evolution of Protein Thermal Stability Using Yeast Surface Display. *Methods Mol. Biol.* **2017**, *1575*, 45–65. [CrossRef]
46. Xu, L.; Kohli, N.; Rennard, R.; Jiao, Y.; Razlog, M.; Zhang, K.; Baum, J.; Johnson, B.; Tang, J.; Schoeberl, B.; et al. Rapid optimization and prototyping for therapeutic antibody-like molecules. *mAbs* **2013**, *5*, 237–254. [CrossRef]
47. Jia, Y.; Ren, P.; Duan, S.; Zeng, P.; Xie, D.; Zeng, F. An optimized yeast display strategy for efficient scFv antibody selection using ribosomal skipping system and thermo resistant yeast. *Biotechnol. Lett.* **2019**, *41*, 1067–1076. [CrossRef]
48. Scott, M.J.; Lee, J.A.; Wake, M.S.; Batt, K.V.; Wattam, T.A.; Hiles, I.D.; Batuwangala, T.D.; Ashman, C.I.; Steward, M. 'In-Format' screening of a novel bispecific antibody format reveals significant potency improvements relative to unformatted molecules. *mAbs* **2016**, *9*, 85–93. [CrossRef]
49. Kim, D.Y.; Hussack, G.; Kandalaft, H.; Tanha, J. Mutational approaches to improve the biophysical properties of human single-domain antibodies. *Biochim. Biophys. Acta* **2014**, *1844*, 1983–2001. [CrossRef]
50. Geddie, M.L.; Kohli, N.; Kirpotin, D.B.; Razlog, M.; Jiao, Y.; Kornaga, T.; Rennard, R.; Xu, L.; Schoerbl, B.; Marks, J.D.; et al. Improving the developability of an anti-EphA2 single-chain variable fragment for nanoparticle targeting. *mAbs* **2017**, *9*, 58–67. [CrossRef]
51. Liu, J.L.; Shriver-Lake, L.C.; Anderson, G.P.; Zabetakis, D.; Goldman, E.R. Selection, characterization, and thermal stabilization of llama single domain antibodies towards Ebola virus glycoprotein. *Microb. Cell Factories* **2017**, *16*, 223. [CrossRef] [PubMed]
52. Kunz, P.; Flock, T.; Soler, N.; Zaiss, M.; Vincke, C.; Sterckx, Y.G.-J.; Kastelic, D.; Muyldermans, S.; Hoheisel, J.D. Exploiting sequence and stability information for directing nanobody stability engineering. *Biochim. Biophys. Acta Gen. Subj.* **2017**, *1861*, 2196–2205. [CrossRef]

53. Baran, D.; Pszolla, M.G.; Lapidoth, G.D.; Norn, C.; Dym, O.; Unger, T.; Albeck, S.; Tyka, M.D.; Fleishman, S.J. Principles for computational design of binding antibodies. *Proc. Natl. Acad. Sci. USA* **2017**, *114*, 10900–10905. [CrossRef] [PubMed]
54. Adolf-Bryfogle, J.; Kalyuzhniy, O.; Kubitz, M.; Weitzner, B.D.; Hu, X.; Adachi, Y.; Schief, W.R.; Dunbrack, R.L. RosettaAntibodyDesign (RAbD): A general framework for computational antibody design. *PLoS Comput. Biol.* **2018**, *14*, e1006112. [CrossRef] [PubMed]
55. Pérez, A.-M.W.; Sormanni, P.; Andersen, J.S.; Sakhnini, L.I.; León, I.R.; Bjelke, J.R.; Gajhede, A.J.; De Maria, L.; Otzen, D.E.; Vendruscolo, M.; et al. In vitro and in silico assessment of the developability of a designed monoclonal antibody library. *mAbs* **2019**, *11*, 388–400. [CrossRef]
56. Soler, M.A.; Medagli, B.; Semrau, M.S.; Storici, P.; Bajc, G.; De Marco, A.; Laio, A.; Fortuna, S. A consensus protocol for the in silico optimisation of antibody fragments. *Chem. Commun.* **2019**, *55*, 14043–14046. [CrossRef] [PubMed]
57. Lee, J.; Der, B.S.; Karamitros, C.S.; Li, W.; Marshall, N.M.; Lungu, O.I.; Miklos, A.E.; Xu, J.; Kang, T.H.; Lee, C.; et al. Computer-based engineering of thermostabilized antibody fragments. *AIChE J.* **2020**, *66*. [CrossRef]
58. Kuroda, D.; Tsumoto, K. Engineering Stability, Viscosity, and Immunogenicity of Antibodies by Computational Design. *J. Pharm. Sci.* **2020**, *109*, 1631–1651. [CrossRef]
59. Lapidoth, G.D.; Baran, D.; Pszolla, G.M.; Norn, C.; Alon, A.; Tyka, M.D.; Fleishman, S.J. AbDesign: An algorithm for combinatorial backbone design guided by natural conformations and sequences. *Proteins* **2015**, *83*, 1385–1406. [CrossRef]
60. Warszawski, S.; Katz, A.B.; Lipsh, R.; Khmelnitsky, L.; Ben Nissan, G.; Javitt, G.; Dym, O.; Unger, T.; Knop, O.; Albeck, S.; et al. Optimizing antibody affinity and stability by the automated design of the variable light-heavy chain interfaces. *PLoS Comput. Biol.* **2019**, *15*, e1007207. [CrossRef]
61. Fischer, N.; Elson, G.; Magistrelli, G.; Dheilly, E.; Fouque, N.; Laurendon, A.; Gueneau, F.; Ravn, U.; Depoisier, J.-F.; Moine, V.; et al. Exploiting light chains for the scalable generation and platform purification of native human bispecific IgG. *Nat. Commun.* **2015**, *6*, 6113. [CrossRef]
62. Amaral, M.; Hölper, S.; Lange, C.; Jung, J.; Sjuts, H.; Weil, S.; Fischer, M.; Radoevic, K.; Rao, E. Engineered Technologies and Bioanalysis of multispecific Antibody Formats. *J. Appl. Bioanal.* **2020**, *6*, 26–51. [CrossRef]
63. Labrijn, A.F.; Meesters, J.I.; Priem, P.; De Jong, R.N.; Bremer, E.T.J.V.D.; Van Kampen, M.D.; Gerritsen, A.F.; Schuurman, J.; Parren, P.W.H.I. Controlled Fab-arm exchange for the generation of stable bispecific IgG1. *Nat. Protoc.* **2014**, *9*, 2450–2463. [CrossRef]
64. Labrijn, A.F.; Meesters, J.I.; De Goeij, B.E.C.G.; Bremer, E.T.J.V.D.; Neijssen, J.; Van Kampen, M.D.; Strumane, K.; Verploegen, S.; Kundu, A.; Gramer, M.J.; et al. Efficient generation of stable bispecific IgG1 by controlled Fab-arm exchange. *Proc. Natl. Acad. Sci. USA* **2013**, *110*, 5145–5150. [CrossRef] [PubMed]
65. Schaefer, W.; Regula, J.T.; Bähner, M.; Schanzer, J.; Croasdale, R.; Dürr, H.; Gassner, C.; Georges, G.; Kettenberger, H.; Imhof-Jung, S.; et al. Immunoglobulin domain crossover as a generic approach for the production of bispecific IgG antibodies. *Proc. Natl. Acad. Sci. USA* **2011**, *108*, 11187–11192. [CrossRef]
66. Merchant, A.M.; Zhu, Z.; Yuan, J.Q.; Goddard, A.; Adams, C.W.; Presta, L.G.; Carter, P. An efficient route to human bispecific IgG. *Nat. Biotechnol.* **1998**, *16*, 677–681. [CrossRef] [PubMed]
67. De Nardis, C.; Hendriks, L.J.A.; Poirier, E.; Arvinte, T.; Gros, P.; Bakker, A.B.H.; De Kruif, J. A new approach for generating bispecific antibodies based on a common light chain format and the stable architecture of human immunoglobulin G1. *J. Biol. Chem.* **2017**, *292*, 14706–14717. [CrossRef] [PubMed]
68. Krah, S.; Schröter, C.; Eller, C.; Rhiel, L.; Rasche, N.; Beck, J.; Sellmann, C.; Günther, R.; Toleikis, L.; Hock, B.; et al. Generation of human bispecific common light chain antibodies by combining animal immunization and yeast display. *Protein Eng. Des. Sel.* **2017**, *30*, 291–301. [CrossRef]
69. Shiraiwa, H.; Narita, A.; Kamata-Sakurai, M.; Ishiguro, T.; Sano, Y.; Hironiwa, N.; Tsushima, T.; Segawa, H.; Tsunenari, T.; Ikeda, Y.; et al. Engineering a bispecific antibody with a common light chain: Identification and optimization of an anti-CD3 epsilon and anti-GPC3 bispecific antibody, ERY974. *Methods* **2019**, *154*, 10–20. [CrossRef]
70. Lewis, S.M.; Wu, X.; Pustilnik, A.; Sereno, A.; Huang, F.; Rick, H.L.; Guntas, G.; Leaver-Fay, A.; Smith, E.M.; Ho, C.; et al. Generation of bispecific IgG antibodies by structure-based design of an orthogonal Fab interface. *Nat. Biotechnol.* **2014**, *32*, 191–198. [CrossRef]

71. Liu, Z.; Leng, E.C.; Gunasekaran, K.; Pentony, M.; Shen, M.; Howard, M.; Stoops, J.; Manchulenko, K.; Razinkov, V.; Liu, H.; et al. A Novel Antibody Engineering Strategy for Making Monovalent Bispecific Heterodimeric IgG Antibodies by Electrostatic Steering Mechanism. *J. Biol. Chem.* **2015**, *290*, 7535–7562. [CrossRef] [PubMed]
72. Wei, H.; Cai, H.; Jin, Y.; Wang, P.; Zhang, Q.; Lin, Y.; Wang, W.; Cheng, J.; Zeng, N.; Xu, T.; et al. Structural basis of a novel heterodimeric Fc for bispecific antibody production. *Oncotarget* **2017**, *8*, 51037–51049. [CrossRef] [PubMed]
73. Froning, K.J.; Leaver-Fay, A.; Wu, X.; Phan, S.; Gao, L.; Huang, F.; Pustilnik, A.; Bacica, M.; Houlihan, K.; Chai, Q.; et al. Computational design of a specific heavy chain/κ light chain interface for expressing fully IgG bispecific antibodies. *Protein Sci.* **2017**, *26*, 2021–2038. [CrossRef]
74. Dillon, M.; Yin, Y.; Zhou, J.; Mccarty, L.; Ellerman, D.; Slaga, D.; Junttila, T.T.; Han, G.; Sandoval, W.; Ovacik, M.A.; et al. Efficient production of bispecific IgG of different isotypes and species of origin in single mammalian cells. *mAbs* **2017**, *9*, 213–230. [CrossRef] [PubMed]
75. Joshi, K.K.; Phung, W.; Han, G.; Yin, Y.; Kim, I.; Sandoval, W.; Carter, P.J. Elucidating heavy/light chain pairing preferences to facilitate the assembly of bispecific IgG in single cells. *mAbs* **2019**, *11*, 1254–1265. [CrossRef]
76. Mullard, A. FDA approves first bispecific. *Nat. Rev. Drug Discov.* **2015**, *14*, 7. [CrossRef]
77. Johnson, S.; Burke, S.; Huang, L.; Gorlatov, S.; Li, H.; Wang, W.; Zhang, W.; Tuaillon, N.; Rainey, J.; Barat, B.; et al. Effector Cell Recruitment with Novel Fv-based Dual-affinity Re-targeting Protein Leads to Potent Tumor Cytolysis and In Vivo B-cell Depletion. *J. Mol. Biol.* **2010**, *399*, 436–449. [CrossRef]
78. Moore, P.A.; Zhang, W.; Rainey, G.J.; Burke, S.; Li, H.; Huang, L.; Gorlatov, S.; Veri, M.C.; Aggarwal, S.; Yang, Y.; et al. Application of dual affinity retargeting molecules to achieve optimal redirected T-cell killing of B-cell lymphoma. *Blood* **2011**, *117*, 4542–4551. [CrossRef]
79. Rader, C. DARTs take aim at BiTEs. *Blood* **2011**, *117*, 4403–4404. [CrossRef]
80. Wu, X.; Sereno, A.J.; Huang, F.; Lewis, S.M.; Lieu, R.L.; Weldon, C.; Torres, C.; Fine, C.; Batt, M.A.; Fitchett, J.R.; et al. Fab-based bispecific antibody formats with robust biophysical properties and biological activity. *mAbs* **2015**, *7*, 470–482. [CrossRef]
81. Gong, S.; Ren, F.; Wu, D.; Wu, X.; Wu, C. Fabs-in-tandem immunoglobulin is a novel and versatile bispecific design for engaging multiple therapeutic targets. *mAbs* **2017**, *9*, 1118–1128. [CrossRef] [PubMed]
82. Wu, C.; Ying, H.; Grinnell, C.; Bryant, S.; Miller, R.; Clabbers, A.; Bose, S.; McCarthy, D.; Zhu, R.-R.; Santora, L.; et al. Simultaneous targeting of multiple disease mediators by a dual-variable-domain immunoglobulin. *Nat. Biotechnol.* **2007**, *25*, 1290–1297. [CrossRef] [PubMed]
83. Shibuya, Y.; Haga, N.; Asano, R.; Nakazawa, H.; Hattori, T.; Takeda, D.; Sugiyama, A.; Kurotani, R.; Kumagai, I.; Umetsu, M.; et al. Generation of camelid VHH bispecific constructs via in-cell intein-mediated protein trans-splicing. *Prot. Eng. Des. Sel.* **2017**, *30*, 15–21.
84. Hemmi, S.; Asano, R.; Kimura, K.; Umetsu, M.; Nakanishi, T.; Kumagai, I.; Makabe, K. Construction of a circularly connected VHH bispecific antibody (cyclobody) for the desirable positioning of antigen-binding sites. *Biochem. Biophys. Res. Commun.* **2020**, *523*, 72–77. [CrossRef] [PubMed]
85. Han, L.; Chen, J.; Ding, K.; Zong, H.; Xie, Y.; Jiang, H.; Zhang, B.; Lu, H.; Yin, W.; Gilly, J.; et al. Efficient generation of bispecific IgG antibodies by split intein mediated protein trans-splicing system. *Sci. Rep.* **2017**, *7*, 1–11. [CrossRef]
86. Han, L.; Zong, H.; Zhou, Y.; Pan, Z.; Chen, J.; Ding, K.; Xie, Y.; Jiang, H.; Zhang, B.; Lu, H.; et al. Naturally split intein Npu DnaE mediated rapid generation of bispecific IgG antibodies. *Methods* **2019**, *154*, 32–37. [CrossRef]
87. Hofmann, T.; Schmidt, J.; Ciesielski, E.; Becker, S.; Rysiok, T.; Schütte, M.; Toleikis, L.; Kolmar, H.; Doerner, A. Intein mediated high throuput screening for bispecific antibodies. *mAbs* **2020**, *12*, 1731938. [CrossRef]
88. Moussa, E.M.; Panchal, J.P.; Moorthy, B.S.; Blum, J.S.; Joubert, M.K.; Narhi, L.O.; Topp, E. Immunogenicity of Therapeutic Protein Aggregates. *J. Pharm. Sci.* **2016**, *105*, 417–430. [CrossRef]
89. Ratanji, K.D.; Derrick, J.P.; Dearman, R.J.; Kimber, I. Immunogenicity of therapeutic proteins: Influence of aggregation. *J. Immunotoxicol.* **2014**, *11*, 99–109. [CrossRef]
90. Perchiacca, J.M.; Bhattacharya, M.; Tessier, P.M. Mutational analysis of domain antibodies reveals aggregation hotspots within and near the complementarity determining regions. *Proteins Struct. Funct. Bioinform.* **2011**, *79*, 2637–2647. [CrossRef]

91. Perchiacca, J.M.; Ladiwala, A.R.A.; Bhattacharya, M.; Tessier, P.M. Aggregation-resistant domain antibodies engineered with charged mutations near the edges of the complementarity-determining regions. *Protein Eng. Des. Sel.* **2012**, *25*, 591–602. [CrossRef]
92. Dudgeon, K.; Rouet, R.; Kokmeijer, I.; Schofield, P.R.; Stolp, J.; Langley, D.B.; Stock, D.; Christ, D. General strategy for the generation of human antibody variable domains with increased aggregation resistance. *Proc. Natl. Acad. Sci. USA* **2012**, *109*, 10879–10884. [CrossRef]
93. Perchiacca, J.M.; Lee, C.C.; Tessier, P.M. Optimal charged mutations in the complementarity-determining regions that prevent domain antibody aggregation are dependent on the antibody scaffold. *Protein Eng. Des. Sel.* **2014**, *27*, 29–39. [CrossRef] [PubMed]
94. Van Der Kant, R.; Karow-Zwick, A.R.; Van Durme, J.; Blech, M.; Gallardo, R.; Seeliger, D.; Aßfalg, K.; Baatsen, P.; Compernolle, G.; Gils, A.; et al. Prediction and Reduction of the Aggregation of Monoclonal Antibodies. *J. Mol. Biol.* **2017**, *429*, 1244–1261. [CrossRef]
95. Chaudhuri, R.; Cheng, Y.; Middaugh, C.R.; Volkin, D. High-Throughput Biophysical Analysis of Protein Therapeutics to Examine Interrelationships Between Aggregate Formation and Conformational Stability. *AAPS J.* **2014**, *16*, 48–64. [CrossRef] [PubMed]
96. Chennamsetty, N.; Voynov, V.; Kayser, V.; Helk, B.; Trout, B.L. Design of therapeutic proteins with enhanced stability. *Proc. Natl. Acad. Sci. USA* **2009**, *106*, 11937–11942. [CrossRef] [PubMed]
97. Chennamsetty, N.; Voynov, V.; Kayser, V.; Helk, B.; Trout, B.L. Prediction of Aggregation Prone Regions of Therapeutic Proteins. *J. Phys. Chem. B* **2010**, *114*, 6614–6624. [CrossRef] [PubMed]
98. Roberts, C.J. Therapeutic protein aggregation: Mechanisms, design, and control. *Trends Biotechnol.* **2014**, *32*, 372–380. [CrossRef] [PubMed]
99. Lee, C.C.; Perchiacca, J.M.; Tessier, P.M. Toward aggregation-resistant antibodies by design. *Trends Biotechnol.* **2013**, *31*, 612–620. [CrossRef]
100. Schaefer, Z.P.; Bailey, L.J.; Kossiakoff, A.A. A polar ring endows improved specificity to an antibody fragment. *Protein Sci.* **2016**, *25*, 1290–1298. [CrossRef]
101. Jones, S.; Thornton, J.M. Protein-protein interactions: A review of protein dimer structures. *Prog. Biophys. Mol. Biol.* **1995**, *63*, 31–65. [CrossRef]
102. Jones, S.; Thornton, J.M. Principles of protein-protein interactions. *Proc. Natl. Acad. Sci. USA* **1996**, *93*, 13–20. [CrossRef] [PubMed]
103. Bogan, A.A.; Thorn, K.S. Anatomy of hot spots in protein interfaces. *J. Mol. Biol.* **1998**, *280*, 1–9. [CrossRef] [PubMed]
104. Sakhnini, L.I.; Greisen, P.J.; Wiberg, C.; Bozoky, Z.; Lund, S.; Perez, A.-M.W.; Karkov, H.S.; Huus, K.; Hansen, J.-J.; Bülow, L.; et al. Improving the Developability of an Antigen Binding Fragment by Aspartate Substitutions. *Biochemistry* **2019**, *58*, 2750–2759. [CrossRef] [PubMed]
105. Brummitt, R.K.; Nesta, D.P.; Chang, L.; Chase, S.F.; Laue, T.M.; Roberts, C.J. Nonnative Aggregation of an IgG1 Antibody in Acidic Conditions: Part 1. Unfolding, Colloidal Interactions, and Formation of High-Molecular-Weight Aggregates. *J. Pharm. Sci.* **2011**, *100*, 2087–2103. [CrossRef] [PubMed]
106. Austerberry, J.; Dajani, R.; Panova, S.; Roberts, D.; Golovanov, A.P.; Pluen, A.; Van Der Walle, C.F.; Uddin, S.; Warwicker, J.; Derrick, J.P.; et al. The effect of charge mutations on the stability and aggregation of a human single chain Fv fragment. *Eur. J. Pharm. Biopharm.* **2017**, *115*, 18–30. [CrossRef]
107. Austerberry, J.I.; Thistlethwaite, A.; Fisher, K.; Golovanov, A.P.; Pluen, A.; Esfandiary, R.; Van Der Walle, C.F.; Warwicker, J.; Derrick, J.P.; Curtis, R. Arginine to Lysine Mutations Increase the Aggregation Stability of a Single-Chain Variable Fragment through Unfolded-State Interactions. *Biochemistry* **2019**, *58*, 3413–3421. [CrossRef]
108. Shan, L.; Mody, N.; Sormani, P.; Rosenthal, K.L.; Damschroder, M.M.; Esfandiary, R.; Sormanni, P. Developability Assessment of Engineered Monoclonal Antibody Variants with a Complex Self-Association Behavior Using Complementary Analytical and in Silico Tools. *Mol. Pharm.* **2018**, *15*, 5697–5710. [CrossRef]
109. Hsu, H.-J.; Lee, K.H.; Jian, J.-W.; Chang, H.-J.; Yu, C.-M.; Lee, Y.-C.; Chen, I.-C.; Peng, H.-P.; Wu, C.Y.; Huang, Y.-F.; et al. Antibody Variable Domain Interface and Framework Sequence Requirements for Stability and Function by High-Throughput Experiments. *Structure* **2014**, *22*, 22–34. [CrossRef]
110. Wörn, A.; Plückthun, A. Stability engineering of antibody single-chain Fv fragments. *J. Mol. Biol.* **2001**, *305*, 989–1010. [CrossRef]

111. Jung, S.; Honegger, A.; Plückthun, A. Selection for improved protein stability by phage display 1 1Edited by J. A. Wells. *J. Mol. Biol.* **1999**, *294*, 163–180. [CrossRef] [PubMed]
112. Wörn, A.; Plückthun, A. Different Equilibrium Stability Behavior of ScFv Fragments: Identification, Classification, and Improvement by Protein Engineering. *Biochemistry* **1999**, *38*, 8739–8750. [CrossRef] [PubMed]
113. Wörn, A.; Plückthun, A. Mutual Stabilization of VLand VHin Single-Chain Antibody Fragments, Investigated with Mutants Engineered for Stability. *Biochemistry* **1998**, *37*, 13120–13127. [CrossRef] [PubMed]
114. Yamauchi, S.; Kobashigawa, Y.; Fukuda, N.; Teramoto, M.; Toyota, Y.; Liu, C.; Ikeguchi, Y.; Sato, T.; Sato, Y.; Kimura, H.; et al. Cyclization of Single-Chain Fv Antibodies Markedly Suppressed Their Characteristic Aggregation Mediated by Inter-Chain VH-VL Interactions. *Molecules* **2019**, *24*, 2620. [CrossRef]
115. Miller, B.R.; Glaser, S.M.; Demarest, S.J. Rapid Screening Platform for Stabilization of scFvs in *Escherichia coli*. *Methods Mol. Biol.* **2009**, *525*, 279–289, xiv.
116. Jain, T.; Sun, T.; Durand, S.; Hall, A.; Houston, N.R.; Nett, J.H.; Sharkey, B.; Bobrowicz, B.; Caffry, I.; Yu, Y.; et al. Biophysical properties of the clinical-stage antibody landscape. *Proc. Natl. Acad. Sci. USA* **2017**, *114*, 944–949. [CrossRef]
117. Bailly, M.; Mieczkowski, C.; Juan, V.; Metwally, E.; Tomazela, D.; Baker, J.; Uchida, M.; Kofman, E.; Raoufi, F.; Motlagh, S.; et al. Predicting Antibody Developability Profiles Through Early Stage Discovery Screening. *mAbs* **2020**, *12*, 1743053. [CrossRef]
118. Clarke, S.C.; Ma, B.; Trinklein, N.D.; Schellenberger, U.; Osborn, M.J.; Ouisse, L.-H.; Boudreau, A.; Davison, L.M.; Harris, K.E.; Ugamraj, H.S.; et al. Multispecific Antibody Development Platform Based on Human Heavy Chain Antibodies. *Front. Immunol.* **2018**, *9*. [CrossRef]
119. Lauer, T.M.; Agrawal, N.J.; Chennamsetty, N.; Egodage, K.; Helk, B.; Trout, B.L. Developability Index: A Rapid in Silico Tool for the Screening of Antibody Aggregation Propensity. *J. Pharm. Sci.* **2012**, *101*, 102–115. [CrossRef]
120. Obrezanova, O.; Arnell, A.; De La Cuesta, R.G.; Berthelot, M.E.; Gallagher, T.R.; Zurdo, J.; Stallwood, Y. Aggregation risk prediction for antibodies and its application to biotherapeutic development. *mAbs* **2015**, *7*, 352–363. [CrossRef]
121. Zhang, C.; Samad, M.; Yu, H.; Chakroun, N.; Hilton, D.; Dalby, P.A. Computational Design to Reduce Conformational Flexibility and Aggregation Rates of an Antibody Fab Fragment. *Mol. Pharm.* **2018**, *15*, 3079–3092. [CrossRef] [PubMed]
122. Wang, X.; Das, T.K.; Singh, S.K.; Kumar, S. Potential aggregation prone regions in biotherapeutics: A survey of commercial monoclonal antibodies. *mAbs* **2009**, *1*, 254–267. [CrossRef]
123. Wang, X.; Singh, S.K.; Kumar, S. Potential Aggregation-Prone Regions in Complementarity-Determining Regions of Antibodies and Their Contribution Towards Antigen Recognition: A Computational Analysis. *Pharm. Res.* **2010**, *27*, 1512–1529. [CrossRef] [PubMed]
124. Christ, D.; Famm, K.; Winter, G. Repertoires of aggregation-resistant human antibody domains. *Protein Eng. Des. Sel.* **2007**, *20*, 413–416. [CrossRef] [PubMed]
125. Wu, S.-J.; Luo, J.; O'Neil, K.T.; Kang, J.; Lacy, E.R.; Canziani, G.; Baker, A.; Huang, M.; Tang, Q.M.; Raju, T.; et al. Structure-based engineering of a monoclonal antibody for improved solubility. *Protein Eng. Des. Sel.* **2010**, *23*, 643–651. [CrossRef] [PubMed]
126. Lee, C.C.; Julian, M.C.; Tiller, K.E.; Meng, F.; Duconge, S.E.; Akter, R.; Raleigh, D.P.; Tessier, P.M. Design and Optimization of Anti-amyloid Domain Antibodies Specific for β-Amyloid and Islet Amyloid Polypeptide. *J. Biol. Chem.* **2016**, *291*, 2858–2873. [CrossRef] [PubMed]
127. Schmitt, M.G.; Rajendra, Y.; Hougland, M.D.; Boyles, J.S.; Barnard, G.C. Polymer-mediated flocculation of transient CHO cultures as a simple, high throughput method to facilitate antibody discovery. *Biotechnol. Prog.* **2017**, *33*, 1393–1400. [CrossRef]
128. Evans, A.R.; Capaldi, M.T.; Goparaju, G.; Colter, D.; Shi, F.F.; Aubert, S.; Li, L.-C.; Mo, J.; Lewis, M.J.; Hu, P.; et al. Using bispecific antibodies in forced degradation studies to analyze the structure-function relationships of symmetrically and asymmetrically modified antibodies. *mAbs* **2019**, *11*, 1101–1112. [CrossRef]
129. Shi, R.L.; Xiao, G.; Dillon, T.M.; Ricci, M.S.; Bondarenko, P.V. Characterization of therapeutic proteins by cation exchange chromatography-mass spectrometry and top-down analysis. *mAbs* **2020**, *12*, 1739825. [CrossRef]

130. Luo, D.; Mah, N.; Krantz, M.; Wilde, K.; Wishart, D.; Zhang, Y.; Jacobs, F.; Martin, L. Vl-linker-Vh orientation-dependent expression of single chain Fv-containing an engineered disulfide-stabilized bond in the framework regions. *J. Biochem.* **1995**, *118*, 825–831. [CrossRef]
131. Young, N.; MacKenzie, C.; Narang, S.A.; Oomen, R.P.; Baenziger, J.E. Thermal stabilization of a single-chain Fv antibody fragment by introduction of a disulphide bond. *FEBS Lett.* **1995**, *377*, 135–139. [CrossRef]
132. Rajagopal, V.; Pastan, I.; Kreitman, R.J. A form of anti-Tac(Fv) which is both single-chain and disulfide stabilized: Comparison with its single-chain and disulfide-stabilized homologs. *Protein Eng.* **1997**, *10*, 1453–1459. [CrossRef] [PubMed]
133. Hao, H.; Jiang, Y.; Zheng, Y.-L.; Ma, R.; Yu, D.-W. Improved stability and yield of Fv targeted superantigen by introducing both linker and disulfide bond into the targeting moiety. *Biochimie* **2005**, *87*, 661–667. [CrossRef] [PubMed]
134. Sheikholvaezin, A.; Sandström, P.; Eriksson, D.; Norgren, N.; Riklund, K.; Stigbrand, T. Optimizing the Generation of Recombinant Single-Chain Antibodies Against Placental Alkaline Phosphatase. *Hybridoma* **2006**, *25*, 181–192. [CrossRef]
135. Zhao, J.; Yang, L.; Gu, Z.-N.; Chen, H.; Tian, F.; Chen, Y.Q.; Zhang, H.; Chen, W. Stabilization of the Single-Chain Fragment Variable by an Interdomain Disulfide Bond and Its Effect on Antibody Affinity. *Int. J. Mol. Sci.* **2010**, *12*, 1. [CrossRef]
136. Huang, Y.-J.; Chen, I.-C.; Yu, C.-M.; Lee, Y.-C.; Hsu, H.-J.; Ching, A.T.C.; Chang, H.-J.; Yang, A.-S. Engineering Anti-vascular Endothelial Growth Factor Single Chain Disulfide-stabilized Antibody Variable Fragments (sc-dsFv) with Phage-displayed sc-dsFv Libraries. *J. Biol. Chem.* **2010**, *285*, 7880–7891. [CrossRef]
137. Weatherill, E.E.; Cain, K.; Heywood, S.P.; Compson, J.E.; Heads, J.T.; Adams, R.; Humphreys, D.T. Towards a universal disulphide stabilised single chain Fv format: Importance of interchain disulphide bond location and vL-vH orientation. *Protein Eng. Des. Sel.* **2012**, *25*, 321–329. [CrossRef]
138. Cao, M.; Wang, C.; Chung, W.K.; Motabar, D.; Wang, J.; Christian, E.; Lin, S.; Hunter, A.; Wang, X.; Liu, D. Characterization and analysis of scFv-IgG bispecific antibody size variants. *mAbs* **2018**, *10*, 1236–1247. [CrossRef]
139. Trexler-Schmidt, M.; Sargis, S.; Chiu, J.; Sze-Khoo, S.; Mun, M.; Kao, Y.-H.; Laird, M.W. Identification and prevention of antibody disulfide bond reduction during cell culture manufacturing. *Biotechnol. Bioeng.* **2010**, *106*, 452–461. [CrossRef]
140. Koterba, K.L.; Borgschulte, T.; Laird, M.W. Thioredoxin 1 is responsible for antibody disulfide reduction in CHO cell culture. *J. Biotechnol.* **2012**, *157*, 261–267. [CrossRef]
141. Chung, W.K.; Russell, B.; Yang, Y.; Handlogten, M.; Hudak, S.; Cao, M.; Wang, J.; Robbins, D.; Ahuja, S.; Zhu, M. Effects of antibody disulfide bond reduction on purification process performance and final drug substance stability. *Biotechnol. Bioeng.* **2017**, *114*, 1264–1274. [CrossRef] [PubMed]
142. Handlogten, M.W.; Zhu, M.; Ahuja, S. Glutathione and thioredoxin systems contribute to recombinant monoclonal antibody interchain disulfide bond reduction during bioprocessing. *Biotechnol. Bioeng.* **2017**, *114*, 1469–1477. [CrossRef] [PubMed]
143. Swope, N.; Chung, W.K.; Cao, M.; Motabar, D.; Liu, D.; Ahuja, S.; Handlogten, M.W. Impact of enzymatic reduction on bivalent bispecific antibody fragmentation and loss of product purity upon reoxidation. *Biotechnol. Bioeng.* **2020**, *117*, 1063–1071. [CrossRef] [PubMed]
144. Dobson, C.L.; Devine, P.W.A.; Phillips, J.J.; Higazi, D.R.; Lloyd, C.; Popovic, B.; Arnold, J.; Buchanan, A.; Lewis, A.; Goodman, J.; et al. Engineering the surface properties of a human monoclonal antibody prevents self-association and rapid clearance in vivo. *Sci. Rep.* **2016**, *6*, 38644. [CrossRef]
145. Geoghegan, J.C.; Fleming, R.; Damschroder, M.; Bishop, S.M.; Sathish, H.A.; Esfandiary, R. Mitigation of reversible self-association and viscosity in a human IgG1 monoclonal antibody by rational, structure-guided Fv engineering. *mAbs* **2016**, *8*, 941–950. [CrossRef]
146. Chow, C.-K.; Allan, B.W.; Chai, Q.; Atwell, S.; Lu, J. Therapeutic Antibody Engineering to Improve Viscosity and Phase Separation Guided by Crystal Structure. *Mol. Pharm.* **2016**, *13*, 915–923. [CrossRef]
147. Du, Q.; Damschroder, M.M.; Pabst, T.M.; Hunter, A.K.; Wang, W.K.; Luo, H. Process optimization and protein engineering mitigated manufacturing challenges of a monoclonal antibody with liquid-liquid phase separation issue by disrupting inter-molecule electrostatic interactions. *mAbs* **2019**, *11*, 789–802. [CrossRef]
148. Raut, A.S.; Kalonia, D.S. Effect of Excipients on Liquid–Liquid Phase Separation and Aggregation in Dual Variable Domain Immunoglobulin Protein Solutions. *Mol. Pharm.* **2016**, *13*, 774–783. [CrossRef]

149. Brereton, H.M.; Taylor, S.D.; Farrall, A.; Hocking, D.; Thiel, M.A.; Tea, M.; Coster, D.J.; Williams, K.A. Influence of format on in vitro penetration of antibody fragments through porcine cornea. *Br. J. Ophthalmol* **2005**, *89*, 1205–1209. [CrossRef]
150. Tesar, D.; Luoma, J.; Wyatt, E.A.; Shi, C.; Shatz, W.; Hass, P.E.; Mathieu, M.; Yi, L.; Corn, J.E.; Maass, K.F.; et al. Protein engineering to increase the potential of a therapeutic antibody Fab for long-acting delivery to the eye. *mAbs* **2017**, *9*, 1297–1305. [CrossRef]
151. Marmor, M.F.; Martin, L.J.; Tharpe, S. Osmotically induced retinal detachment in the rabbit and primate. Electron miscoscopy of the pigment epithelium. *Investig. Ophthalmol. Vis. Sci.* **1980**, *19*, 1016–1029.
152. Rabia, L.A.; Desai, A.A.; Jhajj, H.S.; Tessier, P.M. Understanding and overcoming trade-offs between antibody affinity, specificity, stability and solubility. *Biochem. Eng. J.* **2018**, *137*, 365–374. [CrossRef] [PubMed]
153. Pindrus, M.; Shire, S.J.; Kelley, R.F.; Demeule, B.; Wong, R.; Xu, Y.; Yadav, S. Solubility Challenges in High Concentration Monoclonal Antibody Formulations: Relationship with Amino Acid Sequence and Intermolecular Interactions. *Mol. Pharm.* **2015**, *12*, 3896–3907. [CrossRef]
154. Bethea, D.; Wu, S.-J.; Luo, J.; Hyun, L.; Lacy, E.R.; Teplyakov, A.; Jacobs, S.A.; O'Neil, K.T.; Gilliland, G.L.; Feng, Y. Mechanisms of self-association of a human monoclonal antibody CNTO607. *Protein Eng. Des. Sel.* **2012**, *25*, 531–538. [CrossRef]
155. Benschop, R.J.; Chow, C.-K.; Tian, Y.; Nelson, J.; Barmettler, B.; Atwell, S.; Clawson, D.; Chai, Q.; Jones, B.E.; Fitchett, J.; et al. Development of tibulizumab, a tetravalent bispecific antibody targeting BAFF and IL-17A for the treatment of autoimmune disease. *mAbs* **2019**, *11*, 1175–1190. [CrossRef] [PubMed]
156. Liu, Y.; Caffry, I.; Wu, J.; Geng, S.B.; Jain, T.; Sun, T.; Reid, F.; Cao, Y.; Estep, P.; Yu, Y.; et al. High-throughput screening for developability during early-stage antibody discovery using self-interaction nanoparticle spectroscopy. *mAbs* **2014**, *6*, 483–492. [CrossRef]
157. Sule, S.V.; Dickinson, C.D.; Lu, J.; Chow, C.-K.; Tessier, P.M. Rapid Analysis of Antibody Self-Association in Complex Mixtures Using Immunogold Conjugates. *Mol. Pharm.* **2013**, *10*, 1322–1331. [CrossRef]
158. Estep, P.; Caffry, I.; Yu, Y.; Sun, T.; Cao, Y.; Lynaugh, H.; Jain, T.; Vásquez, M.; Tessier, P.M.; Xu, Y. An alternative assay to hydrophobic interaction chromatography for high-throughput characterization of monoclonal antibodies. *mAbs* **2015**, *7*, 553–561. [CrossRef]
159. Wu, J.; Schultz, J.S.; Weldon, C.L.; Sule, S.V.; Chai, Q.; Geng, S.B.; Dickinson, C.D.; Tessier, P.M. Discovery of highly soluble antibodies prior to purification using affinity-capture self-interaction nanoparticle spectroscopy. *Protein Eng. Des. Sel.* **2015**, *28*, 403–414. [CrossRef]
160. Kingsbury, J.S.; Saini, A.; Auclair, S.M.; Fu, L.; Lantz, M.M.; Halloran, K.T.; Calero-Rubio, C.; Schwenger, W.; Airiau, C.Y.; Zhang, J.; et al. A single molecular descriptor to predict solution behavior of therapeutic antibodies. *Sci. Adv.* **2020**, *6*, eabb0372. [CrossRef]
161. Li, L.; Kantor, A.; Warne, N. Application of a PEG precipitation method for solubility screening: A tool for developing high protein concentration formulations. *Protein Sci.* **2013**, *22*, 1118–1123. [CrossRef] [PubMed]
162. Gibson, T.J.; Mccarty, K.; McFadyen, I.J.; Cash, E.; Dalmonte, P.; Hinds, K.D.; Dinerman, A.A.; Alvarez, J.C.; Volkin, D.B. Application of a High-Throughput Screening Procedure with PEG-Induced Precipitation to Compare Relative Protein Solubility During Formulation Development with IgG1 Monoclonal Antibodies. *J. Pharm. Sci.* **2011**, *100*, 1009–1021. [CrossRef] [PubMed]
163. Yamniuk, A.P.; Ditto, N.; Patel, M.; Dai, J.; Sejwal, P.; Stetsko, P.; Doyle, M.L. Application of a Kosmotrope-Based Solubility Assay to Multiple Protein Therapeutic Classes Indicates Broad Use as a High-Throughput Screen for Protein Therapeutic Aggregation Propensity. *J. Pharm. Sci.* **2013**, *102*, 2424–2439. [CrossRef]
164. Chai, Q.; Shih, J.; Weldon, C.; Phan, S.; Jones, B.E. Development of a high-throughput solubility screening assay for use in antibody discovery. *mAbs* **2019**, *11*, 747–756. [CrossRef] [PubMed]
165. Hofmann, M.; Winzer, M.; Weber, C.; Gieseler, H. Limitations of polyethylene glycol-induced precipitation as predictive tool for protein solubility during formulation development. *J. Pharm. Pharmacol.* **2017**, *70*, 648–654. [CrossRef]
166. Izadi, S.; Patapoff, T.W.; Walters, B.T. Multiscale Coarse-Grained Approach to Investigate Self-Association of Antibodies. *Biophys. J.* **2020**, *118*, 2741–2754. [CrossRef]
167. Sharma, V.K.; Patapoff, T.W.; Kabakoff, B.; Pai, S.; Hilario, E.; Zhang, B.; Li, C.; Borisov, O.; Kelley, R.F.; Chorny, I.; et al. In silico selection of therapeutic antibodies for development: Viscosity, clearance, and chemical stability. *Proc. Natl. Acad. Sci. USA* **2014**, *111*, 18601–18606. [CrossRef]

168. Tomar, D.S.; Li, L.; Broulidakis, M.P.; Luksha, N.G.; Burns, C.T.; Singh, S.K.; Kumar, S. In-silico prediction of concentration-dependent viscosity curves for monoclonal antibody solutions. *mAbs* **2017**, *9*, 476–489. [CrossRef]
169. Calero-Rubio, C.; Saluja, A.; Roberts, C.J. Coarse-Grained Antibody Models for "Weak" Protein–Protein Interactions from Low to High Concentrations. *J. Phys. Chem. B* **2016**, *120*, 6592–6605. [CrossRef]
170. Ferreira, G.M.; Calero-Rubio, C.; Sathish, H.A.; Remmele, R.L.; Roberts, C.J.; Hasige, S. Electrostatically Mediated Protein-Protein Interactions for Monoclonal Antibodies: A Combined Experimental and Coarse-Grained Molecular Modeling Approach. *J. Pharm. Sci.* **2019**, *108*, 120–132. [CrossRef]
171. Wang, G.; Varga, Z.; Hofmann, J.; Zarraga, I.E.; Swan, J.W. Structure and Relaxation in Solutions of Monoclonal Antibodies. *J. Phys. Chem. B* **2018**, *122*, 2867–2880. [CrossRef] [PubMed]
172. Kastelic, M.; Dill, K.A.; Kalyuzhnyi, Y.V.; Vlachy, V. Controlling the viscosities of antibody solutions through control of their binding sites. *J. Mol. Liq.* **2018**, *270*, 234–242. [CrossRef] [PubMed]
173. Tu, C.; Terraube, V.; Tam, A.S.P.; Stochaj, W.; Fennell, B.J.; Lin, L.; Stahl, M.; LaVallie, E.R.; Somers, W.; Finlay, W.J.J.; et al. A Combination of Structural and Empirical Analyses Delineates the Key Contacts Mediating Stability and Affinity Increases in an Optimized Biotherapeutic Single-chain Fv (scFv). *J. Biol. Chem.* **2016**, *291*, 1267–1276. [CrossRef] [PubMed]
174. Tilegenova, C.; Izadi, S.; Yin, J.; Huang, C.S.; Wu, J.; Ellerman, D.; Hymowitz, S.G.; Walters, B.T.; Salisbury, C.; Carter, P.J. Dissecting the molecular basis of high viscosity of monospecific and bispecific IgG antibodies. *mAbs* **2020**, *12*, 1692764. [CrossRef] [PubMed]
175. Li, L.; Kumar, S.; Buck, P.M.; Burns, C.; Lavoie, J.; Singh, S.K.; Warne, N.W.; Nichols, P.; Luksha, N.; Boardman, D. Concentration Dependent Viscosity of Monoclonal Antibody Solutions: Explaining Experimental Behavior in Terms of Molecular Properties. *Pharm. Res.* **2014**, *31*, 3161–3178. [CrossRef]
176. Yadav, S.; Laue, T.M.; Kalonia, D.S.; Singh, S.N.; Shire, S.J. The Influence of Charge Distribution on Self-Association and Viscosity Behavior of Monoclonal Antibody Solutions. *Mol. Pharm.* **2012**, *9*, 791–802. [CrossRef]
177. Buck, P.M.; Chaudhri, A.; Kumar, S.; Singh, S.K. Highly Viscous Antibody Solutions Are a Consequence of Network Formation Caused by Domain–Domain Electrostatic Complementarities: Insights from Coarse-Grained Simulations. *Mol. Pharm.* **2015**, *12*, 127–139. [CrossRef]
178. Nichols, P.; Li, L.; Kumar, S.; Buck, P.M.; Singh, S.K.; Goswami, S.; Balthazor, B.; Conley, T.R.; Sek, D.; Allen, M.J. Rational design of viscosity reducing mutants of a monoclonal antibody: Hydrophobic versus electrostatic inter-molecular interactions. *mAbs* **2015**, *7*, 212–230. [CrossRef]
179. Kumar, S.; Roffi, K.; Tomar, D.S.; Cirelli, D.; Luksha, N.; Meyer, D.; Mitchell, J.; Allen, M.J.; Li, L. Rational optimization of a monoclonal antibody for simultaneous improvements in its solution properties and biological activity. *Protein Eng. Des. Sel.* **2018**, *31*, 313–325. [CrossRef]
180. Raut, A.S.; Kalonia, D.S. Viscosity Analysis of Dual Variable Domain Immunoglobulin Protein Solutions: Role of Size, Electroviscous Effect and Protein-Protein Interactions. *Pharm. Res.* **2016**, *33*, 155–166. [CrossRef]
181. Woldeyes, M.A.; Josephson, L.L.; Leiske, D.L.; Galush, W.J.; Roberts, C.J.; Furst, E.M. Viscosities and Protein Interactions of Bispecific Antibodies and Their Monospecific Mixtures. *Mol. Pharm.* **2018**, *15*, 4745–4755. [CrossRef]
182. Gallivan, J.P.; Dougherty, D.A. A Computational Study of Cation−π Interactions vs. Salt Bridges in Aqueous Media: Implications for Protein Engineering. *J. Am. Chem. Soc.* **2000**, *122*, 870–874. [CrossRef]
183. Apgar, J.; Tam, A.S.P.; Sorm, R.; Moesta, S.; King, A.C.; Yang, H.; Kelleher, K.; Murphy, D.; D'Antona, A.M.; Yan, G.; et al. Modeling and mitigation of high-concentration antibody viscosity through structure-based computer-aided protein design. *PLoS ONE* **2020**, *15*, e0232713. [CrossRef] [PubMed]
184. Agrawal, N.J.; Helk, B.; Kumar, S.; Mody, N.; Sathish, H.A.; Samra, H.S.; Buck, P.M.; Li, L.; Trout, B.L. Computational tool for the early screening of monoclonal antibodies for their viscosities. *mAbs* **2016**, *8*, 43–48. [CrossRef]
185. Liu, J.; Nguyen, M.D.; Andya, J.D.; Shire, S.J. Reversible Self-Association Increases the Viscosity of a Concentrated Monoclonal Antibody in Aqueous Solution. *J. Pharm. Sci.* **2005**, *94*, 1928–1940. [CrossRef] [PubMed]
186. Du, W.; Klibanov, A.M. Hydrophobic salts markedly diminish viscosity of concentrated protein solutions. *Biotechnol. Bioeng.* **2011**, *108*, 632–636. [CrossRef]

187. Kanai, S.; Liu, J.; Patapoff, T.W.; Shire, S.J. Reversible Self-Association of a Concentrated Monoclonal Antibody Solution Mediated by Fab–Fab Interaction That Impacts Solution Viscosity. *J. Pharm. Sci.* **2008**, *97*, 4219–4227. [CrossRef]
188. Inoue, N.; Takai, E.; Arakawa, T.; Shiraki, K. Specific Decrease in Solution Viscosity of Antibodies by Arginine for Therapeutic Formulations. *Mol. Pharm.* **2014**, *11*, 1889–1896. [CrossRef]
189. Ashish; Solanki, A.K.; Boone, C.D.; Krueger, J.K. Global structure of HIV-1 neutralizing antibody IgG1 b12 is asymmetric. *Biochem. Biophys. Res. Commun.* **2010**, *391*, 947–951. [CrossRef]
190. Starr, C.G.; Tessier, P.M. Selecting and engineering monoclonal antibodies with drug-like specificity. *Curr. Opin. Biotechnol.* **2019**, *60*, 119–127. [CrossRef]
191. Jacobs, S.A.; Wu, S.-J.; Feng, Y.; Bethea, D.; O'Neil, K.T. Cross-Interaction Chromatography: A Rapid Method to Identify Highly Soluble Monoclonal Antibody Candidates. *Pharm. Res.* **2010**, *27*, 65–71. [CrossRef] [PubMed]
192. Hötzel, I.; Theil, F.-P.; Bernstein, L.J.; Prabhu, S.; Deng, R.; Quintana, L.; Lutman, J.; Sibia, R.; Chan, P.; Bumbaca, D.; et al. A strategy for risk mitigation of antibodies with fast clearance. *mAbs* **2012**, *4*, 753–760. [CrossRef] [PubMed]
193. Mouquet, H.; Scheid, J.F.; Zoller, M.J.; Krogsgaard, M.; Ott, R.G.; Shukair, S.; Artyomov, M.N.; Pietzsch, J.; Connors, M.; Pereyra, F.; et al. Polyreactivity increases the apparent affinity of anti-HIV antibodies by heteroligation. *Nat. Cell Biol.* **2010**, *467*, 591–595. [CrossRef] [PubMed]
194. Xu, Y.; Roach, W.; Sun, T.; Jain, T.; Prinz, B.; Yu, T.-Y.; Torrey, J.; Thomas, J.; Bobrowicz, P.; Vásquez, M.; et al. Addressing polyspecificity of antibodies selected from an in vitro yeast presentation system: A FACS-based, high-throughput selection and analytical tool. *Protein Eng. Des. Sel.* **2013**, *26*, 663–670. [CrossRef] [PubMed]
195. Kelly, R.L.; Sun, T.; Jain, T.; Caffry, I.; Yu, Y.; Cao, Y.; Lynaugh, H.; Brown, M.; Vásquez, M.; Wittrup, K.D.; et al. High throughput cross-interaction measures for human IgG1 antibodies correlate with clearance rates in mice. *mAbs* **2015**, *7*, 770–777. [CrossRef]
196. Kelly, R.L.; Geoghegan, J.C.; Feldman, J.; Jain, T.; Kauke, M.; Le, D.; Zhao, J.; Wittrup, K.D. Chaperone proteins as single component reagents to assess antibody nonspecificity. *mAbs* **2017**, *9*, 1036–1040. [CrossRef] [PubMed]
197. Kelly, R.L.; Le, D.; Zhao, J.; Wittrup, K. Reduction of Nonspecificity Motifs in Synthetic Antibody Libraries. *J. Mol. Biol.* **2018**, *430*, 119–130. [CrossRef] [PubMed]
198. Kelly, R.L.; Zhao, J.; Le, D.; Wittrup, K.D. Nonspecificity in a nonimmune human scFv repertoire. *mAbs* **2017**, *9*, 1029–1035. [CrossRef] [PubMed]
199. Avery, L.B.; Wade, J.; Wang, M.; Tam, A.; King, A.; Piche-Nicholas, N.; Kavosi, M.S.; Penn, S.; Cirelli, D.; Kurz, J.C.; et al. Establishing in vitro in vivo correlations to screen monoclonal antibodies for physicochemical properties related to favorable human pharmacokinetics. *mAbs* **2018**, *10*, 244–255. [CrossRef]
200. Frese, K.; Eisenmann, M.; Ostendorp, R.; Brocks, B.; Pabst, S. An automated immunoassay for early specificity profiling of antibodies. *mAbs* **2013**, *5*, 279–287. [CrossRef]
201. Li, B.; Tesar, D.; Boswell, C.A.; Cahaya, H.S.; Wong, A.; Zhang, J.; Meng, Y.G.; Eigenbrot, C.; Pantua, H.; Diao, J.; et al. Framework selection can influence pharmacokinetics of a humanized therapeutic antibody through differences in molecule charge. *mAbs* **2014**, *6*, 1255–1264. [CrossRef] [PubMed]
202. Dostalek, M.; Prueksaritanont, T.; Kelley, R.F. Pharmacokinetic de-risking tools for selection of monoclonal antibody lead candidates. *mAbs* **2017**, *9*, 756–766. [CrossRef] [PubMed]
203. Kraft, T.E.; Richter, W.F.; Emrich, T.; Knaupp, A.; Schuster, M.; Wolfert, A.; Kettenberger, H. Heparin chromatography as an in vitro predictor for antibody clearance rate through pinocytosis. *mAbs* **2019**, *12*, 1683432. [CrossRef] [PubMed]
204. Schoch, A.; Kettenberger, H.; Mundigl, O.; Winter, G.; Engert, J.; Heinrich, J.; Emrich, T. Charge-mediated influence of the antibody variable domain on FcRn-dependent pharmacokinetics. *Proc. Natl. Acad. Sci. USA* **2015**, *112*, 5997–6002. [CrossRef] [PubMed]
205. Crowell, S.; Wang, K.; Famili, A.; Shatz, W.; Loyet, K.M.; Chang, V.; Liu, Y.; Prabhu, S.; Kamath, A.V.; Kelley, R.F. Influence of Charge, Hydrophobicity, and Size on Vitreous Pharmacokinetics of Large Molecules. *Transl. Vis. Sci. Technol.* **2019**, *8*, 1. [CrossRef]

206. Schaller, T.H.; Foster, M.W.; Thompson, W.; Spasojevic, I.; Normantaite, D.; Moseley, M.A.; Sanchez-Perez, L.; Sampson, J.H. Pharmacokinetic Analysis of a Novel Human EGFRvIII:CD3 Bispecific Antibody in Plasma and Whole Blood Using a High-Resolution Targeted Mass Spectrometry Approach. *J. Proteome Res.* **2019**, *18*, 3032–3041. [CrossRef]
207. Birtalan, S.; Zhang, Y.; Fellouse, F.A.; Shao, L.; Schaefer, G.; Sidhu, S.S. The Intrinsic Contributions of Tyrosine, Serine, Glycine and Arginine to the Affinity and Specificity of Antibodies. *J. Mol. Biol.* **2008**, *377*, 1518–1528. [CrossRef]
208. Birtalan, S.; Fisher, R.D.; Sidhu, S.S. The functional capacity of the natural amino acids for molecular recognition. *Mol. BioSyst.* **2010**, *6*, 1186. [CrossRef]
209. Tiller, K.E.; Li, L.-J.; Kumar, S.; Julian, M.C.; Garde, S.; Tessier, P.M. Arginine mutations in antibody complementarity-determining regions display context-dependent affinity/specificity trade-offs. *J. Biol. Chem.* **2017**, *292*, 16638–16652. [CrossRef]
210. Wardemann, H.; Yurasov, S.; Schaefer, A.; Young, J.W.; Meffre, E.; Nussenzweig, M.C. Predominant Autoantibody Production by Early Human B Cell Precursors. *Science* **2003**, *301*, 1374–1377. [CrossRef]
211. Datta-Mannan, A.; Thangaraju, A.; Leung, D.; Tang, Y.; Witcher, D.R.; Lu, J.; Wroblewski, V.J. Balancing charge in the complementarity-determining regions of humanized mAbs without affecting pI reduces non-specific binding and improves the pharmacokinetics. *mAbs* **2015**, *7*, 483–493. [CrossRef]
212. Rabia, L.A.; Zhang, Y.; Ludwig, S.D.; Julian, M.C.; Tessier, P.M. Net charge of antibody complementarity-determining regions is a key predictor of specificity. *Protein Eng. Des. Sel.* **2018**, *31*, 409–418. [CrossRef]
213. Zhang, Y.; Wu, L.; Gupta, P.; Desai, A.A.; Smith, M.D.; Rabia, L.A.; Ludwig, S.D.; Tessier, P.M. Physicochemical Rules for Identifying Monoclonal Antibodies with Drug-like Specificity. *Mol. Pharm.* **2020**, *17*, 2555–2569. [CrossRef]
214. Ovacik, M.; Lin, K. Tutorial on Monoclonal Antibody Pharmacokinetics and Its Considerations in Early Development. *Clin. Transl. Sci.* **2018**, *11*, 540–552. [CrossRef]
215. Paci, A.; Desnoyer, A.; Delahousse, J.; Blondel, L.; Maritaz, C.; Chaput, N.; Mir, O.; Broutin, S. Pharmacokinetic/pharmacodynamic relationship of therapeutic monoclonal antibodies used in oncology: Part 1, monoclonal antibodies, antibody-drug conjugates and bispecific T-cell engagers. *Eur. J. Cancer* **2020**, *128*, 107–118. [CrossRef] [PubMed]
216. Datta-Mannan, A.; Croy, J.E.; Schirtzinger, L.; Torgerson, S.; Breyer, M.; Wroblewski, V.J. Aberrant bispecific antibody pharmacokinetics linked to liver sinusoidal endothelium clearance mechanism in cynomolgus monkeys. *mAbs* **2016**, *8*, 969–982. [CrossRef] [PubMed]
217. Yazaki, P.; Lee, B.; Channappa, D.; Cheung, C.-W.; Crow, D.; Chea, J.; Poku, E.; Li, L.; Andersen, J.T.; Sandlie, I.; et al. A series of anti-CEA/anti-DOTA bispecific antibody formats evaluated for pre-targeting: Comparison of tumor uptake and blood clearance. *Protein Eng. Des. Sel.* **2012**, *26*, 187–193. [CrossRef] [PubMed]
218. Rossi, E.A.; Chang, C.-H.; Cardillo, T.M.; Goldenberg, D.M. Optimization of Multivalent Bispecific Antibodies and Immunocytokines with Improved in Vivo Properties. *Bioconjug. Chem.* **2012**, *24*, 63–71. [CrossRef]
219. Datta-Mannan, A.; Brown, R.M.; Fitchett, J.; Heng, A.R.; Balasubramaniam, D.; Pereira, J.; Croy, J.E. Modulation of the Biophysical Properties of Bifunctional Antibodies as a Strategy for Mitigating Poor Pharmacokinetics. *Biochemistry* **2019**, *58*, 3116–3132. [CrossRef]
220. Ghosh, J.G.; Nguyen, A.A.; Bigelow, C.E.; Poor, S.; Qiu, Y.; Rangaswamy, N.; Ornberg, R.; Jackson, B.; Mak, H.; Ezell, T.; et al. Long-acting protein drugs for the treatment of ocular diseases. *Nat. Commun.* **2017**, *8*, 14837. [CrossRef]
221. Sleep, D.; Cameron, J.; Evans, L.R. Albumin as a versatile platform for drug half-life extension. *Biochim. Biophys. Acta* **2013**, *1830*, 5526–5534. [CrossRef] [PubMed]
222. Malm, M.; Bass, T.; Gudmundsdotter, L.; Lord, M.; Frejd, F.; Ståhl, S.; Lofblom, J. Engineering of a bispecific affibody molecule towards HER2 and HER3 by addition of an albumin-binding domain allows for affinity purification and in vivo half-life extension. *Biotechnol. J.* **2014**, *9*, 1215–1222. [CrossRef]
223. Nilvebrant, J.; Åstrand, M.; Georgieva-Kotseva, M.; Björnmalm, M.; Lofblom, J.; Hober, S. Engineering of Bispecific Affinity Proteins with High Affinity for ERBB2 and Adaptable Binding to Albumin. *PLoS ONE* **2014**, *9*, e103094. [CrossRef] [PubMed]

224. Nilvebrant, J.; Alm, T.; Hober, S.; Lofblom, J. Engineering Bispecificity into a Single Albumin-Binding Domain. *PLoS ONE* **2011**, *6*, e25791. [CrossRef]
225. Davé, E.; Adams, R.; Zaccheo, O.; Carrington, B.; Compson, J.E.; Dugdale, S.; Airey, M.; Malcolm, S.; Hailu, H.; Wild, G.; et al. Fab-dsFv: A bispecific antibody format with extended serum half-life through albumin binding. *mAbs* **2016**, *8*, 1319–1335. [CrossRef]
226. Day, S.; Acquah, K.; Mruthyunjaya, P.; Grossman, D.S.; Lee, P.P.; Sloan, F.A. Ocular Complications After Anti–Vascular Endothelial Growth Factor Therapy in Medicare Patients with Age-Related Macular Degeneration. *Am. J. Ophthalmol.* **2011**, *152*, 266–272. [CrossRef] [PubMed]
227. Fernández, L.; Bustos, R.-H.; Zapata, C.; Garcia, J.; Jauregui, E.; Ashraf, G.M.; Rodríguez, R.H.B.L.F. Immunogenicity in Protein and Peptide Based-Therapeutics: An Overview. *Curr. Protein Pept. Sci.* **2018**, *19*, 958–971. [CrossRef]
228. Sauna, Z.E.; Lagassé, D.; Pedras-Vasconcelos, J.; Golding, B.; Rosenberg, A. Evaluating and Mitigating the Immunogenicity of Therapeutic Proteins. *Trends Biotechnol.* **2018**, *36*, 1068–1084. [CrossRef]
229. Yuseff, M.-I.; Pierobon, P.; Reversat, A.; Lennon-Duménil, A.-M. How B cells capture, process and present antigens: A crucial role for cell polarity. *Nat. Rev. Immunol.* **2013**, *13*, 475–486. [CrossRef]
230. Germain, R.N.; Margulies, D.H. The biochemistry and cell biology of antigen processing and presentation. *Annu. Rev. Immunol.* **1993**, *11*, 403–450. [CrossRef]
231. Paul, S.; Grifoni, A.; Peters, B.; Sette, A. Major Histocompatibility Complex Binding, Eluted Ligands, and Immunogenicity: Benchmark Testing and Predictions. *Front. Immunol.* **2020**, *10*, 3151. [CrossRef] [PubMed]
232. Rosenberg, A.; Sauna, Z.E. Immunogenicity assessment during the development of protein therapeutics. *J. Pharm. Pharmacol.* **2017**, *70*, 584–594. [CrossRef] [PubMed]
233. Gunn, G.R.; Sealey, D.C.F.; Jamali, F.; Meibohm, B.; Ghosh, S.; Shankar, G. From the bench to clinical practice: Understanding the challenges and uncertainties in immunogenicity testing for biopharmaceuticals. *Clin. Exp. Immunol.* **2016**, *184*, 137–146. [CrossRef] [PubMed]
234. FDA. Immunogenicity Testing of Therapeutic Protein Products—Developing and Validating Assays for Anti-Drug Antibody Detection. 2019. Available online: https://www.fda.gov/media/119788/download (accessed on 29 August 2020).
235. Shankar, G.; Arkin, S.; Cocea, L.; Devanarayan, V.; Kirshner, S.; Kromminga, A.; Quarmby, V.; Richards, S.; Schneider, C.K.; Subramanyam, M.; et al. Assessment and Reporting of the Clinical Immunogenicity of Therapeutic Proteins and Peptides—Harmonized Terminology and Tactical Recommendations. *AAPS J.* **2014**, *16*, 658–673. [CrossRef]
236. Salazar-Fontana, L.I.; Desai, D.D.; Khan, T.A.; Pillutla, R.C.; Prior, S.; Ramakrishnan, R.; Schneider, J.; Joseph, A. Approaches to Mitigate the Unwanted Immunogenicity of Therapeutic Proteins during Drug Development. *AAPS J.* **2017**, *19*, 377–385. [CrossRef] [PubMed]
237. Tourdot, S.; Hickling, T.P. Nonclinical immunogenicity risk assessment of therapeutic proteins. *Bioanalysis* **2019**, *11*, 1631–1643. [CrossRef]
238. Baumann, A.; Fischmann, S.; Blaich, G.; Friedrich, M. Leverage nonclinical development of bispecifics by translational science. *Drug Discov. Today Technol.* **2016**, *21–22*, 95–102. [CrossRef]
239. Gorovits, B.; Peng, K.; Kromminga, A. Current Considerations on Characterization of Immune Response to Multi-Domain Biotherapeutics. *BioDrugs* **2019**, *34*, 39–54. [CrossRef]
240. Harmsen, M.M.; De Haard, H.J. Properties, production, and applications of camelid single-domain antibody fragments. *Appl. Microbiol. Biotechnol.* **2007**, *77*, 13–22. [CrossRef]
241. Hao, C.-H.; Han, Q.-H.; Shan, Z.-J.; Hu, J.-T.; Zhang, N.; Zhang, X.-P. Effects of different interchain linkers on biological activity of an anti-prostate cancer single-chain bispecific antibody. *Theor. Biol. Med. Model.* **2015**, *12*, 14. [CrossRef]
242. Kibria, G.; Akazawa-Ogawa, Y.; Rahman, N.; Hagihara, Y.; Kuroda, Y. The immunogenicity of an anti-EGFR single domain antibody (VHH) is enhanced by misfolded amorphous aggregation but not by heat-induced aggregation. *Eur. J. Pharm. Biopharm.* **2020**, *152*, 164–174. [CrossRef]
243. Rahman, N.; Islam, M.M.; Unzai, S.; Miura, S.; Kuroda, Y. Nanometer-Sized Aggregates Generated Using Short Solubility Controlling Peptide Tags Do Increase the In Vivo Immunogenicity of a Nonimmunogenic Protein. *Mol. Pharm.* **2020**, *17*, 1629–1637. [CrossRef] [PubMed]

244. Rosenberg, A. Effects of protein aggregates: An immunologic perspective. *AAPS J.* **2006**, *8*, E501–E507. [CrossRef] [PubMed]
245. Broders, O.; Wessels, U.; Zadak, M.; Beckmann, R.; Stubenrauch, K. Novel bioanalytical method for the characterization of the immune response directed against a bispecific F(ab) fragment. *Bioanalysis* **2020**, *12*, 509–517. [CrossRef]
246. Bivi, N.; Moore, T.; Rodgers, G.; Denning, H.; Shockley, T.; Swearingen, C.A.; Gelfanova, V.; Calderon, B.; Peterson, D.A.; Hodsdon, M.E.; et al. Investigation of pre-existing reactivity to biotherapeutics can uncover potential immunogenic epitopes and predict immunogenicity risk. *mAbs* **2019**, *11*, 861–869. [CrossRef] [PubMed]
247. Song, S.; Yang, L.; Trepicchio, W.L.; Wyant, T. Understanding the Supersensitive Anti-Drug Antibody Assay: Unexpected High Anti-Drug Antibody Incidence and Its Clinical Relevance. *J. Immunol. Res.* **2016**, *2016*, 1–8. [CrossRef]
248. Quarmby, V.; Phung, Q.; Lill, J.R. MAPPs for the identification of immunogenic hotspots of biotherapeutics; an overview of the technology and its application to the biopharmaceutical arena. *Expert Rev. Proteom.* **2018**, *15*, 733–748. [CrossRef]
249. Karle, A.C. Applying MAPPs Assays to Assess Drug Immunogenicity. *Front. Immunol.* **2020**, *11*, 698. [CrossRef]
250. Wu, Y.; Li, C.; Xia, S.; Tian, X.; Kong, Y.; Wang, Z.; Gu, C.; Zhang, R.; Tu, C.; Xie, Y.; et al. Identification of Human Single-Domain Antibodies against SARS-CoV-2. *Cell Host Microbe* **2020**, *27*, 891–898.e5. [CrossRef]
251. Waldmann, H. Human Monoclonal Antibodies: The Benefits of Humanization. *Methods Mol. Biol.* **2019**, *1904*, 1–10.
252. Almagro, J.C.; Fransson, J. Humanization of antibodies. *Front. Biosci.* **2008**, *13*, 1619–1633. [PubMed]
253. Safdari, Y.; Farajnia, S.; Asgharzadeh, M.; Khalili, M. Antibody humanization methods—A review and update. *Biotechnol. Genet. Eng. Rev.* **2013**, *29*, 175–186. [CrossRef] [PubMed]
254. Wollacott, A.M.; Xue, C.; Qin, Q.; Hua, J.; Bohnuud, T.; Viswanathan, K.; Kolachalama, V.B. Quantifying the nativeness of antibody sequences using long short-term memory networks. *Protein Eng. Des. Sel.* **2019**, *32*, 347–354. [CrossRef]
255. Schmitz, S.; Soto, C.; Crowe, J.E.; Meiler, J.; Crowe, J.E. Human-likeness of antibody biologics determined by back-translation and comparison with large antibody variable gene repertoires. *mAbs* **2020**, *12*, 1758291. [CrossRef] [PubMed]
256. Peters, B.; Nielsen, M.; Sette, A. T Cell Epitope Predictions. *Annu. Rev. Immunol.* **2020**, *38*, 123–145. [CrossRef]
257. Reynisson, B.; Barra, C.; Kaabinejadian, S.; Hildebrand, W.H.; Peters, B.; Nielsen, M. Improved Prediction of MHC II Antigen Presentation through Integration and Motif Deconvolution of Mass Spectrometry MHC Eluted Ligand Data. *J. Proteome Res.* **2020**, *19*, 2304–2315. [CrossRef]
258. Garde, C.; Ramarathinam, S.H.; Jappe, E.C.; Nielsen, M.; Kringelum, J.V.; Trolle, T.; Purcell, A.W. Improved peptide-MHC class II interaction prediction through integration of eluted ligand and peptide affinity data. *Immunogenetics* **2019**, *71*, 445–454. [CrossRef]
259. Sekiguchi, N.; Kubo, C.; Takahashi, A.; Muraoka, K.; Takeiri, A.; Ito, S.; Yano, M.; Mimoto, F.; Maeda, A.; Iwayanagi, Y.; et al. MHC-associated peptide proteomics enabling highly sensitive detection of immunogenic sequences for the development of therapeutic antibodies with low immunogenicity. *mAbs* **2018**, *10*, 1168–1181. [CrossRef]
260. Barra, C.; Ackaert, C.; Reynisson, B.; Schockaert, J.; Jessen, L.E.; Watson, M.; Jang, A.; Comtois-Marotte, S.; Goulet, J.-P.; Pattijn, S.; et al. Immunopeptidomic Data Integration to Artificial Neural Networks Enhances Protein-Drug Immunogenicity Prediction. *Front. Immunol.* **2020**, *11*, 1304. [CrossRef]

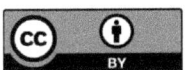

© 2020 by the authors. Licensee MDPI, Basel, Switzerland. This article is an open access article distributed under the terms and conditions of the Creative Commons Attribution (CC BY) license (http://creativecommons.org/licenses/by/4.0/).

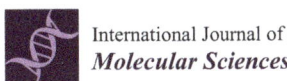

Review

Modular Chimeric Antigen Receptor Systems for Universal CAR T Cell Retargeting

Ashley R. Sutherland [1], Madeline N. Owens [1] and C. Ronald Geyer [2,*]

[1] Department of Biochemistry, Microbiology and Immunology, University of Saskatchewan, Saskatoon, SK S7N 5E5, Canada; ashley.sutherland@usask.ca (A.R.S.); mno167@usask.ca (M.N.O.)
[2] Department of Pathology and Laboratory Medicine, University of Saskatchewan, Saskatoon, SK S7N 5E5, Canada
* Correspondence: ron.geyer@usask.ca

Received: 4 September 2020; Accepted: 29 September 2020; Published: 30 September 2020

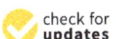

Abstract: The engineering of T cells through expression of chimeric antigen receptors (CARs) against tumor-associated antigens (TAAs) has shown significant potential for use as an anti-cancer therapeutic. The development of strategies for flexible and modular CAR T systems is accelerating, allowing for multiple antigen targeting, precise programming, and adaptable solutions in the field of cellular immunotherapy. Moving beyond the fixed antigen specificity of traditional CAR T systems, the modular CAR T technology splits the T cell signaling domains and the targeting elements through use of a switch molecule. The activity of CAR T cells depends on the presence of the switch, offering dose-titratable response and precise control over CAR T cells. In this review, we summarize developments in universal or modular CAR T strategies that expand on current CAR T systems and open the door for more customizable T cell activity.

Keywords: chimeric antigen receptor (CAR T); universal CAR T; modular CAR T; universal immune receptor; CAR adaptor; adoptive immunotherapy; antibody; split CAR

1. Introduction

Engineering T cells to express chimeric antigen receptors (CARs) has shown wide-ranging potential as a potent anti-cancer therapeutic. Characteristically, CARs consist of an extracellular antigen-binding single-chain antibody variable fragment (scFv) and hinge region linked to transmembrane and intracellular signaling regions. This engineered construct fuses the specificity of an antibody to T cell-effector functions, allowing for target cell lysis, release of cytokines, and T cell proliferation [1,2]. In clinical trials, CAR T cell therapy has shown remarkable success in treating hematological malignancies by targeting B cell antigen CD19. Numerous studies showed high remission rates, rapid tumor eradication, and durable responses in patients with refractory disease, raising expectations for expanding the types of cancers that can be treated with CAR therapy [3–5]. Although these results are encouraging, several challenges exist that inhibit the broad application of this treatment. Firstly, tumor heterogeneity is a complication that hinders CAR T development. Conventional CAR T cells have a fixed, single-antigen targeting ability, making the therapy vulnerable to antigen-loss relapse due to downregulation or antigen deletion [6,7]. CAR T therapy targeting a single antigen may initially demonstrate tumor regression; however, many cases have been reported in clinical trials of antigen-negative relapse after CD19 CAR T therapy due to tumor antigen escape [8,9]. Engineering of CAR T cells against a variety of tumor-associated antigens (TAAs) is a method to overcome tumor immunoediting, yet this approach comes with its own set of challenges. Further clinical success of CARs would necessitate the engineering of T cells tailored for each patient targeting various TAAs. However, significant technical requirements and financial costs involved in the generation and optimization of CARs directed at individual antigens limit this approach's usefulness. To circumvent the technical and economic challenges of individually manufacturing and testing each new CAR, creating a platform using 'universal' redirected T cells against virtually any cell surface antigen is of particular importance for the rapid screening in pre-clinical models and the broad application of CAR T therapy.

The ability to generate modular or universal CARs hinges on the separation of targeting and signaling elements. Modular CAR T cells are not targeted at the tumor antigen itself; instead, the CAR is directed at an adaptor or switch element (Figure 1). This adaptor serves as the targeting element, binding to the tumor antigen, and is required to bridge the immunological synapse. The firing of the CAR T should occur only in the presence of the switch, and swapping out the adaptor molecule allows for redirection of the T cell without the need for re-engineering and time-consuming remanufacturing. This modular treatment approach offers the possibility for flexibility in tumor targeting in the clinic; adapting with the patient's tumor by adjusting treatment based on the cancer's changing antigen expression could be envisioned. Fixed antigen targeting often hinders cancer treatment, with this modular CAR T approach driving an already innovative biological therapy into truly tailored cancer therapy.

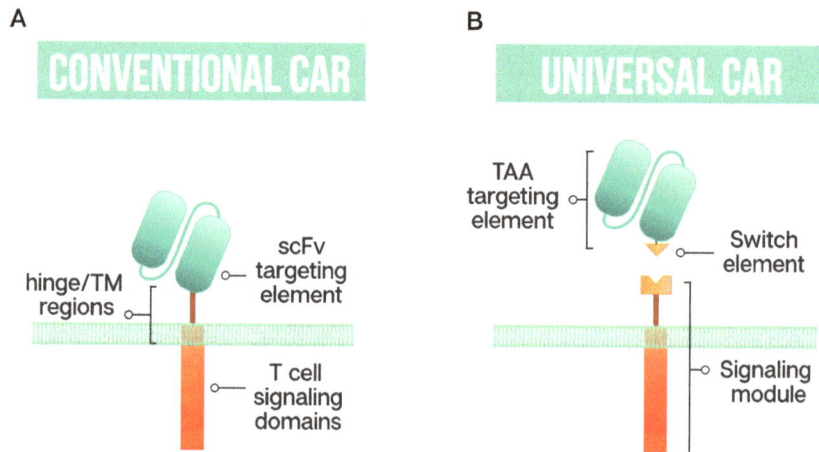

Figure 1. Schematic representation of a conventional CAR T cell and a universal or modular CAR T cell (**A**) Conventional CAR T cells have a single-chain antibody fragment (scFv) targeting element, expressed in tandem with signaling domains derived from the T cell receptor and costimulatory domains such as 4-1BB and CD28 connected through a transmembrane (TM) domain and a flexible spacer or hinge region; (**B**) a universal CAR T cell has a split design containing a tumor-associated antigen (TAA) targeting element, usually derived from a monoclonal antibody, a switch element and the signaling module, consisting of the T cell signaling domains and an extracellular region which interacts with the switch element.

In the toolkit of building modular CARs, the number of adaptors has been increasing, with components such as immunoglobulin (IgG)-based adaptors such as scFvs (single-chain variable fragment), Fabs (antigen-binding fragment), nanobodies, and full-length IgGs being the most established. Both antibody-based and targeting ligand adaptors have been redirected using tags attached either genetically or post-translationally and include peptide tags such as neo-epitopes, SpyTag, leucine zippers, biotin and fluorescein isothiocyanate (FITC). Repurposing clinically approved IgGs and adding redirecting tags could reduce the regulatory hurdles and allow for a suite of targeting elements that clinicians could employ for a wide variety of cancer indications.

Improving the safety profile of CAR T therapy is a rapidly developing area of research with the goal of expanding the therapy to treat a broader range of cancer patients. With the promise of CAR T therapy comes life-threatening side effects, including severe cytokine release syndrome

(CRS), neurological toxicities and organ failure, resulting from the unrestrained proliferation of CAR T cells [10,11]. Toxicities related to on-target off-tumor reactions can occur when low levels of the targeted cancer antigen found on normal tissue are targeted by the engineered T cells. When toxicities become severe enough, administration of high-dose corticosteroids is required, decreasing the T cell numbers [10–12]. Research in the area of 'next-generation' CAR T cells has incorporated methods such as suicide genes or switches as a means to eliminate T cells. These 'emergency stop' methods may avert a lethal outcome to the patient; however, the drawback is that the CAR T cells are eliminated, and with it any therapeutic response—a bad ending for a costly and time-consuming therapy. Universal or modular CAR T strategies that require administration of an adaptor may fit the criteria for better control of engineered T cells. The ability to titrate on adaptors could facilitate the 'turning off' of CAR T cells by halting administration of the adaptor, possibly enhancing their safety profile without the need to destroy the T cells. Additionally, this tunable response could better manage side effects as well as fine tuning of CAR T activity. These approaches for CAR T generation allow for conjugation of the tagged targeting element with the anti-tag CAR T. This enables targeting multiple TAAs and flexibility in administration of the targeting element, a step towards overcoming current clinical limitations of CAR T therapy.

In this review, we summarize emerging systems developed to overcome the limitations of CARs with fixed antigen specificity using universal CAR T strategies. This modular approach using adaptors to 'turn on' CARs enables targeting multiple TAAs with one receptor, imparting near-limitless antigen specificity and fine tuning of CAR activity.

2. Modular CAR T Platforms

2.1. Biotin-Binding Immune Receptors

Exploiting one of nature's strongest non-covalent bonds, the avidin–biotin interaction has been used to generate a universal tumor-targeting system, biotin-binding immunoreceptor (BBIR) (Figure 2A). BBIRs constructed by Urbanska et al. [13] consist of an extracellular modified dimeric avidin (dcAv) linked to an intracellular T cell signaling domain. This split design allows for easy target modification and targeting of multiple antigens. Monomeric avidin was unable to elicit an effector response, most likely due to the decreased affinity between biotin and monomeric avidin.

Tumor cells in vitro are either pre-targeted or co-administered with biotinylated antigen-targeting molecules (IgG antibodies, scFvs, or other tumor-specific ligands), and T cells expressing BBIRs bound specifically to exert effector cell functions. In vitro functioning of dcAv BBIR is comparable to traditional CAR T for cell lysis and cytokine secretion, illustrating this system's utility to target cells and perform effector functions. Significantly, BBIR cells generated a dose-dependent response with the addition of adaptors. When tested against a panel of cells with variable TAAs, BBIRs could target antigens both simultaneously or sequentially, showing the tunability of CAR response and their utility in antigen escape scenarios. Furthermore, the authors proposed a platform using BBIRs to screen candidate antibodies or other targeting elements in vitro for rapid pre-clinical screening. BBIRs performed similarly in vivo in a xenograft mouse model of human ovarian cancer. As CAR safety is essential for moving into the clinic, BBIRs were exposed to supraphysiological levels of biotin and showed no antigen-independent activation. Interestingly, T cells could not be 'pre-armed' with the biotinylated targeting element; the adaptor had to be either pre-targeted to coat the tumor surface or co-administered with BBIR T cells.

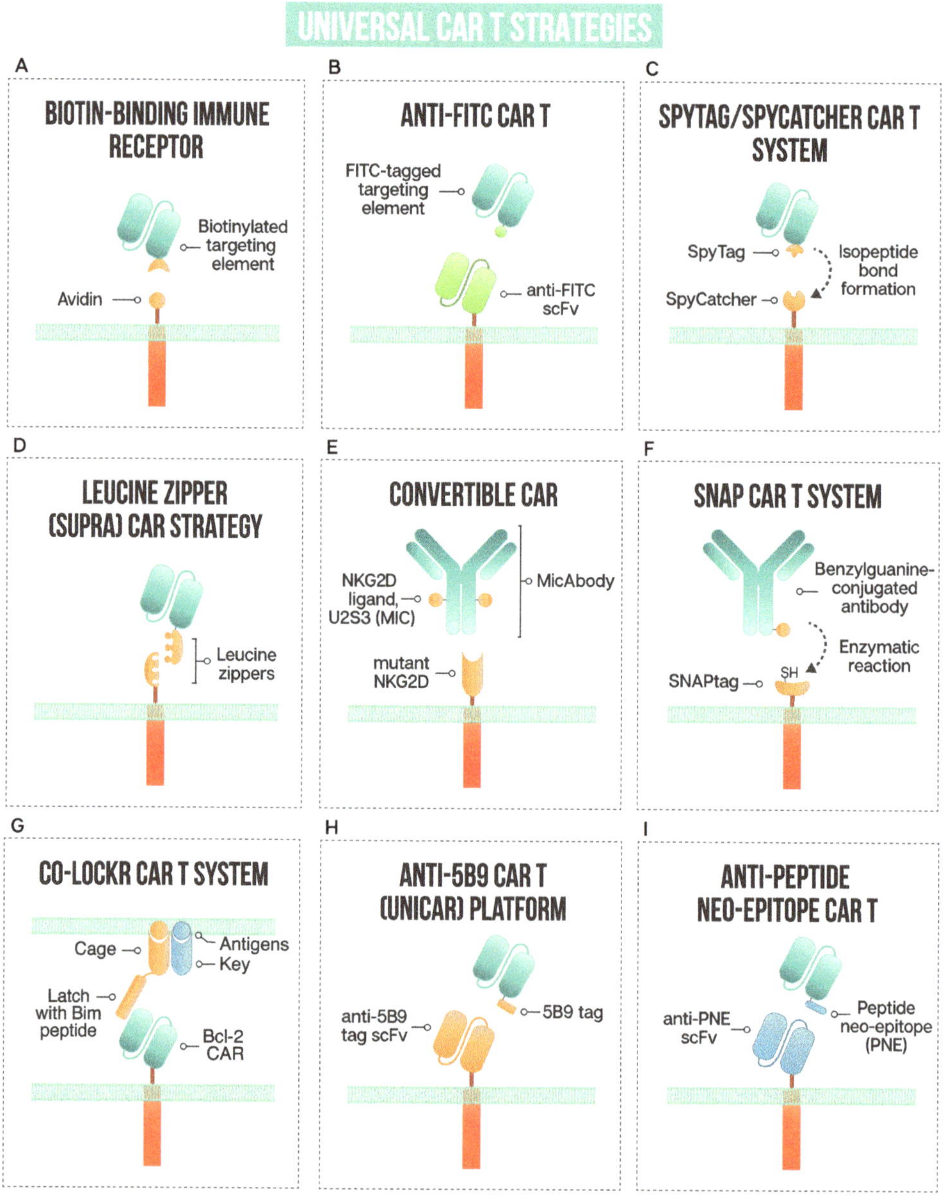

Figure 2. A schematic of strategies used in universal CAR T design: (**A**) biotin-binding immune receptor; (**B**) anti-FITC CAR T; (**C**) the SpyTag/SpyCatcher CAR T system; (**D**) leucine zipper or SUPRA CAR T; (**E**) convertibleCAR or modified NKG2D CAR T; (**F**) SNAP CAR T enzymatic CAR labeling system; (**G**) the co-localization-dependent protein switch (Co-LOCKR) CAR T system; (**H**) UniCAR or anti-5B9 peptide CAR platform; (**I**) anti-peptide neo-epitope (PNE) CAR T.

Lohmueller et al. [14] drew on this system and further affinity enhanced streptavidin, designing a biotin-binding domain where monomeric streptavidin could be used in the CAR system with higher affinity to biotin than the dimeric form. This affinity-enhanced form, mSA2, has a more compact structure than the dimeric form employed previously, possibly increasing the type of antigens able to be targeted by this system. The mSA2 CARs were able to distinguish antigen-positive cells precoated with biotinylated antibody in vitro and produce a specific effector response. Antigen-negative tumor cells did not elicit an effector response, neither did non-binding biotinylated antibody, showing that in order for CAR T cells to be turned on, the antibody must be bound to the target cells. The mSA2 CAR T cells showed potent effector functions; however, its potential immunogenicity could hamper its adoption in the clinic. With the BBIR system, excess biotin does not impart an inhibitory effect, and therefore could not be used as a potential 'off switch' for added safety.

2.2. Anti-FITC CAR Strategy

Fluorescein isothiocyanate (FITC), derived from fluorescein, is a fluorescent label commonly used to tag antibodies. Tamada et al. [15] first exploited this common labeling method and generated anti-FITC CAR T cells able to be directed by FITC-tagged antibodies (Figure 2B). The extracellular portion of the CAR is comprised of an anti-FITC scFv that recognizes FITC-labeled cetuximab (anti-EGFR), trastuzumab (anti-HER2), and rituximab (anti-CD20), antibodies that are already employed clinically. Redirected CAR T cells were found to be effective both in vitro and in vivo to specifically bind their respective tumor cells and exert anti-tumor effects. This system showed effectiveness at targeting multiple TAAs to better address heterogenous cancer populations. Additionally, the use of anti-FITC CAR T cells was shown to restore the usefulness of monoclonal antibodies to additional cancer types. They discuss that in patients with *Kras* mutations, cetuximab does not provide therapeutic benefits; however, when cetuximab is utilized with anti-FITC CAR T cells, anti-tumor effects are shown, as illustrated with the SW480 cell line that containing a *Kras* mutation. The anti-FITC CAR T system was applied using trastuzumab—Cao et al. conjugated FITC to trastuzumab in a site-specific manner compared to another strategy where a peptide neo-epitope (PNE) was fused to trastuzumab [16]. Both antibody tagging methods showed a dose-titratable immune response, capable of completely clearing HER2-positive tumors in vivo. The first clinical use of trastuzumab incorporated into a CAR T resulted in a serious adverse event, with the patient developing on-target, off-tumor toxicity related to the redirection of CAR T cells to lung epithelium, proving fatal [17]. Since this initial trial, many groups have investigated safer ways to target HER2, reviewed by Liu et al. [18], with the modular anti-FITC CAR T technology, a contender to address the safety issues with targeting this cancer-associated antigen.

Expanding the targeting elements to more than full-length antibodies, Zhang et al. employed switchable CAR-engineered T cells using anti-tumor peptides that specifically target integrin $\alpha v \beta 3$ through an 18-amino acid sequence fused to FITC [19]. This peptide adaptor molecule, termed FITC-HM-3, specifically targeted tumor cells and regulated CAR T cell activity. Demonstrating that low-molecular-weight switch molecules can be effective at redirecting engineered T cells, Lee et al. [20] employed a cocktail of small bifunctional molecules in conjunction with anti-fluorescein CAR T cells to target cancer cells in vitro and in vivo. The bifunctional molecules, called CAR T cell adapter molecules (CAMs), consist of fluorescein linked to a tumor-specific ligand through a hydrophilic spacer. The use of a mixture of CAMs enables the targeting of heterogenous solid tumors and broadens the applicability of CAR T cell therapy by using small molecules, which could improve tumor penetration, as opposed to larger full-length antibodies. Additionally, improved safety is offered by the short half-life (~90 min) of small molecules, allowing them to rapidly clear from receptor-negative tissue.

Optimizing the complex between the CAR T cell, switch, and tumor antigen is essential for optimal CAR T activation and cell killing. Using the modular CAR system, Ma et al. [21] utilized anti-FITC CARs to target both CD19 and CD22, whereby antibody fragments were site-specifically modified with FITC through genetically encoded non-canonical amino acids. This allowed for the incorporation of FITC to optimize of the geometry of the immunological synapse. Compared head to head, the optimized anti-FITC CAR T targeting CD19 performed similarly to conventional CD19-targeting CAR T, necessary for moving this technology forward into the clinic. Furthermore, excess FITC at 10 µM was shown to dampen CAR T activity in vitro, a feature that could be used to improve safety in the clinic. Others have shown that the addition of FITC-labeled non-specific antibodies could also be used to attenuate CAR T cells [15].

The targeting of folate receptors using anti-FITC CARs has been demonstrated by several groups [22–24]. Lu et al. [23], using FITC conjugated to folic acid as the switch molecule, modeled severe cytokine release syndrome and determined that CRS could be alleviated through the titration of the folate FITC adaptor or by intermittent dosing. Reversal of severe CRS could be achieved by intravenous sodium fluorescein to transiently interrupt CARs, without destroying the engineered T cells. With the ability to shut down the CAR T response through the addition of FITC [21], FITC labeled non-specific antibodies [15] or sodium fluorescein [23,24], this system with its added 'safety switches' could allow for engineered immune cell deactivation if toxicity develops, possibly being able to salvage the therapy by re-administering the switch molecules. While encouraging, the possible immunogenicity of FITC adaptors in the context of CAR T systems requires further study.

2.3. The SpyTag-SpyCatcher Universal CAR T System

The SpyTag/SpyCatcher protein ligation system employs a unique peptide: protein ligation reaction to link the tagged targeting element to the immune receptor. In 2012, Zackeri et al. reported a fibronectin-binding protein from *Streptococcus pyogenes* that, upon splitting it into two parts, followed by rational engineering, an N-terminal protein fragment (SpyCatcher) and a C-terminal 13-amino acid peptide (SpyTag) were produced [25]. The two parts will spontaneously reconstitute to form an isopeptide bond without the need for co-factors, enzymes, or specific conditions. Minutolo et al. exploited this system to generate a SpyCatcher immune receptor [26] (Figure 2C). This immune receptor contains the SpyCatcher protein as the extracellular domain, linked to intracellular signaling regions. TAA-specific targeting ligands, such as IgG antibodies, are site-specifically labeled with SpyTag. This post-translational covalent assembly allows for the redirection of T cells to multiple TAAs to exert targeted effector cell functions. The SpyCatcher immune receptor activity depends on the presence of both target antigen and SpyTag-labeled targeting element, allowing for titratable control of the engineered T cells. Arming the SpyCatcher CAR T cells with SpyTagged antibodies showed receptor levels decreasing over time, with complete loss observed after 96 h. SpyCatcher CAR T cells were shown to become functional upon the addition of SpyTag targeting element and lyse antigen-expressing target cells in vitro. Using an immunodeficient mouse xenograft model, the authors showed that HER2-positive xenografts could be targeted with SpyCatcher CAR T cells pre-armed with SpyTagged Herceptin. Additional targeting ligand was administered every three days, and administration throughout treatment was shown to be necessary for tumor clearance. The SpyTag/SpyCatcher system was tested using targeting elements against HER2, EGFR, EpCAM and CD20 and Liu et al. expanded the range of targetable antigens by demonstrating SpyCatcher immune receptors could be constructed to target the hepatocellular carcinoma antigen, human glypican-3 (hGPC3) using a SpyTagged anti-hGPC3 scFv [27].

Potential immunogenicity is an issue that may hamper SpyCatcher immune receptor adoption in the clinic. Owing to its bacterial origin, the Tag/Catcher system may be vulnerable to recognition by the patient's immune system. Work has been performed in developing SpyCatcher/SpyTag variants with truncations aimed at reducing potential immunogenicity [28] and tested using immunocompetent mice, but further study is needed to determine the likelihood of adverse reactions in humans.

2.4. Leucine Zippers to Retarget CAR T

Cho and colleagues developed a split, universal, and programmable (SUPRA) CAR system that allows for a modular platform to tune the specificity and activation of CAR T cells [29] (Figure 2D). The system consists of two parts: (1) a universal receptor (zipCAR) expressed on T cell surfaces (2) and a tumor-targeting scFv adaptor (zipFv). The zipCAR component consists of intracellular signaling domains linked through a transmembrane domain to an extracellular leucine zipper. The zipFv is a fusion protein consisting of an scFv and a leucine zipper that can interact with the leucine zipper of the zipCAR.

The split CAR design has several variables that can be manipulated to modify the specificity and adjust the SUPRA CAR T cells' activity. The leucine zipper pairs' affinity correlated with cellular activation as determined by cytokine secretion and target cell killing efficiency. Cells with higher zipCAR expression showed greater cytokine secretion upon activation. The authors showed that SUPRA CAR T cell activity could be inhibited using competitive zipFvs with leucine zipper domains that bind the original zipFv but not the zipCAR, thus preventing the activation of zipCARs. The activation level of SUPRA CAR T cells could be further modified by changing the competitive zipFv's leucine zipper's affinity for the original zipFv. SUPRA CAR T cells can also be used to increase tumor specificity through combinatorial antigen sensing, wherein more than one zipFv is introduced. Different signaling domains could be controlled by orthogonal SUPRA CARs, where zipCARs consisting of different intracellular signaling domains and leucine zipper components to specifically activate certain pathways upon antigen binding. The in vitro and in vivo effectiveness of the zipCAR platform was demonstrated; however, further studies, including clinical trials, are needed to confirm its efficacy and safety.

2.5. ConvertibleCAR Strategy Using Modified NKG2D Extracellular Domain

This modular CAR T cell variant, termed *convertible*CAR T cells, uses an inert form of the NKG2D extracellular domain as the ectodomain of the CAR [30] (Figure 2E). NKG2D, an activating receptor expressed on NK cells and some myeloid and T cells, was mutated in its ectodomain such that it cannot engage naturally occurring ligands. This mutant is deemed inert and referred to as inert NKG2D (iNKG2D). Orthogonal ligands were selected that specifically engaged iNKG2D but not WT NKG2D. Antibodies were fused to the orthogonal ligand, U2S3, to generate bispecific MicAbodies, which can specifically direct and activate iNKG2D-CAR-expressing T cells upon binding the respective antigen on a target cell surface. This modular system allows *convertible*CAR T cells to be redirected to different antigen-positive target cells. Additionally, the U2S3 ligand can be fused to payloads, such as cytokines to be delivered to iNKG2D-CAR-expressing cells, promoting their expansion. Expanding the repertoire of modular CAR T systems to more than cancer, Herzig et al. demonstrated that a *convertible*CAR T approach can be utilized to effectively and specifically kill HIV-infected CD4 cells [31]. Despite the advances in antiretroviral therapy, the primary obstacle to curing HIV-positive individuals is latently infected cells that persist. In an effort to target this reservoir of HIV-infected cells, the authors employed *convertible*CAR T cells armed with anti-HIV antibodies fused to an orthogonal MIC ligand. This allowed for the specific killing of HIV-infected primary CD4 T cells in vitro, only when the *convertible*CAR T cells and MicAbodies were bound. The use of a modified human activating receptor, NKGD2, may reduce the chance of an immunogenic reaction in the clinic, but *convertible*CAR system's safety has yet to be established.

2.6. SNAP CAR Strategy: Enzymatic Self-Labeling CARs

As one of the newest methods to be utilized for the generation of modular CAR Ts, an enzymatic strategy to link adaptor to CAR signaling regions is employed, where the CAR's extracellular domain contains the self-labeling SNAPtag enzyme [32] (Figure 2F). Antibodies are conjugated with benzylguanine (BG), with which the SNAP enzyme can react and form a covalent bond. SNAPtag is a modified human O-6-methylguanine-DNA methyltransferase, engineered to react with BG. Potent effector cell activity was shown when SNAP-CAR T cells were co-cultured with antigen-positive target cells, both with BG-conjugated full-length IgG antibodies and Fab fragment. An advantage to this anti-tag CAR system is the formation of a covalent bond between the SNAP enzyme and the BG moiety on the antibody.

Along with the SpyTag/SpyCatcher system, SNAP CARs are distinct from the other anti-tag systems, which rely on a transient interaction between antibody-tag conjugate and the CAR-modified cells. Additionally, the SNAP protein is of human origin and thus is unlikely to be immunogenic. A similar system was designed using the synthetic Notch receptor (synNotch) instead of the T cell receptor, wherein upon antigen binding, the Notch core protein is cleaved by endogenous proteases and releases a transcription factor from the cell membrane where it then travels to the nucleus to carry out its transcriptional regulation function. The generated self-labeling synNotch receptor, containing the SNAPtag protein covalently fused to the adaptor antibody, similar to the SNAP CAR system, functions as modular platforms for switchable CAR T activity.

2.7. The Co-Localization-Dependent Protein Switch (Co-LOCKR) CAR T System

Utilizing a novel logic-gated system, Lajoie et al. designed a protein switch system termed co-localization-dependent protein switch (Co-LOCKR), whereby the switch is engaged through a conformational change only when conditions are met, allowing for the implementation of AND, OR and NOT logic gates for precision target cell killing [33] (Figure 2G). The switch consists of a 'cage' protein, which sequesters a functional 'latch' peptide in an inactive conformation. The binding of a separate 'key' protein will induce a conformational change such that an effector protein or CAR T cell can interact. The authors employed a Bim-Bcl-2 interacting pair where the CAR contains a Bcl-2 binder which interacts with the Bim contained on the latch peptide. Using designed ankyrin repeat protein (DARPin) domains to target the cage element to HER2 and two key domains to EGFR and EpCAM, only cells that co-express both antigens (either HER2 + EGFR or HER2 + EpCAM) will activate Co-LOCKR. The cage domain containing the latch with Bim peptide will only be exposed once the key element interacts, initiating Bcl-2 CAR binding and subsequent T cell activation. Using target cells that express combinations of HER2, EGFR and EpCAM in a mixed population, a HER2-EpCAM Co-LOCKR showed that it would preferentially kill cells expressing both HER2 and EpCAM, and not those expressing HER2 and EGFR, or only HER2 or only EpCAM. The same experiments were performed with HER2-EGFR Co-LOCKR showing target cell killing by Bcl-2 CAR was restricted to only cells containing both HER2 and EGFR. These experiments demonstrated that CAR T cells were engaged specifically when in the presence of target cells co-expressing the correct pair of antigens and the degree of CAR expansion correlated with the density of antigen. The authors showed that between 2.5 nM and 20 nM of Co-LOCKR could be used without causing off-target CAR T cell killing, and the sensitivity of the switch could be further tuned through altering the cage-latch and cage-key affinities.

This method has the ability to reduce off-target effects and precisely direct CAR T activity towards specific target antigens. Additionally, decoy proteins fused to a targeting domain against an antigen to be avoided could be created, allowing for a CAR T 'off switch', where NOT logic is employed as the decoy sequesters the key, preventing cage activation and CAR T firing. In vivo experimentation is needed to evaluate the system's efficacy, and further studies on the potential immunogenicity of the designed proteins are required to broaden the application of this modular CAR T system.

2.8. Anti-5B9 Tag CAR: The UniCAR Platform

Using a unique peptide derived from an autoantigen to redirect CAR T cells, a novel modular CAR system, termed UniCAR, was developed [34] (Figure 2H). The system consists of two components: (1) a CAR with an anti-La protein scFv and (2) specific targeting modules (TMs) that redirect UniCAR T cells to targeted tumor cells. The anti-La protein recognizes a short non-immunogenic peptide motif of ten aa (5B9 tag) derived from the human nuclear autoantigen La/SS-B. TMs consist of a binding domain, such as a tumor-specific scFv, fused to the 5B9 tag that is recognized by the scFv portion of the UniCAR. UniCAR T cells are inactive when TMs are absent, providing an 'on' and 'off switch' to effector cell activity. The variety of antigens targeted by this system illustrates the flexibility of this approach; CD33, CD98, CD123, FLT3, EGFR, STn, GD2, PSMA, and PSCA [34–43] have all been targeted with the UniCAR platform. An advantage of the UniCAR system is the inherent safety switch by halting the infusion of TMs, and the flexibility that can enable targeting of tumor escape variants by using bispecific targeting agents.

Cartellieri et al. used the UniCAR system to target acute myeloid leukemia (AML), a heterogenous leukemic disease [34]. A previous analysis showed that nearly all AML blasts are positive for

CD33, CD123, or both, and scFv-based TMs were designed to target these antigens. Additionally, a dual-specific TM was engineered to target CD33 and CD123 and was shown in a cytotoxicity assay to lyse AML cell lines more effectively than equal molar ratios of each monospecific TM. Using this bispecific strategy may help reduce the risk of tumor escape variants. In the absence of TMs, the UniCAR T cells remained inert in vivo and did not show signs of toxicity.

As a more 'off-the-shelf' therapeutic approach, Mitwasi et al. demonstrated that UniCAR platform could be adapted to the NK-92 cell line [44]. The TM targeted the disialoganglioside GD2. Two types of TMs were explored: an scFv form as previously described, and a novel homodimeric format wherein the E5B9 epitope is connected to the GD2-specific antibody domain via an IgG4 Fc region. This novel TM format was used due to its longer half-life compared to the scFv version; the longer half-life was desired to be closer to that of the NK-92 lifespan due to their limited in vivo persistence. Therefore, they do not require a fast safety switch and the longer half-life of the adaptor reduces the need for continuous infusion. Both versions of the TM led to efficient and specific cell lysis of GD2+ neuroblastoma cells in vitro and in vivo. The use of the NK-92 cell line provides advantages such as lower side effect risk due to their restricted lifespan. Although the 5B9 peptide is derived from an autoantigen, studies completed examining the immune response against the La autoantigen demonstrated anti-La antibodies were not developed and an immune response was not mounted against the 5B9 peptide, as reviewed by Bachmann [45], which would indicate that UniCAR TMs are likely not immunogenic.

Albert et al. examined whether other antibody derivatives could be employed in the UniCAR platform [37]. They incorporated a nanobody targeting EGFR as the targeting module, which effectively retargeted UniCAR T cells to EGFR+ tumor cells and mediated specific cell lysis in vitro and in vivo. The anti-EGFR nanobody was subsequently radiolabeled with ^{64}Cu and ^{68}Ga, and biodistribution, clearance and stability of the targeting module-UniCAR complex were measured. The experiments established that TMs could be released from the UniCAR and dissociated both in vitro and in vivo in a dose-dependent manner, demonstrating its ability to act as a self-limiting switch. The rapid elimination of the nanobody-based TM could improve its safety profile. This work, along with Loureiro et al. [38] and Ardnt et al. [42], demonstrated the potential for UniCARs to be used for targeted immunotherapy and simultaneously as a PET imaging tool to track CAR T therapy. The PET tracer PSMA-11, which binds prostate-specific membrane antigen, was converted into a UniCAR-TM having a dual function as a CAR retargeting element as well as a non-invasive PET imaging reagent, making this a member of a new class of theranostics.

2.9. Anti-PNE CARs: Redirecting T Cells Using Peptide Neo-Epitope Tagging

Similar to the UniCAR platform, anti-PNE CARs take advantage of a peptide tag to redirect CAR T cells. Rodgers et al. first engineered an antibody-based bifunctional switch to be compatible with anti-peptide neo-epitope (PNE) CAR T cells, called switchable CAR-T cells (sCAR T) [46] (Figure 2I). The switch molecule is a 14 amino acid peptide neo-epitope derived from a yeast transcription factor that was shown to have a low probability of inducing an antibody response. The sCAR T cells form an immunological synapse through a PNE engrafted Fab to specifically direct T cell activity to the targeted cells using an anti-PNE scFv CAR. The authors created sCAR T cells directed against CD19 and CD20 and used the system to target B cell malignancies. The switch molecules were systematically optimized, focusing on spatial interactions, to achieve the most efficacious effector/target cell interaction. The authors show that sCAR-T cell activity is titratable, dose-dependent, and strictly dependent on the presence of the switch molecule; all of these characteristics contribute to improved safety compared to that of conventional CAR T cell therapy. Additionally, the codelivery of anti-CD19 and -CD20 switch molecules may prevent antigen escape to more effectively eliminate heterogenous B cell cancers. Viaud and colleagues further studied CD19-directed switchable CARs by examining the factors determining the induction of memory and expansion of sCAR T cells [47]. The formation of a memory population is important to consider, as a naïve, persistent central memory phenotype has been correlated with prolonged remissions in acute lymphoblastic leukemia patients. Conventional CAR T cell therapy cannot achieve the "rest" period required to stimulate a memory phenotype as they are constitutively "on" and interact with antigen. sCAR T cells targeted against CD19+ B cell lymphomas in a competent murine host showed that the timing and dosage of the anti-CD19 switch molecule could promote the expansion and contraction as well as the phenotype of the sCAR T cell population. It was established that a "rest" period used in conjunction with cyclical dosing of switch molecules could induce the production of a memory population, showing potential for enhancing the efficiency and persistence of CAR engineered T cells.

In addition to hematological cancers, anti-PNE CARs have been developed to target solid tumors expressing HER2 [16,48]. Pancreatic ductal adenocarcinoma (PDAC) was targeted with switchable CAR T cells using an anti-HER2 Fab-based switch molecule engrafted with a PNE tag. Using patient-derived xenografts obtained from patients with advanced stage, difficult-to-treat pancreatic tumors, durable remission was achieved by a single injection of switchable CAR T cells and five doses of the switch molecules. Switch molecules were further administered for 10–14 injections, resulting in long-term remission for all animals involved. Switchable CAR T cells persisted even after switch injections were halted, demonstrating switchable CAR T cells have the potential to be effective in safely treating aggressive and disseminated disease. The ability to modulate the dosage of the switchable CAR T may allow for safer targeting of HER2 and other antigens in the clinic.

3. Conclusions and Future Perspectives

CAR T cell therapy has already proven itself in the clinic as a powerful anti-cancer therapeutic. Needed to further its expansion into a wider array of cancers types is both identification of new targets combined with innovative CAR T design. For CAR T therapy to realize its potential in solid tumors, addressing tumor heterogenicity is paramount to its adoption in the clinic, along with a means to better modulate CAR activity to enhance its safety profile. An adaptable system such as modular CAR Ts conceivably could address these issues by tailoring CARs to a patient's specific cancer and adapting treatment using a toolkit of adaptor targeting elements. Simultaneous or sequential targeting of multiple TAAs through universal CARs could mitigate antigen escape, all without the time-consuming and expensive re-engineering of T cells.

Essential for the success of any CAR T approach is the ability to mitigate side effects. Modular CAR activity can be dialed in for enhanced control of engineered T cells and interruption of switch molecules administration, or in some cases using titratable 'off switches', able to dampen side effects associated with T cell proliferation. The use of adaptors to redirect CAR T cells expands on the repertoire of possible targeting elements such as using full-length IgGs; elements that are not possible through traditional CAR genetic engineering approaches. Although the adaptor format is near-limitless, the expense of generating CAR switch molecules and the requirement of continuous or multiple infusions of adaptors could curb its clinical implementation. CAR switch molecules rely on the addition of exogenous components; infusion of elements with non-endogenous origin could prove immunogenic, and the effect on patients remains untested.

The versatile nature of modular CARs and the ability for intelligent antigen targeting makes it an attractive candidate for CAR T therapy to be accessible to a wider range of cancer indications. Combining modular CAR T technology with new approaches in allogeneic CAR T treatment or natural killer (NK) cell engineering could create an extremely versatile product and a truly "off-the-shelf" therapy. Modular CAR T technology advances precision controllable engineered T cells and offers a more sophisticated approach to an already potent anti-cancer immunotherapy.

Author Contributions: A.R.S., writing—original draft preparation; M.N.O., writing; C.R.G., supervision. All authors have read and agreed to the published version of the manuscript.

Funding: Western Diversification Canada 12939.

Conflicts of Interest: The authors declare no conflict of interest.

Abbreviations

CAR	Chimeric antigen receptor
TAA	Tumor-associated antigen
IgG	Immunoglobulin
Fab	Antigen-binding fragment
scFv	Single-chain variable fragment
FITC	Fluorescein isothiocyanate
CRS	Cytokine release syndrome
BBIR	Biotin-binding immune receptor
dcAv	Dimeric avidin
PNE	Peptide neo-epitope
CAM	CAR T cell adapter molecule
hGPC3	Human glypican-3
SUPRA	Split, universal, and programmable
iNKG2D	Inert NKG2D
BG	Benzylguanine
synNotch	Synthetic Notch receptor
TM	Targeting modules
AML	Acute myeloid leukemia
sCAR T	Switchable CAR T
PDAC	Pancreatic ductal adenocarcinoma
NK	Natural killer

References

1. Sadelain, M.; Brentjens, R.; Rivière, I. The Basic Principles of Chimeric Antigen Receptor Design. *Cancer Discov.* **2013**, *3*, 388–398. [CrossRef]
2. Shirasu, N.; Kuroki, M. Functional Design of Chimeric T-Cell Antigen Receptors for Adoptive Immunotherapy of Cancer: Architecture and Outcomes. *Anticancer Res.* **2012**, *32*, 2377–2383.
3. Brentjens, R.J.; Davila, M.L.; Riviere, I.; Park, J.; Wang, X.; Cowell, L.G.; Bartido, S.; Stefanski, J.; Taylor, C.; Olszewska, M.; et al. CD19-Targeted T Cells Rapidly Induce Molecular Remissions in Adults with Chemotherapy-Refractory Acute Lymphoblastic Leukemia. *Sci. Transl. Med.* **2013**, *5*, 177ra38. [CrossRef]
4. Lee, D.W.; Kochenderfer, J.N.; Stetler-Stevenson, M.; Cui, Y.K.; Delbrook, C.; Feldman, S.A.; Fry, T.J.; Orentas, R.; Sabatino, M.; Shah, N.N.; et al. T cells expressing CD19 chimeric antigen receptors for acute lymphoblastic leukaemia in children and young adults: A phase 1 dose-escalation trial. *Lancet* **2015**, *385*, 517–528. [CrossRef]
5. Kochenderfer, J.N.; Dudley, M.E.; Feldman, S.A.; Wilson, W.H.; Spaner, D.E.; Maric, I.; Stetler-Stevenson, M.; Phan, G.Q.; Hughes, M.S.; Sherry, R.M.; et al. B-cell depletion and remissions of malignancy along with cytokine-associated toxicity in a clinical trial of anti-CD19 chimeric-antigen-receptor–transduced T cells. *Blood* **2012**, *119*, 2709–2720. [CrossRef]
6. Xu, X.; Sun, Q.; Liang, X.; Chen, Z.; Zhang, X.; Zhou, X.; Li, M.; Tu, H.; Liu, Y.; Tu, S.; et al. Mechanisms of Relapse After CD19 CAR T-Cell Therapy for Acute Lymphoblastic Leukemia and Its Prevention and Treatment Strategies. *Front. Immunol.* **2019**, *10*, 2664. [CrossRef]
7. Kailayangiri, S.; Altvater, B.; Wiebel, M.; Jamitzky, S.; Rossig, C. Overcoming Heterogeneity of Antigen Expression for Effective CAR T Cell Targeting of Cancers. *Cancers* **2020**, *12*, 1075. [CrossRef]
8. Maude, S.L.; Laetsch, T.W.; Buechner, J.; Rives, S.; Boyer, M.; Bittencourt, H.; Bader, P.; Verneris, M.R.; Stefanski, H.E.; Myers, G.D.; et al. Tisagenlecleucel in Children and Young Adults with B-Cell Lymphoblastic Leukemia. *N. Engl. J. Med.* **2018**, *378*, 439–448. [CrossRef]
9. Park, J.H.; Rivière, I.; Gonen, M.; Wang, X.; Sénéchal, B.; Curran, K.J.; Sauter, C.; Wang, Y.; Santomasso, B.; Mead, E.; et al. Long-Term Follow-up of CD19 CAR Therapy in Acute Lymphoblastic Leukemia. *N. Engl. J. Med.* **2018**, *378*, 449–459. [CrossRef]

10. Chen, H.; Wang, F.; Zhang, P.; Zhang, Y.; Chen, Y.; Fan, X.; Cao, X.; Liu, J.; Yang, Y.; Wang, B.; et al. Management of cytokine release syndrome related to CAR-T cell therapy. *Front. Med.* **2019**, *13*, 610–617. [CrossRef]
11. Brudno, J.N.; Kochenderfer, J.N. Recent advances in CAR T-cell toxicity: Mechanisms, manifestations and management. *Blood Rev.* **2019**, *34*, 45–55. [CrossRef] [PubMed]
12. Thakar, M.S.; Kearl, T.J.; Malarkannan, S. Controlling Cytokine Release Syndrome to Harness the Full Potential of CAR-Based Cellular Therapy. *Front. Oncol.* **2020**, *9*, 1529. [CrossRef] [PubMed]
13. Urbanska, K.; Lanitis, E.; Poussin, M.; Lynn, R.C.; Gavin, B.P.; Kelderman, S.; Yu, J.; Scholler, N.; Powell, D.J. A Universal Strategy for Adoptive Immunotherapy of Cancer through Use of a Novel T-cell Antigen Receptor. *Cancer Res.* **2012**, *72*, 1844–1852. [CrossRef] [PubMed]
14. Lohmueller, J.J.; Ham, J.D.; Kvorjak, M.; Finn, O.J. mSA2 affinity-enhanced biotin-binding CAR T cells for universal tumor targeting. *OncoImmunology* **2018**, *7*, e1368604. [CrossRef] [PubMed]
15. Tamada, K.; Geng, D.; Sakoda, Y.; Bansal, N.; Srivastava, R.; Li, Z.; Davila, E. Redirecting Gene-Modified T Cells toward Various Cancer Types Using Tagged Antibodies. *Clin. Cancer Res.* **2012**, *18*, 6436–6445. [CrossRef]
16. Cao, Y.; Rodgers, D.T.; Du, J.; Ahmad, I.; Hampton, E.N.; Ma, J.S.Y.; Mazagova, M.; Choi, S.; Yun, H.Y.; Xiao, H.; et al. Design of Switchable Chimeric Antigen Receptor T Cells Targeting Breast Cancer. *Angew. Chem. Int. Ed.* **2016**, *55*, 7520–7524. [CrossRef]
17. Morgan, R.A.; Yang, J.C.; Kitano, M.; Dudley, M.E.; Laurencot, C.M.; Rosenberg, S.A. Case Report of a Serious Adverse Event Following the Administration of T Cells Transduced With a Chimeric Antigen Receptor Recognizing ERBB2. *Mol. Ther.* **2010**, *18*, 843–851. [CrossRef]
18. Liu, X.; Zhang, N.; Shi, H. Driving better and safer HER2-specific CARs for cancer therapy. *Oncotarget* **2017**, *8*, 62730–62741. [CrossRef]
19. Zhang, E.; Gu, J.; Xue, J.; Lin, C.; Liu, C.; Li, M.; Hao, J.; Setrerrahmane, S.; Chi, X.; Qi, W.; et al. Accurate control of dual-receptor-engineered T cell activity through a bifunctional anti-angiogenic peptide. *J. Hematol. Oncol.* **2018**, *11*, 44. [CrossRef]
20. Lee, Y.G.; Marks, I.; Srinivasarao, M.; Kanduluru, A.K.; Mahalingam, S.M.; Liu, X.; Chu, H.; Low, P.S. Use of a Single CAR T Cell and Several Bispecific Adapters Facilitates Eradication of Multiple Antigenically Different Solid Tumors. *Cancer Res.* **2019**, *79*, 387–396. [CrossRef]
21. Ma, J.S.Y.; Kim, J.Y.; Kazane, S.A.; Choi, S.-H.; Yun, H.Y.; Kim, M.S.; Rodgers, D.T.; Pugh, H.M.; Singer, O.; Sun, S.B.; et al. Versatile strategy for controlling the specificity and activity of engineered T cells. *Proc. Natl. Acad. Sci. USA* **2016**, *113*, E450–E458. [CrossRef] [PubMed]
22. Chu, W.; Zhou, Y.; Tang, Q.; Wang, M.; Ji, Y.; Yan, J.; Yin, D.; Zhang, S.; Lu, H.; Shen, J. Bi-specific ligand-controlled chimeric antigen receptor T-cell therapy for non-small cell lung cancer. *Biosci. Trends* **2018**, *12*, 298–308. [CrossRef] [PubMed]
23. Lu, Y.J.; Chu, H.; Wheeler, L.W.; Nelson, M.; Westrick, E.; Matthaei, J.F.; Cardle, I.I.; Johnson, A.; Gustafson, J.; Parker, N.; et al. Preclinical Evaluation of Bispecific Adaptor Molecule Controlled Folate Receptor CAR-T Cell Therapy With Special Focus on Pediatric Malignancies. *Front. Oncol.* **2019**, *9*, 151. [CrossRef] [PubMed]
24. Kim, M.S.; Ma, J.S.Y.; Yun, H.; Cao, Y.; Kim, J.Y.; Chi, V.; Wang, D.; Woods, A.; Sherwood, L.; Caballero, D.; et al. Redirection of Genetically Engineered CAR-T Cells Using Bifunctional Small Molecules. *J. Am. Chem. Soc.* **2015**, *137*, 2832–2835. [CrossRef]
25. Zakeri, B.; Fierer, J.O.; Celik, E.; Chittock, E.C.; Schwarz-Linek, U.; Moy, V.T.; Howarth, M. Peptide tag forming a rapid covalent bond to a protein, through engineering a bacterial adhesin. *Proc. Natl. Acad. Sci. USA* **2012**, *109*, E690–E697. [CrossRef]
26. Minutolo, N.G.; Sharma, P.; Poussin, M.; Shaw, L.C.; Brown, D.P.; Hollander, E.E.; Smole, A.; Rodriguez-Garcia, A.; Hui, J.Z.; Zappala, F.; et al. Quantitative Control of Gene-Engineered T-Cell Activity through the Covalent Attachment of Targeting Ligands to a Universal Immune Receptor. *J. Am. Chem. Soc.* **2020**, *142*, 6554–6568. [CrossRef]
27. Liu, X.; Wen, J.; Yi, H.; Hou, X.; Yin, Y.; Ye, G.; Wu, X.; Jiang, X. Split chimeric antigen receptor-modified T cells targeting glypican-3 suppress hepatocellular carcinoma growth with reduced cytokine release. *Ther. Adv. Med. Oncol.* **2020**, *12*, 1–16. [CrossRef]
28. Liu, Z.; Zhou, H.; Wang, W.; Tan, W.; Fu, Y.-X.; Zhu, M. A novel method for synthetic vaccine construction based on protein assembly. *Sci. Rep.* **2014**, *4*, 7266. [CrossRef]

29. Cho, J.H.; Collins, J.J.; Wong, W.W. Universal Chimeric Antigen Receptors for Multiplexed and Logical Control of T cell Responses. *Cell* **2018**, *173*, 1426–1438. [CrossRef]
30. Landgraf, K.E.; Williams, S.R.; Steiger, D.; Gebhart, D.; Lok, S.; Martin, D.W.; Roybal, K.T.; Kim, K.C. convertibleCARs: A chimeric antigen receptor system for flexible control of activity and antigen targeting. *Commun. Biol.* **2020**, *3*, 296. [CrossRef]
31. Herzig, E.; Kim, K.C.; Packard, T.A.; Vardi, N.; Schwarzer, R.; Gramatica, A.; Deeks, S.G.; Williams, S.R.; Landgraf, K.; Killeen, N.; et al. Attacking Latent HIV with convertibleCAR-T Cells, a Highly Adaptable Killing Platform. *Cell* **2019**, *179*, 880–894. [CrossRef] [PubMed]
32. Lohmueller, J.; Butchy, A.A.; Tivon, Y.; Kvorjak, M.; Miskov-Zivanov, N.; Deiters, A.; Finn, O.J. Post-Translational Covalent Assembly of CAR and Synnotch Receptors for Programmable Antigen Targeting; Synthetic Biology. 2020. Available online: https://www.biorxiv.org/content/10.1101/2020.01.17 (accessed on 28 March 2020).
33. Lajoie, M.J.; Boyken, S.E.; Salter, A.I.; Bruffey, J.; Rajan, A.; Langan, R.A.; Olshefsky, A.; Muhunthan, V.; Bick, M.J.; Gewe, M.; et al. Designed protein logic to target cells with precise combinations of surface antigens. *Science* **2020**, *369*, eaba6527. [CrossRef] [PubMed]
34. Cartellieri, M.; Feldmann, A.; Koristka, S.; Arndt, C.; Loff, S.; Ehninger, A.; von Bonin, M.; Bejestani, E.P.; Ehninger, G.; Bachmann, M.P. Switching CAR T cells on and off: A novel modular platform for retargeting of T cells to AML blasts. *Blood Cancer J.* **2016**, *6*, e458. [CrossRef] [PubMed]
35. Fasslrinner, F.; Arndt, C.; Feldmann, A.; Koristka, S.; Loureiro, L.R.; Schmitz, M.; Jung, G.; Bornhaeuser, M.; Bachmann, M. Targeting the FMS-like Tyrosin Kinase 3 with the Unicar System: Preclinical Comparison of Murine and Humanized Single-Chain Variable Fragment-Based Targeting Modules. *Blood* **2019**, *134*, 5614. [CrossRef]
36. Albert, S.; Arndt, C.; Feldmann, A.; Bergmann, R.; Bachmann, D.; Koristka, S.; Ludwig, F.; Ziller-Walter, P.; Kegler, A.; Gärtner, S.; et al. A novel nanobody-based target module for retargeting of T lymphocytes to EGFR-expressing cancer cells via the modular UniCAR platform. *Oncoimmunology* **2017**, *6*, e1287246. [CrossRef]
37. Albert, S.; Arndt, C.; Koristka, S.; Berndt, N.; Bergmann, R.; Feldmann, A.; Schmitz, M.; Pietzsch, J.; Steinbach, J.; Bachmann, M. From mono- to bivalent: Improving theranostic properties of target modules for redirection of UniCAR T cells against EGFR-expressing tumor cells in vitro and in vivo. *Oncotarget* **2018**, *9*, 25597–25616. [CrossRef]
38. Loureiro, L.R.; Feldmann, A.; Bergmann, R.; Koristka, S.; Berndt, N.; Máthé, D.; Hegedüs, N.; Szigeti, K.; Videira, P.A.; Bachmann, M.; et al. Extended half-life target module for sustainable UniCAR T-cell treatment of STn-expressing cancers. *J. Exp. Clin. Cancer Res.* **2020**, *39*, 77. [CrossRef]
39. Loureiro, L.R.; Feldmann, A.; Bergmann, R.; Koristka, S.; Berndt, N.; Arndt, C.; Pietzsch, J.; Novo, C.; Videira, P.; Bachmann, M. Development of a novel target module redirecting UniCAR T cells to Sialyl Tn-expressing tumor cells. *Blood Cancer J.* **2018**, *8*, 81. [CrossRef]
40. Mitwasi, N.; Feldmann, A.; Bergmann, R.; Berndt, N.; Arndt, C.; Koristka, S.; Kegler, A.; Jureczek, J.; Hoffmann, A.; Ehninger, A.; et al. Development of novel target modules for retargeting of UniCAR T cells to GD2 positive tumor cells. *Oncotarget* **2017**, *8*, 108584–108603. [CrossRef]
41. Feldmann, A.; Arndt, C.; Bergmann, R.; Loff, S.; Cartellieri, M.; Bachmann, D.; Aliperta, R.; Hetzenecker, M.; Ludwig, F.; Albert, S.; et al. Retargeting of T lymphocytes to PSCA- or PSMA positive prostate cancer cells using the novel modular chimeric antigen receptor platform technology "UniCAR". *Oncotarget* **2017**, *8*, 31368–31385. [CrossRef]
42. Arndt, C.; Feldmann, A.; Koristka, S.; Schäfer, M.; Bergmann, R.; Mitwasi, N.; Berndt, N.; Bachmann, D.; Kegler, A.; Schmitz, M.; et al. A theranostic PSMA ligand for PET imaging and retargeting of T cells expressing the universal chimeric antigen receptor UniCAR. *Oncoimmunology* **2019**, *8*, 1659095. [CrossRef] [PubMed]
43. Bachmann, D.; Aliperta, R.; Bergmann, R.; Feldmann, A.; Koristka, S.; Arndt, C.; Loff, S.; Welzel, P.; Albert, S.; Kegler, A.; et al. Retargeting of UniCAR T cells with an in vivo synthesized target module directed against CD19 positive tumor cells. *Oncotarget* **2018**, *9*, 7487–7500. [CrossRef] [PubMed]
44. Mitwasi, N.; Feldmann, A.; Arndt, C.; Koristka, S.; Berndt, N.; Jureczek, J.; Loureiro, L.R.; Bergmann, R.; Máthé, D.; Hegedüs, N.; et al. "UniCAR"-modified off-the-shelf NK-92 cells for targeting of GD2-expressing tumour cells. *Sci. Rep.* **2020**, *10*, 2141. [CrossRef] [PubMed]

45. Bachmann, M. The UniCAR system: A modular CAR T cell approach to improve the safety of CAR T cells. *Immunol. Lett.* **2019**, *211*, 13–22. [CrossRef]
46. Rodgers, D.T.; Mazagova, M.; Hampton, E.N.; Cao, Y.; Ramadoss, N.S.; Hardy, I.R.; Schulman, A.; Du, J.; Wang, F.; Singer, O.; et al. Switch-mediated activation and retargeting of CAR-T cells for B-cell malignancies. *Proc. Natl. Acad. Sci. USA* **2016**, *113*, E459–E468. [CrossRef]
47. Viaud, S.; Ma, J.S.Y.; Hardy, I.R.; Hampton, E.N.; Benish, B.; Sherwood, L.; Nunez, V.; Ackerman, C.J.; Khialeeva, E.; Weglarz, M.; et al. Switchable control over in vivo CAR T expansion, B cell depletion, and induction of memory. *Proc. Natl. Acad. Sci. USA* **2018**, *115*, E10898–E10906. [CrossRef]
48. Raj, D.; Yang, M.-H.; Rodgers, D.; Hampton, E.N.; Begum, J.; Mustafa, A.; Lorizio, D.; Garces, I.; Propper, D.; Kench, J.G.; et al. Switchable CAR-T cells mediate remission in metastatic pancreatic ductal adenocarcinoma. *Gut* **2019**, *68*, 1052–1064. [CrossRef]

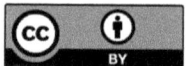

© 2020 by the authors. Licensee MDPI, Basel, Switzerland. This article is an open access article distributed under the terms and conditions of the Creative Commons Attribution (CC BY) license (http://creativecommons.org/licenses/by/4.0/).

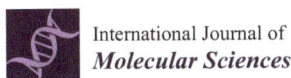 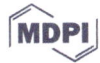

Technical Note

A Simple and Efficient Genetic Immunization Protocol for the Production of Highly Specific Polyclonal and Monoclonal Antibodies against the Native Form of Mammalian Proteins

Julie Pelletier [1], Hervé Agonsanou [1,2], Fabiana Manica [1,2], Elise G. Lavoie [1,2], Mabrouka Salem [1,2], Patrick Luyindula [1,2], Romuald Brice Babou Kammoe [1,2] and Jean Sévigny [1,2,*]

1. Centre de Recherche du CHU de Québec—Université Laval, Quebec City, QC G1V 4G2, Canada; julie.pelletier@crchudequebec.ulaval.ca (J.P.); herveagonsanou@yahoo.fr (H.A.); manicafabiana@gmail.com (F.M.); elise.gaudreau-lavoie@crchudequebec.ulaval.ca (E.G.L.); mabrouka.salem@crchudequebec.ulaval.ca (M.S.); patluyind@yahoo.fr (P.L.); romuald.babou@crchudequebec.ulaval.ca (R.B.B.K.)
2. Département de Microbiologie-Infectiologie et d'Immunologie, Faculté de Médecine, Université Laval, Québec City, QC G1V 0A6, Canada
* Correspondence: jean.sevigny@crchudequebec.ulaval.ca

Received: 14 August 2020; Accepted: 21 September 2020; Published: 25 September 2020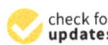

Abstract: We have generated polyclonal and monoclonal antibodies by genetic immunization over the last two decades. In this paper, we present our most successful methodology acquired over these years and present the animals in which we obtained the highest rates of success. The technique presented is convenient, easy, affordable, and generates antibodies against mammalian proteins in their native form. This protocol requires neither expensive equipment, such as a gene gun, nor sophisticated techniques such as the conjugation of gold microspheres, electroporation, or surgery to inject in lymph nodes. The protocol presented uses simply the purified plasmid expressing the protein of interest under a strong promoter, which is injected at intramuscular and intradermal sites. This technique was tested in five species. Guinea pigs were the animals of choice for the production of polyclonal antibodies. Monoclonal antibodies could be generated in mice by giving, as a last injection, a suspension of transfected cells. The antibodies detected their antigens in their native forms. They were highly specific with very low non-specific background levels, as assessed by immune-blots, immunocytochemistry, immunohistochemistry and flow cytometry. We present herein a detailed and simple procedure to successfully raise specific antibodies against native proteins.

Keywords: immunization; antibody; protocol; guinea pig; cDNA

1. Introduction

Antibodies that detect native proteins with high specificity are essential research tools. To obtain these precious immunoglobulins, different types of antigens can be used such as synthetic peptides conjugated to a carrier. The antibodies generated against peptides often do not detect the proteins of interest in their native forms. To circumvent this limitation, purified proteins can be utilized for immunization. However, the techniques necessary to purify proteins are laborious and may denaturate the proteins of interest during the purification steps, especially transmembrane proteins. Furthermore, the level of purity necessary to raise specific antibodies is high as some of the impurities are often immunogenic. A genetic immunization approach represents an interesting alternative [1] but it generally generates sera with low titers.

In genetic immunization, the protein of interest is expressed using a plasmid containing its gene under the control of a strong enhancer-promoter such as the one from cytomegalovirus (CMV) for a high expression level. This construct is injected into the animal where it is taken up by cells and the gene of interest is expressed. As a result, the animal reacts against this "non-self" antigen and produces specific immunoglobulins. This technique has the advantage to produce an antigen 100% pure without any effort. When using the full coding sequence of a mammalian gene, the protein of interest undergoes normal post-translational modifications. Therefore, the antibodies produced are directed against the protein in a normal mammalian form.

Genetic immunization has been used in different species such as rat [2], mouse [3], monkey [4], ferret [4] and rabbit [5]. Thus far, cDNA immunization in the guinea pig was mostly used in models of infectious challenge to verify the protective effect of cDNA vaccine. Most of these cDNA vaccine protocols in the guinea pig have been established using electroporation [6,7], which requires further equipment.

In this study, we summarize our results obtained over the last two decades using cDNA injection in different animal species and we propose an optimized, easy, and convenient protocol for the generation of polyclonal as well as monoclonal antibodies. During this work, we observed that one species in particular produced polyclonal antibodies in a consistent and reproducible manner, namely the guinea pig. Monoclonal antibodies could also be obtained in mice with a similar cDNA immunization procedure, to which we added a final injection constituted of a suspension of cells transiently transfected with the protein of interest for a stronger and faster challenge.

2. Results

2.1. Polyclonal Antibodies

2.1.1. Analysis of the Antibodies Produced

Over the last two decades, we have tested different immunization conditions to raise antibodies. We have tested several conditions that allowed us to identify a protocol that is very convenient and reliable to successfully raise specific antibodies excellent for research purposes. This protocol can be used by laboratories with minimal immunization experience. We will first present some of the immunization procedures that led us to the protocol that we describe at the end of this manuscript.

The sera obtained were tested by western blot, immunocytochemistry and immunohistochemistry after the third injection and compared to their respective pre-immune sera collected immediately before the first injection. We considered that an animal serum was positive when a specific signal was obtained either in western blot, immunohistochemistry or immunocytochemistry, and absent in the pre-immune serum. The best antibodies were also tested by flow cytometry. It is noteworthy that most of the antibodies that we have generated by cDNA immunization detected the native protein with its normal disulfide bridges. Therefore, the antibodies generally did not detect the proteins of interest in western blots under reducing conditions, with either DTT or mercaptoethanol. Broadly speaking, when using this immunization technique, antisera that reacted positively in western blot under non-reducing conditions detected also efficiently the antigens by immunocytochemistry, immunohistochemistry and flow cytometry.

Most of the antibodies documented in this study can now be obtained commercially. The monoclonal and polyclonal antibodies to NTPDases, NPPs and CD73 can be obtained at ectonucleotidases-ab.com. The antibodies to Robo4, Dectin-2 and RANK were licensed to Medimabs and a different monoclonal anti-human RANK was licensed to Millipore, where they can be obtained.

2.1.2. Administration Routes and Electroporation

Most of the immunization protocols were performed by intramuscular (IM) and intradermal (ID) injections, which is easy and convenient. Alternative routes of injection, some of which having been reported to elicit a stronger and more rapid immunization [8], were also tested. Administration in the subscapular area was tested in seven rabbits with different antigens and compared with ID and IM injections on 13 rabbits (see Table 1). Unfortunately, antibodies were produced only in one of those groups with the plasmid expressing mouse NTPDase2. The serum of the animal injected in the subscapular region did not give a better signal than those of the two rabbits injected at ID and IM sites. For the six other plasmids (angiomotin, Bmx/Etk, LCCP, mouse NTPDase8, RANK, RANKL), no antibody was produced either by the rabbits injected ID and IM or by those injected in the subscapular region in addition to ID and IM injections.

The injection of cDNA in lymph nodes has been reported to increase the antibody response with lower levels of cDNAs [8]. We tested the popliteal lymph node route in rabbits injected with plasmids coding for mouse NTPDase3 and rat NTPDase6. Among the rabbits injected with the mouse NTPDase3 expression plasmid, one was injected at IM and ID sites, and the other rabbit received the same amount of cDNA in ID sites as well as in both popliteal lymph nodes (see Table 1). In this assay, the serum of the rabbit that received only IM and ID injection gave a better response by flow cytometry than the serum of the rabbit that received cDNA in the popliteal lymph nodes in addition to ID injections. Meanwhile, as the sera of both of these rabbits showed very high background in western blots (Figure 1D, rabbit "j" and "i", respectively) it is difficult to conclude whether one of those bands actually corresponds to the antigen. Similar results were obtained in another series with the plasmid encoding rat NTPDase6. In these experiments, one rabbit received only IM and ID injections and two rabbits received IM, ID and popliteal lymph node injections. The rabbits injected only at IM and ID sites gave a stronger signal by immunohistochemistry than the two rabbits injected in the popliteal lymph nodes (data not shown).

Although our limited study does not allow us to draw a conclusion on the effectiveness of these two injections routes (subscapular and popliteal lymph nodes), we obtained better responses and reliability by ID and IM immunization in the animals tested. It is noteworthy that popliteal lymph node injection requires a level of surgical technical skills that did not meet our goal of identifying an easy and convenient procedure of immunization. Furthermore, the latter injection protocols were not necessary to obtain a good antibody response. Therefore, as these injections routes were more demanding technically and that they were not improving significantly antibody production with the plasmids tested, we decided to abandon the injections of the subscapular and popliteal lymph nodes.

Electroporation was also reported to increase antibody titer [9,10]. This technique was tested on three guinea pigs and four mice injected with plasmids expressing mouse NTPDase8 and human NTPDase2, respectively. No specific antibodies were obtained using electroporation in guinea pigs while positive antisera were obtained with the same plasmid in 10 out of 11 guinea pigs when injected at ID and IM sites. In our hands, electroporation was very efficient in mice as a host where the sera of all the treated mice showed a positive immune-blotting signal with a better signal versus background ratio than the sera of the two mice that received only ID and IM injections. In agreement with the literature, electroporation induced a more rapid antibody production than that observed in response to ID or IM injections alone [9]. For the mice that received DNA-electroporation, one mouse gave a positive signal in western blot after the second injection, two mice after the third injection and the fourth mouse after the fourth injection. In comparison with the two mice that received the same plasmid at ID and IM sites, one mouse gave a positive signal after the third injection and the other mouse gave a weak positive signal after the fourth injection. Among the animals that gave a positive response with ID and IM immunizations, a positive antiserum was observed after the third injection in 10% (1 out of 10) in mice, 40% (12 out of 30) in guinea pigs and 62% (16 out of 26) in rabbits. The majority of the successful animals responded following four sets of ID and IM injections (60% (six out of 10) in mice, 91% (30 out of 33) in guinea pigs and 100% (28 out of 28) in rabbits).

Since ID and IM injections do not require special surgical skills or specialized apparatus such as an electrical device, and as they have been shown to be very efficient routes of injection thus far, we selected those easy and convenient administration routes for our next assays.

Table 1. Immunization protocol summary.

Species	Number of Animals	Number of Antigens Tested	Administration Route	Number of Site × Volume per Site	DNA Injected per Immunization (µg)	Injection Intervals (Weeks Between Each Injection)	
						Injection 1 to 3	Injection 3 to 6
Rabbit	64	25	ID	6–10 × 50 µL	300–800		
			IM	2–4 × 125–250 µL			
	7	7	ID	6–8 × 50 µL	625–1000	2–4	8–17[a]
			IM	2 × 150–175 µL			
			SS	1 × 350 µL			
	3	2	ID	6–8 × 50 µL	800		
			Pop	1–2 × 150 µL			
			±IM	1 × 250 µL			
Guinea pig	50	17	ID	2 × 50 µL			
			IM	1 × 100 µL			
	2	1	ID	4 × 50 µL	125–200	1.5–4	7–16
	2	1	IM	2 × 100 µL			
	3	1	IM + EP	1 × 100 µL	100–400	5–7	8
Mouse	20	6	ID	2 × 25 µL			
			IM	1 × 50 µL			
	4	1	IM	2 × 50 µL	100	2–3	8–12
	4	1	IM + EP	1 × 30 µL	60	3–8	7–11
Rat	2	1	ID	2 × 50 µL			
			IM	1 × 100 µL			
	2	1	ID	4 × 50 µL	200	2	8–16
	2	1	IM	2 × 100 µL	125–200		
Hamster	2	1	ID	2 × 25 µL			
			IM	1 × 50 µL			
	2	1	ID	4 × 25 µL	100	2	10
	2	1	IM	2 × 50 µL			

EP: electroporation; ID: intradermal; IM: intramuscular; Pop: Popliteal; SS: Subscapular. [a]: for the mouse NTPDase8 antigen injected to three rabbits a total of nine injections were performed at an interval of 4 to 10 weeks for the last three injections.

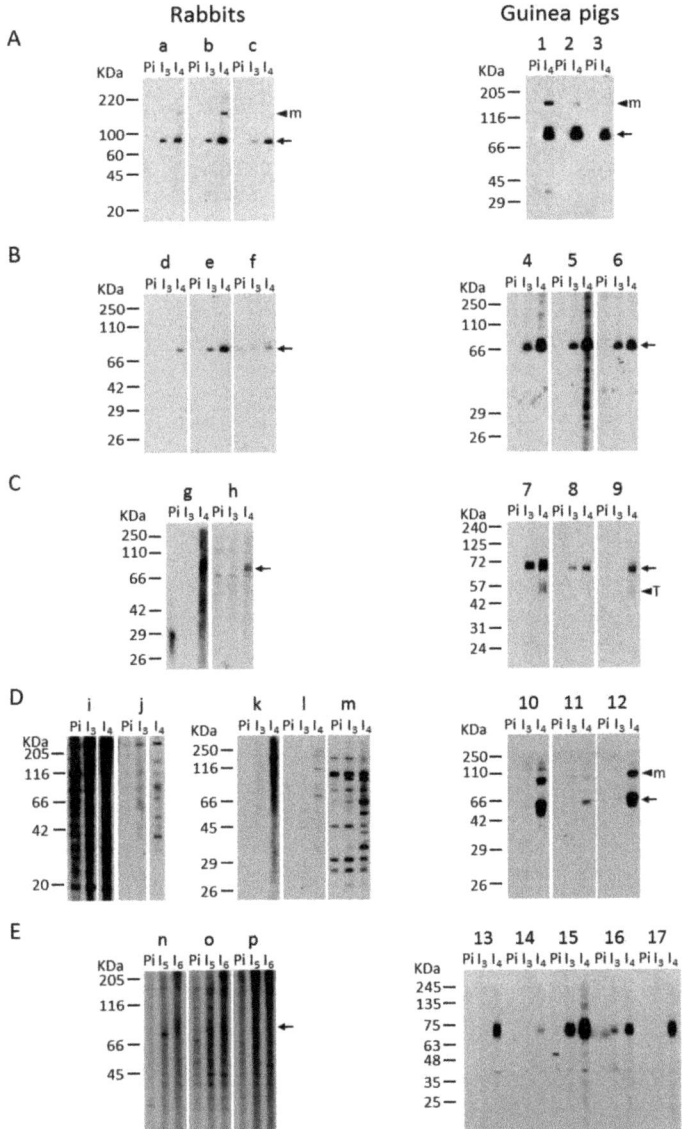

Figure 1. Immuno-blotting-based comparative analysis of rabbit and guinea pig antisera. Lysates for one large well from COS-7 cells or HEK 293T cells transfected with plasmids encoding human ecto-5′-nucleotidase (A), rat ecto-5′-nucleotidase (B), human NTPDase1 (C), mouse NTPDase3 (D) or mouse NTPDase8 (E) were subjected to electrophoresis under non-reducing conditions, electrotransferred to an Immobilon-P membrane and probed with rabbits "a" to "p" (left panels) or guinea pig "1" to "17" (right panels) antisera. The sera presented are the pre-immune (Pi) negative controls and the immune sera collected after the third (I_3), the fourth (I_4), the fifth (I_5) or the sixth (I_6) injection. Specific bands are denoted with an arrow. Multimeric (M) and truncated (T) protein forms are indicated with an arrow head. The antibodies shown were diluted 1:500 except for the rabbit "g" in panel C and rabbits "k," "l" and "m" in panel D that were diluted 1:1000.

2.1.3. Immunization of Different Species

Most antibodies raised in this work were produced in rabbits. We injected 25 plasmids to 74 rabbits. The cDNA immunization in rabbits led to specific antibodies in 35 out of 74 rabbits (47%). Specific antibodies were also efficiently produced in mice, the animal of choice to generate monoclonal antibodies, with a similar ID and IM immunization protocol as that used in rabbits. Among the 28 mice injected with five different plasmids, 16 mice (57%) reacted positively. To compare this cDNA immunization procedure in different species we have also immunized three rabbits, six hamsters, six rats and 11 guinea pigs with the same antigen, a plasmid encoding mouse NTPDase8. No specific antibodies were obtained in three rabbits (Figure 1E) or in six hamsters. A positive signal was obtained in two out of six rats, but only by immuno-cytochemistry (Table 2). In contrast, 10 out of 11 guinea pigs responded to this plasmid. This prompted us to test this species further with the same immunization technique. A majority of the 54 guinea pigs injected with 17 different plasmids produced a positive and specific serum with low background (41 positives out of 54 or 76%) (Table 2).

Table 2. Polyclonal antibodies raised.

Species	Number of Plasmids Tested	Number of Animals Immunized	Responding Animals (number, %)
Rabbit	25	74	35, 47%
Guinea pig	17	54	41, 76%
Mouse	5	28	16, 57%
Rat	1	6	2, 33% *
Hamster	1	6	0

Compilation of animal antisera that were considered positive when a specific signal was obtained in either western blot, immunohistochemistry or immunocytochemistry, and absent in the pre-immune serum. * A positive signal could be detected by immunocytochemistry but not by western blot.

As rabbits and guinea pigs are two species of interest for the production of polyclonal antibodies and as both of these species generated specific antibodies with our protocol, we carried out a systematic comparison between them by injecting the same six plasmids into these two species. For three of those plasmids (those expressing mouse NTPDase1, human ecto-5′-nucleotidase and rat ecto-5′-nucleotidase), antisera with similar signal intensities versus background were obtained in both species. The data are presented for human ecto-5′-nucleotidase and rat ecto-5′-nucleotidase in Figure 1A,B, respectively. On the other hand, for the three other plasmids (human NTPDase1, mouse NTPDase3 and mouse NTPDase8), rabbits failed to produce specific antibodies, while guinea pigs produced, again, highly specific antibodies with low background, as seen by immune blot (Figure 1 and data not shown). Among the 10 rabbits immunized with the latter three plasmids, five rabbits gave a weak positive signal with high background in western blot for the plasmids encoding human NTPDase1 (two/two rabbits), mouse NTPDase3 (three/five rabbits), mouse NTPDase8 (zero/three rabbits). In contrast, among the 17 guinea pigs injected with those three cDNAs, 11 guinea pigs gave a strong signal without background and five other guinea pigs showed a moderate, but clean, signal in western blot: human NTPDase1 (three/three guinea pigs), mouse NTPDase3 (three/three guinea pigs), mouse NTPDase8 (10/11 guinea pigs). Most of the antisera produced are presented in Figure 1. In general, guinea pigs generated antisera with higher titer and lower background than rabbits.

All antisera were also tested by immunocytochemistry and immunohistochemistry, and the positive ones by flow cytometry. Nearly all of the antisera that gave a positive signal by western blot in non-reducing conditions also detected the protein of interest by immunocytochemistry, immunohistochemistry and flow cytometry, and vice versa. The antiserum mN3-3$_c$ against mouse NTPDase3 (rabbit "12" in Figure 1D) is presented as an example in Figure 2 and the specificity for the antisera mN1-1$_c$ and rN3-1$_L$ are presented in Figure 3.

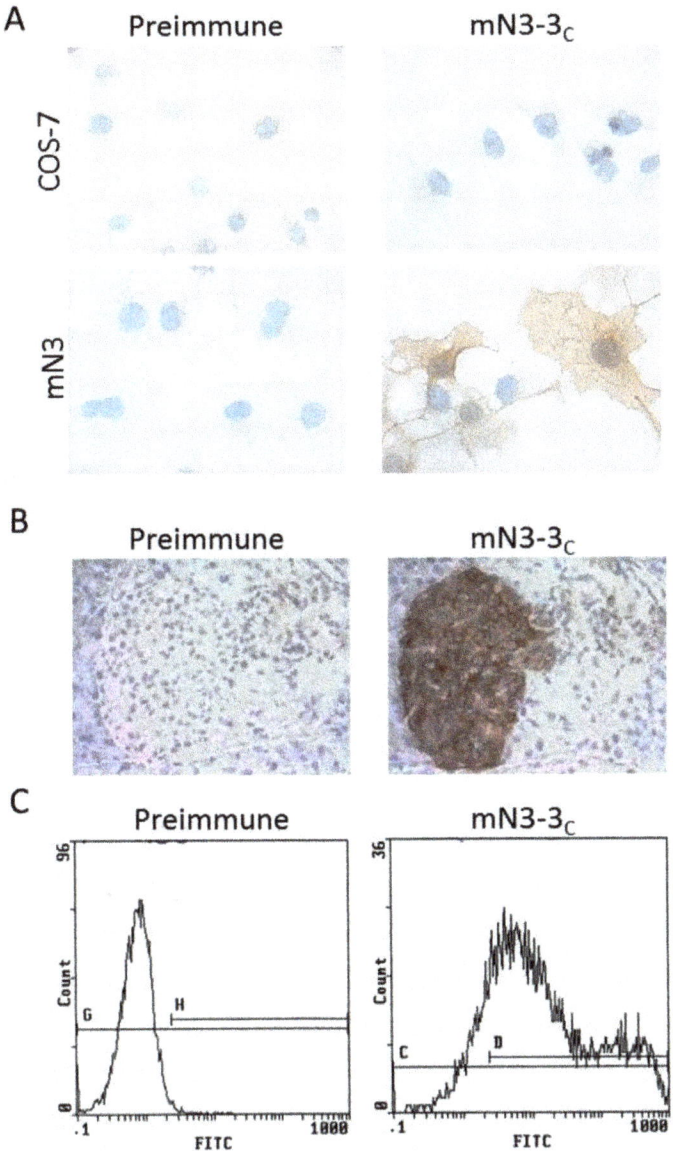

Figure 2. Specificity of the guinea pig anti-mouse NTPDase3 antibody mN3-3$_c$. (**A**) Strong signals in immunocytochemistry of transfected COS-7 cells with a plasmid encoding mouse NTPDase3 (mN3) are only detected with antiserum mN3-3$_c$ (rabbit "12" in Figure 1D). No signals are detected with the pre-immune serum or with the anti-serum on un-transfected cells (COS-7). (**B**) Immuno- histochemistry of serial sections from a mouse pancreas. The antiserum displays a positive reaction on the cells of the Langerhans islets. (**C**) Flow cytometry of transfected HEK 293T cells with a plasmid encoding mouse NTPDase3 shows a rightward shift (right panel) when compared to its pre-immune control (left panel). Nuclei were stained in blue with hematoxylin (**A**,**B**).

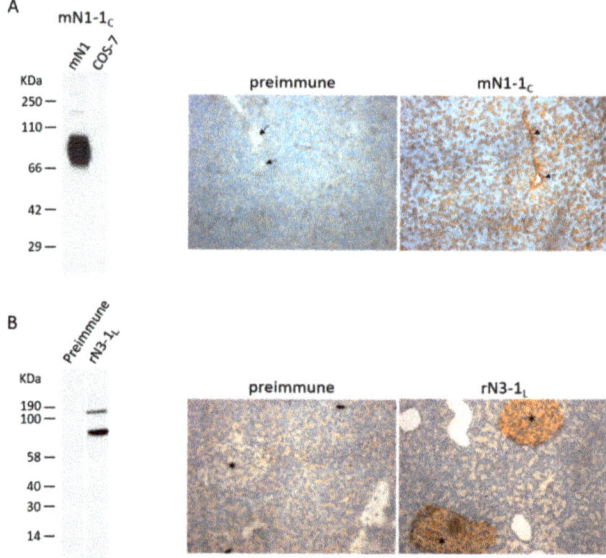

Figure 3. Specificity of the guinea pig anti-mouse NTPDase1 antibody mN1-1$_c$ (**A**) and of the rabbit anti-rat NTPDase3 antibody rN3-1$_L$ (**B**) analyzed by immunoblot (left panels) or by immunohistochemistry (right panels). A) Immunoblot of lysates from COS-7 cells transfected with plasmids encoding mouse NTPDase1 (mN1) or from untransfected COS-7 cells (COS-7). A strong reaction is observed in the transfected cell lysate only. Right panel shows immunohistochemical staining of a mouse pancreas section incubated with the antiserum mN1-1$_c$ or with the pre-immune serum. The antiserum displays a strong positive reaction on blood vessels shown by arrows and on zymogen granules in pancreatic acinar cells. (**B**) Immunoblot of lysates from COS-7 cells transfected with plasmids encoding rat NTPDase3 incubated with the antiserum rN3-1$_L$ or with its pre-immune serum shows a strong reaction only with the antiserum. NTPDase3 is detected as both a monomer and a dimer. Right panels show immunohistochemical staining of rat pancreas sections incubated with the antiserum or the pre-immune serum. The antiserum displays a positive reaction on Langerhans islet cells which are indicated by a star. Nuclei were stained in blue with hematoxylin in immunohistochemistry. The antisera were diluted 1:500 except for mN1-1$_c$ in the immunoblot (**A**) that was diluted 1:5000.

2.2. Mouse Monoclonal Antibodies

We also tested the ability of the above-described cDNA-based immunization technique to generate monoclonal antibodies in the mouse. To produce monoclonal antibodies, we first tested if the ID and IM injections could induce a sufficiently strong immune response to subsequently isolate monoclonal antibodies. The ID and IM injection procedures, with or without electroporation, were unsuccessful. Although electroporation have previously been reported as an immunization technique to produce monoclonal antibodies [11], we did not succeed to get a hybridoma producing a desired immunoglobulin after four to seven injections of cDNA coding for the protein of interest in two rats and two mice. To increase the titers and to get better chances in obtaining positive hybridomas, we injected HEK 293T cells transiently overexpressing human NTPDase2 to a mouse that was injected with the same plasmid encoding human NTPDase2 and that was treated by electroporation. The injection of transfected cells was done with cells never seen by the animal and the ELISA screening assay was performed with another transfected cells lines, COS-7, to eliminate false positives as much as possible. This led to the production of four hybridomas producing excellent monoclonal antibodies [12]. We then tested if the injections of HEK 293T that produces the protein of interest would also be successful in a mouse that received only IM and ID injections. From seven fusions performed in these conditions for human NTPDase1, human NTPDase2, human NTPDase3, human NTPDase8 and human Rank, three fusion procedures allowed us to obtain hybridomas that produced monoclonal antibodies against human NTPDase3 [13,14], human NTPDase8 [15] and human RANK. These data suggest that ID and IM injections, without electroporation, can be sufficient to prime the animals, and that a final injection with the recombinant protein expressed by transfected cells induces a rapid and high production of activated B cells suitable for the isolation of specific hybridomas.

2.3. Protocol Proposed

The above data led us to propose the protocol in Table 3 that we now routinely use for rabbits, guinea pigs and mice. The plasmid containing the protein of interest is injected at ID sites and at IM sites at an interval of 2 to 3 weeks for the first three injections and then at 8 to 10 weeks intervals for the two subsequent injections. For guinea pigs and rabbits, we suggest testing a serum sample after the third and fourth injection to identify the good responders. If a strong immunoreaction is observed after the third injection, rabbits and guinea pigs should be exsanguinated after a fourth and final immunization. If guinea pigs and rabbits do not respond after the fourth injection, they should be sacrificed as they will unlikely respond with more injections. On the other hand, five cDNA immunization procedures should be done in mice before selecting the best one for the final injection before fusion with myeloma cells.

Table 3. Proposed protocol to raise polyclonal and monoclonal antibodies by cDNA immunization.

Species	Route	Number of Sites × Volume per Site	DNA Concentration (mg/mL)	DNA Injected per Immunization (µg)	Injection Intervals (Weeks between Each Injection)		Blood Collection (Days after Injection)	Spleen Collection (Days after Transfected Cell Injection *)	Number of Animals per Antigen
					Injection 1 to 3	Injection 3 to 5 #			
Rabbit	ID	6–10 × 50 µL	0.5–0.8	500–800 &	2–3	8 ¶	13–14	N/A	3–5
	IM	2–4 × 125–250 µL							
Guinea pig	ID	2 × 50 µL	1	200	2–3	8 ¶	12–13	N/A	2–3
	IM	1 × 100 µL							
Mouse	ID	2 × 25 µL	1	100	2–3	7 ¶	12–13	3	5–10
	IM	1 × 50 µL							

The final injection before the fusion with SP2/0 cells should be done with 10 to 18 million HEK 293T transfected cells using a high efficiency transfection system. Other related cell lines can be used for transfection. # If a strong immunoreaction is observed after the third injection, rabbits and guinea pigs should be exsanguinated after a fourth and final immunization. & A lower amount of plasmids (650 ± 50 µg) is suggested for the first four injections, and a higher amount (800 µg) for the last injection. ¶ As the animals remain primed for several weeks to months, the intervals between the last injections can be longer.

As reliability to get antibodies is better in the guinea pig species, we suggest a lower number of guinea pigs (two or three) than rabbits (three to five) or mice (five to 10). Indeed, we obtained similar excellent antisera in all responding guinea pigs tested, which was not the case for the two other species. As mice exhibited a highly variable response from animal to animal (57% of the mice responded positively) while not requiring large amounts of plasmids, and having low housing costs, it would be wise to use two cages of mice (eight–10 mice) in order to get a better probability in obtaining a high responder in the first four or five injections to be selected for the final injection with transfected cells and for fusion with myeloma cells. The final injection can be done with 10 to 18 million HEK 293T cells transfected with the same plasmid used for the ID and IM injections. We recommend collecting the spleen three days later to perform the fusion with SP2/0 myelomas cells.

3. Discussion

We produced in the last two decades several antibodies using cDNA immunization techniques. We tested different strategies that finally led us to propose the protocol presented in Table 3 that we now use routinely in guinea pigs. When larger amount of serum or when antibodies from different species are necessary, or in the rare case where guinea pigs do not respond, we also use rabbits. Obviously, when a monoclonal antibody is necessary, we do it in mice with a similar protocol, also presented in Table 3, with the difference that we perform a final injection with the recombinant proteins to elicit a faster and stronger response using an expression cell system that has never been seen by the immunized animals. Indeed, the injection of HEK 293T cells expressing the protein of interest three days before the fusion procedure was more successful to obtain clones expressing the monoclonal antibodies of interest than injecting only DNA for all immunization steps. Other groups have also come to the same conclusion [16,17]. Obviously, this last injection would be inappropriate when generating polyclonal antibodies as the background would be expected to increase, which is not an issue when producing monoclonal antibodies as the desired B cells are cloned. Along the same line, it may be advantageous to transfect a mouse cell line for the final injection to reduce the number of false positive clones, but this might trigger a weaker immunological response and cause lower chances in getting hybridomas. This could be a subject for future improvement.

Guinea pigs are often the only species that we now immunize as they are high responders to this protocol and the response is generally similar from one animal to the other, which was not the case with mice and rabbits. There is therefore no need to inject five or six guinea pigs with our technique, as is often suggested in immunization protocols for most animals. Another advantage of using guinea pigs over rabbits is the much lower amount of DNA necessary (three–four times less) to trigger an antibody response. Depending of the animal facilities, housing costs for guinea pigs are also generally less expensive than rabbits.

Antibody response has been reported to be increased when injecting the cDNA in lymph nodes, or when using electroporation, but as plasmids can be easily produced in large amount, and with an extremely high purity, it is much easier to produce more plasmids to inject at ID and IM sites rather than to inject in the lymph nodes to save some plasmids. This is especially important when the surgery skills are not at hand. The same situation applies when comparing the technique that we present in Table 3 with other techniques using expensive technologies such as the injection of gold or tungsten conjugated particles with a gene gun. As the technique presented in Table 3 is efficient and easy to perform, there is no need to buy expensive equipment or to use unnecessarily sophisticated techniques.

cDNA immunization technique, as presented here, elicited an antibody response that reacted against the antigen in its native form. This is of interest when using plasmids encoding mammalian protein antigens to immunize guinea pigs, rabbits or mice that will perform mammalian post-translational modifications, although they can differ slightly between mammalian species. As post-translational modifications are different in non-mammalian species, the protocol proposed here might not be as efficient to raise antibodies against antigens in their native forms when they originate from non-mammalian sources, such as for antigens from prokaryotes or plants. This will depend on the epitope(s) selected by the host animal. Another issue, especially when using non mammalian antigens, is to make sure that the expression level of the gene is adequate in the host animal. This can be corrected or ameliorated by codon optimization of the gene of interest. In agreement with this idea, an increased antibody response was reported by a few groups after optimizing the codon sequences of some HIV genes [18–21]. Post-translational modifications and codon optimization could therefore represent a subject for future amelioration of cDNA immunization.

Another point to consider when using this technique is the protein location after its expression from the plasmid. Indeed, as we did in this paper, cDNA immunization has mostly been used to produce antibodies against transmembrane proteins. Several groups have also reported some success in generating antibodies against intracellular and secreted proteins by gene gun [22,23] or electroporation [24–26]. Efficiency to produce antibodies against an intracellular protein by injecting cDNA at ID or IM sites differs from group to group. Few studies have compared the same intracellular protein with or without a signal peptide to mediate protein secretion. In one of these studies, a plasmid with or without such a signal sequence was injected IM and a similar antibody response was reported for both plasmids [27]. Other studies reported a better efficiency when a signal sequence was added to a gene coding for an intracellular antigen [28,29]. In the results presented here, the majority of the plasmids encoded a transmembrane protein which led to specific antibody in 80% (41 out of 51) in guinea pigs, 60% (33 out of 55) in rabbits and 57% (16 out of 28) in mice. In our study, we did not succeed to raise antibodies in rabbits (zero out of 11) injected with a plasmid coding for an intracellular protein. The immune responses to an antigen encoded by plasmids coding for secreted proteins were slightly stronger. Although we did not succeed in guinea pigs (zero out of three) a few rabbits (two out of eight) produced antibodies against a secreted protein. Another alternative to get antibodies to soluble proteins is to modify the protein by adding a transmembrane domain to direct the protein to the external surface of the plasma membrane. We tested this idea with one plasmid, which successfully produced antibodies in one out of five mice (unpublished data in collaboration with Dr J. Fietto, Universidade federal de Viçosa, Brazil). This is another avenue of study to make cDNA immunization more efficient for more protein types.

As there is no immunization technique that works all the time, when should we stop to immunize an animal with our protocol presented on Table 3? We observed that when there was no positive signal after the fourth injection in guinea pigs and in rabbits, there was limited chance to obtain a good antiserum by doing additional injections. Indeed, the few times that a fifth injection was positive for the guinea pigs, the titer was too low to be useful for a research purpose. Therefore, we now sacrifice all guinea pigs and rabbits that do not give a good response in the first four immunizations. On the other hand, injecting a good responder too many times might not be beneficial, and on the contrary, the antibody response might decrease and the background signals may increase. Accordingly, when a rabbit or a guinea pig responds well at the third injection, it should be exsanguinated after the fourth injection. Our observations were different in mice as we observed some mice that did not react at the fourth injection but gave an interesting response after the fifth injection. But as this was seen only in a few mice (four out of 10) with the same plasmid, we cannot draw any definitive conclusions at the moment concerning this point. Nevertheless, it might be safer to try a fifth DNA injection before sacrificing mice. Indeed, according to our results, mice often required five cDNA injections to get a strong positive signal.

4. Materials and Methods

4.1. Materials

Hypoxanthine-aminopterin-thymidine solution, hypoxanthine-thymidine solution, poly-ethylene glycol and bovine serum albumin were purchased from Sigma-Aldrich (Oakville, ON, Canada). Dulbecco's modified Eagle's medium and Lipofectamine were obtained from Life Technologies (Burlington, ON, Canada). Fetal bovine serum (FBS), phosphate-buffered saline (PBS), antibiotic/antimycotic and HCell-100 hybridomas media were purchased from Wisent (St-Bruno, QC, Canada). Secondary antibodies conjugated to horseradish peroxidase (HRP) were obtained from: goat anti-mouse IgG (H + L) from Jackson ImmunoResearch Laboratories Inc. (West Grove, PA, USA), goat anti-guinea pig from Santa Cruz Biotechnology (Dallas, TX, USA), donkey anti-rabbit from GE Healthcare Life Sciences (Baie d'Urfe, QC, Canada). The secondary goat anti-guinea pig antibody conjugated to biotin was from Jackson ImmunoResearch Laboratories Inc. (West Grove, PA, USA). Enhanced K-Blue® Substrate was from Neogen Corporation (Lansing, MI, USA).

4.2. Animals

Female New Zealand rabbits (4 months), Hartley guinea pigs (6–7 weeks), BALB/c mice (4–6 weeks), Sprague-Dawley rats (7 weeks), LVG Golden Syrian hamsters (7 weeks), were obtained from Charles River Laboratories (St-Constant, QC, Canada). For two antigen series, rabbits (four) were 9–10 weeks old. All procedures were approved by the Canadian Council on Animal Care and the Université Laval Animal Welfare Committee (protocol number: 2001-120; 2004-179; 2007-124; 2010-102; 2013-108; 2017-109).

4.3. Immunization

Complementary DNA (cDNA) was prepared using Endofree plasmid kits from Qiagen (Toronto, ON, Canada) and diluted in PBS 0.8× at a concentration range of 0.5–1 mg/mL. Intradermal (ID) or intramuscular (IM) injections were performed in the dorsal skin or in a thigh, respectively. Two groups of rabbits received the cDNA in the popliteal lymph node(s). This injection route was performed once during the injection schedule and the rabbits received ID and IM injections for the other injections. In one of these groups, rabbits received DNA coding for mouse NTPDase3 in popliteal lymph nodes of both legs at the second injection in addition to ID injections. In the second group, rabbits received DNA coding for rat NTPDase6 in a popliteal lymph node of one leg at the first injection, in addition to ID and IM injection. Specific information related to the number of sites, amount injected and injection schedule is reported in Table 1. Each animal received at least five series of immunization to assure adequate priming. In some cases, animal received up to nine series of immunization.

4.4. Electroporation

Mice and guinea pigs received DNA followed by an electroporation as previously described [9,12]. Briefly, an IM injection of DNA diluted in Hank's balanced salt solution or in PBS, for the mouse or the guinea pig, respectively, was made in the tibialis anterior. After application of an electrode cream on the skin, electroporation was carried out at the site of DNA injection with two electrode plates connected to an electroporator according to the following parameters: seven pulses of 100 $V.cm^{-1}$ and a duration of 20 ms.

4.5. Blood Collection

Blood was collected before the first injection and 11 to 15 days after the second injection when an electroporation was performed, or after each injection after the third one. Blood was collected in spray-coated silica tubes with or without gel separator or in regular microcentrifuge tubes. Tubes were let in the upright position for 1–2 h at room temperature (RT) to allow clot formation, and were then centrifuged at 1500× *g* for 10–30 min depending on the blood volume. A final concentration of 10% glycerol was added to the serum which was then aliquoted and stored at −80 °C until needed.

4.6. Monoclonal Antibodies Raised in Mice

After four to six DNA injections with or without electroporation, as described in Table 1, some mice received a final injection of DNA, and others an injection of human embryonic kidney (HEK 293T) transfected cells. These cells were transfected with Lipofectamine as previously described [30] with the same plasmid used for the previous immunization procedures. Then, 2 days after transfection, the cells were washed twice with PBS and the cells were detached by a 2–5 min incubation at 37 °C in a citric saline solution (135 mM potassium chloride, 15 mM sodium citrate). Cells were centrifuged, resuspended in PBS and counted. The mouse received a final intraperitoneal injection of 10 to 18 million of transfected HEK 293T. The fusion procedure was performed either 6–7 days, or 3 days, after this final injection of DNA, or the cell suspension, respectively. Blood and spleen cells were collected after this final injection and fusion with SP2/0 cells was done as described [13]. The supernatant was screened by ELISA and the positive hybridomas were cloned by limiting dilution. In a few assays, a hybridomas optimized medium, Hcell-100, was used for the clone isolation procedures. The produced immunoglobulins were purified on Protein A Sepharose CL-4B column as described [13].

4.7. ELISA

ELISA was performed as previously described [15]. In brief, protein extract (500 ng per well) from untransfected African green monkey kidney (COS-7) cells or transiently transfected with the plasmid used for immunization diluted in PBS was distributed in a 96 well ELISA plate and incubated overnight at 4 °C. The wells were then washed with PBS-Tween 0.05% (PBS-T) and incubated for 1 h at 37 °C in a blocking solution (0.5% bovine serum albumin diluted in PBS-T). After washing, the supernatant from each hybridoma was added to a well and incubated for 2 h at RT, followed by four washing steps. Then, a goat anti-mouse IgG (H + L)-HRP (1:2500) diluted in the blocking solution was incubated for 2 h at RT, followed by four washing steps. The Enhanced K-Blue® Substrate was then added for 15 min and the reaction was stopped by the addition of an equal volume of 2 N sulphuric acid. The absorbance at 450 nm was then recorded.

4.8. Isotyping

Mouse Immunoglobulin Isotyping ELISA Kit (BD Bioscience, Mississauga, ON, Canada) was used to determine the isotypes produced by the hybridomas, according to the manufacturer's instruction and as previously described [15]. In brief, monoclonal rat anti-mouse IgG1, IgG2a, IgG2b, IgG3, IgA and IgM were coated O/N in 96-well plates. A blocking treatment was performed after washing steps, and then each monoclonal antibody was transferred to the wells. After four washing steps, rat anti-mouse Igs conjugated to HRP was added to each well, and revealed with a substrate provided in the kit. The plate was then read at 450 nm.

4.9. Western Blot

COS-7 cells and HEK 293T cells were cultured and transiently transfected with the indicated cDNA construct as described previously [30]. For western blot assays, lysates from transfected COS-7 cells or HEK 293T cells were resuspended in NuPAGE LDS sample buffer, separated on NuPAGE 4–12% Bis-Tris gels under non-reduced conditions, and transferred to an Immobilon-P membrane (Millipore, Bedford, MA, USA) by electroblotting according to the manufacturer's recommendation and as previously described [15]. Membranes were then blocked with 2.5% non-fat milk in PBS containing 0.15% Tween20 (pH 7.4) O/N at 4°C and subsequently probed with the primary antibodies using the Mini-Protean II multiscreen apparatus (Bio-Rad Laboratories Ltd., Mississauga, ON, Canada) in which 20 antibodies can be tested on one gel. Appropriate secondary HRP-conjugated antibodies were used, and the membranes developed with the western Lightning^{TM} Plus-ECL system (PerkinElmer Life and Analytical Sciences, Waltham, MA, USA).

4.10. Immunocytochemistry and Immunohistochemistry

Immunocytochemistry and immunohistochemistry were performed as previously described [15]. Tissues were frozen in Tissue-Tek®O.C.T.^{TM} Compound (Sakura Finetek, Torrance, CA, USA). COS-7 cells or tissue sections (6 μm thick) were fixed with cold acetone and 10% phosphate-buffered formalin (Fisher Scientific, Ottawa, ON, Canada) (19:1) and blocked in a PBS solution containing 7% normal goat serum for 30 min. COS-7 cells and tissue sections were incubated with the indicated primary antibody at 4 °C or pre-immune serum as a negative control. COS-7 cells and tissue sections were then treated with 0.15% H_2O_2 in PBS for 10 min to inactivate endogenous peroxidase, and with an avidin/biotin solution (Avidin/Biotin Blocking kit; Vector Laboratories, Burlington, ON, Canada) to prevent non-specific staining due to endogenous biotin. This step was followed by incubation with an appropriate biotin-conjugated secondary antibody at a dilution of 1:1000. The avidin–biotinylated HRP complex (VectaStain Elite ABC kit; Vector Laboratories) was added to optimize the reaction. Peroxidase activity was revealed with DAB as the substrate. Nuclei were counterstained with aqueous hematoxylin (Biomeda, Foster City, CA, USA) in accordance with the manufacturer's instructions.

4.11. Flow Cytometry

Flow cytometry was performed as previously described [15]. Briefly, HEK 293T cells transfected with the plasmid expressing the antigen were detached from the plates with a citric saline solution (135 mM potassium chloride, 15 mM sodium citrate). Cells were washed with an ice-cold PBS solution containing 1% FBS and 0.1% NaN_3 (fluorescence-activated cell sorting (FACS) buffer) followed by incubation with the immune serum or the pre-immune serum in FACS buffer for 1 h. After washes with FACS buffer solution, the cells were incubated with the appropriate FITC-conjugated secondary antibody (Jackson ImmunoResearch Laboratories Inc., West Grove, PA, USA) for 30 min on ice, washed with FACS buffer, and analyzed by flow cytometry (BD LSR II, BD Biosciences, San Jose, CA USA).

5. Conclusions

In this paper we propose a detailed protocol for cDNA immunization in guinea pigs and rabbits for the production of polyclonal antibodies and in mice for the generation of monoclonal antibodies. The procedure does not require any sophisticated technical expertise nor any specialized equipment. This protocol works especially well in guinea pigs which produce antisera with high specificity and extremely low background in a consistent manner, allowing the use of fewer animals per antigen to reduce effective costs, especially when comparing with larger animals. To generate monoclonal antibodies in mice, we propose to perform the last injection with a suspension of cells expressing the recombinant protein at a high level.

Author Contributions: Conceptualization, J.S.; Methodology, J.P., E.G.L. and J.S.; Validation, J.P., H.A., F.M., E.G.L., M.S., P.L., R.B.B.K. and J.S.; Formal analysis, J.P.; Investigation, J.S.; Resources, J.S.; Data Curation, J.P., E.G.L. and J.S.; Writing—Original Draft Preparation, J.P.; Writing—Review and Editing, J.S.; Visualization, J.P.; Supervision, J.S.; Project Administration, J.S.; Funding Acquisition, J.S. All authors have read and agreed to the published version of the manuscript.

Funding: This work was supported by grants to J. Sévigny from the Natural Sciences and Engineering Research Council of Canada (NSERC; RGPIN-2016-05867). J.S. was also a recipient of a "Chercheur National" Scholarship from the Fonds de Recherche du Québec-Santé (FRQS). H. Agonsanou was a recipient of a scholarship from the Ministère de la Santé publique du Bénin, F. Manica of a scholarship from The Canadian Bureau for International Education, E.G. Lavoie and M. Salem of a scholarship from the FRQS, P. Luyindula of a scholarship from the Canadian Francophonie Scholarship Program and R.B. Babou Kammoe of a studentship from Université Laval.

Acknowledgments: The authors thank the following research teams with whom some of the antibodies presented here were generated and characterized: Paul H. Naccache, Maria J. Fernandes, Patrice E. Poubelle, Sylvain G. Bourgoin (Québec, Canada), Simon C. Robson (Boston, USA) and Herbert Zimmermann (Frankfurt am Main, Germany). We also thank Aileen F. Knowles (San Diego, USA; human NTPDase2), Terence L. Kirley (Cincinnati, USA; human NTPDase3 and human NTPDase6), James W. Goding (Victoria, Australia; human NPP1), Kimihiko Sano (Kobe, Japan; human NPP2 and human NPP3) and Mathieu Bollen (Leuven, Belgium; mouse NPP1) for providing the indicated expression plasmids used in this study. We are also grateful to Paul H. Naccache for editing this manuscript.

Conflicts of Interest: The authors declare no conflict of interest.

Abbreviations

cDNA	Complementary DNA
COS-7	African green monkey kidney cells
DAB	3, 3′ diaminobenzidine
ELISA	Enzyme-linked immunosorbent assay
FBS	Fetal bovine serum
FRQS	Fonds de Recherche du Québec – Santé
HEK 293T	Human embryonic kidney 293T cells
HRP	Horseradish peroxidase
ID	Intradermal
IM	Intramuscular
PBS	Phosphate-buffered saline
PBS-T	PBS-Tween
Pi	Pre-immune serum
RT	Room temperature
NSERC	Natural Sciences and Engineering Research Council of Canada

References

1. Tang, D.C.; DeVit, M.; Johnston, S.A. Genetic immunization is a simple method for eliciting an immune response. *Nature* **1992**, *356*, 152–154. [CrossRef] [PubMed]

2. Aoyama, T.; Kamata, K.; Yamanaka, N.; Takeuchi, Y.; Higashihara, M.; Kato, S. Characteristics of polyclonal anti-human nephrin antibodies induced by genetic immunization using nephrin cDNA. *Nephrol. Dial. Transplant.* **2006**, *21*, 1073–1081. [CrossRef] [PubMed]
3. Morel, P.A.; Falkner, D.; Plowey, J.; Larregina, A.T.; Falo, L.D. DNA immunisation: Altering the cellular localisation of expressed protein and the immunisation route allows manipulation of the immune response. *Vaccine* **2004**, *22*, 447–456. [CrossRef] [PubMed]
4. Donnelly, J.J.; Friedman, A.; Martinez, D.; Montgomery, D.L.; Shiver, J.W.; Motzel, S.L.; Ulmer, J.B.; Liu, M.A. Preclinical efficacy of a prototype DNA vaccine: Enhanced protection against antigenic drift in influenza virus. *Nat. Med.* **1995**, *1*, 583–587. [CrossRef]
5. Diestre, C.; Martínez-Lorenzo, M.; Bosque, A.; Naval, J.; Larrad, L.; Anel, A. Generation of rabbit antibodies against death ligands by cDNA immunization. *J. Immunol. Methods* **2006**, *317*, 12–20. [CrossRef]
6. Schultheis, K.; Schaefer, H.; Yung, B.S.; Oh, J.; Muthumani, K.; Humeau, L.; Broderick, K.E.; Smith, T.R. Characterization of guinea pig T cell responses elicited after EP-assisted delivery of DNA vaccines to the skin. *Vaccine* **2016**, *35*, 61–70. [CrossRef]
7. Cashman, K.A.; Wilkinson, E.R.; Wollen-Roberts, S.E.; Shamblin, J.D.; Zelko, J.M.; Bearss, J.J.; Zeng, X.; Broderick, K.E.; Schmaljohn, C.S. DNA vaccines elicit durable protective immunity against individual or simultaneous infections with Lassa and Ebola viruses in guinea pigs. *Hum. Vaccines Immunother.* **2017**, *13*, 3010–3019. [CrossRef]
8. Maloy, K.J.; Erdmann, I.; Basch, V.; Sierro, S.; Kramps, T.A.; Zinkernagel, R.M.; Oehen, S.; Kündig, T.M. Intralymphatic immunization enhances DNA vaccination. *Proc. Natl. Acad. Sci. USA* **2001**, *98*, 3299–3303. [CrossRef]
9. Widera, G.; Austin, M.; Rabussay, D.; Goldbeck, C.; Barnett, S.W.; Chen, M.; Leung, L.; Otten, G.R.; Thudium, K.; Selby, M.J.; et al. Increased DNA vaccine delivery and immunogenicity by electroporation in vivo. *J. Immunol.* **2000**, *164*, 4635–4640. [CrossRef]
10. Sardesai, N.Y.; Weiner, D.B. Electroporation delivery of DNA vaccines: Prospects for success. *Curr. Opin. Immunol.* **2011**, *23*, 421–429. [CrossRef]
11. Yang, L.; Cheong, N.; Wang, D.Y.; Lee, B.W.; Kuo, I.C.; Huang, C.H.; Chua, K.Y. Generation of monoclonal antibodies against Blot 3 using DNA immunization with in vivo electroporation. *Clin. Exp. Allergy* **2003**, *33*, 663–668. [CrossRef] [PubMed]
12. Pelletier, J.; Agonsanou, H.; Delvalle, N.; Fausther, M.; Salem, M.; Gulbransen, B.; Sévigny, J. Generation and characterization of polyclonal and monoclonal antibodies to human NTPDase2 including a blocking antibody. *Purinergic Signal.* **2017**, *13*, 293–304. [CrossRef]
13. Munkonda, M.N.; Pelletier, J.; Ivanenkov, V.V.; Fausther, M.; Tremblay, A.; Kunzli, B.; Kirley, T.L.; Sévigny, J. Characterization of a monoclonal antibody as the first specific inhibitor of human NTP diphosphohydrolase-3: Partial characterization of the inhibitory epitope and potential applications. *FEBS J.* **2009**, *276*, 479–496. [CrossRef] [PubMed]
14. Saunders, D.C.; Brissova, M.; Phillips, N.; Shrestha, S.; Walker, J.T.; Aramandla, R.; Poffenberger, G.; Flaherty, D.K.; Weller, K.P.; Pelletier, J.; et al. Ectonucleoside triphosphate diphosphohydrolase-3 antibody targets adult human pancreatic beta cells for in vitro and in vivo analysis. *Cell Metab.* **2018**, *29*, 745–754. [CrossRef] [PubMed]
15. Pelletier, J.; Salem, M.; Lecka, J.; Fausther, M.; Bigonnesse, F.; Sévigny, J. Generation and characterization of specific antibodies to the murine and human ectonucleotidase NTPDase8. *Front. Pharmacol.* **2017**, *8*, 115. [CrossRef]
16. Nagata, S.; Salvatore, G.; Pastan, I. DNA immunization followed by a single boost with cells: A protein-free immunization protocol for production of monoclonal antibodies against the native form of membrane proteins. *J. Immunol. Methods* **2003**, *280*, 59–72. [CrossRef]
17. Chu, T.T.; Halverson, G.R.; Yazdanbakhsh, K.; Øyen, R.; Reid, M. A DNA-based immunization protocol to produce monoclonal antibodies to blood group antigens. *Br. J. Haematol.* **2001**, *113*, 32–36. [CrossRef]
18. André, S.; Seed, B.; Eberle, J.; Schraut, W.; Bültmann, A.; Haas, J. Increased immune response elicited by DNA vaccination with a synthetic gp120 sequence with optimized codon usage. *J. Virol.* **1998**, *72*, 1497–1503. [CrossRef]

19. Deml, L.; Bojak, A.; Steck, S.; Graf, M.; Wild, J.; Schirmbeck, R.; Wolf, H.; Wagner, R. Multiple effects of codon usage optimization on expression and immunogenicity of DNA candidate vaccines encoding the human immunodeficiency virus type 1 gag protein. *J. Virol.* **2001**, *75*, 10991–11001. [CrossRef]
20. Megede, J.Z.; Chen, M.-C.; Doe, B.; Schaefer, M.; Greer, C.E.; Selby, M.; Otten, G.R.; Barnett, S.W. Increased expression and immunogenicity of sequence-modified human immunodeficiency virus type 1 gag gene. *J. Virol.* **2000**, *74*, 2628–2635. [CrossRef]
21. Wang, S.; Farfan-Arribas, D.J.; Shen, S.; Chou, T.H.W.; Hirsch, A.; He, F.; Lu, S. Relative contributions of codon usage, promoter efficiency and leader sequence to the antigen expression and immunogenicity of HIV-1 Env DNA vaccine. *Vaccine* **2006**, *24*, 4531–4540. [CrossRef] [PubMed]
22. García, J.F.; García, J.F.; Maestre, L.; Lucas, E.; Sánchez-Verde, L.; Romero-Chala, S.; Piris, M.Á.; Roncador, G. Genetic immunization: A new monoclonal antibody for the detection of BCL-6 protein in paraffin sections. *J. Histochem. Cytochem.* **2006**, *54*, 31–38. [CrossRef] [PubMed]
23. Maestre, L.; Fontán, L.; Martinez-Climent, J.A.; Garcia, J.F.; Cigudosa, J.C.; Roncador, G. Generation of a new monoclonal antibody against MALT1 by genetic immunization. *Hybridoma* **2007**, *26*, 86–91. [CrossRef] [PubMed]
24. Leinonen, J.; Niemelä, P.; Lövgren, J.; Bocchi, L.; Pettersson, K.; Nevanlinna, H.; Stenman, U.-H. Characterization of monoclonal antibodies against prostate specific antigen produced by genetic immunization. *J. Immunol. Methods* **2004**, *289*, 157–167. [CrossRef] [PubMed]
25. Chen, Y.; Zhang, T.; Li, T.; Han, W.; Zhang, Y.; Ma, D. Preparation and characterization of a monoclonal antibody against CKLF1 using DNA immunization with in vivo electroporation. *Hybridoma* **2005**, *24*, 305–308. [CrossRef]
26. Daftarian, P.; Chowdhury, R.; Ames, P.; Wei, C.; King, A.D.; Vaccari, J.P.D.R.; Dillon, L.; Price, J.; Leung, H.; Ashlock, B.; et al. In vivo electroporation and non-protein based screening assays to identify antibodies against native protein conformations. *Hybridoma* **2011**, *30*, 409–418. [CrossRef]
27. Haddad, D.; Liljeqvist, S.; Stahl, S.; Andersson, I.; Perlmann, P.; Berzins, K.; Ahlborg, N. Comparative study of DNA-based immunization vectors: Effect of secretion signals on the antibody responses in mice. *FEMS Immunol. Med. Microbiol.* **1997**, *18*, 193–202.
28. Svanholm, C.; Bandholtz, L.; Lobell, A.; Wigzell, H. Enhancement of antibody responses by DNA immunization using expression vectors mediating efficient antigen secretion. *J. Immunol. Methods* **1999**, *228*, 121–130. [CrossRef]
29. Inchauspé, G.; Vitvitski, L.; Major, M.E.; Jung, G.; Spengler, U.; Maisonnas, M.; Trepo, C. Plasmid DNA expressing a secreted or a nonsecreted form of hepatitis C virus nucleocapsid: Comparative studies of antibody and T-helper responses following genetic immunization. *DNA Cell Biol.* **1997**, *16*, 185–195. [CrossRef]
30. Kukulski, F.; Lévesque, S.A.; Lavoie, É.G.; Lecka, J.; Bigonnesse, F.; Knowles, A.F.; Robson, S.C.; Kirley, T.L.; Sévigny, J. Comparative hydrolysis of P2 receptor agonists by NTPDases 1, 2, 3 and 8. *Purinergic Signal.* **2005**, *1*, 193–204. [CrossRef]

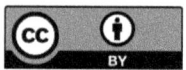

© 2020 by the authors. Licensee MDPI, Basel, Switzerland. This article is an open access article distributed under the terms and conditions of the Creative Commons Attribution (CC BY) license (http://creativecommons.org/licenses/by/4.0/).

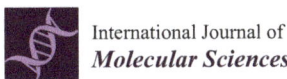 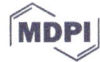

Article

Engineered Fragments of the PSMA-Specific 5D3 Antibody and Their Functional Characterization

Zora Novakova [1,*], Nikola Belousova [1], Catherine A. Foss [2], Barbora Havlinova [1], Marketa Gresova [1], Gargi Das [1], Ala Lisok [2], Adam Prada [1], Marketa Barinkova [1], Martin Hubalek [3], Martin G. Pomper [2] and Cyril Barinka [1,*]

1. Laboratory of Structural Biology, Institute of Biotechnology of the Czech Academy of Sciences, BIOCEV, Prumyslova 595, 252 50 Vestec, Czech Republic; nikolabelousova@gmail.com (N.B.); barbora.havlinova@ibt.cas.cz (B.H.); marketa.gresova@ibt.cas.cz (M.G.); gargi.das@ibt.cas.cz (G.D.); adamprada@gmail.com (A.P.); marketabarinkova@gmail.com (M.B.)
2. The Russell H. Morgan Department of Radiology and Radiological Science, Johns Hopkins Medical Institutions, 1550 Orleans St, Baltimore, MD 21231, USA; cfoss1@jhmi.edu (C.A.F.); alisok1@jhmi.edu (A.L.); mpomper@jhmi.edu (M.G.P.)
3. Mass Spectrometry Group, Institute of Organic Chemistry and Biochemistry of the Czech Academy of Sciences, IOCB & Gilead Research Center, Flemingovo náměstí 542/2, 160 00 Prague, Czech Republic; martin.hubalek@uochb.cas.cz
* Correspondence: zora.novakova@ibt.cas.cz (Z.N.); cyril.barinka@ibt.cas.cz (C.B.); Tel.: +42-0325-873-736 (Z.N.); +42-0325-873-777 (C.B.)

Received: 18 August 2020; Accepted: 9 September 2020; Published: 12 September 2020

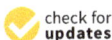

Abstract: Prostate-Specific Membrane Antigen (PSMA) is an established biomarker for the imaging and experimental therapy of prostate cancer (PCa), as it is strongly upregulated in high-grade primary, androgen-independent, and metastatic lesions. Here, we report on the development and functional characterization of recombinant single-chain Fv (scFv) and Fab fragments derived from the 5D3 PSMA-specific monoclonal antibody (mAb). These fragments were engineered, heterologously expressed in insect S2 cells, and purified to homogeneity with yields up to 20 mg/L. In vitro assays including ELISA, immunofluorescence and flow cytometry, revealed that the fragments retain the nanomolar affinity and single target specificity of the parent 5D3 antibody. Importantly, using a murine xenograft model of PCa, we verified the suitability of fluorescently labeled fragments for in vivo imaging of PSMA-positive tumors and compared their pharmacokinetics and tissue distribution to the parent mAb. Collectively, our data provide an experimental basis for the further development of 5D3 recombinant fragments for future clinical use.

Keywords: prostate-specific membrane antigen; in vivo imaging; prostate cancer; monoclonal antibody; antibody fragment; glutamate carboxypeptidase II; NAALADase

1. Introduction

The increasing length of the human lifespan brings about higher incidence of various health problems including cancer. Prostate cancer (PCa) holds a prominent position among tumor-associated diseases among elderly men in industrial countries due to its high incidence and associated mortality rates of metastatic disease [1–3]. To improve PCa prognosis, a combination of precise diagnosis of the tumor stage and specifically designed treatment plans is required. In the clinic today, PCa is routinely detected using imaging techniques such as bone scintigraphy, computed tomography, ultrasound, and magnetic resonance imaging (reviewed in [4]). However, there is still an untapped potential in PCa diagnostics and staging in terms of sensitivity and specificity. Thus, new PCa-specific reagents are extensively researched.

Antibody fragments are considered to be an excellent platform being developed for cancer-related diagnostic and therapeutic approaches, particularly for targeted therapy (reviewed by [5]). Single-chain variable fragments (scFv), Fab fragments and nanobodies are the primary medicinally relevant antibody fragments. They may serve as antigen-targeting moieties in various conjugates, fusion proteins, and bispecific molecules. In contrast to whole immunoglobulin complexes, fragments feature enhanced tumor penetration, fast blood clearance, optimal half-life and biodistribution, low immunogenicity, and low imaging background [6]. Due to these qualities, fragments promote the uptake of drugs by tumor cells, increase the specificity of anti-tumor drug delivery and reduce undesirable cytotoxic side effects in healthy tissues. Furthermore, they can trigger anti-tumor immune responses and collectively modulate the function of immune cells, as well as inhibit the proliferation of tumorigenic cells [7–10]. Coupled with radionuclides, fluorescent dyes, or nanoparticles, antibody fragments serve as imaging modalities for noninvasive detection and staging of tumors, and the evaluation of the surface molecule portfolio of cancer cells. Moreover, fragment-based imaging provides additional information beneficial for treatment including real-time fluorescence-guided surgery [11–14].

Prostate-specific membrane antigen (PSMA) is one of the leading PCa-specific biomarkers strongly expressed on PCa cells [15]. The specific presence of PSMA in primary, high-grade, androgen-independent, and metastatic PCa tumors predetermines the enzyme as a prime tool for PCa imaging and therapy [16–19]. Consequently, PSMA-specific antibodies are being developed as new PCa-targeting theranostics. Various constructs have already been tested in vitro on PSMA-expressing cells [20] as well as in vivo in relevant xenograft models [16,21–25]. Notably, PCa imaging in human patients has also been performed using a PSMA-specific ^{89}Zr-IAB2M minibody [26].

Several PSMA-targeting entities are being developed as PCa therapeutics. Site-specific delivery of Notch1-specific siRNA by an anti-PSMA scFv was documented to inhibit PCa tumor growth [27]. Multimeric structures derived from anti-PSMA scFv and bispecific molecules, namely anti-PSMA/anti-CD3 fusions, have been used in preclinical immunotherapy models [28–34]. Immunotoxin fusions derived from PSMA-specific scFvs showed efficient control of PCa xenografts and enhanced anti-tumor activity of cytotoxic drugs [35–38]. Interestingly, PSMA-specific antibody fragments were documented to direct the cytotoxicity of chimeric antigen receptor T cells (CAR-T cells) not only to PCa but also to ovarian cancer [39,40]. In virotherapy approaches, oncolytic viruses targeted to cancer cells via anti-PSMA scFv revealed potential to induce PCa regression [41,42].

In this report, we exploit the superior features of our newly developed 5D3 mAb, including sub-nanomolar affinity and a high specificity for native PSMA [43]. These characteristics make the 5D3 mAb particularly suitable for in vivo applications [44–46]. Here, we cloned, heterologously expressed, purified, and characterized engineered scFv and Fab fragments of 5D3. Affinity and specificity of the recombinant fragments comparable to the parent antibody, along with the demonstrated applicability for in vivo imaging suggests that the binding site remained intact and the function of the recombinant proteins was retained throughout the engineering process. The study shows a high potential for the further development of 5D3-based engineered molecules, which could enter clinical trials for PCa imaging and therapy.

2. Results

2.1. Identification of Nucleotide and Amino Acid Sequences of the 5D3 mAb

Using N-terminal amino acid sequencing, we identified DIQMTQTNS and EVQPQVSKTMA peptides to be N-termini of light and heavy chains of the 5D3 mAb, respectively. This information was then used to design degenerated PCR primers to amplify sequences encoding the light and heavy chain of the 5D3 Fab fragment using a cDNA template isolated from 5D3 hybridomas. The primary amino acid sequences of 5D3 Fab, as derived from the amplified nucleotide sequences, were then matched against mass spectrometry data of peptides from tryptic and chymotryptic digests of purified full-length 5D3 mAb. Thanks to the complete sequence coverage and 100% match between the predicted and experimental primary amino acid sequences, we verified that the amplified genes really encode the 5D3 mAb that can be used for further engineering efforts.

2.2. Characterization of 5D3 Antibody Fragments Produced in E. coli

To assess whether 5D3 recombinant antibody fragments retained the specificity and high affinity of the original 5D3 antibody, we cloned Fab and scFv fragments into vectors used for heterologous protein expression in the *E. coli* periplasmic space. For Fab production, sequences encoding 5D3 variable domains were cloned into a pASK85 bicistronic expression plasmid that carries genes for constant domains of mouse Cκ and CH1γ1 subclasses (Figure 1) [47,48]. In the case of scFvs, their folding and function is affected by the order of variable domains, the length of the linker between domains, the type of a signal sequence, and the presence and position of purification tags. Consequently, we designed two scFv constructs differing in the order of variable domains, denoted LH and HL, the position of a 6xHis-tag and the sequence of a secretion signal (Figure 1). An identical 18-mer linker was inserted between the heavy and light chain domains in both variants and constructs cloned into the pASK85 vector backbone. All recombinant proteins were secreted into the *E. coli* periplasmic space and purified by a single step nickel chelating affinity chromatography using established protocols [49]. Large scale expressions yielded on average 20–30 µg protein/liter culture with an estimated purity of >90% (Figure 2A).

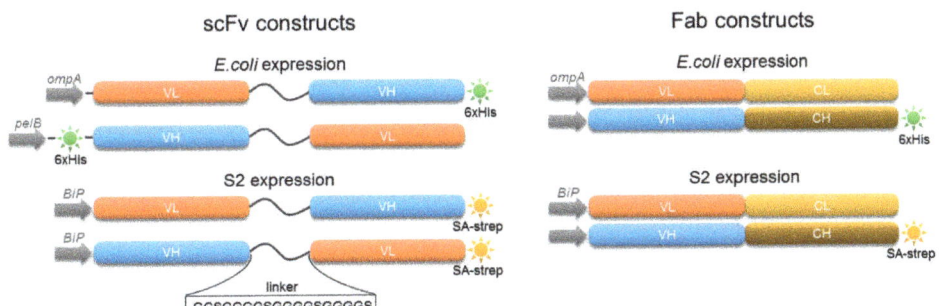

Figure 1. Schematic representation of 5D3 scFvs and Fab expressed by *E. coli* and insect S2 cells. Variants differ in the order of domains, the signal sequence and the type and position of an affinity tag. Signal sequences ompA, pelB, and BiP were inserted N-terminally to allow protein secretion. The SA-strep and 6× His tag positioned at either the N- or C-terminus were added for affinity purification. Variable domains of light (VL) and heavy (VH) chain were separated by an 18-mer linker identical in all scFv variants. Each Fab construct was composed of light (L) and heavy (H) chain consisting of variable (V) and constant (C) domain.

The specificity of purified antibody derivatives was evaluated by indirect immunofluorescence (IF) microscopy and flow cytometry using HEK293T cells overexpressing PSMA [43] and PCa-derived cell lines DU145 (PSMA-negative) and LNCaP (PSMA-positive). The flow cytometry analysis revealed a specific fluorescence signal on PSMA-positive LNCaP cells, while DU145 (PSMA-negative) cells were not labeled. Additionally, signal intensities for both scFv variants as well as the recombinant Fab fragment were comparable to staining with parent 5D3 mAb suggesting that all engineered fragments retained high affinity and specificity for PSMA (Figure 2B). In a complementary IF microscopy approach, a specific signal was also detectable only in samples of PSMA-positive cells—on the surface of non-permeabilized cells, and on the surface and in the cytoplasm of Triton-permeabilized cells (Figure 2C). It shall be noted that a weak non-specific signal was visible in the nuclear region in all samples permeabilized by Triton X-100. This signal is linked to cross-reactivity of the anti-6× His antibody (used as a detection reagent) towards polyhistidine sequences present in nuclear proteins [50].

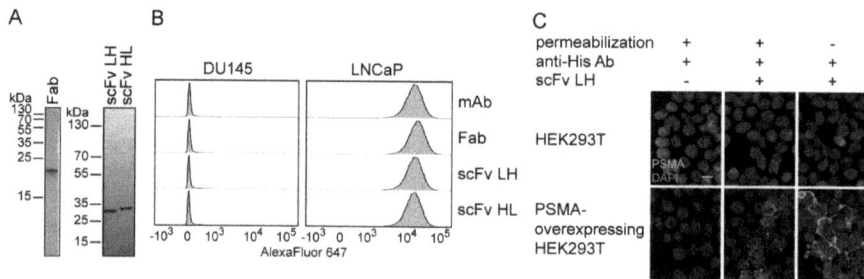

Figure 2. Characterization of 5D3 antibody fragments expressed in *E. coli*. (**A**) Purity of recombinant proteins was estimated from SDS-PAGE gel stained by Coomassie Brilliant Blue G-250 (CBB). (**B**) Binding of 5D3 variants on live cells was estimated by flow cytometry using anti-6× His antibody together with an anti-mouse IgG-Alexa Fluor 647 conjugate. All molecules used at saturating concentrations showed specific staining of PSMA-positive LNCaP cells with similar signal intensity. PSMA-negative DU145 cells were used as a control. (**C**) Indirect immunofluorescence microscopy using 5D3 scFv LH. PSMA-overexpressing HEK293T cells and the parent HEK293T cell line (a negative control) were fixed with/without permeabilization by Triton X-100 and incubated with 5D3 scFv LH. The fragment was then detected by anti-6× His Ab combined with anti-mouse Alexa Fluor 488 conjugate (green channel). Cell nuclei were counterstained by DAPI (blue channel). The scale bar represents 25 µm.

2.3. Expression of Fab and scFv Fragments in Insect S2 Cells

As yields of 5D3 fragments expressed in *E. coli* were rather low and would not allow us to carry out their detailed in vitro/in vivo characterization, we directed the expression of the fragments to insect S2 cells. Genes encoding 5D3 fragments were recloned into a pMT expression vector in frame with a BiP secretion signal sequence and the SA-strep tag sequence was added to the C-terminus of the Fab heavy chain and scFv variants (Figure 1). In the case of Fab, expression vectors containing individual light and heavy Fab chains were co-transfected to Schneider's S2 insect cells at a 2:1 ratio.

Engineered fragments were purified from the conditioned media by a combination of Streptactin affinity and size exclusion chromatography (SEC) and predominant monomeric protein species were observed during SEC runs as expected (Figure 3). Dimers of scFv variants represented <7% of the monomer peak (Figure 3B,C, fractions 3 and 4, respectively). All preparations were highly pure (>95%) with final yields of the Fab and scFv HL variants in the range of 10–20 mg/L culture, whereas the yield of the scFv LH variant was approximately 1 mg/L.

Surprisingly, SDS-PAGE analysis of purified fragments revealed an extra band of a higher molecular weight (app. 2 kDa) in all samples (Figure 3). Subsequent MS analysis identified slower migrating bands as fusions with the uncleaved signal peptide (Figure S1). Apparently, the S2 secretion system can be overwhelmed by robust production of recombinant proteins, and a fraction of secreted proteins is thus not processed properly. However, as shown in the following experiments, the presence of the uncleaved signal peptide does not have any negative influence on the performance of engineered fragments.

2.4. In Vitro Characterization of S2-Produced 5D3 Variants

In a preliminary set of experiments, we determined the stability, specificity, and affinity of S2-produced 5D3 fragments in vitro. Thermal stability of the engineered variants was determined by differential scanning fluorimetry (nanoDSF) and the results are shown in Figure 4A. scFv HL and LH variants unfolded at similar melting temperatures (Tm) of 53.4 °C and 52.5 °C, respectively, while the stability of the Fab fragment was higher as evidenced by Tm = 71.3 °C. The melting temperature of the engineered Fab fragment was similar to the Tm of the intact parent antibody (Tm = 70.7 °C) and the data are in line with results on the stability of mouse IgG1 published previously [51].

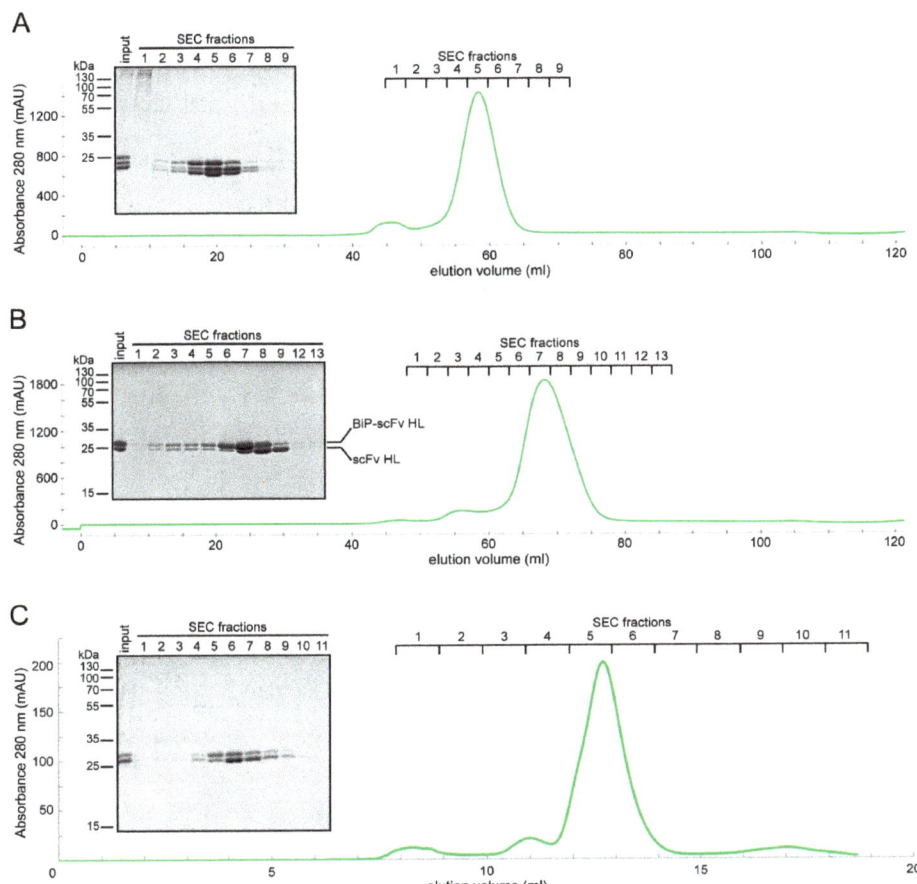

Figure 3. Purification of 5D3 fragments overexpressed in insect cells. Secreted variants were purified by the combination of Streptactin affinity chromatography and size exclusion chromatography (SEC). CBB-stained SDS-PAGE gels and SEC elution profiles are shown for Fab (**A**), scFv HL (**B**) and scFv LH (**C**) variants.

To evaluate the specificity of the variants, we used indirect immunofluorescence microscopy and flow cytometry in setups similar to those described above for variants produced in E. coli. The most notable technical difference was the use of an anti-Strep monoclonal antibody for the detection of the 5D3 fragments. As expected, the staining pattern in the IF microscopy experiment was virtually identical to the one performed on E. coli-expressed variants revealing specific plasma membrane/cytoplasmic staining in Triton-treated samples (Figure 4B). Likewise, only PSMA-positive (LNCaP, PC-3 PIP and CW22Rv1) cells were labeled in flow cytometry experiments, while the fluorescence signal for PSMA-negative cell lines (DU145 and PC-3) was close to background (Figure 4C and Figure S1).

Finally, the affinity of engineered molecules was evaluated by native ELISA and flow cytometry. For native ELISA, purified biotinylated PSMA was immobilized on streptavidin-coated plates and probed using a 2-fold dilution series (1600 nM–0.76 pM) of the recombinant fragments. Apparent dissociation constants (appK$_D$) calculated for Fab, scFv HL and scFv LH were 1.0, 2.3 and 2.4 nM, respectively (Figure 4D and Table 1). An expected decrease in PSMA-binding affinity compared to that of the parent mAb (appK$_D$ = 0.23 nM) most likely results from the monovalent versus divalent binding modes of fragments and full-length mAb, respectively. As affinities of both scFv variants for PSMA were virtually identical, the HL variant was directed to in vivo experiments because of approximately 10-fold higher expression yields. Affinity measurements were additionally performed using PSMA in its native environment on the surface of LNCaP cells by flow cytometry. The data were close to the result of native ELISA measurements revealing appK_D of Fab, scFv HL and LH to be 1.5, 1.5 and 1.3 nM, respectively (Figure 4E and Table 1).

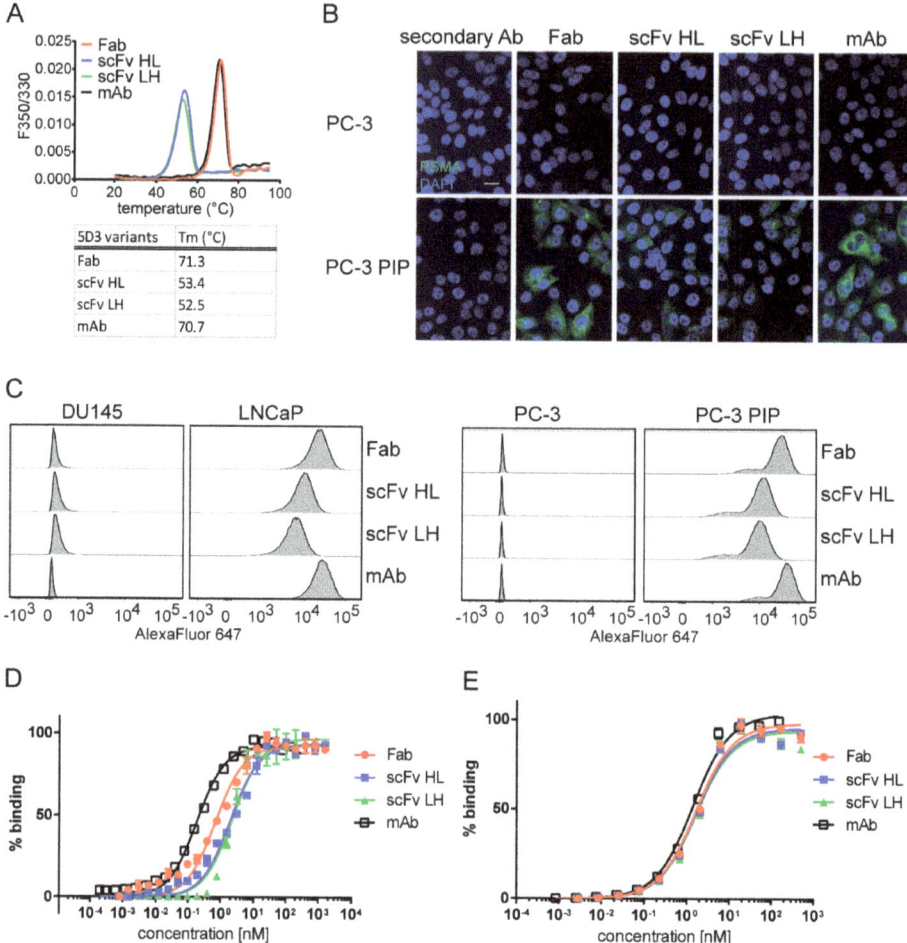

Figure 4. Functional characterization of S2-expressed 5D3 variants. (**A**) Thermal stability was determined using nanoDSF. Melting temperature curves and corresponding numerical values are shown. (**B**) Specificity of 5D3 variants evaluated by indirect immunofluorescence microscopy. PC-3 PIP (PSMA-positive) and parent PC-3 (PSMA-negative) cells were fixed by formaldehyde and permeabilized by Triton X-100 prior to incubation with recombinant 5D3 variants and secondary antibodies (green channel). Cell nuclei were counterstained with DAPI (blue channel). The scale bar represents 25 µm. (**C**) Flow cytometry analysis of PSMA-positive (PC-3 PIP, LNCaP) and negative (PC-3, DU145) cells stained by 100 nM purified 5D3 variants. Each gated population represents approximately 30,000 viable cells. (**D,E**) Determination of binding affinity of 5D3 variants by native ELISA (**D**) and flow cytometry (**E**) using purified PSMA and live LNCaP cells, respectively. PBS and DU145 cells were used as negative controls for ELISA and flow cytometry samples, respectively, and corresponding background signals were subtracted.

Table 1. Apparent K_D of antibody fragments determined by native ELISA and flow cytometry.

5D3 Variants	appK$_D$ (nM)	
	ELISA	Flow Cytometry
Fab	1.0 ± 0.7	1.5 ± 0.2
scFv HL	2.3 ± 1.7	1.5 ± 0.1
scFv LH	2.4 ± 0.1	1.3 ± 0.5
mAb	0.23 ± 0.1	0.85 ± 0.8

Overall, the above in vitro experiments show that the engineered fragments recapitulate excellent characteristics of the parent 5D3 antibody well and can be thus used for further studies targeting PSMA.

2.5. In Vivo PSMA Imaging in an Experimental PCa Mouse Model

For in vivo experiments, engineered fragments were labeled by IRDye680RD amine reactive dye using a recently described protocol [43]. The dye-to-protein ratios of Fab, scFv HL, and mAb conjugates, as determined by ratiometric absorbance measurements, were 0.7, 1.3, and 1.8, respectively. The affinity of conjugates was evaluated by ELISA against immobilized PSMA and no noticeable decrease was observed in the affinity of conjugated proteins compared to their non-conjugated counterparts (Figure S1).

Tumors in the mouse xenograft model of PCa were formed after subcutaneous injection of PSMA-positive (PC-3 PIP) and PSMA-negative (PC-3 FLU) cells behind the front legs. Conjugated 5D3 variants were administered by intravenous injection and conjugates were localized using a fluorescence imager taking longitudinal data.

Reminiscent of full-length 5D3 mAb, conjugates of antibody fragments revealed specific localization in PSMA-positive tumors only (Figure 5). At 24 h post-injection (p.i.), conjugates of antibody fragments were cleared from the PSMA-negative tumor (PSMA−) and inner organs and a fluorescence signal was restricted to the PSMA-positive tumor only (PSMA+). Note that the signal in the gastrointestinal tract originating from chlorophyll in feed was not related to the signal of antibody molecules. Accumulation of Fab in the PSMA-positive tumor was first visible approximately 2.5 h p.i., whereas that of the scFv fragment was visible in the PSMA-positive tumor 1 h p.i. (Figure 5A). A significant difference in the signal:noise ratio of fluorescence in PSMA-positive and -negative tumors was observed 2.5 h p.i. for both fragments. However, the nonspecific signal of circulating Fab and scFv HL conjugates was cleared from the PSMA-negative tumor at 7 and 4 h p.i., respectively. This slight difference in clearance between Fab and scFv fragment was confirmed by scans of tumors and organs in situ (Figure S2) and may be related to their different molecular weights (50 and 27 kDa, respectively). The signal intensity of Fab remained unchanged until 24 h p.i., whereas the scFv conjugate was partially cleared from the PSMA-positive tumor at 24 h p.i. (Figure 5). Similarly to both antibody fragments, the 5D3 IgG was accumulated specifically in the PSMA-positive tumor without any detectable non-specific binding to the PSMA-negative tumor once the circulating conjugate was cleared. However, the conjugate of the full-length mAb penetrated tissues slowly and remained in circulation significantly longer than fragments thus revealing the specific localization of PSMA-positive tumor no earlier than 24 h post-injection. The full-length 5D3 conjugate revealed accumulation in the PSMA-positive tumor, signal:noise ratio peaking at 4–6 days post-injection. The signal persisted in the PSMA-positive tumor until 15 days p.i. (Figure S3). The IgG1 isotype control conjugated to IRDye800CW was injected together with 5D3 mAb-IRDye680RD. At 24 h p.i. The signal of both conjugates was detectable in the PSMA-positive tumor due to slow blood pool clearance. However, unbound circulating conjugates were already cleared out at day 3 p.i. and no accumulation of the isotype conjugate was detectable in the PSMA-positive tumor (Figure S4). This finding confirmed the uptake of 5D3 into the PSMA-positive tumor via its specific binding to the target PSMA antigen.

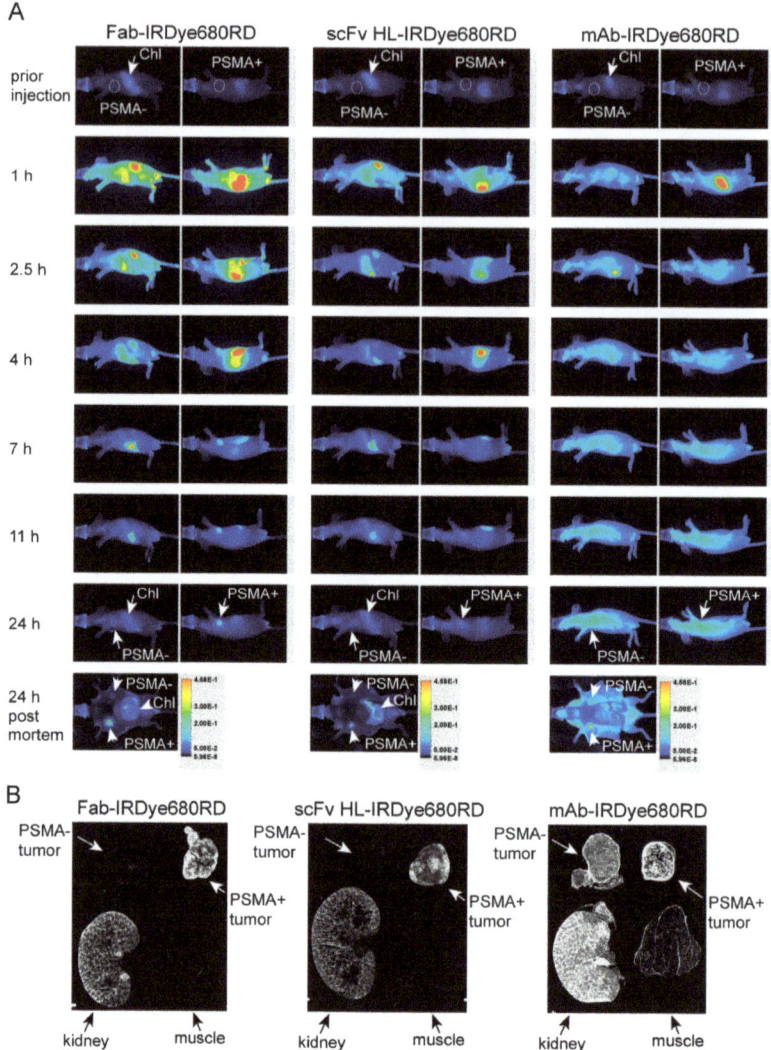

Figure 5. Pharmacokinetics of 5D3 variants and ex vivo NIRF imaging. (**A**) Mice bearing a PSMA-positive (PSMA+, right side) and PSMA-negative (PSMA−, left side) xenograft (location of tumor marked by dashed circle), were intravenously injected with 5D3 variants conjugated to IRDye680RD and images collected at various times post-injection with identical exposure settings. Both Fab and scFv fragments revealed specific localization to the PSMA-positive tumor already after 2.5–4 h p.i., while non-specific binding was still observed for 5D3 mAb at 24 h p.i. due to high levels of the circulating conjugate. At 24 h p.i. mice were sacrificed, and the ventral part dissected, and mice were scanned. The fluorescent signal in the gastrointestinal tract originates from chlorophyll (Chl) present in feed. Figures are representative images from triplicate runs for each 5D3 variant. (**B**) Sections of tumors, kidney and skeletal muscle (24 h p.i.) were scanned ex vivo. The specific signal for scFv and Fab was localized mainly to the rim of PSMA-positive tumors and to the kidney whereas PSMA-negative tumors and skeletal muscle did not show any significant signal. 5D3 mAb showed a strong signal in both tumors as well as kidney, and also observable signal in the PSMA-negative tumor and skeletal muscle.

The specificity of each conjugate was further assessed in dissected tumors and organs in situ following euthanasia 24 h p.i. (Figure 5A). In line with in vivo imaging data, the specific signal of both antibody fragments was detectable in cryosections of PSMA-positive tumors, preferentially at the tumor rim and in renal proximal tubules, which are known to express high levels of PSMA and play a major role in conjugate clearance (Figure 5B). PSMA-negative tumors did not reveal any signal that would significantly differ from the background represented by a skeletal muscle. The full-length mAb conjugate signal was detectable in both tumors as well as in the kidney and a weak signal was also observed in the skeletal muscle due to blood pool content of intact immunoglobulin at 24 h p.i. as observed for in vivo images.

3. Discussion

In our pilot experiments, we opted for a periplasmic prokaryotic expression as this well-established system offers a simple, inexpensive, and speedy production of fully folded and functional mAb fragments [49]. Under optimized fermenter conditions, final yields of recombinant mAb fragments can be up to 5 g/L [52]. However, under our non-optimized testing conditions in shaking flasks, fragment yields were disappointing and would not allow us to carry out planned in vitro/in vivo experiments. Consequently, we turned to the insect S2 system allowing production of tens to hundreds of milligrams of secreted proteins per liter of media [53–55]. While bicistronic or IRES-containing plasmids can, in principle, be used for the co-expression of two genes in S2 cells [56], in the case of Fab production, we chose co-transfection of individual heavy- and light-chain encoding plasmids. In this experimental setup, one can adjust the ratio between the two plasmids to maximize yields of "complete" Fab fragments as expression levels of light and heavy chains can differ markedly [57]. In the case of 5D3 Fab, we found that the 2:1 ratio of expression plasmids resulted in the highest yield, exceeding 20 mg/L.

While recombinant Fab fragments are found almost exclusively in a monomeric form, scFvs frequently exist as a monomer/homodimer mixture. Dimerization is strongly dependent on the length of the interdomain linker and in extreme cases of short linkers (4–12 amino acids) diabodies, i.e., dimeric scFv forms, are formed preferentially [58,59]. Additionally, the length and composition of the linker has been shown to affect stability and thus functional properties of scFvs [60–62]. For 5D3 scFv construction, we utilized an 18-mer [Gly$_4$Ser] linker, which is at the upper limit of the typically used 15–18 AA range [63], with an amino acid composition conveniently following a highly flexible sequence derived from a filamentous bacteriophage protein [64,65]. As documented by all biophysical and functional characteristics (monodispersity, temperature stability, binding affinity) the selected linker length is very well suited in the case of 5D3 scFvs.

SDS-PAGE analysis combined with mass spectrometry revealed that a significant portion of S2-expressed fragments is fused to the signal peptide upon secretion. The compromised cleavage of the signal peptide has been reported earlier and is linked to the specific features in signal sequence and timing of the cleavage (reviewed by [66]). To exclude potential negative effects of the signal sequence on the function of engineered mAb fragments, we used native ELISA to determine appK_D values of the Fab/scFv variant from SEC runs comprising predominantly either fusions with the signal peptide or variants with the signal peptide cleaved. All tested fractions revealed very similar appK_D values independently of the cleaved to uncleaved variant ratio (Figure S5). Overall, these data showed that the presence of the signal peptide does not have a significant effect on the affinity of fragments for PSMA, and the signal sequence does not therefore interfere with antibody–antigen interactions. Consequently, mixtures of uncleaved and cleaved fragments were used for all experiments without any additional purification steps. At the same time, however, heterogenous protein preparation would not meet requirements of clinical trials. Therefore, further development of 5D3 fragments should include the use of an expression system that provides a homogeneous preparation of the target protein, such as *E. coli* or mammalian-based systems used in the field. Alternatively, an enzymatic cleavage site could be inserted into constructs N-terminally to the antibody sequence to eliminate the signal peptide from the antibody fusion.

Compared to the parent intact 5D3 antibody, our engineered fragments have approximately a 5- to 10-fold lower binding strength (affinity for fragments; avidity for the whole mAb) for PSMA as determined by native ELISA. As the avidity of an antibody depends on the affinity of its binding site together with its valency, it is expected that the binding strength of monovalent mAb fragments is lower compared to bivalent parent molecules. Indeed, a decrease in affinity up to 100-fold has been documented for monovalent antibody fragments [60,61,67,68]. Importantly, our nanoDSF data show that the thermal stability of 5D3 Fab corresponds well to the stability of the original 5D3 mAb, suggesting that differences in their respective binding strengths likely stem from valency rather than lower folding stability and compactness of the Fab fragment. An optimal binding strength of antibodies, which is critical for efficient tumor uptake, is believed to be in the range of 1–10 nM [69–71]. Accordingly, our engineered fragments are in this desired range and can thus be used safely for further clinical development. Moreover, 5D3 fragments showed very similar characteristics to other PSMA-specific recombinant proteins. For example, a cytotoxic conjugate of scFv D7 derived from 3/F11 has appK_D = 6–10 nM [35]. Similarly, the RRa92 and gy1 clones of scFv were selected by phage and yeast display with an apparent affinity to recombinant PSMA of 5 nM and 1–4 nM, respectively [72,73]. scFvs derived from mouse antibodies D2B and J591 revealed appK_D = 9 nM and >3 nM, respectively [72,74,75]. A recombinant Fab fragment of the D2B antibody showed 9 nM affinity [23]. However, binding affinity could be enhanced by the use of a bivalent molecule. Therefore, further development of 5D3 fragments toward clinical applications could involve generation of minibody, diabody or (Fab)$_2$ variants that might further improve binding characteristics.

Recombinant antibody fragments showed significantly faster clearance compared to 5D3 mAb thus confirming previously published data from a pepsin-cleaved 5D3 Fab fragment [43]. At 24 h p.i., the background fluorescence of both fragments is completely clear, whereas the mAb still shows a significant background in the whole-body scan. Consistent with data from recombinant fragments of other antibodies [67], 5D3 Fab shows the peak of specific accumulation in the PSMA-positive tumor slightly later (2.5 h p.i.) in comparison to scFv (peaking already at 1 h p.i.). Moreover, scFv starts to clear from the PSMA-positive tumor by 11 h p.i. whereas Fab is not cleared from the antigen-presenting tumor throughout the 24 h post-injection. Our data thus show standard behavior of 5D3 recombinant fragments in vivo that matches fragments of the same type derived from different anti-PSMA antibodies. For example, PSMA-directed scFv gy1 and scFv derived from the D2B Ab showed a very similar timeline of accumulation in the PSMA-positive tumor and clearance from other tissues as scFv 5D3 [72,74]. At the same time, ^{111}In-D2B Fab peaks its accumulation in the PSMA-positive tumor at 48 h p.i., i.e., slightly later compared to our 5D3 fragment, suggesting the possible influence of labeling chemistry on Fab pharmacokinetics [23]. Similarly to other PSMA-specific antibody fragments [72,76], we observed signal originated from 5D3 conjugates in kidneys and liver that is connected with metabolism and clearance of recombinant proteins. Described distribution should be carefully followed particularly in future development of radionuclide or cytotoxic drug 5D3 conjugates because of potential risk of kidney toxicity [45]. The behavior of original 5D3 mAb in long time lapse was also similar to other high-affinity mouse antibodies [77], as the mAb revealed the peak of accumulation at days 4–6 p.i. and was still detectable in the antigen-presenting tumor at day 15 post-injection.

In summary, the biochemical characterization combined with data from in vivo imaging clearly show that 5D3 recombinant fragments retain an intact binding site of the original 5D3 mAb. The efficient and highly specific binding of PSMA in vivo predetermines 5D3 antibody fragments for further clinical development. This could be directed in parallel to development of other PSMA-specific tools such as bispecific molecules and fusions with toxins and immunological molecules combined alternatively with antimitotic drugs [35,78], conjugates with fluorescent dyes or radioisotopes [16,20,72], and multimeric molecules with potential to activate immune cells [31].

4. Materials and Methods

4.1. Chemicals and Reagents

All chemicals were purchased from Sigma–Aldrich (Steinheim, Germany) unless stated otherwise. Restriction enzymes, Antarctic phosphatase and ligase were purchased from New England Biolabs (Ipswich, MA, USA).

4.2. N-Terminal Amino Acid Sequencing

The purified antibody was mixed with the Laemmli sample buffer and individual antibody chains were separated by SDS PAGE. Proteins were transferred onto a PVDF membrane by electroblotting and visualized by staining with Coomassie Brilliant Blue G-250 (CBB). Pyroglutamate was removed from the N-terminus of the heavy chain prior SDS PAGE according to the published protocol [79]. Briefly, 5 µg of antibody was treated with 0.25 mU pyroglutamate aminopeptidase (Takara, Shiga, Japan) for 6 h at 75 °C in Reaction Buffer supplied by the producer and supplemented with 0.08% Tween-20. N-terminal amino acid sequences were determined by Edman degradation using the Procise Protein Sequencing System (494 cLC Protein Sequencer, Applied Biosystems, Foster City, CA, USA). Briefly, in each cycle, an N-terminal amino acid of an antibody chain was modified by phenylisothiocyanate, released from the polypeptide chain and converted to its stable phenylthiohydantoin derivative. The amino acid sequence was then identified by sequential analysis of amino acid derivatives using reversed-phase HPLC.

4.3. RNA Isolation and cDNA Synthesis

Approximately 1×10^7 5D3 hybridoma cells were homogenized in a QIAshredder spin column (Qiagen, Hilden, Germany). Total RNA was isolated by the RNeasy Mini Kit (Qiagen) according to the manufacturer's protocol. DNase treatment was included in the isolation procedure to avoid any contamination by genomic DNA. A quantity of 1 µg of isolated RNA combined with random hexamers (30 ng/µL, Qiagen) was denatured at 65 °C for 5 min and hybridized at 4 °C for 2 min. The first cDNA strand was synthesized by mixing the hybridized template with SuperScript III reverse transcriptase (10 U/µL, Invitrogen, Thermo Fisher Scientific, Carlsbad, CA, USA), RNase inhibitor RNase OUT (1 U/µL, Invitrogen), 5 mM dithiothreitol (Fermentas, Thermo Fisher Scientific, Carlsbad, CA, USA) and 750 µM deoxynucleotide mix. Synthesis of cDNA was carried out at 50 °C for 60 min followed by inactivation at 70 °C for 15 min.

4.4. Antibody Cloning

Nucleotide sequences of both antibody chains encoding the 5D3 Fab fragment were amplified by PCR from the first cDNA strand using a mixture of degenerated forward primers combined with constant region-specific reverse primers. Degenerated primers were designed based on the amino acid sequence of antibody N-termini, whereas reverse primers covering C-termini of CL and CH1 domains were designed according to published antibody sequences of mouse IgG light kappa (GenBank Q58EU8) and heavy chains (GenBank U04352.1), respectively (Table S1). Individual chains were amplified from the cDNA template (1 ng/µL) by PfuUltra II Hotstart PCR Master Mix (Agilent, Santa Clara, CA, USA) in the presence of 0.8 µM primers. Amplification was done in 35 cycles comprising denaturation (95 °C for 30 s), annealing (30 s) and extension (72 °C for 1 min) followed by final extension at 72 °C for 10 min. The annealing temperature was set to 55 and 57.5 °C for the light and heavy chain, respectively.

The pUC19 vector (Invitrogen) was linearized by the SmaI restriction enzyme, dephosphorylated by antarctic phosphatase and purified by extraction from an agarose gel using the Zymoclean Gel DNA Recovery Kit (Zymo Research, Irvine, CA, USA). Blunt-end PCR products were ligated into a linearized pUC19 vector by Blunt/TA Ligase and sequences of antibody chains were determined by Sanger sequencing (GATC Biotech, Ebersberg, Germany).

4.5. Mass Spectrometry Analysis of the Antibody Sequence

The amino acid sequence of the 5D3 mAb was identified by the procedure described in detail elsewhere [80]. Briefly, the protein solution was treated with dithiothreitol and iodoacetamide. After solvent removal, proteins were digested by trypsin and chymotrypsin in separate reactions. Peptides were analyzed by the UltiMate 3000 RSLCnano system (Dionex, Thermo Fisher Scientific, Rockford, IL, USA) coupled with a TripleTOF 5600 mass spectrometer with a NanoSpray III source (Sciex, Framingham, MA, USA) operated by Analyst TF 1.7 software (Sciex). The peptides were trapped, desalted and separated on an Acclaim PepMap100 column. The 125-min elution gradient at the constant flow of 300 nL/min was set to 5% of phase B (0.1% formic acid in 99.9% acetonitrile, phase A 0.1% formic acid) for first 5 min, then with gradient elution by increasing concentration of acetonitrile. Protein Pilot 4.5 (Sciex) was used for protein identification using a database consisting of proposed antibody sequences and common contaminants.

For the identification of the recombinant fragment sequence, Coomassie-stained protein bands were cut out from the gel and treated sequentially by acetonitrile, dithiothreitol and iodoacetamide. Proteins were digested by trypsin (Promega, Madison, WI, USA) in a bicarbonate buffer at 37 °C overnight. Peptides mixed with a γ-α-Cyano-4-hydroxycinnamic acid matrix were subjected to MALDI-TOF analysis (Autoflex Speed MALDI TOF/TOF, Bruker Daltonik, Bremen, Germany). Data were processed by mMass software [81].

4.6. Construction of Recombinant Antibody Expression Vectors

To construct an expression vector for the secretion of Fab in the bacterial periplasm, variable domain sequences were amplified via PCR using conditions identical to those for the parent antibody (see above). We used sequence-specific primers (Table S1) and an annealing temperature of 55 and 60 °C for the light- and heavy-chain variable domain, respectively. Amplified genes were ligated into a pASK85 bicistronic vector [47] containing constant domain sequences of mouse Fab tagged with a 6× Histidine anchor at the C-terminus of the heavy chain. The insertion of the light- and heavy-chain into the vector backbone was done sequentially using Eco53kI/XhoI and PstI/BstEII restriction enzyme pairs, respectively. Nucleotide strings encoding scFv variants were custom-made (Thermo Fisher Scientific). Genes were digested by the XbaI/HindIII pair and ligated into the pASK85 vector.

For S2 cell-based expression vectors, sequences from the pASK85 vector were PCR amplified using sequence-specific primers and an annealing temperature of 60 °C. PCR products were ligated via BglII/AfeI sites individually into a pMT expression vector containing a BiP signal sequence (pMT-BiP), which enabled the secretion of the target protein into the cultivation media. C-termini of genes, except the Fab light chain, were fused to the SA-strep tag. The identity of all constructed expression vectors was verified by Sanger sequencing. Primer sequences are shown in Table S1.

4.7. Cell Lines

Schneider's S2 insect cells (Invitrogen) were grown at 26 °C in Insect Xpress medium (Lonza, Basel, Switzerland) supplemented with 2 mM L-glutamine. PC-3 and DU145 cells were obtained from the American Type Culture Collection, PC-3 PIP and PC-3 FLU cells were generously provided by Dr. Warren Heston (Cleveland Clinic, Cleveland, OH, USA), and LNCaP and CW22Rv1 cells were kindly provided by Z. Hodny (IMG, Prague, Czech Republic) and R. Lapidus (University of Maryland, Baltimore, MD, USA), respectively. Human cell lines were grown in RPMI-1640 medium (Sigma-Aldrich) supplemented with 10% fetal bovine serum and 2 mM L-glutamine under a humidified 5% CO_2 atmosphere at 37 °C, PC3-PIP cells were continuously selected by puromycin (20 µg/mL; InvivoGen, San Diego, CA, USA). Cells used for animal treatment were evaluated as mycoplasma-negative using MycoAlert PLUS mycoplasma detection kit (Lonza).

4.8. Generation of Stably Transfected Insect Cells

Schneider's S2 cells were cultured in a medium supplemented with 10% fetal bovine serum in 24-well non-treated polystyrene plates. Cells were co-transfected by 500 ng pMT-BiP expression vector in combination with 30 ng pCoBlast selection vector (Invitrogen) using an Effectene transfection reagent (Qiagen). pMT-BiP vectors containing heavy- and light-chain of Fab were co-transfected simultaneously at a 1:2 molar ratio. Blasticidin (40 µg/mL; InvivoGen) was added to cell cultures two days after transfection and cells were maintained in the selection medium (changed every fourth day) till the selection of a stable transfected cell culture (approximately three weeks).

4.9. Expression and Purification of Engineered Fragments Produced in E. coli

Heterologous expression and extraction from the E. coli periplasm was done similarly as published earlier [82]. Briefly, JM83 cells [83] were cultured in the 2× YT medium and protein expression was induced by anhydrotetracycline (200 µg/L; stock dissolved in dimethylformamide; Acros Organics, Geel, Belgium) at 22 °C for 4 h. Proteins were extracted from the periplasm by treating cells with a periplasmic extraction buffer (500 mM sucrose, 100 mM Tris, 1 mM EDTA, pH 8) at 4 °C for 30 min. The extract was centrifuged at 5000× g for 15 min and the supernatant was then cleared by a second centrifugation step at 40,000× g at 4 °C for 30 min. Target proteins were purified by affinity chromatography using a NiNTA Superflow resin (IBA, Gottingen, Germany) equilibrated with 50 mM Tris-HCl, 150 mM NaCl, 10 mM KCl, 10% glycerol, pH 8.0. Proteins were eluted from the resin by a stepwise gradient of imidazole, elution fractions were pooled, concentrated, flash frozen in liquid nitrogen, and stored at −80 °C.

4.10. Expression and Purification of Engineered Fragments Produced in Insect Cells

Stable S2 transfectants were expanded to a large volume (700 mL) to the density of 3×10^7 cells/mL and overexpression was induced with 0.7 mM $CuSO_4$ for 7 days. The conditioned medium was harvested by centrifugation at 500× g followed by centrifugation of the supernatant at 10,000× g. The supernatant was supplemented with protease inhibitors (Roche, Basel, Switzerland) and concentrated to 30 mL using an ultrafiltration cell equipped with an Ultracel 10 kDa ultrafiltration disc (Millipore, Merck, Burlington, MA, USA). Streptavidin (8 mg/L) was added to the retentate to complex free biotin present in the culture medium. Target proteins were purified by affinity chromatography using a StrepTactin XT resin (IBA) equilibrated with 50 mM Tris-HCl, 150 mM NaCl, 10 mM KCl, 10% glycerol, pH 8.0, and eluted with 5 mM D-biotin (VWR, Radnor, PA, USA) in the equilibration buffer. Pooled elution fractions were subjected to size exclusion chromatography using a Superdex 75 column (GE Healthcare Bio-Sciences, Uppsala, Sweden) connected to an NGC Chromatography System (Bio-Rad Laboratories, Hercules, CA, USA), PBS/3% glycerol was used as the mobile phase. Fractions containing target proteins were pooled, concentrated, flash frozen in liquid nitrogen and stored at −80 °C.

4.11. Purification of PSMA Extracellular Domain

The expression and purification of the extracellular domain of human PSMA (residues 44–750) that comprised an N-terminal Avi-tag (Avi-PSMA) run according to protocol published earlier [54,84]. Briefly, the recombinant protein was expressed by stably transfected Schneider S2 cells and purified by the combination of affinity chromatography (Streptavidin Mutein Matrix, Roche) and size-exclusion chromatography on a Superdex 200 column (GE Healthcare Bio-Sciences). Concentrated PSMA stock was stored at −80 °C until further use.

4.12. SDS Polyacrylamide Electrophoresis and Western Blotting

Samples were mixed with Laemmli buffer supplemented with 100 mM dithiothreitol, heated to 95 °C and analyzed by sodium dodecyl sulfate polyacrylamide gel electrophoresis (SDS-PAGE) with CBB staining. For Western blotting, an SDS-PAGE gel was electroblotted onto a PVDF membrane in

Tris-CAPS/10% methanol buffer (Bio-Rad Laboratories) using a Trans-Blot SD Semi-Dry Transfer Cell (Bio-Rad Laboratories). The PVDF membrane was blocked in 5% non-fat dry milk/PBS/0.05% Tween-20 for 45 min followed by a 45 min incubation with the Precision Protein StrepTactin-HRP (horseradish peroxidase) Conjugate (Bio-Rad Laboratories) or an anti-6× His tag antibody conjugated to HRP (both conjugates diluted 10,000× in 5% non-fat dry milk/PBS/0.05% Tween-20). Following five washes with PBS/0.05% Tween-20, the signal was developed using Luminata Forte chemiluminescence substrate (Millipore) and visualized by an ImageQuant LAS4000 Imaging System (GE Healthcare Bio-Sciences). Figures were processed using the Adobe CS4 Photoshop software (Adobe Systems, San Jose, CA, USA).

4.13. Indirect Immunofluorescence Microscopy

Cells were passaged on glass slides coated with poly-L-lysine and left to adhere for 24 h. Fixation was done in 3.7% formaldehyde/PBS at RT for 20 min, followed by extensive washing with PBS. Nonpermeabilized samples were directly incubated with tested antibody variants, whereas cells intended to be permeabilized were treated with 0.1% Triton X-100/PBS for 20 min and washed with PBS beforehand. Antibody variants were diluted to 14 µg/mL in PBS and incubated with slides at 4 °C overnight. Binding was detected using either anti-6× His tag antibody (2 µg/mL in PBS for 1 h; Sigma) or anti-Strep tag Ab (2 µg/mL in PBS 2 h; Immo, IBA) combined with a goat anti-mouse IgG Alexa Fluor 488 conjugate (4 µg/mL in PBS/0.05% Tween-20 1 h; Thermo Fisher Scientific). All incubation steps were followed by extensive washes with PBS/0.05% Tween-20. Finally, cells were counterstained with 6-diamidino-2-phenylindole (DAPI; 1 µg/mL) for 5 min and mounted in VectaShield (Vector Laboratories, Burlingame, CA, USA). The fluorescence signal was visualized by an Eclipse E400 fluorescence microscope (Nikon, Tokyo, Japan) equipped with a 20× and 40× magnifying dry objective. Images were taken by a ProgRes MF CCD camera (Jenoptik Optical Systems GmbH, Jena, Germany) and processed in Adobe Photoshop software.

4.14. ELISA

A 384-well MaxiSorp plate was coated with 20 µL/well of recombinant streptavidin (5 µg/mL in TBS) at 4 °C overnight. All further steps were carried out at RT and incubations run on a shaking platform at 700 RPM. The coating solution was discarded, and the plate blocked with 5% BSA dissolved in PBS (80 µL/well) for 2 h. Following three washes with PBS/0.05% Tween-20, Avi-PSMA (5 µg/mL) was immobilized for 1 h. After three washes, a 2-fold dilution series of antibody fragments (1600 nM–0.76 pM) and the parent 5D3 (320 nM–0.15 pM) were pipetted into the plate and incubated for 1 h. The plate was then repeatedly washed and incubated with 20 µL of a StrepMAB Classic HRP conjugate (IBA) diluted 10,000× in PBS for 45 min. TMB (3,3′,5,5′-tetramethylbenzidine) was dissolved in DMSO and further diluted in a 50 mM citrate-phosphate buffer, 0.006% H2O2, pH 5, to the working concentration of 100 µg/mL. The substrate solution (40 µL) was applied to each well and incubated for 5 min. The reaction was stopped by adding 20 µL 3 M H_2SO_4, and absorbance was measured at 450 nm using a ClarioStar microplate reader (BMG Labtech, Ortenberg, Germany). Data were processed in Prism 6 software (GraphPad, San Diego, CA, USA).

4.15. Flow Cytometry

Cells were harvested using 0.025% Trypsin/0.01% EDTA in PBS followed by a wash with 5% fetal bovine serum in PBS. Cells were then extensively washed with PBS/0.5% gelatin from cold water fish skin and incubated with antibody variants. Full-length antibodies were detected by a goat anti-mouse secondary antibody conjugated to Alexa Fluor 647 (4 µg/mL; Thermo Fisher Scientific), whereas recombinant fragments expressed by *E. coli* and insect cells were visualized by an anti-6× His tag antibody (10 µg/mL, Sigma) and an anti-Strep tag antibody (1 µg/mL, Immo, IBA), respectively, followed by incubation with a goat anti-mouse secondary antibody conjugated to Alexa Fluor 647. A three-fold dilution series of tested variants spanned the concentration of range 150 nM–0.85 pM and 500 nM–2.8 pM for mAb and fragments, respectively. All incubations were carried out in PBS supplemented with 0.5% gelatin in a total volume of 20–50 µL at 4 °C for 30 min. Incubations were followed by extensive washes using PBS/0.5% gelatin. Finally, Hoechst 33258 was added to cell suspensions to estimate cell viability. Cell samples were immediately analyzed using the LSRFortessa flow cytometer (BD Biosciences, San Jose, CA, USA). A minimum of 50,000 viable cells underwent subsequent analysis with the FlowJo software (FlowJo, LLC, Ashland, OR, USA).

4.16. Nanoscale Differential Scanning Fluorimetry

Standard capillaries were filled with 0.3 mg/mL protein solutions in PBS/3% glycerol. A 1.5 °C/min temperature gradient of 20–95 °C was applied to samples using a Prometheus NT.48 fluorimeter (NanoTemper Technologies, München, Germany). Melting temperatures were calculated from intrinsic protein fluorescence curves at 330 and 350 nm.

4.17. Fluorescence Dye Conjugation

The labeling of antibody variants was done as reported by Novakova et al. [43] with minor modifications described below. Ten micrograms of IRDye680RD-NHS or IRDye800CW-NHS esters (LI-COR Biosciences, Lincoln, NE, USA; 5 mg/mL dissolved in DMSO) were mixed with 120–160 µg proteins. Reaction mixtures were incubated at RT for 25 min and proteins were separated from the free dye using a Sephadex G-25 size-exclusion column (GE Healthcare Bio-Sciences). The presence of residual free dye in the conjugated protein solution was estimated using silica gel HLF (Analtech, Newark, DE, USA) scanned by a Pearl Impulse imager (LI-COR Biosciences) and quantified by Pearl Impulse Software (LI-COR Biosciences). The number of fluorophores conjugated per one protein molecule was calculated from protein absorbance measured at 280 nm and values of IRDye680RD and IRDye800CW absorbance measured at 672 and 780 nm, respectively. Conjugated proteins were diluted in sterile 0.9% NaCl to a final concentration of 150 µg/mL prior to injection.

4.18. In Vivo Imaging Using Near-Infrared Fluorescence (NIRF)

All animal studies were conducted in full compliance with the protocol approved by the Johns Hopkins University Animal Care and Use Committee. Single subcutaneous xenografts were formed in five-week old intact male athymic nude mice (Taconic Biosciences, Hudson, NY, USA) after a single injection of 3×10^6 PSMA-positive PC-3 PIP cells behind a front leg and the injection of PSMA-negative PC-3 FLU cells on the opposite side [85]. Cells were inoculated subcutaneously in 100 µL of Hanks buffered saline solution. When tumors reached 4–6 mm in diameter, fluorescently labeled antibody variants (30 µg) were applied in a single dose of 200 µL into the tail vein. Mice were scanned under 2–2.5% isoflurane anesthesia in oxygen (2 L/min) at the stated time points using a Pearl Impulse imager (LI-COR Biosciences) equipped with 700 nm and 800 nm emission channels. All images were normalized to a single image in each set in Pearl Impulse software allowing for identical acquisition time and thresholding to manage comparison among time points, treatments, and animals. Immediately after the last scan, mice were euthanized using isoflurane-anesthetized cervical dislocation, the ventral side was opened, and uncovered tumors and inner organs were scanned.

4.19. Ex Vivo Imaging

Tumors, a kidney, and a skeletal muscle were dissected, embedded in O.C.T. compound (Sakura Finetek, Torrance, CA, USA) and frozen on dry ice immediately after euthanasia. Frozen tissues were sectioned by a Microm HM550 cryostat (Thermo Fisher Scientific) to 20 µm slides that were placed onto a positively charged glass slide and let thaw at room temperature. Dry sections were scanned by an Odyssey imager (LI-COR Biosciences) using a 700 nm emission channel and images were processed in Adobe Photoshop software.

Supplementary Materials: Supplementary Materials can be found at http://www.mdpi.com/1422-0067/21/18/6672/s1.

Author Contributions: Conceptualization, Z.N. and C.B.; methodology, Z.N., N.B., C.A.F. and C.B.; validation, Z.N., C.A.F. and B.H.; formal analysis, Z.N., N.B., C.A.F., B.H., M.G., A.P., M.B., G.D. and M.H.; investigation, Z.N., N.B., C.A.F., B.H., M.G., G.D., A.L., A.P., M.B. and M.H.; resources, Z.N., C.A.F., M.H., M.G.P. and C.B.; data curation, Z.N., N.B., C.A.F., B.H., G.D., M.H. and C.B.; writing—original draft preparation, Z.N. and C.B.; writing—review and editing, N.B., C.A.F., B.H., M.G., G.D., A.L., A.P., M.B., M.H., M.G.P. and C.B.; visualization, Z.N., N.B., M.G.P. and C.B.; supervision, Z.N., C.A.F., M.G.P. and C.B.; project administration, Z.N., C.A.F., M.G.P. and C.B.; funding acquisition, Z.N., M.G.P. and C.B. All authors have read and agreed to the published version of the manuscript.

Funding: This research was supported by project from MEYS CR (LTAUSA18196), Czech Science Foundation (18-04790S), the CAS (RVO: 86652036), and the project 'BIOCEV' (CZ.1.05/1.1.00/02.0109) from the ERDF. We acknowledge the Imaging Methods Core Facility at BIOCEV, institution supported by the Czech-BioImaging large RI projects (LM2015062 and CZ.02.1.01/0.0/0.0/16_013/0001775, funded by MEYS CR) and the Biophysics facility of CMS supported by MEYS CR (LM2015043) for instrumental support. We also acknowledge CA134675, EB024495 and CA194228.

Acknowledgments: We thank I. Jelinkova and P. Baranova for the excellent technical assistance, P. Pompach for mass spectrometry analysis and Z. Voburka for Edman sequencing.

Conflicts of Interest: The authors declare no conflict of interest.

Abbreviations

appK_D	Apparent dissociation constant
BSA	Bovine serum albumin
CBB	Coomassie Brilliant Blue G-250
ELISA	Enzyme-linked immunosorbent assay
HL	Heavy-to-light
IF	Indirect immunofluorescence
LH	Light-to-heavy
mAb	Monoclonal antibody
MALDI-TOF	Matrix assisted laser desorption/ionization–time-of-flight
NAALADase	N acetylated-alpha-linked acidic dipeptidase
nanoDSF	Differential scanning fluorimetry
p.i.	Post-injection
PBS	Phosphate buffered saline
PCa	Prostate cancer
PSMA	Prostate-specific membrane antigen
PVDF	Polyvinylidene fluoride
SEC	Size exclusion chromatography
scFv	Single chain variable fragment
Tm	Melting temperature

References

1. Ferlay, J.; Colombet, M.; Soerjomataram, I.; Dyba, T.; Randi, G.; Bettio, M.; Gavin, A.; Visser, O.; Bray, F. Cancer incidence and mortality patterns in Europe: Estimates for 40 countries and 25 major cancers in 2018. *Eur. J. Cancer* **2018**, *103*, 356–387. [CrossRef] [PubMed]
2. Pernar, C.H.; Ebot, E.M.; Wilson, K.M.; Mucci, L.A. The Epidemiology of Prostate Cancer. *Cold Spring Harb. Perspect. Med.* **2018**, *8*, a030361. [CrossRef] [PubMed]
3. Siegel, R.L.; Miller, K.D.; Jemal, A. Cancer statistics, 2016. *CA Cancer J. Clin.* **2016**, *66*, 7–30. [CrossRef] [PubMed]
4. Maurer, T.; Eiber, M.; Schwaiger, M.; Gschwend, J.E. Current use of PSMA-PET in prostate cancer management. *Nat. Rev. Urol.* **2016**, *13*, 226–235. [CrossRef]
5. Zhao, X.; Ning, Q.; Mo, Z.; Tang, S. A promising cancer diagnosis and treatment strategy: Targeted cancer therapy and imaging based on antibody fragment. *Artif. Cells Nanomed. Biotechnol.* **2019**, *47*, 3621–3630. [CrossRef]
6. Batra, S.K.; Jain, M.; Wittel, U.A.; Chauhan, S.C.; Colcher, D. Pharmacokinetics and biodistribution of genetically engineered antibodies. *Curr. Opin. Biotechnol.* **2002**, *13*, 603–608. [CrossRef]

7. Bauerschlag, D.; Meinhold-Heerlein, I.; Maass, N.; Bleilevens, A.; Brautigam, K.; Al Rawashdeh, W.; Di Fiore, S.; Haugg, A.M.; Gremse, F.; Steitz, J.; et al. Detection and Specific Elimination of EGFR(+) Ovarian Cancer Cells Using a Near Infrared Photoimmunotheranostic Approach. *Pharm. Res.* **2017**, *34*, 696–703. [CrossRef]
8. Yuan, X.; Yang, M.; Chen, X.; Zhang, X.; Sukhadia, S.; Musolino, N.; Bao, H.; Chen, T.; Xu, C.; Wang, Q.; et al. Characterization of the first fully human anti-TEM1 scFv in models of solid tumor imaging and immunotoxin-based therapy. *Cancer Immunol. Immunother.* **2017**, *66*, 367–378. [CrossRef]
9. Rabenhold, M.; Steiniger, F.; Fahr, A.; Kontermann, R.E.; Ruger, R. Bispecific single-chain diabody-immunoliposomes targeting endoglin (CD105) and fibroblast activation protein (FAP) simultaneously. *J. Control. Release* **2015**, *201*, 56–67. [CrossRef]
10. Rafiq, S.; Yeku, O.O.; Jackson, H.J.; Purdon, T.J.; van Leeuwen, D.G.; Drakes, D.J.; Song, M.; Miele, M.M.; Li, Z.; Wang, P.; et al. Targeted delivery of a PD-1-blocking scFv by CAR-T cells enhances anti-tumor efficacy in vivo. *Nat. Biotechnol.* **2018**, *36*, 847–856. [CrossRef]
11. Zhang, M.; Kobayashi, N.; Zettlitz, K.A.; Kono, E.A.; Yamashiro, J.M.; Tsai, W.K.; Jiang, Z.K.; Tran, C.P.; Wang, C.; Guan, J.; et al. Near-Infrared Dye-Labeled Anti-Prostate Stem Cell Antigen Minibody Enables Real-Time Fluorescence Imaging and Targeted Surgery in Translational Mouse Models. *Clin. Cancer Res.* **2019**, *25*, 188–200. [CrossRef] [PubMed]
12. Knowles, S.M.; Tavare, R.; Zettlitz, K.A.; Rochefort, M.M.; Salazar, F.B.; Jiang, Z.K.; Reiter, R.E.; Wu, A.M. Applications of immunoPET: Using 124I-anti-PSCA A11 minibody for imaging disease progression and response to therapy in mouse xenograft models of prostate cancer. *Clin. Cancer Res.* **2014**, *20*, 6367–6378. [CrossRef] [PubMed]
13. Boonstra, M.C.; Tolner, B.; Schaafsma, B.E.; Boogerd, L.S.; Prevoo, H.A.; Bhavsar, G.; Kuppen, P.J.; Sier, C.F.; Bonsing, B.A.; Frangioni, J.V.; et al. Preclinical evaluation of a novel CEA-targeting near-infrared fluorescent tracer delineating colorectal and pancreatic tumors. *Int. J. Cancer* **2015**, *137*, 1910–1920. [CrossRef]
14. Debie, P.; Hernot, S. Emerging Fluorescent Molecular Tracers to Guide Intra-Operative Surgical Decision-Making. *Front. Pharmacol.* **2019**, *10*, 510. [CrossRef] [PubMed]
15. Wright, G.L., Jr.; Haley, C.; Beckett, M.L.; Schellhammer, P.F. Expression of prostate-specific membrane antigen in normal, benign, and malignant prostate tissues. *Urol. Oncol.* **1995**, *1*, 18–28. [CrossRef]
16. Frigerio, B.; Franssen, G.; Luison, E.; Satta, A.; Seregni, E.; Colombatti, M.; Fracasso, G.; Valdagni, R.; Mezzanzanica, D.; Boerman, O.; et al. Full preclinical validation of the 123I-labeled anti-PSMA antibody fragment ScFvD2B for prostate cancer imaging. *Oncotarget* **2017**, *8*, 10919–10930. [CrossRef]
17. Czerwinska, M.; Bilewicz, A.; Kruszewski, M.; Wegierek-Ciuk, A.; Lankoff, A. Targeted Radionuclide Therapy of Prostate Cancer-From Basic Research to Clinical Perspectives. *Molecules* **2020**, *25*, 1743. [CrossRef]
18. Foss, C.A.; Mease, R.C.; Cho, S.Y.; Kim, H.J.; Pomper, M.G. GCPII imaging and cancer. *Curr. Med. Chem.* **2012**, *19*, 1346–1359. [CrossRef]
19. Barinka, C.; Rojas, C.; Slusher, B.; Pomper, M. Glutamate carboxypeptidase II in diagnosis and treatment of neurologic disorders and prostate cancer. *Curr. Med. Chem.* **2012**, *19*, 856–870. [CrossRef]
20. Nawaz, S.; Mullen, G.E.D.; Blower, P.J.; Ballinger, J.R. A 99mTc-labelled scFv antibody fragment that binds to prostate-specific membrane antigen. *Nucl. Med. Commun.* **2017**, *38*, 666–671. [CrossRef]
21. Mazzocco, C.; Fracasso, G.; Germain-Genevois, C.; Dugot-Senant, N.; Figini, M.; Colombatti, M.; Grenier, N.; Couillaud, F. In vivo imaging of prostate cancer using an anti-PSMA scFv fragment as a probe. *Sci. Rep.* **2016**, *6*, 23314. [CrossRef] [PubMed]
22. Frigerio, B.; Morlino, S.; Luison, E.; Seregni, E.; Lorenzoni, A.; Satta, A.; Valdagni, R.; Bogni, A.; Chiesa, C.; Mira, M.; et al. Anti-PSMA (124)I-scFvD2B as a new immuno-PET tool for prostate cancer: Preclinical proof of principle. *J. Exp. Clin. Cancer Res.* **2019**, *38*, 326. [CrossRef] [PubMed]
23. Lutje, S.; van Rij, C.M.; Franssen, G.M.; Fracasso, G.; Helfrich, W.; Eek, A.; Oyen, W.J.; Colombatti, M.; Boerman, O.C. Targeting human prostate cancer with 111In-labeled D2B IgG, F(ab')2 and Fab fragments in nude mice with PSMA-expressing xenografts. *Contrast Media Mol. Imaging* **2015**, *10*, 28–36. [CrossRef] [PubMed]
24. Wong, P.; Li, L.; Chea, J.; Delgado, M.K.; Crow, D.; Poku, E.; Szpikowska, B.; Bowles, N.; Channappa, D.; Colcher, D.; et al. PET imaging of (64)Cu-DOTA-scFv-anti-PSMA lipid nanoparticles (LNPs): Enhanced tumor targeting over anti-PSMA scFv or untargeted LNPs. *Nucl. Med. Biol.* **2017**, *47*, 62–68. [CrossRef] [PubMed]

25. Viola-Villegas, N.T.; Sevak, K.K.; Carlin, S.D.; Doran, M.G.; Evans, H.W.; Bartlett, D.W.; Wu, A.M.; Lewis, J.S. Noninvasive Imaging of PSMA in prostate tumors with (89)Zr-Labeled huJ591 engineered antibody fragments: The faster alternatives. *Mol. Pharm.* **2014**, *11*, 3965–3973. [CrossRef] [PubMed]
26. Pandit-Taskar, N.; O'Donoghue, J.A.; Ruan, S.; Lyashchenko, S.K.; Carrasquillo, J.A.; Heller, G.; Martinez, D.F.; Cheal, S.M.; Lewis, J.S.; Fleisher, M.; et al. First-in-Human Imaging with 89Zr-Df-IAB2M Anti-PSMA Minibody in Patients with Metastatic Prostate Cancer: Pharmacokinetics, Biodistribution, Dosimetry, and Lesion Uptake. *J. Nucl. Med.* **2016**, *57*, 1858–1864. [CrossRef] [PubMed]
27. Su, Y.; Yu, L.; Liu, N.; Guo, Z.; Wang, G.; Zheng, J.; Wei, M.; Wang, H.; Yang, A.G.; Qin, W.; et al. PSMA specific single chain antibody-mediated targeted knockdown of Notch1 inhibits human prostate cancer cell proliferation and tumor growth. *Cancer Lett.* **2013**, *338*, 282–291. [CrossRef]
28. Baum, V.; Buhler, P.; Gierschner, D.; Herchenbach, D.; Fiala, G.J.; Schamel, W.W.; Wolf, P.; Elsasser-Beile, U. Antitumor activities of PSMAxCD3 diabodies by redirected T-cell lysis of prostate cancer cells. *Immunotherapy* **2013**, *5*, 27–38. [CrossRef]
29. Friedrich, M.; Raum, T.; Lutterbuese, R.; Voelkel, M.; Deegen, P.; Rau, D.; Kischel, R.; Hoffmann, P.; Brandl, C.; Schuhmacher, J.; et al. Regression of human prostate cancer xenografts in mice by AMG 212/BAY2010112, a novel PSMA/CD3-Bispecific BiTE antibody cross-reactive with non-human primate antigens. *Mol. Cancer Ther.* **2012**, *11*, 2664–2673. [CrossRef]
30. Hernandez-Hoyos, G.; Sewell, T.; Bader, R.; Bannink, J.; Chenault, R.A.; Daugherty, M.; Dasovich, M.; Fang, H.; Gottschalk, R.; Kumer, J.; et al. MOR209/ES414, a Novel Bispecific Antibody Targeting PSMA for the Treatment of Metastatic Castration-Resistant Prostate Cancer. *Mol. Cancer Ther.* **2016**, *15*, 2155–2165. [CrossRef]
31. Jachimowicz, R.D.; Fracasso, G.; Yazaki, P.J.; Power, B.E.; Borchmann, P.; Engert, A.; Hansen, H.P.; Reiners, K.S.; Marie, M.; von Strandmann, E.P.; et al. Induction of in vitro and in vivo NK cell cytotoxicity using high-avidity immunoligands targeting prostate-specific membrane antigen in prostate carcinoma. *Mol. Cancer Ther.* **2011**, *10*, 1036–1045. [CrossRef] [PubMed]
32. Leconet, W.; Liu, H.; Guo, M.; Le Lamer-Dechamps, S.; Molinier, C.; Kim, S.; Vrlinic, T.; Oster, M.; Liu, F.; Navarro, V.; et al. Anti-PSMA/CD3 Bispecific Antibody Delivery and Antitumor Activity Using a Polymeric Depot Formulation. *Mol. Cancer Ther.* **2018**, *17*, 1927–1940. [CrossRef] [PubMed]
33. Zhang, Q.; Helfand, B.T.; Carneiro, B.A.; Qin, W.; Yang, X.J.; Lee, C.; Zhang, W.; Giles, F.J.; Cristofanilli, M.; Kuzel, T.M. Efficacy Against Human Prostate Cancer by Prostate-specific Membrane Antigen-specific, Transforming Growth Factor-beta Insensitive Genetically Targeted CD8(+) T-cells Derived from Patients with Metastatic Castrate-resistant Disease. *Eur. Urol.* **2018**, *73*, 648–652. [CrossRef] [PubMed]
34. Li, J.; Franek, K.J.; Patterson, A.L.; Holmes, L.M.; Burgin, K.E.; Ji, J.; Yu, X.; Wagner, T.E.; Wei, Y. Targeting foreign major histocompatibility complex molecules to tumors by tumor cell specific single chain antibody (scFv). *Int. J. Oncol.* **2003**, *23*, 1329–1332. [CrossRef] [PubMed]
35. Michalska, M.; Schultze-Seemann, S.; Bogatyreva, L.; Hauschke, D.; Wetterauer, U.; Wolf, P. In vitro and in vivo effects of a recombinant anti-PSMA immunotoxin in combination with docetaxel against prostate cancer. *Oncotarget* **2016**, *7*, 22531–22542. [CrossRef] [PubMed]
36. Noll, T.; Schultze-Seemann, S.; Kuckuck, I.; Michalska, M.; Wolf, P. Synergistic cytotoxicity of a prostate cancer-specific immunotoxin in combination with the BH3 mimetic ABT-737. *Cancer Immunol. Immunother.* **2018**, *67*, 413–422. [CrossRef]
37. Baiz, D.; Hassan, S.; Choi, Y.A.; Flores, A.; Karpova, Y.; Yancey, D.; Pullikuth, A.; Sui, G.; Sadelain, M.; Debinski, W.; et al. Combination of the PI3K inhibitor ZSTK474 with a PSMA-targeted immunotoxin accelerates apoptosis and regression of prostate cancer. *Neoplasia* **2013**, *15*, 1172–1183. [CrossRef]
38. Meng, P.; Dong, Q.C.; Tan, G.G.; Wen, W.H.; Wang, H.; Zhang, G.; Wang, Y.Z.; Jing, Y.M.; Wang, C.; Qin, W.J.; et al. Anti-tumor effects of a recombinant anti-prostate specific membrane antigen immunotoxin against prostate cancer cells. *BMC Urol.* **2017**, *17*, 14. [CrossRef]
39. Hassani, M.; Hajari Taheri, F.; Sharifzadeh, Z.; Arashkia, A.; Hadjati, J.; van Weerden, W.M.; Abdoli, S.; Modarressi, M.H.; Abolhassani, M. Engineered Jurkat Cells for Targeting Prostate-Specific Membrane Antigen on Prostate Cancer Cells by Nanobody-Based Chimeric Antigen Receptor. *Iran. Biomed. J.* **2020**, *24*, 81–88. [CrossRef]

40. Santoro, S.P.; Kim, S.; Motz, G.T.; Alatzoglou, D.; Li, C.; Irving, M.; Powell, D.J., Jr.; Coukos, G. T cells bearing a chimeric antigen receptor against prostate-specific membrane antigen mediate vascular disruption and result in tumor regression. *Cancer Immunol. Res.* **2015**, *3*, 68–84. [CrossRef]
41. Menotti, L.; Avitabile, E.; Gatta, V.; Malatesta, P.; Petrovic, B.; Campadelli-Fiume, G. HSV as A Platform for the Generation of Retargeted, Armed, and Reporter-Expressing Oncolytic Viruses. *Viruses* **2018**, *10*, 352. [CrossRef] [PubMed]
42. Liu, C.; Hasegawa, K.; Russell, S.J.; Sadelain, M.; Peng, K.W. Prostate-specific membrane antigen retargeted measles virotherapy for the treatment of prostate cancer. *Prostate* **2009**, *69*, 1128–1141. [CrossRef] [PubMed]
43. Novakova, Z.; Foss, C.A.; Copeland, B.T.; Morath, V.; Baranova, P.; Havlinova, B.; Skerra, A.; Pomper, M.G.; Barinka, C. Novel Monoclonal Antibodies Recognizing Human Prostate-Specific Membrane Antigen (PSMA) as Research and Theranostic Tools. *Prostate* **2017**, *77*, 749–764. [CrossRef] [PubMed]
44. Banerjee, S.R.; Kumar, V.; Lisok, A.; Plyku, D.; Novakova, Z.; Brummet, M.; Wharram, B.; Barinka, C.; Hobbs, R.; Pomper, M.G. Evaluation of (111)In-DOTA-5D3, a Surrogate SPECT Imaging Agent for Radioimmunotherapy of Prostate-Specific Membrane Antigen. *J. Nucl. Med.* **2019**, *60*, 400–406. [CrossRef]
45. Huang, C.T.; Guo, X.; Barinka, C.; Lupold, S.E.; Pomper, M.G.; Gabrielson, K.; Raman, V.; Artemov, D.; Hapuarachchige, S. Development of 5D3-DM1: A Novel Anti-Prostate-Specific Membrane Antigen Antibody-Drug Conjugate for PSMA-Positive Prostate Cancer Therapy. *Mol. Pharm.* **2020**, *17*, 3392–3402. [CrossRef]
46. Hapuarachchige, S.; Huang, C.T.; Donnelly, M.C.; Barinka, C.; Lupold, S.E.; Pomper, M.G.; Artemov, D. Cellular Delivery of Bioorthogonal Pretargeting Therapeutics in PSMA-Positive Prostate Cancer. *Mol. Pharm.* **2020**, *17*, 98–108. [CrossRef]
47. Schiweck, W.; Skerra, A. Fermenter production of an artificial fab fragment, rationally designed for the antigen cystatin, and its optimized crystallization through constant domain shuffling. *Proteins* **1995**, *23*, 561–565. [CrossRef]
48. Skerra, A. Use of the tetracycline promoter for the tightly regulated production of a murine antibody fragment in Escherichia coli. *Gene* **1994**, *151*, 131–135. [CrossRef]
49. Schlapschy, M.; Fiedler, M.; Skerra, A. *Purification and Characterization of His-Tagged Antibody Fragments in Antibody Engineering*, 2nd ed.; Springer: Berlin, Germany, 2010; pp. 279–291. [CrossRef]
50. Chilumuri, A.; Markiv, A.; Milton, N.G. Immunocytochemical staining of endogenous nuclear proteins with the HIS-1 anti-poly-histidine monoclonal antibody: A potential source of error in His-tagged protein detection. *Acta Histochem.* **2014**, *116*, 1022–1028. [CrossRef]
51. Vermeer, A.W.; Bremer, M.G.; Norde, W. Structural changes of IgG induced by heat treatment and by adsorption onto a hydrophobic Teflon surface studied by circular dichroism spectroscopy. *Biochi. Biophys. Acta* **1998**, *1425*, 1–12. [CrossRef]
52. Gupta, S.K.; Shukla, P. Microbial platform technology for recombinant antibody fragment production: A review. *Crit. Rev. Microbiol.* **2017**, *43*, 31–42. [CrossRef] [PubMed]
53. De Jongh, W.A.; Salgueiro, S.; Dyring, C. The use of Drosophila S2 cells in R&D and bioprocessing. *Pharm. Bioprocess.* **2013**, *1*, 197–213.
54. Tykvart, J.; Sacha, P.; Barinka, C.; Knedlik, T.; Starkova, J.; Lubkowski, J.; Konvalinka, J. Efficient and versatile one-step affinity purification of in vivo biotinylated proteins: Expression, characterization and structure analysis of recombinant human glutamate carboxypeptidase II. *Protein Expr. Purif.* **2012**, *82*, 106–115. [CrossRef] [PubMed]
55. Ventini-Monteiro, D.; Dubois, S.; Astray, R.M.; Castillo, J.; Pereira, C.A. Insect cell entrapment, growth and recovering using a single-use fixed-bed bioreactor. Scaling up and recombinant protein production. *J. Biotechnol.* **2015**, *216*, 110–115. [CrossRef]
56. Daniels, R.W.; Rossano, A.J.; Macleod, G.T.; Ganetzky, B. Expression of multiple transgenes from a single construct using viral 2A peptides in Drosophila. *PLoS ONE* **2014**, *9*, e100637. [CrossRef]
57. Mori, K.; Hamada, H.; Ogawa, T.; Ohmuro-Matsuyama, Y.; Katsuda, T.; Yamaji, H. Efficient production of antibody Fab fragment by transient gene expression in insect cells. *J. Biosci. Bioeng.* **2017**, *124*, 221–226. [CrossRef]
58. Holliger, P.; Prospero, T.; Winter, G. "Diabodies": Small bivalent and bispecific antibody fragments. *Proc. Natl. Acad. Sci. USA* **1993**, *90*, 6444–6448. [CrossRef]

59. Viti, F.; Tarli, L.; Giovannoni, L.; Zardi, L.; Neri, D. Increased binding affinity and valence of recombinant antibody fragments lead to improved targeting of tumoral angiogenesis. *Cancer Res.* **1999**, *59*, 347–352.
60. Bird, R.E.; Hardman, K.D.; Jacobson, J.W.; Johnson, S.; Kaufman, B.M.; Lee, S.M.; Lee, T.; Pope, S.H.; Riordan, G.S.; Whitlow, M. Single-chain antigen-binding proteins. *Science* **1988**, *242*, 423–426. [CrossRef]
61. Huston, J.S.; Levinson, D.; Mudgett-Hunter, M.; Tai, M.S.; Novotny, J.; Margolies, M.N.; Ridge, R.J.; Bruccoleri, R.E.; Haber, E.; Crea, R.; et al. Protein engineering of antibody binding sites: Recovery of specific activity in an anti-digoxin single-chain Fv analogue produced in Escherichia coli. *Proc. Natl. Acad. Sci. USA* **1988**, *85*, 5879–5883. [CrossRef]
62. Whitlow, M.; Bell, B.A.; Feng, S.L.; Filpula, D.; Hardman, K.D.; Hubert, S.L.; Rollence, M.L.; Wood, J.F.; Schott, M.E.; Milenic, D.E.; et al. An improved linker for single-chain Fv with reduced aggregation and enhanced proteolytic stability. *Protein Eng.* **1993**, *6*, 989–995. [CrossRef] [PubMed]
63. Olafsen, T.; Kenanova, V.E.; Wu, A.M. *Generation of Single-Chain Fv Fragments and Multivalent Derivatives scFv-Fc and scFv-CH3 (Minibodies) in Antibody Engineering*, 2nd ed.; Springer: Berlin, Germany, 2010; pp. 69–84. [CrossRef]
64. Kellmann, S.J.; Dubel, S.; Thie, H. A strategy to identify linker-based modules for the allosteric regulation of antibody-antigen binding affinities of different scFvs. *MAbs* **2017**, *9*, 404–418. [CrossRef] [PubMed]
65. Muller, D. *scFv by Two-Step Cloning in Antibody Engineering*, 2nd ed.; Springer: Berlin, Germany, 2010; pp. 55–59. [CrossRef]
66. Martoglio, B.; Dobberstein, B. Signal sequences: More than just greasy peptides. *Trends Cell Biol.* **1998**, *8*, 410–415. [CrossRef]
67. El-Sayed, A.; Bernhard, W.; Barreto, K.; Gonzalez, C.; Hill, W.; Pastushok, L.; Fonge, H.; Geyer, C.R. Evaluation of antibody fragment properties for near-infrared fluorescence imaging of HER3-positive cancer xenografts. *Theranostics* **2018**, *8*, 4856–4869. [CrossRef] [PubMed]
68. Pavlinkova, G.; Beresford, G.W.; Booth, B.J.; Batra, S.K.; Colcher, D. Pharmacokinetics and biodistribution of engineered single-chain antibody constructs of MAb CC49 in colon carcinoma xenografts. *J. Nucl. Med.* **1999**, *40*, 1536–1546.
69. Adams, G.P.; Schier, R.; Marshall, K.; Wolf, E.J.; McCall, A.M.; Marks, J.D.; Weiner, L.M. Increased affinity leads to improved selective tumor delivery of single-chain Fv antibodies. *Cancer Res.* **1998**, *58*, 485–490.
70. Adams, G.P.; Schier, R.; McCall, A.M.; Simmons, H.H.; Horak, E.M.; Alpaugh, R.K.; Marks, J.D.; Weiner, L.M. High affinity restricts the localization and tumor penetration of single-chain fv antibody molecules. *Cancer Res.* **2001**, *61*, 4750–4755.
71. Zhou, Y.; Goenaga, A.L.; Harms, B.D.; Zou, H.; Lou, J.; Conrad, F.; Adams, G.P.; Schoeberl, B.; Nielsen, U.B.; Marks, J.D. Impact of intrinsic affinity on functional binding and biological activity of EGFR antibodies. *Mol. Cancer Ther.* **2012**, *11*, 1467–1476. [CrossRef]
72. Han, D.; Wu, J.; Han, Y.; Wei, M.; Han, S.; Lin, R.; Sun, Z.; Yang, F.; Jiao, D.; Xie, P.; et al. A novel anti-PSMA human scFv has the potential to be used as a diagnostic tool in prostate cancer. *Oncotarget* **2016**, *7*, 59471–59481. [CrossRef]
73. Rezaei, J.; RajabiBazl, M.; Ebrahimizadeh, W.; Dehbidi, G.R.; Hosseini, H. Selection of Single Chain Antibody Fragments for Targeting Prostate Specific Membrane Antigen: A Comparison Between Cell-based and Antigen-based Approach. *Protein Pept. Lett.* **2016**, *23*, 336–342. [CrossRef]
74. Frigerio, B.; Fracasso, G.; Luison, E.; Cingarlini, S.; Mortarino, M.; Coliva, A.; Seregni, E.; Bombardieri, E.; Zuccolotto, G.; Rosato, A.; et al. A single-chain fragment against prostate specific membrane antigen as a tool to build theranostic reagents for prostate cancer. *Eur. J. Cancer* **2013**, *49*, 2223–2232. [CrossRef] [PubMed]
75. Parker, S.A.; Diaz, I.L.; Anderson, K.A.; Batt, C.A. Design, production, and characterization of a single-chain variable fragment (ScFv) derived from the prostate specific membrane antigen (PSMA) monoclonal antibody J591. *Protein Expr. Purif.* **2013**, *89*, 136–145. [CrossRef] [PubMed]
76. Kampmeier, F.; Williams, J.D.; Maher, J.; Mullen, G.E.; Blower, P.J. Design and preclinical evaluation of a 99mTc-labelled diabody of mAb J591 for SPECT imaging of prostate-specific membrane antigen (PSMA). *EJNMMI Res.* **2014**, *4*, 13. [CrossRef] [PubMed]
77. Brown, B.A.; Comeau, R.D.; Jones, P.L.; Liberatore, F.A.; Neacy, W.P.; Sands, H.; Gallagher, B.M. Pharmacokinetics of the monoclonal antibody B72.3 and its fragments labeled with either 125I or 111In. *Cancer Res.* **1987**, *47*, 1149–1154. [PubMed]

78. Fortmuller, K.; Alt, K.; Gierschner, D.; Wolf, P.; Baum, V.; Freudenberg, N.; Wetterauer, U.; Elsasser-Beile, U.; Buhler, P. Effective targeting of prostate cancer by lymphocytes redirected by a PSMA x CD3 bispecific single-chain diabody. *Prostate* **2011**, *71*, 588–596. [CrossRef] [PubMed]
79. Werner, W.E.; Wu, S.; Mulkerrin, M. The removal of pyroglutamic acid from monoclonal antibodies without denaturation of the protein chains. *Anal. Biochem.* **2005**, *342*, 120–125. [CrossRef] [PubMed]
80. Lubyova, B.; Hodek, J.; Zabransky, A.; Prouzova, H.; Hubalek, M.; Hirsch, I.; Weber, J. PRMT5: A novel regulator of Hepatitis B virus replication and an arginine methylase of HBV core. *PLoS ONE* **2017**, *12*, e0186982. [CrossRef]
81. Strohalm, M.; Hassman, M.; Kosata, B.; Kodicek, M. mMass data miner: An open source alternative for mass spectrometric data analysis. *Rapid Commun. Mass Spectrom.* **2008**, *22*, 905–908. [CrossRef]
82. Gebauer, M.; Skerra, A. Anticalins small engineered binding proteins based on the lipocalin scaffold. *Methods Enzymol.* **2012**, *503*, 157–188. [CrossRef]
83. Yanisch-Perron, C.; Vieira, J.; Messing, J. Improved M13 phage cloning vectors and host strains: Nucleotide sequences of the M13mp18 and pUC19 vectors. *Gene* **1985**, *33*, 103–119. [CrossRef]
84. Barinka, C.; Ptacek, J.; Richter, A.; Novakova, Z.; Morath, V.; Skerra, A. Selection and characterization of Anticalins targeting human prostate-specific membrane antigen (PSMA). *Protein Eng. Des. Sel.* **2016**, *29*, 105–115. [CrossRef] [PubMed]
85. Banerjee, S.R.; Foss, C.A.; Castanares, M.; Mease, R.C.; Byun, Y.; Fox, J.J.; Hilton, J.; Lupold, S.E.; Kozikowski, A.P.; Pomper, M.G. Synthesis and evaluation of technetium-99m- and rhenium-labeled inhibitors of the prostate-specific membrane antigen (PSMA). *J. Med. chem.* **2008**, *51*, 4504–4517. [CrossRef] [PubMed]

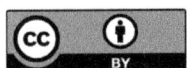

© 2020 by the authors. Licensee MDPI, Basel, Switzerland. This article is an open access article distributed under the terms and conditions of the Creative Commons Attribution (CC BY) license (http://creativecommons.org/licenses/by/4.0/).

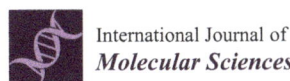

Article

Selection and Characterization of YKL-40-Targeting Monoclonal Antibodies from Human Synthetic Fab Phage Display Libraries

Kyungjae Kang [1,†], Kicheon Kim [2,†,‡], Se-Ra Lee [1], Yoonji Kim [1], Joo Eon Lee [1], Yong Sun Lee [2], Ju-Hyeon Lim [1], Chung-Su Lim [1], Yu Jung Kim [1], Seung Il Baek [1], Du Hyun Song [1], Jin Tae Hong [2,*] and Dae Young Kim [1,*]

1. New Drug Development Center, Osong Medical Innovation Foundation, Cheongju-si, Chungcheongbuk-do 28160, Korea; kyungjae@kbiohealth.kr (K.K.); srlee@kbiohealth.kr (S.-R.L.); yoon555@kbiohealth.kr (Y.K.); jooeona@kbiohealth.kr (J.E.L.); sinistemcells@kbiohealth.kr (J.-H.L.); opern88@kbiohealth.kr (C.-S.L.); yjkim@kbiohealth.kr (Y.J.K.); bsi022013@kbiohealth.kr (S.I.B.); biosong@kbiohealth.kr (D.H.S.)
2. College of Pharmacy, Chungbuk National University, Cheongju-si, Chungcheongbuk-do 28160, Korea; k.kicheon@gmail.com (K.K.); kallintz@gmail.com (Y.S.L.)
* Correspondence: jinthong@chungbuk.ac.kr (J.T.H.); kimdae@kbiohealth.kr (D.Y.K.); Tel.: +82-43-261-2813 (J.T.H.); Tel.: +82-43-200-9521 (D.Y.K.)
† These authors contributed equally to this work.
‡ Current address: National Center for Efficacy Evaluation of Respiratory Disease Product, Korea Institute of Toxicology, 30 Baekhak1-gil, Jeongeup, Jeollabuk-do 53212, Korea.

Received: 11 June 2020; Accepted: 28 August 2020; Published: 1 September 2020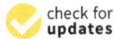

Abstract: YKL-40, also known as chitinase-3-like 1 (CHI3L1), is a glycoprotein that is expressed and secreted by various cell types, including cancers and macrophages. Due to its implications for and upregulation in a variety of diseases, including inflammatory conditions, fibrotic disorders, and tumor growth, YKL-40 has been considered as a significant therapeutic biomarker. Here, we used a phage display to develop novel monoclonal antibodies (mAbs) targeting human YKL-40 (hYKL-40). Human synthetic antibody phage display libraries were panned against a recombinant hYKL-40 protein, yielding seven unique Fabs (Antigen-binding fragment), of which two Fabs (H1 and H2) were non-aggregating and thermally stable (75.5 °C and 76.5 °C, respectively) and had high apparent affinities (K_D = 2.3 nM and 4.0 nM, respectively). Reformatting the Fabs into IgGs (Immunoglobulin Gs) increased their apparent affinities (notably, for H1 and H2, K_D = 0.5 nM and 0.3 nM, respectively), presumably due to the effects of avidity, with little change to their non-aggregation property. The six anti-hYKL-40 IgGs were analyzed using a trans-well migration assay in vitro, revealing that three clones (H1, H2, and H4) were notably effective in reducing cell migration from both A549 and H460 lung cancer cell lines. The three clones were further analyzed in an in vivo animal test that assessed their anti-cancer activities, demonstrating that the tumor area and the number of tumor nodules were significantly reduced in the lung tissues treated with H1 (IgG). Given its high affinity and desirable properties, we expect that the H1 anti-hYKL-40 mAb will be a suitable candidate for developing anti-cancer therapeutics.

Keywords: YKL-40; CHI3L1; monoclonal antibody; phage display; lung metastasis

1. Introduction

YKL-40, also known as chitinase 3-like 1 (Chi3L1), is a 40 kDa secreted glycoprotein belonging to the family of chitinase-like proteins (CLPs) [1]. It is a highly conserved chitin-binding protein and its crystallographic three-dimensional structures reveal the typical fold of the chitinase family protein but lacks chitinase activity due to mutation of an essential amino acid residue in its catalytic domain [2]. YKL-40 is overexpressed in cancers and tumor-associated macrophages, and its serum levels are elevated in patients with metastatic cancers and in various chronic inflammatory diseases, implicating pathological role of YKL-40 in cancer progression, metastasis, and inflammation [1,3–6].

While many things remain to be understood regarding the molecular nature of its action mechanism, a number of studies have verified YKL-40 as a promising therapeutic target for the treatment of various cancers and inflammatory diseases [1]. In various cancer cells, the YKL-40 signaling cascades are triggered by the membrane receptors such as syndecan-1, integrin αvβ5, VEGF receptor 2, and RAGE, leading to the increased expression levels of VEGF, MMP9, CCL2, and CXCL2 through FAK and ERK1/2-MAPK activity which result in the elevation of angiogenesis and tumor proliferation [7–9]. YKL-40-inhibiting small compounds such as caffeine, theophylline, chitin (β-(1-4)-poly-N-acetyl D-glucosamine), and siRNA complex are known to be effective in reducing tumor growth and metastasis in diverse kinds of cancers through down-regulation of signaling pathways, including PI3K/AKT, STAT3, and NF-kB, downstream of YKL-40 [10–15]. YKL-40 is also associated with various inflammatory diseases including atherosclerosis, liver injury, and rheumatoid arthritis. The pro-inflammatory signaling pathways such as STAT3, caspase 3, and NF-κB, are induced by YKL-40–mediated RAGE activation. Intriguingly, YKL-40 is able to regulate apoptotic cell death depending on the association of TMEM219 with IL13Rα2, a known YKL-40 cellular receptor. That is, apoptotic cell death is reduced through the activation of the Erk1/2 and Akt signaling pathway when YKL-40 binds a YKL-40 receptor complex composed of TMEM219 and IL13Rα2, while YKL-40 binding to IL-13Rα2 in the absence of TMEM219 induces apoptotic cell death by stimulating the Wnt/β-catenin signaling [16–18]. YKL-40-inhibiting shRNA and miR-590-3p are known to reduce rheumatoid arthritis via downregulation of IL-18 production through PI3K/AKT pathway, while a proteasome inhibitor, Bortezomib, is found to suppress the expression of YKL-40, resulting in the reduction of pro-inflammatory and pro-fibrotic factors via down-regulation of NF-kB pathway [19,20]. Moreover, YKL-40 is associated with Alzheimer's disease (AD) which is one of the inflammatory diseases. The expression of YKL-40 is induced by pro-inflammatory cytokines such as IL-1β and IL-6 through a STAT3 signaling pathway in astrocytes and the inflammation-induced YKL-40 activates the MAPK, β-catenin, and NF-κB signaling pathways via RAGE [16,21]. K284-6111, a YKL-40 inhibitor, reduces the expression of neuroinflammatory genes such as COX-2, iNOS, and GFAP in AD animal model through downregulation of NF-kB pathway, resulting in attenuation of memory dysfunction [22]. In addition to YKL-40-inhibiting small compounds, anti-YKL-40 antibodies were also found to attenuate angiogenesis via inhibition of tumor vascularization in brain and breast cancers [23–25].

As antibody-based therapeutics, full-length monoclonal antibodies (mAbs) have proven successful as drugs and remain unrivaled so far in spite of their drawback such as costly and time-consuming production in mammalian cell lines. In fact, most approved mAbs and those in regulatory review are canonical IgG antibodies [26,27]. Among numerous methods to identify human mAbs, phage display is a powerful tool that enables to display proteins and peptides on the surface of phage, which can be applied to study protein-protein interactions, define epitopes, identify enzyme inhibitors, screen antibody libraries, and to identify agonists and antagonists of cellular receptors [28–30]. In particular, phage display antibody libraries, generated in either naïve or synthetic antibody (mostly in Fab (Antigen-binding fragment) or scFv forms) formats, have proven to be highly successful for the selection of human mAbs against wide ranges of therapeutic targets ranging from cancers and inflammatory diseases to infectious diseases [31–39].

In this study, we panned synthetic human Fab phage display libraries against human YKL-40 (hYKL-40) and obtained monoclonal antibodies (mAbs) with high affinities and desirable biophysico-chemical properties for hYKL-40. We also described their activities interfering migration and proliferation of cancer cells, resulting in a selection of a candidate mAb, H1. We anticipate the

H1 mAb can be further developed as a promising biologic in various pathological circumstances including cancers.

2. Results

2.1. Selection of Human Anti-hYKL-40 Fabs

We have recently constructed some synthetic human antibody phage display libraries (size, $\approx 1 \times 10^{10}$ for all): two synthetic human Fab phage display libraries (KFab-I and KFab-II, built on a human VH3/Vk1 and a VH1/Vk1 framework (FR), respectively) and a synthetic human scFv phage display library (KscFv-I, built on the same FR as the KFab-I library) (unpublished data). In order to isolate human antibodies that specifically recognize hYKL-40, the KFab-I library was panned against a recombinant hYKL-40 immobilized on immunotubes, and 94 monoclonal phages from each of the third and fourth rounds of the panning were evaluated by ELISA (Figure 1a and Figure S1). Of the 94 individual clones from the third round, 26 had ELISA read-outs that were clearly higher than those of the background level (no immobilized hYKL-40 control) and were considered to be potential binders, while 86% (81 out of the 94) of the clones from the fourth round were determined to be positives based on their ELISA read-outs. The clones from the third round were sequenced, and 22 clones were determined to be complete and in-frame. The remaining clones contained mutations, such as frameshifts. By analyzing the CDR sequences of the 22 clones, 2 unique Fab clones (H1 (Fab) and H2 (Fab)) were identified. The H1 (Fab) was dominantly selected via panning (73% of sequences (16 out of the 22)), while the H2 (Fab) was present at a lower frequency (27% (6 out of the 22)) (Figure 1b). Since they already seemed quite enriched in the third round, the clones from the fourth round were not further analyzed (Figure S1).

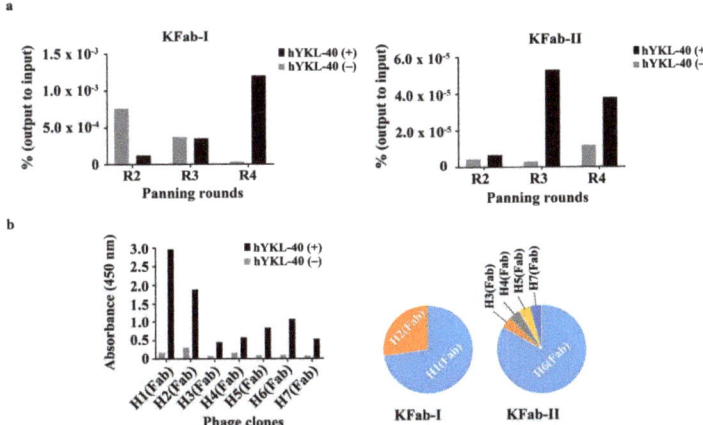

Figure 1. Panning of the phage-displayed synthetic Fab libraries on hYKL-40. (**a**) Monitoring of the phage titers over three rounds (R2–R4) of panning. Black and gray bars indicate the ratio of the phage output to the input titers, presented as a percentage (%), from panning on immobilized hYKL-4 (black, hYKL-40(+)) and non-immobilized hYKL-40 (gray, hYKL-40(−)) surfaces. The ratio of the output to the input (%) = (phage output titer ÷ phage input titer) × 100. (**b**) Phage ELISA performed on the immobilized hYKL-40 surfaces of seven Fab phage clones (left) and their selection frequency (%) over the panning (right). The selection frequency of a unique clone (%) = (Number of unique clones ÷ Total number of phage ELISA positives) × 100. Fab: Antigen-binding fragment; ELISA: enzyme-linked immunosorbent assay.

In parallel, the other Fab phage display library, KFab-II, was also panned on a recombinant immobilized hYKL-40 surface, yielding 13 and 12 ELISA positives out of 94 individual clones from each of the third and fourth rounds of the panning, respectively, with relatively lower ELISA read-outs compared to those of the clones from the KFab-I library (Figure 1a and Figure S1). The clones were sequenced, and 23 clones were determined to be complete and in-frame. The remaining clones contained mutations, such as a stop codon (data not shown). By analyzing the CDR sequences of the 23 clones, 5 clones (H4 (Fab), H6 (Fab), and H7 (Fab) from the third round; H3 (Fab) and H5 (Fab) from the fourth round) were identified. H6 (Fab) was found to be the most dominant clone, with 83% of the sequences (19 out of 23), and the rest of the clones were selected by 1 out of the 23 clones (≈4%) (Figure 1b).

2.2. Production and Characterization of Human Anti-hYKL-40 Fabs

To produce and characterize the binders as Fab proteins, the selected sequences were next cloned into an in-house bacterial expression vector (pKFAB). The Fabs were expressed in bacteria and subsequently purified. The resulting Fabs were highly pure, with protein yields of 1.8 mg/L, 0.2 mg/L, 0.2 mg/L, 0.5 mg/L, and 0.6 mg/L for H1 (Fab), H2 (Fab), H3 (Fab), H4 (Fab), and H7 (Fab), respectively (Figure 2a). H5 (Fab) and H6 (Fab) yielded little soluble protein.

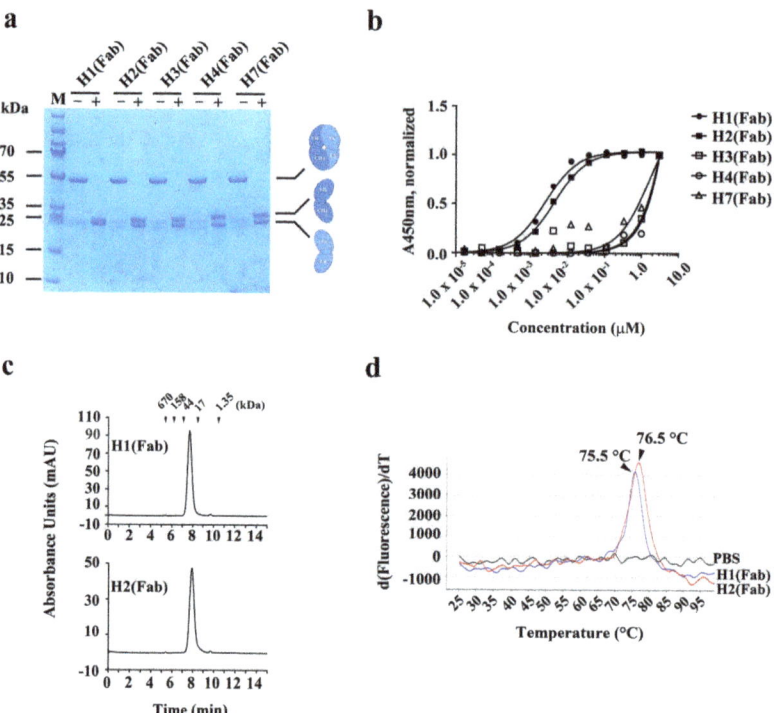

Figure 2. Production and characterization of human anti-hYKL-40 Fabs. (**a**) SDS-PAGE analysis of two human anti-hYKL-40 Fabs, H1 (Fab) and H2 (Fab), purified from periplasmic extracts of *E. coli* transformed with the indicated expression vectors. + and − indicate with and without the reducing reagent (β-mercaptoethanol), respectively. (**b**) Soluble ELISA of serially diluted H1 (Fab) and H2 (Fab) on immobilized hYKL-40 surfaces to measure their apparent affinities (EC_{50}, nM). (**c**) Size-exclusion chromatography analysis of H1 (Fab) and H2 (Fab). The positions of the molecular mass markers, shown as kDa, on the retention time x-axis are shown above the peaks. (**d**) Protein thermal shift assay of H1 (Fab) and H2 (Fab) to determine their thermal stability (T_m, °C). Fab: antigen-binding fragment; SDS-PAGE: sodium dodecyl sulfate-polyacrylamide gel electrophoresis; M: molecular mass marker.

The apparent affinities of the 5 Fabs for hYKL-40 were assessed using ELISA (EC_{50}, nM) (Figure 2b). While the 3 Fabs (H3 (Fab), H4 (Fab), and H7 (Fab)) had very low apparent affinities for hYKL-40 (not fittable), the remaining Fabs, H1 (Fab) and H2 (Fab), showed notably higher apparent affinities (2.3 nM and 4.0 nM, respectively) (Figure 2b). The two Fab proteins H1 (Fab) and H2 (Fab) were observed to be monomeric, with no visible high-molecular-weight (HWM) aggregates found through size-exclusion chromatography (Figure 2c). In order to assess their thermal stability, the melting temperatures (T_m, °C) of the 2 Fab proteins were measured using a protein thermal shift (PTS) assay. The results showed that H1 (Fab) and H2 (Fab) were stable, with a T_m of 75.5 °C and 76.5 °C, respectively (Figure 2d).

2.3. Production and Characterization of Human Anti-hYKL-40 IgGs

In order to produce and characterize the Fab binders in an IgG form, the individual VH and VL sequences from each of the Fab clones were cloned into heavy (IgG1 Fc) and light chain (Ck1) expression vectors, respectively. IgGs were expressed transiently in Expi293 cells and subsequently purified. As shown in Figure 3, the resulting IgGs were highly pure, with protein yields of 0.8 mg/L, 5.9 mg/L, 21.5 mg/L, 1.0 mg/L, 1.7 mg/L, and 17.4 mg/L for H1 (IgG), H2 (IgG), H4 (IgG), H5 (IgG), H6 (IgG), and H7 (IgG), respectively (Figure 3a). H3 (IgG) could not be purified due to its aggregating nature.

To determine whether the apparent affinities of the IgGs for hYKL-40 were changed by reformatting the Fabs into IgGs, the apparent affinities of the IgGs were determined using ELISA (EC_{50}, nM). As shown in Figure 3, the two clones, H1 (IgG) and H2 (IgG), which had high apparent affinities to the Fab forms, showed 5 to 14 fold-increased apparent affinities for H1 (IgG) and H2 (IgG), respectively, compared to their Fab formats (Figure 3b and Table 1), which is possibly due to an avidity effect [40]. The avidity effects were even more remarkable in the remaining IgGs. As shown in Table 1, the apparent affinity of H4 (IgG) was greatly increased to ≈14 nM from having 'not fittable' as its Fab form (Figure 3b), indicating that a significant avidity occurred. Next, to determine whether the IgGs were free of aggregates, they were analyzed using size-exclusion chromatography, revealing that the IgGs did not form any HMW aggregates (Figure 3b). H1 (IgG) was further analyzed using BLI (Bio-layer Interferometry) and a PTS (protein thermal shift) assay, showing that its apparent K_D and thermal stability (T_m) were 5.0×10^{-11} M and 73.7 °C, respectively (Figure S2).

Table 1. Physicochemical properties of human anti-hYKL-40 monoclonal antibodies (mAbs).

Clones	Yield (mg/L Culture)	T_m (°C)	Monomericity (Mon/Agg.)	EC_{50} (nM)	K_D (M)
H1 (Fab)	1.8	76.5	Mon.	2.3	n.d.
H2 (Fab)	0.2	75.5	Mon.	4.0	n.d.
H3 (Fab)	0.2	n.d.	n.d	n.f.	n.d.
H4 (Fab)	0.5	n.d.	n.d	n.f.	n.d.
H7 (Fab)	0.6	n.d.	n.d	n.f.	n.d.
H1 (IgG)	0.8	73.7	Mon.	0.5	5.0×10^{-11}
H2 (IgG)	5.9	n.d.	Mon.	0.3	n.d.
H4 (IgG)	21.5	n.d.	Mon.	13.6	n.d.
H5 (IgG)	1.0	n.d.	Mon.	327.4	n.d.
H6 (IgG)	1.7	n.d.	Mon.	69.4.	n.d.
H7 (IgG)	17.4	n.d.	Mon.	371.3	n.d.

Fab: Antigen-binding fragment; IgG: immunoglobulin G; n.d.: not determined; T_m: melting temperature; EC_{50}: half maximal effective concentration; K_D: equilibrium dissociation constant; Mon.: monomer; Agg.: Aggregate; n.f.: not fittable.

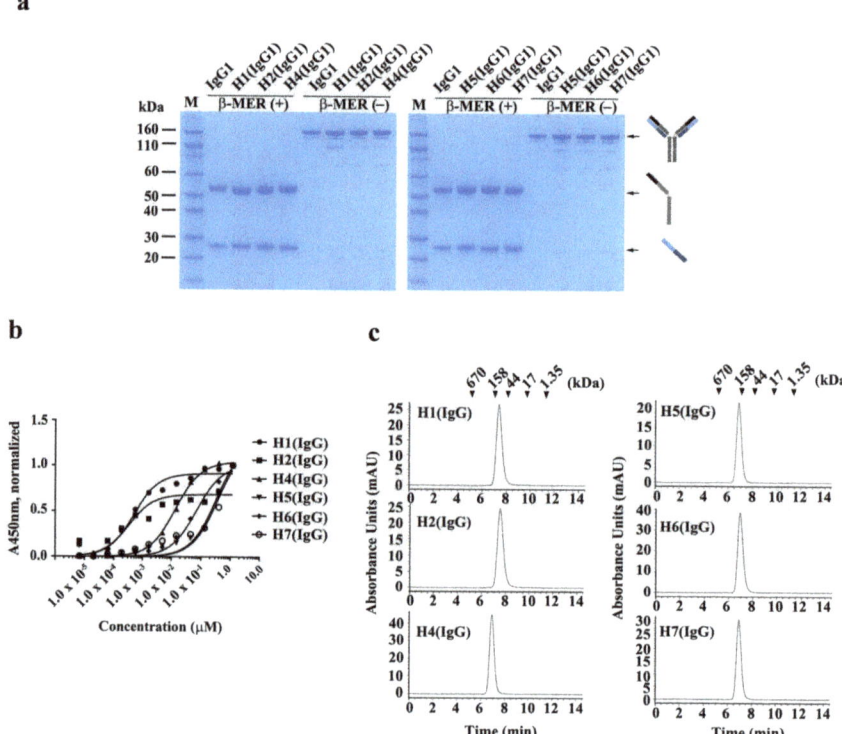

Figure 3. Production and characterization of anti-hYKL-40 IgGs. (**a**) SDS-PAGE analysis of three human anti-hYKL-40 IgGs, H1 (IgG), H2 (IgG), and H4 (IgG), purified from the culture media of Expi293F cells, which were transiently transfected with heavy- and light-chain expression vectors. β-MER (+) and β-MER (−) indicate with and without the reducing reagent (β-mercaptoethanol), respectively. (**b**) Soluble ELISA of serially diluted H1 (IgG), H2 (IgG), and H4 (IgG) on immobilized hYKL-40 surfaces to measure their apparent affinities (EC_{50}, nM). (**c**) Size-exclusion chromatography analysis of H1 (IgG), H2 (IgG), and H4 (IgG). The positions of the molecular mass markers, shown as kDa, on the retention time x-axis are shown above the peaks.

2.4. Trans-Well Migration Assay

Based on our previous study, which revealed that the knock-down of YKL-40 suppressed cancer metastasis in lung cancer cell lines, A549 and H460) [41], we firstly wanted to know whether the anti-hYKL-40 IgGs could mimic the knock-down phenotype by antagonizing the activity of hYKL-40 in cancer cell migration. To address this, we adopted an in vitro trans-well migration assay to investigate their anti-metastatic activity in two different human lung cancer cell lines, A549 and H460 (Figure 4a,b, respectively). We found that all 6 anti-hYKL-40 IgGs significantly inhibited the migration in both the A549 and H460 cell lines. As shown in Figure 4a, 405 ± 21 cells/mm^2 migrated to the lower side of the trans-well in the PBS-treated control group of A549 cells, while 124 ± 5, 132 ± 8, 124 ± 9, 220 ± 22, 263 ± 16, and 229 ± 27 cells/mm^2 migrated to the H1 (IgG)-, H2 (IgG)-, H4 (IgG)-, H5 (IgG)-, H6 (IgG)-, and H7 (IgG)-treated groups, respectively. In Figure 4b, 529 ± 14 cells/mm^2 migrated to the lower side of the trans-well in the PBS-treated control group of H460 cells. However, 112 ± 12, 117 ± 14, 114 ± 11, 158 ± 20, 349 ± 20, and 208 ± 28 cells/mm^2 migrated to the H1 (IgG)-, H2 (IgG)-, H4 (IgG)-, H5 (IgG)-, H6 (IgG)-, and H7 (IgG)-treated groups, respectively. In order to further the in vivo study, we selected 3 anti-hYKL-40 IgGs (H1 (IgG), H2 (IgG), and H4 (IgG)), which showed a significantly higher degree of inhibition in the migration of the lung cancer cells. The 6 anti-hYKL-40 IgGs were further characterized on B16F10 mouse melanoma cells to assess their inhibitory effects in the migration of the melanoma cells prior to an in vivo assay on B16F10 cells. It was revealed that they all inhibited the migration in B16F10 cells as observed on the human lung cancer cells among which the 3 anti-hYKL-40 IgGs (H1, H2, and H4) were playing better compared to the others in antagonizing the cell migration (Figure S3).

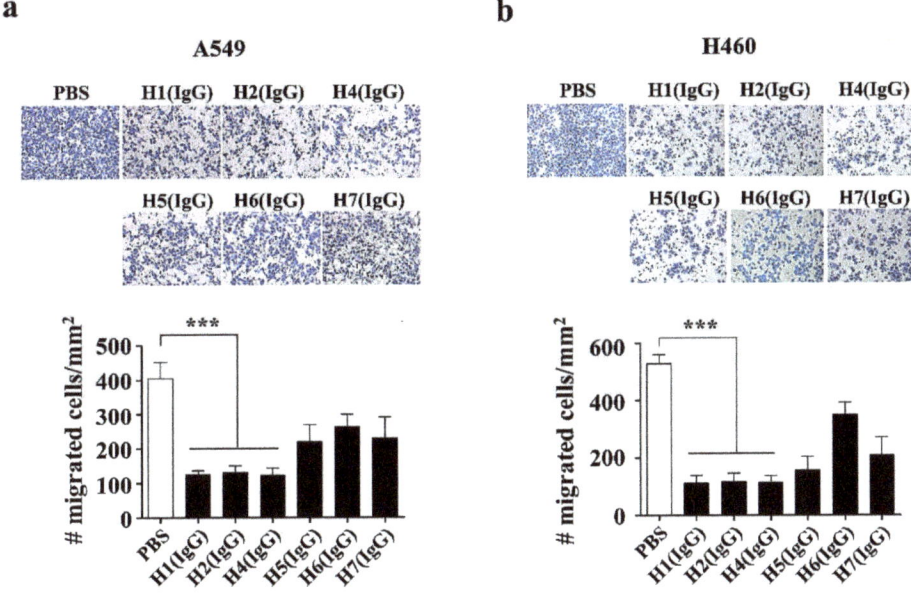

Figure 4. Trans-well migration assay of human anti-hYKL-40 IgGs. (**a**,**b**) Trans-well migration assay of human anti-hYKL-40 IgGs (H1 (IgG), H2 (IgG), H4 (IgG), H5 (IgG), H6 (IgG), and H7 (IgG)) on A549 (**a**) and H460 (**b**) cells to assess their inhibitory effects in cell migration. The number of migrated cells per square mm (mm^2) was counted, plotted and compared to that of a negative control (PBS (phosphate-buffered saline)-treated). The data are presented as the mean ± SE (SEM). *** $p < 0.001$.

2.5. In Vivo Anti-Cancer Effect of hYKL-40 IgGs

To investigate the in vivo anti-cancer effect of the three anti-hYKL-40 IgGs (H1 (IgG), H2 (IgG), and H4 (IgG)), which showed significant inhibitory activities in the in vitro assay on the human lung cancer cells and a mouse melanoma cell (B16F10) (Figure 4 and Figure S3), we considered the differences between applying and not applying the treatments of the anti-hYKL-40 IgGs, in terms of the tumor area and the number of tumor nodules on the lung tissues, to mice injected with B16F10 mouse melanoma cells (Figure 5). To address this, we measured the area of the tumor and total lung tissues of each mouse using a calipus, as described in the materials and methods. As shown in the Figure 5a, the tumor occupied 41.3 ± 5.0% of the surface of the lung tissues in the PBS-treated control group (with no treatment of anti-hYKL-40 IgG), while the tumor area on the surface of the lung tissues was significantly decreased to 7 ± 1.2% with the treatment of H1 (IgG). Unlike H1 (IgG), however, the tumor areas of the lung surfaces treated with H2 (IgG) and H4 (IgG) were 32.3 ± 2.2% and 54 ± 11.0%, respectively, which are not significantly different from the percentages of the PBS-treated control group. Furthermore, the average number of tumor nodules (38.7 ± 4.9) on the lung surface of the PBS-treated mice was significantly decreased to 3.8 ± 0.4 in H1 (IgG)-treated mice (Figure 5b). To see if H1 (IgG) is localized on the lung tissue, we performed an ex vivo imaging and revealed that H1 (IgG) is indeed present on the lung tissue (Figure S4). Moreover, a western blot analysis revealed that H1 (IgG) is able to recognize both recombinant human and mouse YKL-40s, and native YKL-40s from human and murine cells including human and mouse lung cells as well (Figure S5).

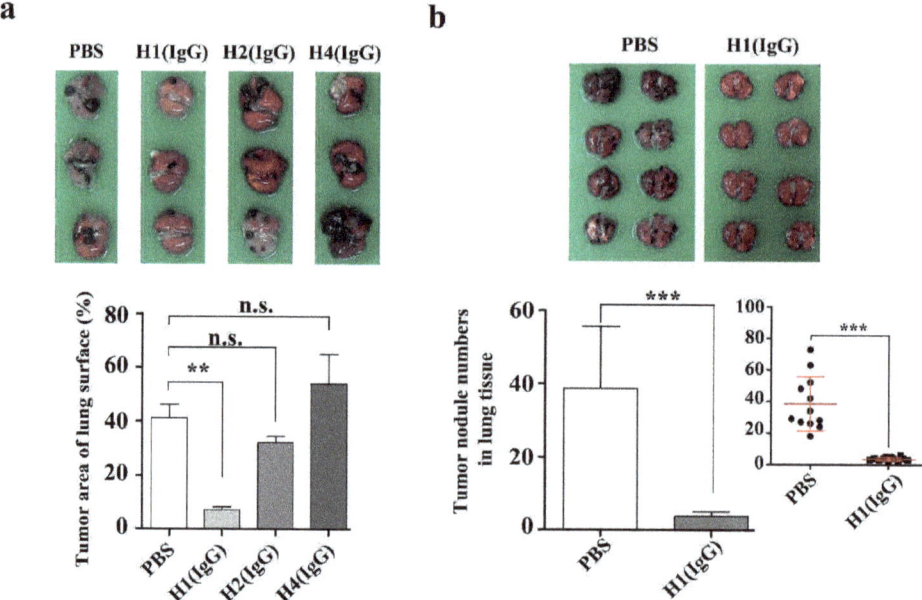

Figure 5. Anti-metastatic effect of anti-hYKL-40 IgGs. (**a**) A plot comparing the inhibitory effects of H1 (IgG), H2 (IgG), and H4 (IgG) by the tumor area on lung tissue. (**b**) A plot revealing the inhibitory effect of H1 (IgG) by the number of tumor nodules on the lung tissue. The original plot, showing the mean value and the standard error of the mean (SEM) marked in red lines, is shown as the inlet. The closed circles indicate the individual lung tissues examined. ** $p < 0.01$, *** $p < 0.001$. n.s.: not significant.

3. Discussion

We report the selection of human mAbs specific to hYKL-40 using human synthetic Fab phage display libraries. In vitro display technologies, such as phage and yeast display, have been successful for therapeutic applications against a variety of target antigens [36,42,43]. In particular, phage display is a powerful tool that has been proved to be highly effective for the selection of human antibodies through diverse human phage display libraries, mostly in either a naïve format generated from human peripheral blood mononuclear cells (PBMCs) or a semi-synthetic format constructed on a selected VH and VL scaffold by randomizing their CDRs [31–34]. Given the increased therapeutic value of YKL-40, many studies employing antibodies targeting hYKL-40 have been performed and reported that the antibodies are effective to modulate the biological processes that YKL-40 is involved, such as growth, differentiation, and metastasis of cancer cells [23–25] but most of the studies were performed with antibodies from mouse hybridoma and thus this is believed to be the first report of human antibodies targeting hYKL-40 identified from a human synthetic antibody phage display library. Moreover, human antibodies had desirable biophysical properties in terms of affinity, thermal stability, and non-aggregation, which are essential for the development of therapeutics.

Over the antibody selection with the phage display libraries employed, the KFab-I library, an in house human synthetic Fab phage display library constructed on a V_H3 and a V_k1 framework by randomizing their CDRs, yielded two anti-hYKL-40 mAb clones (H1 and H2) with high affinity of which H1 was selected dominantly (~73%) and found to be effective to inhibit growth and migration of cancer cells. Although more binders were identified from KFab-II, the other human synthetic Fab phage display library built on a V_H1 and a V_k1 framework, those clones were far below the two binders from KFab-I in their affinity and efficacy. Since the two libraries were built with CDRs designed by the same randomization scheme, we reasoned that the framework could make the difference. Previous studies have shown that among human V_H families, human V_H3 has the highest stability and yield of soluble protein and its germline usage is about 43% (out of 51 germline segments) which is far above other human V_H families [44]. Indeed, it was revealed that a considerable number of antibodies selected from various antibody libraries including the Griffiths library and the HuCAL library belong to the V_H3 family (74% for the Griffiths library and 36% for the HuCAL) [45,46]. This indicates that the V_H3 framework is highly favored due to its desirable properties. However, since our phage display selections were performed separately with each Fab library but not with a mixture of both V_H3 and V_H1 frameworks from KFab-I and KFab-II, it is hard to say that the V_H3 was indeed preferred to the V_H1 framework for human YKL-40 over the phage display selections. More intriguingly, the scFv library we used did not yield any binder for hYKL-40 from the phage display selection. Since the scFv library is built on the same frameworks (V_H3 and V_k1) as the KFab-I library, it seems not due to the framework itself, but rather due to sub-optimal orientation of CDRs in the scFv form toward a binding region (i.e., epitope) on the human YKL-40 protein.

We showed that the H2, one of the two Fabs selected from KFab-I, had an affinity close to that of the H1 and had desirable properties as well, but the H2 turned out to be non-functional in the in vivo set of assay performed. Since the serum terminal half-life ($t_{1/2}$) of human IgG1 in mice has been known to be about 9.5 days [47], we ruled out the possibility that it could be due to a short half-life of the human mAb in mice serum. Indeed, our pharmacokinetic analysis of H1 (IgG) in mice revealed a $t_{1/2}$ of ~11 days which is comparable to the previous report (Figure S6 and Table S1) and we believe that other anti-hYKL-40 mAbs including H2 (IgG) and H4 (IgG) would have similar serum half-lives in mice as observed on H1 (IgG), since they all were built on the same framework (V_H3 and V_k1) and showed similar non-aggregation properties. Next, we reasoned that the two anti-hYKL-40 mAbs might recognize different epitopes so the epitope recognized by the H1 might play a more critical role in the neutralization. Indeed, an ELISA to test whether the two mAbs could compete on hYKL-40 immobilized on a surface revealed that the binding of H1 (Fab) with hYKL-40 seemed not to interfere with the presence of the H2 (Fab), suggesting that the two anti-hYKL-40 mAbs' epitopes might not be overlapped (data not shown). However, we believe that this needs to be further confirmed with other methods such as BLI (Octet). We are currently undergoing to analyze the molecular detail of the association through a tertiary structure of the hYKL-40-H1 (Fab) complex using an X-ray crystallography (PDB deposit number 7CJ2), which should lead us to gain better understanding of how the association of the H1 with the epitope can lead to the anti-cancer activity. In addition, the structural understanding will possibly allow to further engineer the H1 to improve its affinity, and also to design and select small molecules including synthetic compounds and peptides. Moreover, recent studies showed that YKL-40 negatively regulates Th1 cells and cytotoxic T lymphocyte (CTL) activity and so its reduction by siRNA could increase the anti-cancer T cell population in lung metastasis [13], and somehow IL-13Rα2, a putative receptor of YKL-40, might play a role in their interplay with T cells [17,48]. Thus, it would be interesting to know if the H1 acts by antagonizing the interaction of YKL-40 with IL-13Rα2, and more interestingly how the H1 will interplay with YKL-40 in the T cell immunity in lung metastasis, which may shed a light on its possible interaction with PD-1, a well-known immune-checkpoint [13,49].

In conclusion, we have selected high-affinity human anti-hYKL-40 mAbs from human synthetic Fab phage display libraries. We characterized the resulting Fabs and IgGs to observe their desirable biophysical properties such as high affinity, non-aggregation, and thermal stability. We tested those in an in vitro and an in vivo assay to assess their anti-cancer activities and identified a clone, H1, which demonstrated its exceptional ability to inhibit growth and migration of cancer cells in vivo. Further refinement of the H1 mAb should warrant the development of a promising anti-cancer biologics.

4. Materials and Methods

4.1. Library Panning

Two human synthetic Fab phage display libraries produced in-house (KFab-I and KFab-II, built on a human VH3/Vk1 and a human VH1/Vk1 germline-based scaffold, with randomized complementarity-determining regions (CDRs), respectively) and a human synthetic scFv phage display library (KscFv-I, built on a human VH3/Vk1 germline-based scaffold, with randomized complementarity-determining regions (CDRs)) were used for the selection of specific binders against a recombinant human YKL-40 protein (hYKL-40) (Sino Biological, Beijing, China). hYKL-40 was immobilized in immunotubes (Nunc, Rochester, NY, USA) at a concentration of 10 µg/mL in PBS (phosphate-buffered saline, pH 7.4) at 4 °C for 18 h. After rinsing them twice with tap water, the immunotubes were blocked with 5% skim milk in PBS for 1 h at room temperature (RT). At the same time, the phage library was incubated in 2% skim milk in PBS for 1 h at room temperature (RT). Blocked phages were transferred to the immunotubes coated with hYKL-40 and incubated for 1 h at 37 °C, before being washed three times with PBS-T (PBS containing 0.05% Tween 20). Bound phages were eluted from immunotubes with 100 mM triethylamine for 10 min at RT, followed by neutralization with 1 M Tris-HCl (pH 7.4). Neutralized eluted phages were transferred to mid-log-phage *Escherichia coli* (*E. coli*) TG1 cells and incubated for 1 h at 37 °C with gentle rotation (120 rpm). The infected TG1 cells were spread on 2× YT agar plates supplemented with 2% glucose and 100 µg/mL ampicillin and incubated overnight at 37 °C. The colonies were collected by scraping with 6 mL of a 2× YT medium. A total of 50 mL of 2× YT supplemented with 2% glucose and 100 µg/mL ampicillin were inoculated with the scraped cells to yield an OD_{600} of 0.05 to 0.1 and incubated at 37 °C with shaking (220 rpm) until the OD_{600} reached 0.5. Then, the culture was infected with a VCSM13 helper phage (provided by Dr. Hong from Kangwon National University, Chuncheon-si, Gangwon-do, Korea) at a multiplicity of infection (M.O.I.) of 20:1. After incubation for 1 h at 37 °C with gentle rotation (120 rpm), kanamycin was added to a final concentration of 70 µg/mL, and the culture was grown overnight at 30 °C with shaking (220 rpm). Cells were then centrifuged at $24,793\times g$ for 30 min, and the supernatant was passed through a 0.22 µm filter. Phage particles were precipitated using one-fifth of the volume of the precipitation buffer (20% PEG8000, 15% NaCl) for 30 min on ice. The precipitated phages were pelleted by centrifugation at 12,000 rpm for 30 min and resuspended in PBS. The phage suspension was used for the next round of panning. For stringent selections, the number of washing steps was gradually increased, and the amount of antigen for immobilization was decreased: first round: 10 µg/mL; second round: 5 µg/mL; third and fourth rounds: 1 µg/mL in PBS (1 mL).

4.2. Monoclonal Phage ELISA

A monoclonal phage ELISA was performed after three rounds of panning. Several 96-Well Half-Area Microplates (Corning, New York, NY, USA) were coated overnight at 4 °C, with 30 µL per well of 1 µg/mL hYKL-40, and each well was blocked with 5% skim milk in PBS for 1 h at RT. The amplified phages of individual clones from the third round of panning were added and incubated for 1 h at 37 °C. After washing four times with PBS-T, horseradish peroxidase (HRP)-conjugated anti-M13 antibody (1:5000, Sino Biological, Beijing, China) was incubated for 1 h at 37 °C. After washing it four times with PBS-T, a TMB substrate solution (Sigma-Aldrich, St. Louis, MO, USA) was added for 8 min, and the reaction was stopped with 1 N sulfuric acid (Merck, Darmstadt, Germany). The absorbance was measured at 450 nm using a SpectraMax 190 Microplate Reader (Molecular Devices, Sunnydale, CA, USA).

4.3. Production of Fab Proteins

An in-house bacterial expression vector (pKFAB) was used to construct the Fab expression vectors. The Fab fragments were amplified by a polymerase chain reaction (PCR). The PCR products were purified using a QIAquick PCR Purification Kit (QIAGEN, Hilden, Germany) and digested with *SfiI*

(New England Biolabs, Ipswich, MA, USA). The digestion products were separated on a 1% agarose gel, and the single band was purified with a QIAquick Gel Extraction Kit (QIAGEN, Hilden, Germany). The fragments were inserted into vector fragments digested using the same restriction enzymes with a T4 DNA ligase (New England Biolabs, Ipswich, MA, USA), and *E. coli* DH5α competent cells (Enzynomics, Daejeon, Korea) were transformed with the ligation mixtures. The individual colonies of the transformed cells were isolated, and the sequences of the isolated clones were verified. Top10F' Competent Cells (Invitrogen, Carlsbad, CA, USA) were transformed with the Fab expression vectors, and the transformants were grown in 200 mL of TB (Terrific Broth) media supplemented with 100 μg/mL ampicillin at 37 °C with shaking (220 rpm) until the OD_{600} reached 0.5. The log-phase cultures were then induced with 0.5 mM isopropyl β-D-1-thiogalactopyranoside (IPTG) and incubated overnight at 30 °C with shaking (220 rpm). The cells were collected and resuspended in 16 mL of 1× TES (50 mM Tris-HCl, 1 mM EDTA, 20% Sucrose, pH 8.0). After incubation for 30 min on ice, 24 mL of 0.2× TES was added and incubated for 1 h on ice. The periplasmic fractions were collected after centrifugation at 12,000 rpm for 30 min and filtered through a 0.22 μm filter. The periplasmic extracts were loaded on a column packed with 0.5 mL of Strep-Tactin XT (IBA, Goettingen, Germany). The column was washed with 10 column volumes (CVs) of Buffer W (IBA, Goettingen, Germany) and eluted with 5 CVs of Buffer BXT (IBA, Goettingen, Germany). The eluted proteins were concentrated and buffer-exchanged with PBS using Amicon Ultra-15 Centrifuge Filter Units (Milipore, Carrigtwohill, Co., Cork, Ireland).

4.4. Determination of Apparent Affinity by ELISA

Several 96-Well Half-Area Microplates were coated overnight at 4 °C, with 30 μL per well of 2 μg/mL hYKL-40. After rinsing them twice with tap water, the wells were blocked with 5% skim milk in PBS for 1 h at RT. Serially diluted anti-hYKL-40 Fabs were added and incubated for 1 h at 37 °C. After washing the plates four times with PBS-T, the HRP-conjugated StrepMAB-Classic (1:10,000, IBA, Goettingen, Germany) was added to the plates and incubated for 1 h at 37 °C. After washing the plates four times with PBS-T, a TMB substrate solution was incubated for 8 min, and the reaction was stopped with 1 N sulfuric acid. The absorbance was measured at 450 nm using a SpectraMax 190 Microplate Reader. A plot was created using a non-linear curve fit algorithm with Graphpad Prism 7 (GraphPad Software, San Diego, CA, USA), and half-maximal effective concentration (EC_{50}) values were determined accordingly.

4.5. Determination of Melting Temperature by a Protein Thermal Shift (PTS) Assay

To each well of a MicroAmp Fast Optical 96-Well Reaction Plate (Applied Biosystems, Foster City, CA, USA), 18 μL of anti-hYKL-40 Fab and 2 μL of Protein Thermal Shift Dye (10×, Applied Biosystems, Foster City, CA, USA) were added. As a negative control, PBS was mixed with the Protein Thermal Shift Dye. The plate was sealed with a MicroAmp Optical Adhesive Film (Applied Biosystems, Foster City, CA, USA) and centrifuged at 142× *g* for 1 min. The measurement was performed using a real-time PCR instrument. The instrument was set up according to the manufacturer's instructions. All the experiments were performed at least in triplicate.

4.6. Size-Exclusion Chromatography (SEC) and Intact Mass Analysis

The separation of the antibodies using size-exclusion chromatography was conducted using a Waters Alliance 2695 (Waters, Milford, MA, USA) connected to a Biosuite high-resolution SEC column (7.5 mm × 300 mm, 10 μm particle size, Waters, Milford, MA, USA). The separation was performed using an isocratic elution with PBS, pH 7.4, at a flow rate of 1 mL/min. The effluent was detected using a UV/Vis detector 2489 at 280 nm.

4.7. Determination of Affinity by Bio-Layer Interferometry (BLI)

BLI (Bio-layer Interferometry) experiments were performed on an Octet QK384 (ForteBio, Menlo Park, CA, USA) instrument. The hYKL-40 protein was immobilized at 15 μg/mL in a 10 mM sodium acetate buffer (pH 5.0) and dispensed into a 96-well tilted-bottom microplate (200 µL per well) (Greiner bio-one, Monroe, NC, USA). Eight vertical wells were used at the same concentration. A second 96-well microplate contained the hYKL40-H1 antibody at 8 different concentrations (50 nM~0 nM, in 2-fold serial dilutions) and 1× PBS (supplemented with 0.09% (v/v) Tween 20) for baseline stabilization. Before the binding measurements, the AR2G (Amine reactive 2nd generation; ForteBio, Menlo Park, CA, USA) sensor tips were pre-hydrated in dH$_2$O for 10 min, activated in a 1:1 mixture of 0.1 M N-Hydroxysuccinimide (NHS)/0.4 M 1-Ethyl-3-(3-dimethylaminopropyl)-carbodiimide (EDC) for 300 s and incubated in a binding buffer for 300 s (loading step). After a 180 s baseline dip in 1× PBS (supplemented with 0.09% (v/v) Tween 20), the binding kinetics were measured by dipping the hYKL-40-coated sensors into wells containing the H1 (IgG) antibody at various concentrations. The binding interactions were monitored over a 350 s association step, followed by a 500 s dissociation step, in which the sensors were dipped into new wells containing 1 × PBS (supplemented with 0.09% (v/v) Tween 20). Non-specific binding was assessed using sensor tips without the hYKL-40 protein. Data analysis was performed using Octet Data Analysis Software v6.4 (ForteBio, Menlo Park, CA, USA). The data were fitted to a 1:1 binding model to determine the association rate (k_a) and dissociation rate (k_d), and the equilibrium dissociation constant (K_D, M) was calculated as follows: $K_D = k_d \div k_a$.

4.8. Conversion to IgG and Production of IgG Proteins

The light- and heavy-chain vectors (pcDNA3.3 and pOptiVEC, respectively) used for the Herceptin expression were used as IgG1 backbone vectors. The VL, VH, and CL (Light-chain variable domain, heavy-chain variable domain, and light-chain constant domain, respectively) genes were individually amplified by a polymerase chain reaction (PCR), and then VL and CL were used in an overlap extension PCR. The PCR products (VL-CL and VH) were purified with a QIAquick PCR Purification Kit (QIAGEN, Hilden, Germany) and digested with the following restriction enzymes (New England Biolabs, Ipswich, MA, USA): VL-CL: *Sfi*I and *Eco*RI; VH: *Sfi*I and *Nhe*I. The digestion products were separated on a 1% agarose gel, and the single band was purified with a QIAquick Gel Extraction Kit (QIAGEN, Hilden, Germany). The fragments were inserted into vector fragments digested with the same restriction enzymes using a T4 DNA ligase (New England Biolabs, Ipswich, MA, USA), and *E. coli* DH5α competent cells (Enzynomics, Daejeon, Korea) were transformed with the ligation mixtures. Individual colonies of the transformed cells were isolated, and the sequences of isolated clones were verified.

Expi293F cells were cultured in an Expi293F Expression Medium (Thermo Fisher Scientific, Waltham, MA, USA) in a humidified 8% CO$_2$ incubator at 37 °C with shaking at 125 rpm. On the day of transfection, the Expi293F cell density was approximately 2.9×10^6 cells/mL. Expi293F transfections were performed using an ExpiFectamine 293 transfection reagent (Thermo Fisher Scientific, Waltham, MA, USA), according to the manufacturer's protocol. IgG antibodies were purified using HiTrap MabSelect SuRe (GE Healthcare, Pittsburgh, PA, USA) columns. Briefly, equilibration was carried out using buffer A (PBS, pH 7.4). The sample was loaded onto the equilibrated column. Following sample loading, the column was washed with buffer A, until a stable baseline was established. Following the washing step, the protein was eluted with buffer B (0.1 M glycine, pH 2.7). Following the elution, the IgG was brought to a neutral pH using a 1 M Tris base, pH 9.0, and dialyzed into PBS gels (Thermo Fisher Scientific, Waltham, MA, USA). Purified and buffer-exchanged IgG samples were separated on 4–12% Bis-Tris gels (Thermo Fisher Scientific, Waltham, MA, USA) and stained with a Sun-Gel Staining Solution (LPS Solution, Deajeon, Korea).

4.9. Cell Culture

B16F10, A549, and H460 NSCLC cells were obtained from the American Type Culture Collection (Manassas, VA, USA). A549 and H460 cells were cultured in an RPMI 1640 medium supplemented with 10% heat-inactivated fetal bovine serum (FBS), 100 U/mL penicillin, and 100 µg/mL streptomycin. B16F10 skin melanoma cells were cultured in DMEM (supplemented with 10% heat-inactivated FBS,

100 U/mL penicillin, and 100 µg/mL streptomycin). Cell cultures were maintained in a humidified 5% CO_2 incubator at 37 °C.

4.10. In Vitro Trans-Well Migration Assay

The migration of human lung cancer cells (A549 and H460) and mouse melanoma cells (B16F10) was quantitatively performed on permeable inserts (8 µm pore trans-well; Corning, New York, NY, USA). The cells treated with 1 µg/mL of anti-hYKL-40 IgGs were plated at 2.0×10^4 cells per well (for A549 and H460) and 2.5×10^5 cells (for B16F10) per well and incubated in a humidified 5% CO_2 incubator at 37 °C for 17 h. After incubation, the cells were fixed with 3.7% formaldehyde for 2 min and then washed with PBS twice. Next, the cells were permeated with 100% methanol for 15 min at RT and stained with trypan blue for 20 min. Non-migrated cells on the inside of the wells were removed with a cotton swab, and the images, captured under a light microscope (Olympus, Tokyo, Japan) at 200× magnification, were analyzed, using NIH ImageJ software (imagej.nih.gov/ij/download/).

4.11. In Vivo Anti-Tumorigenic Assay

The study was conducted on random-bred, 6–7-week-old male C57BL/6 mice, with a body weight of 24–28 g. Animals were maintained under controlled conditions of temperature and light (Light:dark, 10 h:14 h.). They were provided standard mice feed (procured from Daehan Biolink, Eumsung, Korea) and water ad libitum. To induce metastasis, B16F10 mouse melanomas were injected intravenously into tail vein (3.75×10^4 tumor cells/200 µL in phosphate-buffered saline (PBS) with a 27-gauge needle) of 8-week-old C57BL/6 mice [50,51]. After 4 days, 0.5 mpk (mg per kg body weight) of anti-hYKL-40 IgGs were inoculated through intravenous injection and these injections were performed every week for three weeks enough to maintain the concentration of IgG during this study period. Mice were sacrificed by 4 weeks after the injection of B16F10 cells to investigate the metastatic tumor nodule number and tumor area on the lung surface. The percentage of tumor area on the lung surface was measured with 2 pictures taken back and forth using NIH ImageJ software. The diameter of tumor nodules counted in this study was over 0.2 mm. All protocols involving mice in this study were reviewed and approved by the Chungbuk National University Institutional Animal Care and Use Committee (IACUC) on the date of 13 March 2017 and complied with the Korean National Institute of Health Guide for the Care and Use of Laboratory Animals (CBNUA-1073-17-01).

4.12. Ex Vivo Imaging of ICG-Labeled H1 (IgG)

H1 (IgG) was conjugated to ICG (Indocyanine green) using the ICG labeling kit (Dojindo, Kumamoto, Japan), according to the manufacturer's instructions. ICG-labeled H1 (IgG) (1 mg/kg) was intravenously injected into C57BL/6 mice via the tail vein. Fifteen mins after administration, lungs were isolated and washed with PBS. Fluorescence intensity was analyzed by the VISQUE In vivo Optical Imager System (VIEWORKS, Gyeonggi, Korea). The NIR filter set (Excitation: 740 to 790 nm; Emission: 810 nm to 860 nm) was used for ICG fluorescence. A negative control was performed with lungs from PBS-treated mice.

4.13. Statistical Analysis

Statistical analysis was carried out using SPSS version 18.0 (IBM SPSS, New York, NY, USA). All error bars reported are the standard error of the mean (±SEM), unless otherwise indicated. Pairwise comparisons were conducted using a one-way Student's *t*-test. Multiple comparisons were conducted using a one-way analysis of variance, followed by Tukey's tests. Differences between groups are considered significant at *p*-values below 0.05 (* $p < 0.05$; ** $p < 0.01$; *** $p < 0.001$).

5. Conclusions

We have selected high-affinity human anti-hYKL-40 mAbs from human synthetic Fab phage display libraries. We characterized the resulting Fabs and IgGs to observe their desirable biophysical properties, such as their high affinity, non-aggregation, and thermal stability. We conducted in vitro and in vivo assays to assess their anti-cancer activities and identified a clone, H1, which demonstrated an exceptional ability to inhibit the growth and migration of cancer cells in vivo. A further refinement of the H1 mAb should allow for the development of a promising biological anti-cancer therapeutic.

6. Patents

We are in the process of obtaining a patent for the data on the human anti-hYKL-40 Fabs and IgGs in Korea (patent application number 10-2019-0112572; application date 11 September 2019).

Supplementary Materials: Supplementary materials can be found at http://www.mdpi.com/1422-0067/21/17/6354/s1. Figure S1: Phage ELISA on an immobilized hYKL-40 surface with phages from each of the 3rd round and 4th round of the panning using KFab-I and KFab-II libraries; Figure S2. Determination of the affinity and melting temperature (T_m) of H1 (IgG) using BLI (Octet); Figure S3. Trans-well migration assay of human anti-hYKL-40 IgGs on B16F10 melanoma cells; Figure S4. Ex vivo imaging of H1 (IgG) on the lung tissue; Figure S5. Western blot analysis on recombinant YKL-40 and cell lysates; Figure S6. The concentration-time profile of H1 (IgG) in C57BL/6 mice after intravenous administration (5 mg/kg); Table S1. Pharmacokinetic parameters of H1 (IgG).

Author Contributions: Conceptualization and experiment design, J.T.H. and D.Y.K.; investigation, K.K. (Kyungjae Kang), K.K. (Kicheon Kim), S.-R.L., Y.K., J.E.L., Y.S.L., J.-H.L., C.-S.L., Y.J.K. and S.I.B.; supervision, J.T.H. and D.Y.K.; project administration and data curation, D.H.S.; writing—original draft preparation, D.Y.K.; writing—review and editing, K.K. (Kicheon Kim), Y.S.L., J.T.H., and D.Y.K.; funding acquisition, J.T.H. and D.Y.K. All authors have read and agreed to the published version of the manuscript.

Funding: This research was funded by the Chungcheongbuk-do Value Creation Program (no grant number issued).

Acknowledgments: We thank Hong-Hyo Jeong (Kangwon National University, Gangwon-do, Korea) for her work in constructing the human Fab synthetic phage display library. We are also grateful to Tae Gyu Lee, the President of the New Drug Development Center, for his support throughout the research.

Conflicts of Interest: K.J.K., Y.K., S.-R.L., J.T.H., and D.Y.K. are inventors with the Korean patent application number 10-2019-0112572 (application date September 11, 2019). The authors declare no other conflict of interest.

Abbreviations

mAb	Monoclonal antibody
CHI3L1	Chitinase-3-like 1
CLP	Chitinase-like protein
ELISA	Enzyme-linked immunosorbent assay
EC_{50}	Half maximal effective concentration
IgG	Immunoglobulin G
Fab	Antigen-binding fragment
scFv	Single-chain variable fragment
SEC	Size-exclusion chromatography
PTS	Protein thermal shift
T_m	Melting temperature
K_D	Equilibrium dissociation constant
IPTG	Isopropyl β-D-1-thiogalactopyranoside
PBS	Phosphate-buffered saline
SDS-PAGE	Sodium dodecyl sulfate-polyacrylamide gel electrophoresis
CDR	Complementarity-determining region
FR	Framework
VH	Heavy-chain variable domain
VL	Light-chain variable domain
CL	Light-chain constant domain
BLI	Bio-layer Interferometry

References

1. Yeo, I.J.; Lee, C.-I.; Han, S.-B.; Yun, J.; Hong, J.T. Roles of chitinase 3-like 1 in the development of cancer, neurodegenerative diseases, and inflammatory diseases. *Pharmacol. Ther.* **2019**, *203*, 107394–107413. [CrossRef] [PubMed]
2. Fusetti, F.; Pijning, T.; Kalk, K.H.; Bos, E.; Dijkstra, B.W.; Houston, D.R. Crystal Structure and Carbohydrate-Binding Properties of the Human Cartilage glycoprotein-39. *J. Biol. Chem.* **2003**, *278*, 37753–37760. [CrossRef] [PubMed]
3. Johansen, J.S.; Christensen, I.J.; Jørgensen, L.N.; Olsen, J.; Rahr, H.B.; Nielsen, K.T.; Laurberg, S.; Brünner, N.; Nielsen, H.J.; Johansen, J.S. Serum YKL-40 in Risk Assessment for Colorectal Cancer: A Prospective Study of 4,496 Subjects at Risk of Colorectal Cancer. *Cancer Epidemiol. Biomark. Prev.* **2015**, *24*, 621–626. [CrossRef] [PubMed]
4. Wang, X.W.; Cai, C.-L.; Xu, J.-M.; Jin, H.; Xu, Z.-Y. Increased expression of chitinase 3-like 1 is a prognosis marker for non-small cell lung cancer correlated with tumor angiogenesis. *Tumor Biol.* **2015**, *36*, 901–907. [CrossRef] [PubMed]
5. Lal, A.; Lash, A.E.; Altschul, S.F.; Velculescu, V.; Zhang, L.; McLendon, R.E.; Marra, M.A.; Prange, C.; Morin, P.J.; Polyak, K.; et al. A Public Database for Gene Expression in Human Cancers. *Cancer Res.* **1999**, *59*, 5403–5407. [PubMed]
6. Lau, S.H.; Sham, J.S.T.; Xie, D.; Tzang, C.-H.; Tang, D.; Ma, N.; Hu, L.; Wang, Y.; Wen, J.-M.; Xiao, G.; et al. Clusterin plays an important role in hepatocellular carcinoma metastasis. *Oncogene* **2006**, *25*, 1242–1250. [CrossRef]
7. Kawada, M.; Seno, H.; Kanda, K.; Nakanishi, Y.; Akitake, R.; Komekado, H.; Kawada, K.; Sakai, Y.; Mizoguchi, E.; Tsutomu Chiba, T. Chitinase 3-like 1 promotes macrophage recruitment and angiogenesis in colorectal cancer. *Oncogene* **2012**, *31*, 3111–3123. [CrossRef]
8. Francescone, R.A.; Scully, S.; Faibish, M.; Taylor, S.L.; Oh, D.; Moral, L.; Yan, W.; Bentley, B.; Shao, R. Role of YKL-40 in the Angiogenesis, Radioresistance, and Progression of Glioblastoma. *J. Biol. Chem.* **2011**, *286*, 15332–15343. [CrossRef]
9. Kzhyshkowska, J.; Yin, S.; Liu, T.; Riabov, V.; Mitrofanova, I. Role of chitinase-like proteins in cancer. *Biol. Chem.* **2016**, *397*, 231–247. [CrossRef]
10. Ma, J.-Y.; Li, R.-H.; Huang, K.; Tan, G.; Li, C.; Zhi, F.-C. Increased expression and possible role of chitinase 3-like-1 in a colitis-associated carcinoma model. *World J. Gastroenterol.* **2014**, *20*, 15736–15744. [CrossRef]
11. Wang, Y.; Wong, C.W.; Yan, M.; Li, L.; Liu, T.; Or, P.M.-Y.; Tsui, S.K.-W.; Waye, M.M.-Y.; Chan, A.M.-L. Differential Regulation of the Pro-Inflammatory Biomarker, YKL-40/CHI3L1, by PTEN/Phosphoinositide 3-kinase and JAK2/STAT3 Pathways in Glioblastoma. *Cancer Lett.* **2018**, *429*, 54–65. [CrossRef] [PubMed]
12. Peng, H.; Su, Q.; Lin, Z.-C.; Zhu, X.-H.; Peng, M.-S.; Lv, Z.-B. Potential suppressive effects of theophylline on human rectal cancer SW480 cells in vitro by inhibiting YKL-40 expression. *Oncol. Lett.* **2018**, *15*, 247–252. [CrossRef]
13. Kim, D.-H.; Park, H.-J.; Lim, S.; Koo, J.-H.; Lee, H.-G.; Choi, J.O.; Oh, J.H.; Ha, S.-J.; Kang, M.-J.; Lee, C.-M.; et al. Regulation of chitinase-3-like-1 in T cell elicits Th1 and cytotoxic responses to inhibit lung metastasis. *Nat. Comm.* **2018**, *9*, 503–516. [CrossRef] [PubMed]
14. Libreros, S.; Garcia-Areas, R.; Iragavarapu-Charyulu, V. CHI3L1 plays a role in cancer through enhanced production of pro-inflammatory/pro-tumorigenic and angiogenic factors. *Immunol. Res.* **2013**, *57*, 99–105. [CrossRef]
15. Lee, D.H.; Han, J.H.; Lee, Y.S.; Jung, Y.S.; Roh, Y.S.; Yun, J.S.; Han, S.-B.; Hong, J.T. Chitinase-3-like-1 Deficiency Attenuates Ethanol-Induced Liver Injury by Inhibition of Sterol Regulatory Element Binding Protein 1-dependent Triglyceride Synthesis. *Metabolism* **2019**, *95*, 46–56. [CrossRef]
16. Low, J.Y.; Subramaniam, R.; Lin, L.; Aomatsu, T.; Mizoguchi, A.; Ng, A.; DeGruttola, A.K.; Lee, C.G.; Elias, J.A.; Andoh, A.; et al. Chitinase 3-like 1 induces survival and proliferation of intestinal epithelial cells during chronic inflammation and colitis-associated cancer by regulating S100A9. *Oncotarget* **2015**, *6*, 36535–36550. [CrossRef]
17. He, C.H.; Lee, C.G.; Cruz, C.S.D.; Lee, C.-M.; Zhou, Y.; Ahangari, F.; Ma, B.; Herzog, E.L.; Rosenberg, S.A.; Li, Y.; et al. Chitinase 3-like 1 regulates cellular and tissue responses via IL-13 receptor α2. *Cell Rep.* **2013**, *4*, 830–841. [CrossRef] [PubMed]

18. Lee, C.-M.; He, C.H.; Nour, A.M.; Zhou, Y.; Ma, B.; Park, J.W.; Kim, K.H.; Cruz, C.D.; Sharma, L.; Nasr, M.L.; et al. IL-13Rα2 uses TMEM219 in chitinase 3-like-1-induced signalling and effector responses. *Nat. Comm.* **2016**, *7*, 13541–13552. [CrossRef]
19. Bhardwaj, R.; Yester, J.W.; Singh, S.K.; Biswas, D.D.; Surace, M.J.; Waters, M.R.; Hauser, K.F.; Yao, Z.; Boyce, B.F.; Kordula, T. RelB/p50 complexes regulate cytokine-induced YKL-40 expression. *J. Immunol.* **2016**, *194*, 2862–2870. [CrossRef]
20. Choi, J.Y.; Yeo, J.J.; Kim, K.C.; Choi, W.R.; Jung, J.-K.; Han, S.-B.; Hong, J.T. K284-6111 prevents the amyloid beta-induced neuroinflammation and impairment of recognition memory through inhibition of NF-κB-mediated CHI3L1 expression. *J. Neuroinflamm.* **2018**, *15*, 224–236. [CrossRef]
21. Li, T.-M.; Liu, S.-L.; Huang, Y.-H.; Huang, C.-C.; Hsu, C.-J.; Tsai, C.-H.; Wang, S.-W.; Tang, C.-H. YKL-40-Induced Inhibition of miR-590-3p Promotes Interleukin-18 Expression and Angiogenesis of Endothelial Progenitor Cells. *Int. J. Mol. Sci.* **2017**, *18*, 920. [CrossRef] [PubMed]
22. Miyata, H.; Ashizawa, T.; Iizuka, A.; Kondou, R.; Nonomura, C.; Sugino, T.; Urakami, K.; Asai, A.; Hayashi, N.; Mitsuya, K.; et al. Combination of a STAT3 Inhibitor and an mTOR Inhibitor Against a Temozolomide-resistant Glioblastoma Cell Line. *Cancer Genom. Proteom.* **2017**, *14*, 83–92. [CrossRef] [PubMed]
23. Ngernyuang, N.; Shao, R.; Suwannarurk, K.; Limpaiboon, T. Chitinase 3 Like 1 (CHI3L1) Promotes Vasculogenic Mimicry Formation in Cervical Cancer. *Pathology* **2018**, *50*, 293–297. [CrossRef] [PubMed]
24. Faibish, M.; Francescone, R.; Bentley, B.; Yan, W.; Shao, R. A YKL-40 neutralizing antibody blocks tumor angiogenesis and progression: A potential therapeutic agent in cancers. *Mol. Cancer Ther.* **2011**, *10*, 742–751. [CrossRef]
25. Shao, R.; Francescone, R.; Ngernyuang, N.; Bentley, B.; Taylor, S.L.; Moral, L.; Yan, W. Anti-YKL-40 antibody and ionizing irradiation synergistically inhibit tumor vascularization and malignancy in glioblastoma. *Carcinogenesis* **2014**, *35*, 373–382. [CrossRef]
26. Reichert, J.M.; Dhimolea, E. The Future of Antibodies as Cancer Drugs. *Drug Discov. Today* **2012**, *17*, 954–963. [CrossRef]
27. Kaplon, H.; Muralidharan, M.; Schneider, Z.; Reichert, J.M. Antibodies to watch in 2020. *mAbs* **2020**, *12*, 1703531–1703554. [CrossRef]
28. Smith, G.P. Filamentous Fusion Phage: Novel Expression Vectors That Display Cloned Antigens on the Virion Surface. *Science* **1985**, *228*, 1315–1317. [CrossRef]
29. Pande, J.; Szewczyk, M.M.; Grover, A.K. Phage display: Concept, innovations, applications and future. *Biotechnol. Adv.* **2010**, *28*, 849–858. [CrossRef]
30. Paschke, M. Phage display systems and their applications. *Appl. Microbiol. Biotechnol.* **2006**, *70*, 2–11. [CrossRef]
31. de Haard, H.J.; van Neer, N.; Reurs, A.; Hufton, S.E.; Roovers, R.C.; Henderikx, P.; de Bruine, A.P.; Arends, J.-W.; Hoggenboom, H.R. A large non-immunized human Fab fragment phage library that permits rapid isolation and kinetic analysis of high affinity antibodies. *J. Biol. Chem.* **1999**, *274*, 18218–18230. [CrossRef]
32. Ward, E.S.; Güssow, D.; Griffiths, A.D.; Jones, P.T.; Winter, G. Binding Activities of a Repertoire of Single Immunoglobulin Variable Domains Secreted From Escherichia Coli. *Nature* **1989**, *341*, 544–546. [CrossRef]
33. Sidhu, S.S. Phage display in pharmaceutical biotechnology. *Curr. Opin. Biotechnol.* **2000**, *11*, 610–616. [CrossRef]
34. Hoogenboom, H.R. Selecting and screening recombinant antibody libraries. *Nat. Biotechnol.* **2005**, *23*, 1105–1116. [CrossRef]
35. Winter, G.; Griffiths, A.D.; Hawkins, R.E.; Hoogenboom, H.R. Making antibodies by phage display technology. *Ann. Rev. Immunol.* **1994**, *12*, 433–455. [CrossRef]
36. Bradbury, A.R.M.; Sidhu, S.; Dübel, S.; McCafferty, J. Beyond natural antibodies: The power of in vitro display technologies. *Nat. Biotechnol.* **2011**, *29*, 245–254. [CrossRef] [PubMed]
37. Saw, O.E.; Song, E.-W. Phage display screening of therapeutic peptide for cancer targeting and therapy. *Prot. Cell.* **2019**, *10*, 787–807. [CrossRef] [PubMed]
38. Sclavons, C.; Burtea, C.; Boutry, S.; Laurent, S.; Elst, L.V.; Muller, R.N. Phage Display Screening for Tumor Necrosis Factor-α-Binding Peptides: Detection of Inflammation in a Mouse Model of Hepatitis. *Int. J. Pep.* **2013**, *2013*, 348409–348417. [CrossRef] [PubMed]

39. Huang, J.X.; Bishop-Hurley, S.L.; Cooper, M.A. Development of anti-infectives using phage display: Biological agents against bacteria, viruses, and parasites. *Antimicrob. Agents Chemother.* **2012**, *56*, 4569–4582. [CrossRef] [PubMed]
40. Kim, Y.; Lee, H.; Park, K.; Park, S.; Lim, J.-H.; So, M.K.; Woo, H.-M.; Ko, H.; Lee, J.-M.; Lim, S.H.; et al. Selection and characterization of monoclonal antibodies targeting Middle East respiratory syndrome coronavirus through a human synthetic Fab phage display library panning. *Antibodies* **2019**, *8*, 42. [CrossRef]
41. Kim, K.C.; Yun, J.; Son, D.J.; Kim, J.Y.; Jung, J.-K.; Choi, J.S.; Kim, Y.R.; Song, J.K.; Kim, S.Y.; Kang, S.K.; et al. Suppression of metastasis through inhibition of chitinase 3-like 1 expression by miR-125a-3p-mediated up-regulation of USF1. *Theranostics* **2018**, *8*, 4409–4428. [CrossRef]
42. FitzGerald, K. In vitro display technologies – new tools for drug discovery. *Drug Disc. Today* **2000**, *5*, 253–258. [CrossRef]
43. Rothe, A.; Hosse, R.J.; Power, B.E. In vitro display technologies reveal novel biopharmaceutics. *FASEB J.* **2006**, *20*, 1599–1610. [CrossRef] [PubMed]
44. Ewert, S.; Huber, T.; Honegger, A.; Pluckthün, A. Biophysical properties of human antibody variable domains. *J. Mol. Biol.* **2003**, *325*, 531–553. [CrossRef]
45. Griffiths, A.D.; Williams, S.C.; Hartley, O.; Tomlinson, I.M.; Waterhouse, P.; Crosby, W.L.; Kontermann, R.E.; Jones, P.T.; Low, N.M. Isolation of high affinity human antibodies directly from large synthetic repertoires. *EMBO J.* **1994**, *13*, 3245–3260. [CrossRef] [PubMed]
46. Knappik, A.; Ge, L.; Honegger, A.; Pack, P.; Fischer, M.; Wellnhofer, G.; Hoess, A.; Wolle, J.; Pluckthün, A.; Virnekas, B. Fully synthetic human combinatorial antibody libraries (HuCAL) based on modular consensus frameworks and CDRs randomized with trinucleotides. *J. Mol. Biol.* **2000**, *296*, 57–86. [CrossRef] [PubMed]
47. Unverdorben, F.; Richter, F.; Hutt, M.; Seifert, O.; Malinge, P.; Fischer, N.; Kontermann, R.E. Pharmacokinetic properties of IgG and various Fc fusion proteins in mice. *mAbs* **2016**, *8*, 120–128. [CrossRef]
48. Cohen, N.; Shani, O.; Raz, Y.; Sharon, Y.; Hoffman, D.; Abramovitz, L. Fibroblasts drive an immunosuppressive and growth-promoting microenvironment in breast cancer via secretion of Chitinase 3-like 1. *Oncogene* **2017**, *36*, 4457–4468. [CrossRef]
49. Sharpe, A.H.; Pauken, K.E. The Diverse Functions of the PD1 Inhibitory Pathway. *Nat. Rev. Immunol.* **2018**, *18*, 153–167. [CrossRef]
50. Malik, G.; Knowles, L.M.; Dhir, R.; Xu, S.; Yang, S.; Ruoslahti, E.; Pilch, J. Plasma fibronectin promotes lung metastasis by contributions to fibrin clots and tumor cell invasion. *Cancer Res.* **2010**, *70*, 4327–4334. [CrossRef]
51. Fu, Q.; Zhang, Q.; Lou, Y.; Yang, J.; Nie, G.; Chen, Q.; Chen, Y.; Zhang, J.; Wang, J.; Wei, T.; et al. Primary tumor-derived exosomes facilitate metastasis by regulating adhesion of circulating tumor cells via SMAD3 in liver cancer. *Oncogene* **2018**, *37*, 6105–6118. [CrossRef] [PubMed]

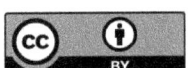

© 2020 by the authors. Licensee MDPI, Basel, Switzerland. This article is an open access article distributed under the terms and conditions of the Creative Commons Attribution (CC BY) license (http://creativecommons.org/licenses/by/4.0/).

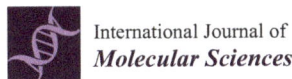 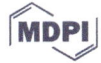

Review

Evolution of *Escherichia coli* Expression System in Producing Antibody Recombinant Fragments

Annamaria Sandomenico *, Jwala P. Sivaccumar and Menotti Ruvo *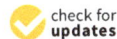

Istituto di Biostrutture e Bioimmagini, CNR, via Mezzocannone, 16, 80134 Napoli, Italy; jwala.priyadarsini@gmail.com
* Correspondence: annamaria.sandomenico@cnr.it (A.S.); menotti.ruvo@unina.it (M.R.)

Received: 26 July 2020; Accepted: 25 August 2020; Published: 31 August 2020

Abstract: Antibodies and antibody-derived molecules are continuously developed as both therapeutic agents and key reagents for advanced diagnostic investigations. Their application in these fields has indeed greatly expanded the demand of these molecules and the need for their production in high yield and purity. While full-length antibodies require mammalian expression systems due to the occurrence of functionally and structurally important glycosylations, most antibody fragments and antibody-like molecules are non-glycosylated and can be more conveniently prepared in *E. coli*-based expression platforms. We propose here an updated survey of the most effective and appropriate methods of preparation of antibody fragments that exploit *E. coli* as an expression background and review the pros and cons of the different platforms available today. Around 250 references accompany and complete the review together with some lists of the most important new antibody-like molecules that are on the market or are being developed as new biotherapeutics or diagnostic agents.

Keywords: antibody fragment; Fab; scFv; *E. coli*

---

1. Introduction

Antibody fragments are widely utilized in therapeutic and diagnostic applications as well as in basic life science research [1]. Unlike conventional immunoglobulins, these smaller biomolecules take several pharmacokinetics advantages over whole antibodies including better penetration into tissues, faster clearance for imaging purposes and generally lower immunogenicity. On the other hand, the absence of the Fc domain and the small size results in a shorter half-life compared to full-length antibodies [2].

In accordance with the antibody's structure–activity relationship, the prerequisite for generating active and smaller antibody-mimicking molecules is the presence of the "antigen-binding site", the tridimensional pocket arising from the variable domains of heavy (VH) and light (VL) chains. The target specificity is mediated by three peptide loops at the tip of each V-domain, designated as complementarity determining region (CDR). Together, these six CDR loops form the target-binding paratope or idiotype of an antibody. For proper target binding, the two V-domains need to pair up in the proper orientation so that the CDR loops jointly form a specific paratope.

Despite that several alternative antibody-like formats derived from different Ig-like domain combinations are continuously developed and proposed [1] such as single-domain antibody fragments (dAbs), the antigen-binding fragments (Fab) and single-chain variable fragments (scFv) are those most used and widespread.

Owing to the lack of glycosylation and their size, these small antibody-like molecules can be readily produced in active and functional recombinant forms via *E. coli* prokaryotic expression systems which enable easier production and with low costs compared to other available expression platforms like yeasts, insect cell lines, mammalian cells and transgenic plants and animals [3].

Single-domain antibody fragments (dAbs), also known as nanobodies, consist of VH or VL domains of 12–15 kDa and are the smallest functional antibody fragments that retain full antigen-binding specificity. Given their high-affinity, solubility and stability also in absence of the partner VL domain, the camelid VH domains (VHH) [4] and the shark VH domains called V-NAR (New Antigen Receptor) [5], are currently used as templates to generate highly efficient and stable new antibody fragments collectively termed nanobodies [6–8]. The natural evolution of VHH and V-NAR Ig domains, derived from the respective HCAbs (heavy-chain Abs that lack light chains), is to deliver new structural solutions for overcoming limitations such as Ig folding stability and antigen affinity. This can be achieved through the design of recombinant "super stable" Ab-fragments, optimizing the hydrophobic VH/VL interfaces and the CDR loops [9,10]. Compared to the VH domains, the VHH and V-NAR domains contain more hydrophilic residues on the surface that interfaces with the VL domains, and some hydrophobic residues, that are fixed in the sequences, are analogous to those at the VH/VL interface and are used for interacting with hydrophobic residues in the CDR3 loop [11,12]. Moreover, the high-affinity binding of VHH and V-NAR domains is likely supported by an increased length of the majority of the CDR3 loops (3–28 amino acids) compared to that of the VH domains [13]. The extended CDR3 loop of nanobodies has the capacity to form a finger-like structure with greater structural flexibility which, in turn, is likely fixed in one single conformation upon antigen-binding [14,15].

The single-chain fragment variable (scFv) domains consist of a single polypeptide (25 kDa) in which the variable regions of the light (VL) and heavy chains (VH) are joined by a flexible linker resistant to endopeptidases. The sequence and length of the ideal linkers may differ between scFvs in order to optimize the affinity for the antigen, reduce the oligomerization and increase the thermostability [16]. It has been largely demonstrated that the linker length influences the oligomeric state. Linkers greater than 15 residues generally lead to monomers while linkers of 6–15 residues can be utilized to deliberately favor the formation of stable dimers and trimers [17,18]. Linkers with fewer than five residues result in the generation of higher-order multimeric molecules [19,20]. The length and amino acid sequence of the peptide linker are, therefore, crucial for proper domain orientation and for regulating their intramolecular or intermolecular interactions. In the presence of short linkers, one antibody fragment's VL or VH domain interacts with another molecule's complimentary domain through a mechanism known as "domain swapping" generating dimers or higher-order oligomers [21]. De facto, short or even medium linkers (up to 15 residues) hamper the proper rotation and intramolecular alignment of the covalently linked complimentary Ig domains preventing the formation of the correct interface. This configuration promotes a swap of the Ig domains leading to the intermolecular association between two, three or even four molecules of scFvs and the generation of the so-called diabodies, triabodies or tetrabodies, respectively. An interesting application of the Ig domain swapping in scFv molecules is the development of bispecific diabodies, especially as antitumor biotherapeutics [22,23]. One such diabody is Blinatumomab, a bispecific T-cell engager (BiTEs) which combines one binding site against CD3, occurring on T cells, and a second anti-CD19 site, specific for cancerous B cells. Blinatumomab is an FDA-approved drug used for treating B-ALL (B cell precursor acute lymphoblastic leukemia, ALL). In cancer immunotherapy, the scFv technology has been also adopted for the development of the CAR T cells (chimeric antigen receptor) technology. Both these strategies use scFvs to recruit cytotoxic T lymphocytes (CTL) in proximity of target tumoral cells that express specific surface antigens (i.e., CD19) and facilitate the polyclonal T-cell response to tumor antigens [24]. The most common linkers used for the generation of scFvs are glycine- and serine-rich amino acidic stretches having sequences (GGGGS)$_3$ of 15 aa, or (GGGGS)$_4$, of 20 aa. These linkers are widely used to keep the carboxy terminus of one variable domain and the amino terminus of the other at a distance that favors the correct folding and the formation of the antigen-binding site while minimizing, at the same time, the oligomerization [25,26]. Some reports have performed the screening of linkers in terms of length and amino acid composition in order to optimize the scFv fragments solubility and activity [27–29]. The order in which the heavy and light domains are fused to build the scFv varies throughout the literature. In some cases, VL-linker-VH [30] rather than VH-linker-VL shows favorable biophysical characteristics, while in other cases, the reverse is true [31]. In some cases, the two different formats exhibited the same antigen-binding activities [32].

Despite the relatively simple structure of scFv fragments, their practical use is limited by the aggregation propensity and consequent low homogeneity. This is due to their dynamic structural features (open and closed state) depending on interchain VH-VL interactions. To suppress this dynamic equilibrium the introduction of a disulfide bond at the VH-VL interface has been attempted. It has been found that the replacement of residues vH44 and vL100 leads to one of the most favorable disulfide configurations [33]. In this instance, the phage display method has been used to generate stable mutants [29,34]. Recently, the use of cyclic scFvs variants has been also successfully reported as an innovative strategy to suppress their intrinsic oligomerization tendency and to optimize the production of stable and active products in bacterial cytoplasm [35,36].

The Fab fragment is a heterodimeric and monovalent antibody fragment (50 kDa) composed of an antibody light chain (VL + CL domains) linked by a disulfide bond to the antibody heavy chain (VH + CH1 domains). Usually, Fab fragments are biochemically more stable than scFv counterparts due to the mutual stabilization that occurs between the VH/VL and CH1/CL interfaces [37]. In addition to the possible aggregation and degradation issues, also the production of Fab fragments in *E. coli* hosts results challenging. It is indeed necessary to achieve the "optimum" expression rather than the "maximum" expression of both chains because the best ratio of HC and LC and protein folding rates are needed and the separately expressed light and heavy chains must assemble correctly to constitute the functional heterodimer with four intrachain and one interchain disulfide bond [38].

In this field, significant efforts have been made to obtain satisfactory expression levels and to identify optimal processing and folding procedures. A comprehensive and progressive better understanding of the mechanisms by which the Ig domains fold and retain their native/functional conformation and of the stability and solubility in "host-environmental conditions" is however still required to improve the production and quality of antibody-based biomolecules. This is the first step towards large-scale productions for clinical applications. In the last decade, several tools including innovative cloning, expression and purification strategies have been explored to increase the production of functional antibody-like fragments using *E. coli* microbial platforms. Due to the ability of *E. coli* to grow at high cell densities, these biomolecules can be produced in high cell density cultures grown in stirred tank reactors using fed-batch methods. Moreover, in the case of scFvs and nanobodies, the reduced size and the single polypeptide nature make antibody fragments readily amenable to high-throughput selection technologies such as phage display, cell display, yeast display and ribosomal display [39]. Finally, these biomolecules obtained as recombinant proteins can be ad hoc engineered and specifically tuned to optimize serum half-lives, tumor penetration and clearance features by controlling their size through chemical or genetic modifications. These technologies include: (i) PEGylation, used for example to obtain certolizumab pegol, or Cimzia®, a marketed PEGylated anti-TNFα Fab for rheumatoid arthritis [40]; (ii) conjugation to the Fc domain of conventional antibodies; (iii) coupling to highly abundant and safe serum proteins such as human serum albumin (HSA), apolipoprotein L1 and β-Lactamase [41]; (iv) site-specific tagging for the generation of drug conjugated antibody fragments that promote tumor homing [42]; (v) generation of multifunctional and multispecific bigger molecules such as diabody (60 kDa), triabodies (90 kDa), tetrabodies (120 kDa), Fab dimers (100 kDa) and Fab trimers F(ab')3 (150 kDa) [1].

The aim of this review is to revisit the current protein expression approaches using *E. coli* as host for the production of recombinant antibody-like fragments, especially Fab and scFv, and to address the development of new strategies based on both cell-based and cell-free systems. A brief survey of antibody fragments produced in *E. coli*, which are FDA-approved or are in the clinical phases, is also provided.

2. *E. coli* as Microbial Expression Stem for the Production of Antibody Fragments

E. coli is one of the most well-established cell factories for the production of recombinant proteins (RPP) [43]. Currently, many molecular tools and protocols are available for the high-level production of heterologous proteins, including a vast catalog of expression plasmids and of engineered strains and many cultivation strategies. From a theoretical point of view, the steps needed for obtaining a recombinant protein are pretty straightforward. The gene of interest (GOI) is cloned in whatever available expression vector, is transformed into the host of choice, expression is induced and the protein is then ready for purification and biochemical, structural and functional characterization. Practically, however, many things can go wrong such as poor growth of the host, inclusion body (IB) formation, protein inactivity, and even lack of protein expression. Choosing the perfect combination is not possible *a priori*, thereby multiple conditions should be empirically tested to obtain a soluble and active recombinant protein.

2.1. Features, Advantages and Disadvantages of the E. coli Microbial Expression System

Given the fast growth rate (doubling time is 20 min), the low cost (the medium is inexpensive), the easiness of genetic manipulation, the well-known molecular features, the good productivity and the simple fermentation process development for manufacturing scale-up, this microorganism represents an affordable expression system for recombinant protein [43–46]. In shake flasks, *E. coli* generally produces a low amount of proteins (mg/L). However, in fermenters, several grams in a liter (g/L) can be achieved [47]. Besides the above-mentioned benefits, there are some main and general drawbacks that can arise, like the lack of proper post-translational modifications (PTMs), the formation of inclusion bodies (IB), codon bias, metabolic burden (acetate accumulation) [48] and occurrence of proteins degradation.

In the last decades, numerous *E. coli* strains engineered to improve their efficiency in the production of recombinant proteins have been developed [49–53] and have been also largely used for the preparation of recombinant antibody-like fragments [54–56]. Some of them have also become the gold standard for biopharmaceutical applications while others have remained only tools for basic research [44]. Of interest, the "bacterial glycoengineering" is emerging as an advanced biotechnological approach that harnesses prokaryotic glycosylation systems for the generation of recombinantly glycosylated proteins using *E. coli* host [57]. In a recent exhaustive review, Harding and coworkers have described the oligosaccharyltransferase (OTase)-dependent (periplasmic) and OTase-independent (cytoplasmic) pathways which are recombinantly introduced into *E. coli* to produce N- or O-glycosylated recombinant proteins, including glycoconjugated vaccines and therapeutic proteins. The same approach can be potentially applied for N-glycosylation of monoclonal antibodies and antibody-related fragments [58,59].

Recently, Kulmala and coworkers have demonstrated that the "harmonized versions" of Fab fragments rather than the classic "over-optimized" one increases the expression from negligible levels to 10 mg/L [60]. Following the "codon harmonization" method [61], they have redesigned codon-optimized synthetic human Fab genes by making synonymous codon substitutions to only five segments of the Fab gene framework. Furthermore, they have also explored the effect of synonymous codon mutation of the pelB leader peptide in Fab periplasmic expression by a combinatorial approach [62].

The Progen company has instead developed the new expression vector pOPE101 [63] which is employed for the production of soluble and functional scFvs as well as for the generation of small fragment antibody libraries in *E. coli* [64]. The cassette vector pOPE101 contains a strong IPTG-inducible synthetic promoter, a pelB leader and a c-myc/His tag sequence for the secretion of functional recombinant proteins into the periplasmic space and to facilitate their detection and purification. The VH and VL genes are joined by a DNA-fragment coding for a flexible 18 amino acid linker containing the first six amino acids of the CH1 constant region domain and the hydrophilic pig brain alpha-tubulin peptide sequence EEGEFSEAR. This linker represents a valuable alternative amino acid sequence with respect to the classic Gly-Ser motifs used to get active and soluble scFv fragments [64].

Other reliable and controllable systems for positively regulating the expression of recombinant proteins in bacteria are based on L-arabinose or L-rhamnose operons. These systems are characterized by a slow response with very low basal transcriptional activity, which can be a great advantage for the production of proteins that are detrimental to the host cell.

In the pBAD vector systems [65], the GOI is placed downstream of the araBAD promoter. Its expression is activated in response to stimulation with L-arabinose and is inhibited by D-glucose that suppresses the basal expression due to a reduction in cellular cAMP levels. Similarly to the pBAD system, the L-rhamnose-inducible promoter pRha has also been successfully used for developing the Expresso ® Rhamnose expression system to obtain high-level recombinant protein expression in the presence of L-rhamnose [66].

Protein expression using pBAD and pRha vectors is more tightly controlled compared to other expression systems such as pET vectors. The precise control of expression levels, based on catabolite repression, makes these systems ideal for producing problematic proteins, such as proteins with toxicity or insolubility issues. As a consequence of more stringent regulation of target gene expression, the attainable yields are relatively lower compared to those reached using pET systems. Through the literature, several attempts have been carried out to improve the production and yield of recombinant antibody fragments using these two vectors. Signal peptide sequences for these vectors have been also optimized following a stress minimization approach [67,68]. Karyolaimos and coworkers have obtained a yield of around 0.2 g/L of a functional scFv fragment in the periplasm using the OmpA signal peptide and 100 µM rhamnose as inductor [68].

Additionally, the Lemo system ™ [20], where the expression is under the tight control of the T7 RNAP activity and the target gene expression level is modulated by L-rhamnose, has been used for the production of soluble and properly folded scFv fragments [69,70].

For the first time, Petrus and coworkers have reported a robust scalable expression system for the production of scFvs in the periplasmic space based on the use of the innovative pSAR-2 vector. The pSAR-2 is an ad hoc engineered expression vector containing a rhamnose-inducible promoter (prhaBAD) and an N-terminal pelB signal peptide. The HIV-neutralizing PGT135 scFv antibody fragment was obtained with an outstanding yield of 1.2 g/L after 48 h of induction at 25 °C using 15 mM L-rhamnose in shake flasks [71].

Ten years ago, a novel tightly regulated expression system based on the chemical inducer cumate (4-isopropylbenzoate) was developed for high protein production in E. coli [72]. The corresponding pNEW vector contains in the expression cassette the regulatory elements of the Pseudomonas putida F1 cym and cmt operons. These two operons control the expression of the target gene at the transcriptional level by means of cumate. The constitutive expression of the desired gene is achieved through switching of the cumate-regulated gene that contains a partial T5-phage promoter merged with a synthetic operator and the repressor protein cymR. In the presence of cumate, the pNEW vector is able to increase the production yield of recombinant proteins by two to three-fold compared to pET-based IPTG-inducible systems. No specific examples of antibody fragment production have been so far reported; however, on the basis of the high-expression yields of the target protein, the tight regulation, the rheostatic control, and the homogenous high-expression bacterial culture, this vector promises to be the basis for innovative strategies to improve the production of antibody-like fragments.

In general, the plasmid-based expression systems exhibit some drawbacks, including the continuous amplification of the plasmid copy number in prolonged cultivations and loss of plasmids over time, propagating the generation of a plasmid-free subpopulation during induction [73]. In this context, the combination of plasmid-free [74] and cell-free approaches [71,75,76] represent new potential strategies for optimizing E. coli expression platforms (see the next section: New Platforms and new technologies for E. coli-based cell-free expression systems).

2.2. Inclusion Bodies

E. coli loses the spatiotemporal control of its own protein synthesis machinery when an exogenous gene is introduced. On the other hand, the newly synthesized recombinant polypeptide is expressed in the microenvironment of the host that may differ from that of the original source in terms of pH, osmolarity, redox potential, cofactors, and folding mechanisms. High local concentrations of the nascent heterologous protein together with an insufficient amount of folding-promoting chaperons may lead to partially folded or misfolded protein intermediates that give rise to the formation, in both the cytoplasm and periplasm, of insoluble protein aggregates known as inclusion bodies, IBs [77]. Usually, these intermediates expose on their surface hydrophobic patches that interact with similar regions and together with the formation of uncorrected disulfide bonds can lead to protein aggregation and precipitation Protein recovery strategies from inclusion bodies via solubilization and refolding processes are laborious, time-consuming and expensive, although various refolding procedures have been developed for therapeutic proteins and applied for antibody fragments [78–80]. An introduction to the IB refolding procedure [81] is outside the scope of this review. Rather, we will look at other more profitable and convenient strategies such as periplasmic and extracellular expression strategies and also co-expression with molecular chaperons for improving solubility and proper folding of antibody-like fragments, even on a laboratory scale.

2.3. Overcoming Drawbacks in Small-Scale Productions

After the transformation of the gene coding for the desired protein in the selected *E. coli* strain, a process development starts through small-scale cultures for the screening of expression conditions using plates and shake flasks. Various cultivation parameters, such as media composition, pH, agitation, aeration, temperature, cell density, concentration of inducers, induction time and strategies affect the protein expression level depending upon expression system [82]. The widely used standard procedures for shake flask cultures are described in the molecular cloning laboratory manual ("Sambrook protocol") [83]. The most popular and suitable media for growing *E. coli* are Luria-Bertani (LB), Terrific Broth (TB) and Super Broth (SB) media that are easily prepared through different combinations of yeast extract, peptones and essential growth factors and vitamins. In the Studier's autoinduction medium [84], the growth is supported at the beginning by glucose, and when glucose is exhausted protein expression is autoinduced by a diauxic shift to lactose utilization, while glycerol is also coutilized as a major carbon source during expression. The most recent EnBase® medium (EnPresso, GmbH, Berlin, Germany), in which glucose, as a primary carbon source, is gradually provided from a soluble polysaccharide by biocatalytic degradation [85], has been successfully used for high-yield cytoplasmic and periplasmic expression of several proteins including antibody fragments [86–89]. Several studies have demonstrated that the yield of recombinant antibody fragments in *E. coli* significantly improves at growth temperature below 30 °C, likely due to the reduction of translation rate that favors proper Ig-like folding and reduces aggregation [90–92].

To overcome the limitations of operating parameters, a slower protein synthesis approach, named "stress minimization" has been developed with positive effects on the yield and solubility of correctly folded recombinant proteins [93]. From an experimental point of view, this approach consists of the careful management of variables such as growth temperature, inducer concentration and time point of induction, whereby growth and RPP proceed concurrently at slower rates. Stress minimization results in the increased viability of cells and process robustness [70,94]. In the so-called Design of Experiments (DoE) setting [95] the optimization of the expression of recombinant Fab and scFv fragments in stress minimization conditions has been successfully achieved through the selection of media [70,88,96,97], screening of signal peptide sequences [67,68,75,98] and optimization of co-expressing chaperone proteins [56,88,99–102]. At the transcriptional level, the concept of "codon harmonization", a sophisticated version of the codon usage optimization, has largely improved the expression of antibodies fragments [60,103].

To overcome the variations deriving from different plasmid vectors a very recent benchmark study has introduced the use of the gene integration (GI) approach to improve the production of Fabs expressed in the *E. coli* periplasmic space in fed-batch fermentations [104]. Recently, Hausjell and coworkers [74] have reported the use of a plasmid-free expression technique for Fab antibody fragments using the BL21 (DE3) expression system. According to the "Recombineering approach", the genes codifying for the heavy and light chains of a Fab fragment were encoded under the control of the T7 promoter and integrated into the genome at the attTN7 site [105]. They have demonstrated that in genome-integrated T7 expression systems, IPTG results in a better inductor compared to lactose in terms of cell fitness and Fab fragment productivity, as opposed to the known toxic effects of IPTG in plasmid-based T7 expression systems [106].

2.4. Protein Localization in E. coli

E. coli cells, like other Gram-negative bacteria, possess an inner and outer membrane that separates the organism into two main subcellular compartments: the cytoplasm and the periplasm. The most common choice for the production of recombinant proteins is the cytoplasm; however, the periplasmic space or the extracellular environment are more suitable when disulfide bonds are required for correct protein folding. As the disulfide bridges cannot be efficiently formed in the reducing conditions of the cytoplasm, antibody fragments are most commonly engineered with a signal sequence that directs them to the more oxidizing bacterial periplasm for proper folding. Folded fragments may further leak from the periplasm into the culture medium (extracellular localization) from which they can be purified without cell lysis. In *E. coli*'s cytoplasm, cysteine-rich polypeptides result mostly in nonfunctional aggregates. Alternative strategies including redox mutant strains with more oxidizing cytoplasm conditions and the coexpression of molecular chaperones could be employed to facilitate the correct folding also in the cytoplasmic space.

In the next sections, the most significant progress achieved in the production of Fabs and scFvs in three different compartments are gathered, analyzed, and matched according to the influence that critical parameters have on the improvement of the quality and recovery of recombinant antibody-like fragments.

2.5. Cytoplasmic Expression

The bacterial cytoplasm provides ample space for protein accumulation and is generally well-suited for the expression of most soluble recombinant proteins [107]. However, the production of homogenously folded disulfide-bonded proteins like antibody fragments is hampered by the cytoplasm reducing conditions and by the lack of suitable molecular chaperons. The excessive production of recombinant proteins in the bacterial cytosol often forces partially folded proteins to interact with each other resulting in protein aggregation and IB formation. The cytoplasmic reducing environment also contributes to protein misfolding and IB formation by inhibiting the intradisulfide bond formation capability.

The cytoplasm has a negative redox potential and this reducing environment is also populated by the thioredoxin–thioredoxin reductase (trxB) and the glutaredoxin–glutaredoxin reductase (gor) systems. Several enzymes like ribonucleotide reductase (RNR), methionine sulfoxide reductase (MsrA), phosphoadenosine phosphosulfate (PAPS) reductase, arsenate reductase (ArsC) and hydrogen peroxide-inducible gene activator (OxyR) continuously regenerate the active thiol sites following a catalytic cycle that is efficiently managed by these reducing pathways [108]. The use of redox-altered mutants of strains such as SHuffle and Origami and others restores an oxidizing environment in the bacterial cytoplasm, thereby their use significantly facilitates the production of soluble cytoplasmic recombinant proteins containing disulfide bonds.

Recently, it has been reported that the expression of an scFv against HER2 derived from Trastuzumab (drug bank number DB00072) in SHuffle at 30 °C resulted in enhanced solubility and a higher expression level of the molecule as compared to its expression in BL21 (DE3) at 37 °C [109–112].

The final production yield of the anti-HER2 scFv was 147 mg/L, under optimal expression conditions (24 h after induction with 0.05 mM IPTG at 30 °C, LB medium, SHuffle strain). The coexpression of molecular chaperones has also been attempted to improve the folding and stability of scFvs and Fabs into the cytoplasm [113–115]. Currently, several plasmids such as pG-KJE8 (dnaK-dnaJ-grpE, groES-groEL), pGr07 (groES-groEL), pKJE7 (dnaK-dnaJ-grpE), pG-Tf2 (groES-groEL-tig) and pTf16 (tig) have become commercially available for the expression of the most widely used cytoplasmic chaperone systems [116,117] such as DnaK-DnaJ-GrpE, trigger factor (TF) and GroEL-GroES. Some comparative studies have demonstrated that the levels of functional Fabs and scFvs have been largely improved in the presence of these cytoplasmic chaperones [113,114]. Recently, Liu and coworkers [102] have reported the cytoplasmic expression of a soluble and active scFv with a yield up to 12.8 mg/L. They have strategically mimicked the oxidizing environment by a combination of the SHuffle strain and by the coexpression of the chaperone proteins GroEL, GroES, DnaK, DnaJ, GrpE and trigger factor (TF) [102]. Through a systematic screening of chaperones, they have identified the GroEL-GroES system as the best performing for the preparation of scFv fragments cloned in pET28 and bearing an N-terminus hexahistidine tag. Plasmids were transformed in two Shuffle-derived strain cells, one containing pG-KJE8 and the other containing pG-Tf2 vectors, and a large-scale preparation was efficiently achieved using the SHuffle strain containing pG-KJE8 in TB medium following induction with 1 mM IPTG at 15 °C o.n. These results suggest that, since the coexpression of chaperones is a critical variable for enhancing the expression yield of soluble scFv/Fab proteins in the *E. coli* cytoplasm, there is not a universal methodology for overcoming the folding problems. Thereby, the successful combination of molecular chaperones and target proteins is identified by a trial and error process. Recently, the same research group reported the use of cyclic scFv variants to overcome the aggregation propensity mediated by interchain VH-VL interactions [35,36]. Cyclic scFvs have been obtained by both covalently connecting the N-terminus and the C-terminus using sortase A and through the split intein-mediated in vivo protein ligation techniques. Accordingly, they optimized the production of soluble cyclic scFv (2.8 mg/L) in bacterial cytoplasm by a combination of chaperone coexpression and SHuffle strain [36].

Several reports have also suggested that the use of fusion partners such as GST [118], maltose-binding protein (MBP) [119,120], small ubiquitin-related modifier (SUMO) [87,121] and thioredoxin (Trx) [122] to the target proteins, especially to scFv fragments, results in solubility-enhancing properties and in increased yields of soluble and active products. However, the fusion partners must be cleaved as big tags usually interfere with the folding of the target protein and with its activity. The entire process of tags removal is however costly and laborious and not often utilized in production processes [123].

The SUMO fusion technology has been successfully applied to the cytosolic production of Fabs in *E. coli*. The highest yield of correctly folded and biologically active SUMO-tagged Fab, 12 mg/L, was recovered from cells harvested after a 16 h growth at 30 °C post-induction with 0.5 mM IPTG using the SHuffle strain and the EnBase medium [87].

Recently, the research group of Nakano has reported the use of a small tag, referred as the SKIK sequence (serine-lysine-isoleucine-lysine), that is able to improve the cytoplasmic expression of Fab fragments in the *E. coli* SHuffle T7 Express strain using the LB medium at 16 °C for 24 h [124,125]. They also described an *ad hoc* engineered Fab fragment bearing a leucine zipper (LZ) pair at the C-termini of both the heavy and light chains, a construct named Zipbody. These extensions would enhance the chain pairing in the active form in both the *E. coli* cytoplasm expression and in the cell-free protein synthesis systems, a technology named Ecobody [124–126].

To overcome the limitations of *E. coli* cytoplasm expression, Gaciarz and coworkers [54,55] have developed the CyDisCo (Cytoplasmic Disulphide bond formation in *E. coli*) system. It is based on the co-expression of a catalyst of disulfide bond formation, usually a sulfhydryl-oxidase such as Erv1p, DsbB or VKOR, plus a catalyst of disulfide bond isomerization like DsbC or PDI. The CyDisCo has been exploited as an efficient route for the production of scFv and Fab fragments derived from known antibodies of different classes and from different organisms (human, mouse and humanized) in the cytoplasm of the KEIO (collection parental K12) *E. coli* strain in shake flasks [127]. The production of an anti-HER2 scFv with CyDisCo was 251 mg/L using EnPresso B media [54] which is 50.3% higher than the yield obtained without CyDisCo using only EnPresso B (167 mg/L) and 70.5% higher than that obtained in SHuffle using the LB medium (147 mg/L) [109]. Additionally, unlike the ΔtrxB/Δgor strains (SHuffle or Origami), CyDisCo, preserving the native cytoplasm environment, results also amenable to large-scale cultivation in chemically defined minimal media as demonstrated by the high-expression yield (139 mg/L) of the scFv of an IgA1 [55]. Collectively, these results highlight the enormous potential of the SHuffle strain for the production of soluble fragments of active antibodies in the *E. coli* cytoplasm, especially scFv. Its use in combination with different chaperones or fusion tags and with the Enpresso B medium, therefore, paves the way to the large-scale production of antibody fragments through cytoplasmic expression also on a lab scale [128]. With such high-expression yields in the flasks, the production of antibody fragments would not require a scale-up to bioreactors during the drug development process [129].

2.6. Periplasmic Expression

The *E. coli* periplasm provides the natural oxidizing conditions for disulfide bond formation and isomerization due to the presence of enzymes and specific chaperones and foldases that facilitate the production of soluble and active proteins containing disulfide bonds [130]. All proteins in *E. coli* are initially synthesized in the cytoplasm as precursors carrying a cleavable N-terminal signal sequence that directs them to the general secretion pathways at the inner membrane. Like other Gram-negative bacteria, *E. coli* exploits three main pathways for protein translocation to the periplasm: the SecB-dependent, the SRP-mediated and the twin-arginine transport (TAT) translocation pathways [131–133]. The SecB and SRP pathways employ the SecYEG complex, a pore in the inner membrane that transports the unfolded polypeptide chains from the cytoplasm to the periplasm.

The SecB pathway is post-translational and the polypeptide chains are translocated after the translation is complete. The SRP pathway instead is co-translational because the translocation occurs while the polypeptide chain is still being translated by the ribosome.

The third mechanism, the twin-arginine transport (TAT) system pathway, consists of a larger pore made up of the TatABC proteins, which transport the fully folded proteins into the periplasm. Proteins with slow folding rates are generally translocated via the SecB pathway, while rapidly folding proteins favor the TAT pathway. Although the TAT system has been successfully used in many cases [134] the majority of recombinant proteins (>90%) translocating to the periplasm are directed via the SecB and SRP pathways. Targeting of the polypeptide chains to the periplasm via SecB, SRP or TAT requires an N-terminal signal peptide that specifically interacts with components of the three secretory pathways. This signal peptide is then opportunely cleaved from the polypeptide chain by proteases during the translocation in the periplasm.

Once they reach the periplasm, the newly exported mature proteins are folded and assembled. Periplasmic proteins may encounter two types of protein folding catalysts: protein disulfide isomerases (Dsb proteins), which catalyze the formation of disulfide bonds, and peptidyl-prolyl isomerases (PPIase), which catalyze the cis-trans isomerization of peptidyl bonds.

The Dsb protein system is composed of five members: DsbA, DsbB, DsbC, DsbD, DsbG [135]. The DsbA/DsbB system assists the formation of disulfide bonds but the process may result in incorrect cysteine pairing and in the trapping of the target protein in non-native conformations. Isomerases DsbC and DsbG promote the rearrangement of the scrambled disulfide bonds assisted by the integral inner membrane enzyme DsbD, which constantly reduces these latter isomerases by transferring the electrons made available by the cytoplasmic thioredoxin. In addition, DsbA, DsbC and DsbG may also have a chaperone activity that favors the recognition and interaction with substrates necessitating disulfide isomerization [136]. The process leading to correct protein folding in the *E. coli* periplasm is further completed and checked by the activity of PPIases such as SurA, FkpA, PpiA, PpiD, Skp, and DegP that leads to protein misfolding and aggregation also in the periplasm. So far, the Cpx two-component system (2CST system CpxRA) and the heat shock σE pathway have been well-characterized as two regulatory transduction pathways of Envelope stress responses (ESRs) systems for preventing any perturbation in the periplasmic protein folding [143].

Another common drawback is related to the leakage of antibody fragments in the medium. The metabolic stress leads to a high accumulation of antibody fragments in the periplasm saturating the secretory machinery. This event generates a more permeable membrane structure that, after sufficient product accumulation in the periplasm, allows a higher diffusive leakage of the periplasm proteins outside the cells [86,144]. However, the optimization of extracellular secretion is becoming another valid option to produce active folded recombinant antibody fragments in E. coli. To overcome the issues associated with protein extracellular effusion and loss, careful optimization is required to match recombinant expression rate with the secretion capacity of the host to optimize translocation and folding efficiency. Protein secretion can be effectively modulated at the transcriptional level by modifying the promoters in the expression vector [145]. Additionally, the choice of the signal peptide sequence [146–149] and the co-expression with chaperons can affect the secretion and folding (see Figure 1).

2.8. Choice of Peptide Signal for Antibody Fragment Expression

Signal peptides act as zip codes marking the protein secretion pathway as well as the protein target location. The choice of the signal peptide has a strong impact on recombinant protein production rate and yield in the periplasm. Recently, Kulmala and coworkers have investigated the effect of synonymous codon pairs and mRNA secondary structures on the pelB peptide sequence for the periplasmic expression of a Fab fragment [62]. By screening a combinatorial library through ad hoc developed time-resolved fluorescence immunoassays [60], they firstly evaluated the effects of synonymous codon mutations in the n-, hydrophobic and c-region of the pelB signal sequences of the light and heavy chains cloned into a bicistronic vector under the control of a Lac promoter. Then the effects of codon usage and mRNA secondary structures were further evaluated for improving the Fab periplasmic expression. The use of an optimal nucleotide triplet coding for leucine in position 5 of the pelB sequence of the light chain resulted in a reduction of the expression level. These results confirmed that the presence of rare codons present in Sec signal peptides is not casual, but is highly important to ensure an efficient interaction of the export proteins with the components of the secretory machinery and also to prevent their degradation [150,151]. Furthermore, bioinformatic analyses related to mRNA secondary structures at the translation initiation regions of the light and heavy chains supported their role on the expression levels [152]. The reduced folding energy of the mRNA secondary structures at the translation initiation region of the light chain and the presence of rare codons in the signal peptides coincided with increased Fab expression.

Sophisticated bioinformatic tools can also be used for the *in silico* prediction of signal peptide sequences and for their cleavage positions also in bacterial amino acid sequences. These include the consolidated PrediSi platform [153] and the more recent Signal_P5 [154] and Mature P [155].

Beyond pelB, other N-terminal signal sequences derived from the outer membrane protein A (OmpA) or from alkaline phosphatase A (PhoA) have been utilized to transport antibody-like fragments to the periplasmic space of *E. coli* via the Sec pathway and the SRP-dependent pathway [146,147,156]. The 22 amino acids long PelB (pectate lyase B) signal sequence from *Erwinia carotovora* [157] is the most frequently used for transportation of the Fabs [88,96] and scFvs [30,101,158,159]. Recently, the expression of an scFv antibody fragment has been used as a showcase for validating the efficacy of the novel vector pSAR-2 containing the pelB leader sequence and the rhamnose-inducible expression promoter, obtaining a yield of 1.2 g/L [71]. A number of other methods and tools have been also devised for exploring the different features of signal peptides and their ability to modulate the expression of scFvs [67,68,98] and Fabs [56,60,88,90,96,99].

(see Figure 1) [137–140]. PPI are enzymes that catalyze the cis-trans isomerization of peptidyl bonds and their activity is the rate-limiting step of the protein folding.

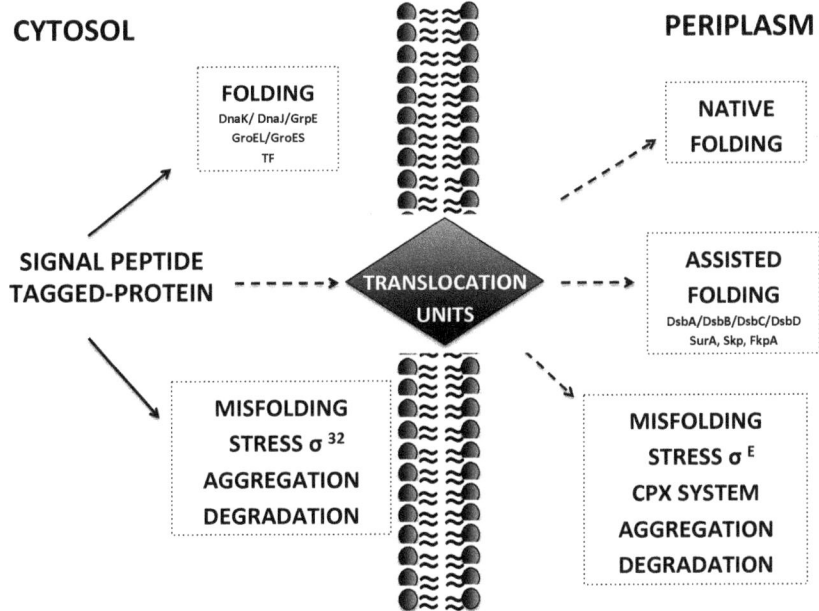

Figure 1. Schematic representation of optional folding and misfolding pathways for periplasmic recombinant protein.

2.7. Advantages and Disadvantages of the E. coli Expression Systems

In addition to the peculiarity of providing a natural oxidizing environment that promotes the formation of disulfide bonds, the secretion of recombinant proteins in the periplasmic space offers other potential advantages. For example, the translocation reduces the exposure of the recombinant protein to host cytoplasmic proteases, reducing the degradation. Additionally, recombinant proteins are produced with a true N-terminus, thus without an N-terminal methionine. For proteins expressed in the periplasm the downstream processing is also simplified because it contains only around 4% to 8% of the natural *E. coli* cellular proteins and the outer membrane can be stripped away applying an osmotic shock or mild heat treatments. In spite of the above-mentioned benefits, the production of recombinant proteins into the *E. coli* periplasmic compartment is limited by the periplasm size and by the secretion capacity of the cell.

The periplasmic compartment accounts for less than 20% of the total cell volume. Depending on the strain, on the signal peptide used for secretion and on the protein of interest, there is a threshold of the protein amount that can be exported into the periplasmic compartment. Above a certain optimal rate of translation, secretion rates can rapidly decrease. Indeed, when the expression is too high, the translocation is slowed down by poorly exported proteins or by defective signal peptides, thereby metastable precursors may accumulate in the cytoplasm promoting inclusion bodies formation that affects protein yields and cell viability [141,142]. This excess of precursors of secretory proteins in the cytoplasm induces the up-regulation of heat shock proteins, which is mediated by the sigma factor 32 (σ32) [141], promoting inclusion bodies formation, reducing protein yields and cell viability (increased cell toxicity). Furthermore, it is not surprising that an excessive *E. coli* stress response could generate increased demand for protein folding and induce an uncharacterized metabolic burden on the cells

For instance, Kasli and coworkers [67] have evaluated the influence of the secretory pathways in scFv periplasmic recovery by comparing the use of the pelB signal peptide (directing to the periplasm via the post-translational SecB pathway) and the DsbA signal peptide (targeting to the periplasm via the cotranslational SRP route). The pelB signal sequence resulted largely superior over the DsbA signal peptide in terms of scFv solubility and cell physiology [67].

An innovative β-lactamase screening system for the optimization of signal peptides has been developed using pelB as scaffold [98]. In this work, a preliminary screening production of the scFv 13R4 in the periplasm driven by the arabinose-inducible pBAD promoter (pLBAD2 vector) using STII, DsbA and PelB signal peptides was performed. pelB was selected and used as the starting point for constructing both an epPCR library (random mutagenesis signal peptide library) and a chemically synthesized (CS) peptide library. According to the signal related to β-lactamase activities, two new peptides were selected from the libraries as improving the periplasmic production of active 13R4 by ~40% compared to the expression obtained using the wild type pelB [98].

Kumar and coworkers have obtained a yield of 25 mg/L of a periplasmic Fab fragment in shake flasks by using the rhamnose-inducible promoter (rhaBAD) and the *mal* and pelB secretion sequences for the heavy and light chains, respectively. The highest biomass and expression was obtained using BL21 (DE3) *E. coli* cells induced with 50 mM rhamnose at 30 °C for 8 h in the Champion medium [96]. A similar periplasmic recovery (30 mg/L) of functional Fab was reported using pelB and induction with 0.1 mM IPTG at 30 °C o.n. when coexpressed with the DsbA/C chaperones in shake flasks [88]. In another study, a recovery of 10 mg/mL of highly immunoreactive Fabs was obtained by using pelB, the BL21 strain and the SB medium in combination with a harmonizing DNA approach [60].

In another study, the use of the heat-stable enterotoxin II (STII) signal peptide led to an expression yield of 332 mg/L of soluble Fab. Here, a gross nitrogen flow was supplied (6.91 g/L) in a 5L scale fermentation at 25 °C using an ad hoc engineered W3110 (ilvG$^{+/+}$ ΔphoA) *E. coli* strain. These results indicate that supplementing a nitrogen source at low temperature is critical for Fab productivity in *E. coli* fermentations [90]. Of note, the alkaline phosphatase (phoA) promoter and the heat-stable enterotoxin II (STII) leader sequence have been also described as a positive combination to facilitate the *E. coli* extracellular production of Fab fragments [160].

Karyolaimos and coworkers [68] have successfully demonstrated that a combinatorial screening of different signal peptides in a titratable system that tunes protein production rates was a valuable and effective approach to enhance scFv recombinant production yields in the periplasm of *E. coli*. The gene encoding for an scFv bearing at the C-terminus a His6-tag was fused to DsbAsp, Hbpsp, OmpAsp, and PhoAsp signal peptides and, in turn, inserted into the rhamnose promoter-based expression vector pRha. This enabled tuning of the protein production rates by varying the rhamnose concentration and avoiding the saturation of the Sec-translocon capacity. For the expression, plasmids were transformed into the *E. coli* strain W3110Δ rha Δlac [161]. The highest periplasmic production yield of an scFv was 0.2 g/L of culture and was achieved using the OmpA signal peptide, LB medium and induction with 100 μM rhamnose at 30 °C in a shake flask [68]. Additionally, Fab fragments bearing the OmpA signal peptide were efficiently produced as soluble periplasmic products by coexpression with DnaK/DnaJ/GrpE in shake flasks using the LB medium and inducing with 0.1 mM IPTG at 25 °C for 8 h [99]. When the same Fab was coexpressed with DsbC in fermentation scale using the ad hoc genetically modified *E. coli* strain deficient in the Tail specific protease (Tsp) and SRP, an optimal recovery of 2.4 g/L was reached [56]. Recently, the OmpA-leader sequence (MKKTAIAIAVALAGFATVAQA) was also selected as the best in plasmid-free expression systems (GI) for the production of a functional Fab fragment [74,104].

2.9. Enhancement of Fab/scFv Secretion into the E. coli Periplasm by Coexpression with Chaperones

The periplasmic localization of several proteins' folding factors and chaperones able to catalyze the proper assembly and folding of functional Fab and scFv antibody fragments has been largely studied. In particular, the correct folding of scFv and Fab fragments has been found to be highly dependent on the activity of PPIases [162]. Following the formation of the intrachain disulfide bonds of variable and constant domains, peptidyl-prolyl cis-trans isomerization reactions drive the folding of Fabs into native conformations. The PPIase activity favors the adoption of correct Ig-like folds playing a crucial role in the prevention of misfolding/aggregation events of antibody fragments. Notably, the kappa light chain variable domains (Vκ) contain two conserved prolines in the cis conformation at positions L8 and L95 (Kabat numbering), unlike the heavy-chain variable (VH) and lambda light chain variable (Vλ) antibody domains [163]. Pioneering studies reported by Plückthun and coworkers [164,165] on the aggregation properties of scFv fragments, demonstrated that the slow isomerization of the peptide bond preceding Pro-L95 is important because it must be in the cis conformation for the formation of the native VH/VL interface. A cis-trans isomerization at Pro-L95 is a rate-limiting step in the folding of the Vκ domains and is essential for the VL/VH docking and, therefore, for the adoption of native protein conformations. The lack of proper peptidyl-prolyl isomerization activity can drive the formation of off-pathway folding intermediates that promote aggregation. Later, the same group also reported that the coexpression of FkpA (a periplasmic PPIase of *Escherichia coli*) resulted in a significant improvement of secretion into the bacterial periplasm of functional scFv fragments containing either Vκ chains, which contain cis-prolines, or Vλ chains which do not contain cis-prolines, suggesting that it has both molecular chaperone and PPIase enzymatic activities [166]. Several groups have attempted with varying degrees of success to improve the bacterial production of antibody fragments also by coexpressing them with molecular chaperones or folding catalysts [122,167,168].

Currently, among the different periplasmic chaperones and/or folding catalysts, the DsbA and DsbC thiol-disulfide oxidoreductases, and two PPIases with chaperone activity, FkpA and Skp, result the most used in coexpression settings. Beyond the basic concept of filling up with chaperones their natural cellular compartments, several groups have also adopted an "interchangeable approach" where the effect of chaperones, both cytoplasmic and periplasmic, has been evaluated in an interchangeable manner both in terms of site of action (making the periplasmic ones devoid of the signal sequence) and in terms of localization of the production of the recombinant antibody fragments.

For instance, Dariushnejad and coworkers have reported that the coexpression of DnaK/DnaJ/GrpE (DnaKJE) results in a 2.5-fold increase in the periplasmic expression level of an anti-TNF-α Fab in shake flasks, using LB medium and BL21(DE3) strains [99,100]. No relevant improvements were detected using the Shuffle strain. Following comparative studies, the authors found that also other chaperones have the ability to increase the solubility of Fab fragments but the DnaKJE chaperone system resulted in the best in terms of activity. This evidence sheds light on the importance of evaluating the activity of soluble antibody fragments to confirm the correct Ig-like folding. As already mentioned above in the cytoplasmic expression paragraph, it has been reported that the coexpression of the periplasmic chaperone DsbC significantly increased the Fab antibody fragment expression in the bacterial cytoplasm using the Origami (DE3) strain [113]. Taken together these data suggest that DsbC overexpression in the cytoplasm exerts a positive effect on the solubility of cytoplasmic proteins [113] not on the recombinant proteins that are targeted to the periplasmic space [99].

The effect of coexpression of cytoplasmic chaperones such as GroEL, DnaJ, Tig, GroES, DnaK and GrpE (see Figure 1) has been evaluated also on the expression of an anti-CD20 human scFv [27]. This scFv fragment was cloned into the pET22b vector containing the pelB sequence and was systematically cotransformed with five commercial plasmids containing different chaperone combinations in BL21 (DE3). Cells were cultured in LB broth and the enhancement of expression was evaluated after induction with 1 mM IPTG for 4 h at 25 °C. Importantly, the coexpression of the pKJE7 plasmid containing GrpE/DnaK/DnaJ had the highest outcome (up to 50%) on solubility compared to other chaperone combinations. Similarly, Sonoda and coworkers [122,167] have reported that the coexpression of DnaKJE with GroELS had negative effects on recombinant protein production in the cytoplasm thus suggesting that there is no cooperativity between GroELS and DnaKJE chaperone systems.

In another report, the cytoplasmic variant of chaperone FkpA (cyt-FkpA) was sucessfully used for improving the periplasmic expression of a Fab fragment [169]. The expression was optimized using commercial TG1 cells harboring the Fab and chaperone plasmid constructs in 2xYT, growth media containing 0.2% arabinose (w/v), and inducing with 1mM IPTG overnight at 30 °C. According to the experimental evidence, authors speculated that the cyt-FkpA has an instrumental cytoplasmic role that improves folding and Fab assembly. It indeed isomerizes key prolines of the kappa light chains prior to the periplasmic export thus preventing a folding bottleneck and favoring the translocation of the heterologously expressed polypeptide chains into the oxidizing periplasmic environment. The strategy improved the levels of soluble periplasmic Fab from 0.4–2.5 mg/L to 3.5–14.2 mg/L.

The synergistic effect of DsbA/DsbC has been next successfully assessed as an effective way to improve the soluble expression of Fabs [56,88] and scFvs [170] in the *E. coli* periplasmic space. In this regard, Rodriguez and coworkers have reported a significant improvement in functional Fab expression into the *E. coli* periplasm (30 mg/L) as a result of its coexpression with the wild type periplasmic DsbA/C [88]. In this case, the BL21 strain harboring the pLac-Fab3F3 and the pBAD-DsbA plasmids was cultivated in EnBase medium [85]. Similarly, Ellis and coworkers developed a novel approach based on the coexpression of Fab fragments with DsbC in ad hoc engineered *E. coli* strain (Tsp spr strains) achieving a very high yield of periplasmic Fab approaching over 2.4 g/L in fermentation scale after 40 h post-induction [56]. The Fab expression was achieved using the pTTO plasmid [171] containing a strong IPTG-inducible tac promoter and the OmpA signal peptide. The lack of the Tsp protease and its extragenic suppressor *spr* in *E. coli* host cells resulted in a recovery of the "wild type" cell viability thus favoring the expression of the Fab and its correct folding in the presence of the Dsb chaperone.

Sun and coworkers reported a yield of 33 mg/L of a soluble and active scFv in shaking-flask cultures by using BL21 (DE3) cells, 2xYT media and following induction with 0.2 mM IPTG for 4 h at 30 °C [170]. For the periplasmic expression, the scFv was cloned into a commercial pET-26b(+) vector whereas Dsb proteins were cloned into the pACYC-Duet-Ara plasmid, a modified version of the pACYC-Duet-1 plasmid (Novagen), where two T7 promoters are replaced by an arabinose-inducible araBAD promoter. These results suggested that the pACYC-Duet-Dsb coexpression vector might be a useful tool for the production of soluble and functional scFv antibody fragments.

In another study, the coexpression of an scFv with the periplasmic chaperones FkpA and Skp significantly improved the cytoplasmic solubility of the scFv and cell viability [168,172].

2.10. Extracellular Secretion

A third option and collateral way to produce recombinant antibody fragments is their recovery directly from the surrounding *E. coli* culture medium. In general, a target protein fused to an N-terminal secretion tag can be recognized and translocated by the Sec machinery to the periplasm but it could further cross the outer membrane reaching the extracellular medium giving rise to a secretory protein. Extracellular protein expression holds several advantages over intracellular production such as the more oxidative and ample environment for effective protein folding, a higher titer of recombinant protein expression, and straightforward downstream purification process. The extracellular expression also enables the direct harvesting of proteins from the culture supernatant, sparing the procedures of cell lysis and reducing the process-related impurities, such as host cell DNA and endotoxins. Furthermore, extracellular secretion can prevent the accumulation of insoluble inclusion bodies in the cytosol or periplasm as well as the toxic effects exerted by some target proteins on the host upon their intracellular expression. The extracellular secretion can be successfully achieved by optimizing the induction starting point and by adding chemical agents that promote outer cell membrane permeability [131,148,173]. To date, the supplementation of Triton X-100 or glycine to the culture medium facilitates the extracellular secretion of target proteins from *E. coli* cells in periplasmic expression settings. Indeed, while glycine induces the swelling of *E. coli* cells and enlargement of the periplasmic space by interfering with the synthesis of peptidoglycans, Triton X-100 disrupts the integrity of the outer membrane [174]. In this way, a functional recombinant scFv has been efficiently recovered (2.86 mg/L) from the extracellular medium by adding 0.25% Triton X-100 [159]. An experimental setting for the efficient secretion of Fab fragments in *E. coli* in shake flasks has been recently described by Luo and coworkers [160]. They have demonstrated that the use of the alkaline phosphatase promoter (phoA) in combination with the heat-stable enterotoxin II (STII) signal peptide (phoA-STII system) is a promising strategy for the extracellular production of Fab fragments, reaching up to 10 mg/L [160]. The authors carefully assessed and compared the effects of promoters, *E. coli* strains and signal peptides on the extracellular expression of a panel of five recombinant Fab fragments. Of interest, they found that the secretion efficiency of the STII signal peptide could be further improved by the coexpression of TolC, the major efflux pump in gram-negative bacteria. The ST signal peptide is translocated across the outer membrane via the TolC/MacAB system [175,176]. Therefore, the overexpression of TolC dramatically enhanced the Fab recovery from the extracellular medium.

Given the undeniable advantages of the production of recombinant protein directly in the extracellular space, several technology platforms have been developed for the large-scale production of these biotherapeutics in *E. coli* supernatants. A graphical overview of the general procedures adopted for obtaining antibody fragments following expression in *E. coli* is reported in Figure 2.

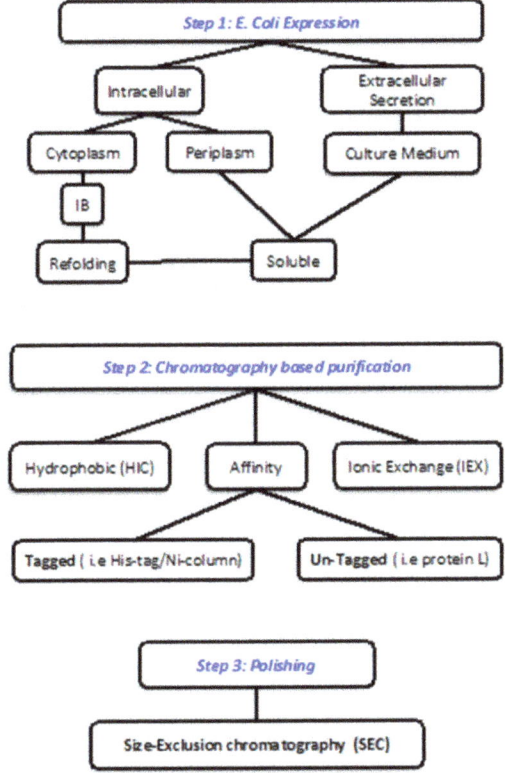

Figure 2. Three step procedure for obtaining purified recombinant antibody fragments following the expression in *E. coli*.

2.11. New Platforms and E. coli-based Cell-Free Expression System

Currently, the *E. coli*-based ESETEC Wacker's secretion technology is one of the most efficient and cost-effective platforms. It relies on the use of the K12 modified strain that enables yields up to 4.0 g/L for Fab fragments and 3.5 g/L for scFvs into the fermentation broth (https://www.wacker.com/cms/en-us/products/brands/esetec/esetec.html).

The RiboTite gene expression control is another innovative technology for protein expression in the cell supernatants (https://gtr.ukri.org/resources/contact.html). It is based on the dual transcriptional–translational gene expression control where a dual Lac-operator/repressor promoter and an orthogonal riboswitch modulate both T7 RNAP and the GOI. In general, a riboswitch is a segment in a messenger RNA that folds into intricate structures that prevent the expression of target genes by interfering with the translation. The binding of an effector molecule induces a conformational change that post-transcriptionally regulates the protein expression. The Dixon lab has developed this system by combining the pETORS expression vector (pET vector engineered with orthogonal riboswitch sequence (ORS) sequence) and ad hoc engineered strains named BL21(IL3) and BL21(LV2) [75,177]. In addition to the IPTG-induced translational control, an orthogonal riboswitch sequence (ORS) controls at the transcriptional level the expression of both chromosomal copies of T7 RNAP and the episomal copies of the recombinant gene of interest. The riboswitch sequence, a modified version of the adenine-sensing A-riboswitch from *Vibrio vulnificus*, is controlled by pyrimido-pyrimidine-2,4-diamine (PPDA) [178], thereby the expression of the target gene occurs only in the presence of both IPTG and PPDA, which effectively reduces the leaky expression to almost undetectable levels.

Batavia Biosciences has developed its own platform technology for cost-effective protein production in *E. coli*, called SCOPE® technology (https://www.bataviabiosciences.com/scope-technology). SCOPE enables the generation of proteins expressed in *E. coli* strains with high yields and tight control of protein expression. In particular, by using the pSAR2 plasmid with a rhamnose promoter, the scFv PGT135 antibody fragment was successfully produced in the periplasmic space. Amounts up to about 1.2 g/L of the biologically active scFv PGT135 were recovered [71].

In recent years, the cell-free protein synthesis systems (CFPS) have been used as an alternative approach to overcome the limitations associated with cell-based expression methods. The well-known and innovative Ecobody technology [179] enables an efficient and cost-effective production of functional proteins including monoclonal antibodies and related fragments [76,180–182]. Taking advantage of the CFPS systems, *E. coli* extracts are used to produce Fabs derived from single B cells. The Zipbody and the SKIK peptide tag technologies have been developed to improve the *de novo* synthesis of soluble and functional Fab fragments [124,126]. Recently, the Ecobody technology has been successfully employed to produce two Fab fragments needed to set up a rapid ELISA assay for the detection of swine influenza virus [183].

Furthermore, Sutro Biopharma has recently developed a novel and flexible Xpress CF platform (Cell-free platform) (https://www.sutrobio.com/technology/xpress-cf/) for the expression of multispecific antibody and antibody–drug conjugates (ADC) in the CFPS modality. The process produces single proteins at g/L yields in 8–10 h at any scale. In particular, the XpressCF+™ technology, through the insertion of non-natural amino acids, provides therapeutic proteins with site-specific conjugation groups. For example, the technology has been used to produce the Sutro's clinical ADC products STRO-001 and STRO-002, in which a cytotoxin is conjugated to an antibody containing non-natural amino acids (STR001—Clinical Trial: NCT03424603. Available online: https://clinicaltrials.gov/ct2/show/NCT03424603).

3. Antibody Fragments as Biotherapeutics and Theranostic Agents

Thanks to their improved pharmacokinetics and their structural and functional flexibility, the three main antibody surrogates, single-domain antibodies (dAbs), scFv and Fabs, are continuously developed and reformatted into bispecific/multi-specific molecules or cytotoxic/radioactive drug carriers to achieve a desired biological efficacy and for multiple clinical applications [1]. In Table 1, most of the classic and ad hoc engineered antibody fragments currently under clinical development or FDA-approved are summarized. We briefly review here five of these that are recombinantly produced in *E. coli* and used for therapeutic intervention.

Certolizumab pegol (CIMZIA®) is a PEGylated Fab' fragment of a humanized anti-TNFα monoclonal antibody. It was developed and manufactured by UCB Pharma and first approved by the FDA in 2008 for treating rheumatoid arthritis. The drug received new therapeutic indications on 28 March 2019 (https://www.drugbank.ca/drugs/DB08904#reference-A176606).

Ranibizumab is a recombinant humanized Fab fragment derived from the parent full-length monoclonal antibody Bevacizumab (Avastin®). It reduces angiogenesis by blocking the activity of the vascular endothelial growth factor A (VEGF-A). Ranibizumab is marketed under the trade name Lucentis®and is indicated for the treatment of macular edema after retinal vein occlusion, age-related macular degeneration (AMD wet), and diabetic macular edema (https://www.drugbank.ca/drugs/DB01270).

Brolucizumab, whose trade name is Beovu®, is a humanized scFv fragment that acts as vascular endothelial growth factor (VEGF) inhibitor, reducing the proliferation of endothelial cells, vascularization of the tissue, and permeability of the vasculature. It is approved for the treatment of neovascular age-related macular degeneration (wet AMD). Brolucizumab was granted FDA approval in October 2019 (https://www.drugbank.ca/drugs/DB14864).

Caplacizumab (trade name Cablivi®) is a humanized sdAb immunoglobulin anti-von Willebrand factor consisting of two identical humanized variable domains genetically linked by a three-alanine linker. Capacizumab is approved for the treatment of adults experiencing episodes of acquired thrombotic thrombocytopenic purpura (aTTP) in conjunction with plasma exchange and immunosuppression in patients 18 years or older. Caplacizumab was developed by Ablynx (a Sanofi company) and FDA-approved on 6 February 2019. The drug was previously approved in the EU in October 2018 as a combination therapy with plasma exchange and immunosuppression. (https://www.drugbank.ca/drugs/DB06081).

Moxetumab pasudotox (MxP), also named BL22, was initially referred to as an scFv fragment derived from the monoclonal antibody RFB4 which specifically binds to CD22 (a lineage-restricted B cell antigen). Then, it has been used to generate a recombinant immunotoxin in which an affinity optimized and stabilized Fv segment has been fused by a disulfide bond to the Pseudomonas exotoxin A (PE38) which has no cell-binding portion. The related drug LUMOXITI™ was developed by Astra Zeneca and FDA-approved on September 13, 2018 (https://www.drugbank.ca/drugs/DB12688).

In recent years, antibody fragments have also achieved encouraging successes as theranostic agents contributing to the development of new personalized and more effective medicine. Their tunable pharmacokinetic properties together with the unique ability to detect with high-affinity and specificity biomarkers in vitro and in vivo, making them excellent agents for tumor imaging [184,185].

An ever-growing number of arrays of antibody fragments serve also as vectors and targeting moieties in "active targeted drug delivery systems" for tumor homing through Antibody-Drug Conjugates (ADC) [186], for reducing the radiation-related toxicity of radioimmunoconjugates used in radioimmunotherapy (RIT)) [187], for nanomedicines applications [188] and also more recently for addressing CAR T cells [189,190].

Table 1. Antibody fragments and formats under clinical development and FDA-approved. Sources: European Medicines Agency public assessment reports, United States Food and Drug Administration (drugs@fda), the international ImMunoGeneTics Information System®(www.imgt.org/mAb-DB/index), Animal Cell Technology Industrial Platform (www.actip.org).

Application [Radiolabeled/Conjugated/Fused]	International Nonproprietary Name	Common Name	Receptor Identification (Species)	Clinical Indication	Development Status (NCT Number)
Therapeutic	Abciximab	c7E3	Fab-G1-kappa [Chimeric]	Acute myocardial infarction [191]	Phase III [NCT00299377]
				Antiplatelet prevention of blood clots in the setting of high risk percutaneous transluminal coronary angioplasty [192]	Phase M FDA Approval, 1994
				Refractory unstable angina when percutaneous coronary intervention is planned [193]	Phase M FDA Approval, 1997
				Acute coronary syndrome (ACS) [194]	Phase IV [NCT00133003]
Therapeutic	Abrezekimab	CDP7766, UCB4144, UCB4144, VR-942	Fab-G1-kappa [Humanized]	Asthma [195]	Phase I [NCT02473939]
Therapeutic [conjugated with pegol]	Alacizumab pegol	CDP791, g165 DFM-PEG	di-Fab′ [Humanized]	Cancers [196]	Phase II [NCT00152477]

Table 1. Cont.

Application [Radiolabeled/Conjugated/Fused]	International Nonproprietary Name	Common Name	Receptor Identification (Species)	Clinical Indication	Development Status (NCT Number)
Therapeutic [fused with CD28 (COTM-CY1) - CD247 (CY2) (1:1)]	Axicabtagene Ciloleucel	Autologous T cells transduced with FMC63 scFv-28Z CAR (FMC63 scFv-CD28-CD247 (CD3Z), KTE-C19, PG13-CD19-H3, FMC63 CD28z, Axi-cel)	scFv-kappa-heavy [Chimeric]	Diffuse large B cell Lymphoma [197]	Phase M FDA Approval, 2017
				Acute lymphocytic leukemia [198]	Phase I/II
				Follicular lymphoma [199]	Phase II
Therapeutic [fused with Homo sapiens IL2 (interleukin 2, IL-2) Pr21-153 (100%) (1:1), noncovalent dimer]	Bifikafusp alfa	L19-IL-2, L19-IL2, L19IL2	scFv-heavy-kappa [Homo sapiens]	Solid Tumor [200]	Phase I/II [NCT02086721]
				Metastatic Melanoma [201]	Phase III [NCT02076633]
Therapeutic	Blinatumomab	AMG103, BITE MT-103, MEDI-538, MT103, bscCD19xCD3	(scFv-kappa-heavy)-(scFv-heavy-kappa) [Mus musculus]	B cell Non-Hodgkin Lymphoma [202]	Phase II [NCT02910063]
				Diffuse large B cell Lymphoma [203]	Phase II [NCT01741792]
				B cell acute lymphoblastic leukemia [204]	Phase M FDA approval, 2014
Therapeutic	Brolucizumab	ESBA-1008, ESBA1008, RTH258	scFv-kappa-heavy [Humanized]	Neovascular Age-related macular degeneration [205]	Phase III [NCT03930641]
Therapeutic	Caplacizumab	ALX-0081, PMP12A2h1-linker AAA-PMP12A2h, caplacizumab-yhdp	VH-VH [Humanized]	Acquired Thrombotic thrombocytopenia purpura [206]	Phase M FDA approval, 2019
Therapeutic	Cibisatamab	CEA TCB, CEA-TCB, RG-7802, RG7802, RO-6958688, RO6958688	IgG1 - kappa/lambda with domain crossover, trivalent [Humanized]	Colorectal cancer [207]	Phase I [NCT03866239]

149

Table 1. Cont.

Application [Radiolabeled/Conjugated/Fused]	International Nonproprietary Name	Common Name	Receptor Identification (Species)	Clinical Indication	Development Status (NCT Number)
Therapeutic [conjugated with pegol]	Certolizumab pegol	CDP870, PHA-738144	Fab'-G1-kappa [Humanized]	Crohn's disease [208]	Phase M FDA approval, 2008
				Psoriasis [209]	Phase III [NCT02326298]
				Rheumatoid arthritis [210,211]	Phase M
				Ankylosing spondylitis	Phase M
				Psoriatic arthritis	Phase M
				Juvenile Idiopathic Arthritis	Phase III [NCT01550003]
				Interstitial cystitis [211]	Phase III [NCT02497976]
Therapeutic [fused with GAA (glucosidase alpha, acid, lysosomal alpha-glucosidase) (Pr67-952) (1:2) Enzyme substitute]	Clervonafusp alfa	VAL-1221	F(ab')2-G1-kappa [Humanized]	Glycogen storage disease type II (GSD-II, Pompe disease [212]	Phase I/II [NCT02898753]
Therapeutic [conjugated with pegol]	Dapirolizumab pegol	CDP7657	Fab'-G1-kappa [Humanized]	Systemic lupus erythematosus [213]	Phase II [NCT02804763]
Therapeutic [fused with Ricinus communis ricin A]	Dorlimomab aritox	4197X-RA, MDX-RA (ricin A chain) immunotoxin	F(ab')2-nd-nd [Mus musculus]	Secondary cataract [214]	Phase III
Therapeutic	Efgartigimod alfa	ARGX-113, ARGX113	Fc-gamma1 [Homo sapiens]	Myasthenia Gravis [215]	Phase II [NCT02965573]
Therapeutic	Faricimab	RG7716, RO6867461	IgG1-kappa-lambda with half-IG VL-CH1/VH-CK crossover [Homo sapiens Humanized]	Neovascular Age-related macular degeneration	Phase II [NCT02484690]
				Diabetic macular edema [216]	Phase II [NCT02699450]
Therapeutic	Flotetuzumab	MGD-006, MGD006, RES234, S80880	V-Lambda-VH _ V-Kappa-VH' [Mus musculus Humanized]	Acute myeloid leukemia	Phase I [NCT04158739]
				Myelodysplastic syndromes	Phase I [NCT02152956]

Table 1. Cont.

Application [Radiolabeled/Conjugated/fused]	International Nonproprietary Name	Common Name	Receptor Identification (Species)	Clinical Indication	Development Status (NCT Number)
Therapeutic	Gancotamab	MM-302	scFv-heavy-lambda [Homo sapiens]	Breast Cancers [217]	Phase I [NCT01304797]
Therapeutic	Glenzocimab	ACT-017, ACT017	Fab-G1-kappa [Humanized]	Ischemic stroke [218]	Phase I/II [NCT03803007]
Therapeutic	Gontivimab	ALX-0171, VR-465	VH-VH-VH [Lama glama]	Respiratory Syncytial Virus Lower Respiratory Tract Infection [219]	Phase II [NCT02979431]
Therapeutic	Gremubamab	MEDI3902	[VH-CH1-scFv-VH-VK-h-CH2-CH3_L-kappa]2 [Homo sapiens Humanized]	P. Aeruginosa nosocomial pneumonia [220]	Phase I [NCT02255760]
Therapeutic [conjugated with pegol]	Lulizumab pegol	BMS-931699	V-kappa [Humanized]	Lupus [221]	Phase II [NCT02265744]
Therapeutic	Lutikizumab	ABT-981	[VH-VH'-H-Gamma1-VL-VL'-C-kappa]-dimer [Humanized]	Osteoarthritis [222]	Phase II [NCT02087904]
Therapeutic [fused with Pseudomonas aeruginosa exotoxin A]	Moxetumomab pasudotox	CAT-8015, GCR-8015, HA22, moxetumomab pasudotox -tdfk	Fv-disulfide stabilized [Mus musculus]	Chronic lymphocytic leukemia [223]	Phase I [NCT01030536]
				Hairy cell leukemia [224]	Phase M FDA approval 2018
				Acute lymphoblastic leukemia [225]	Phase I [NCT00659425]
Therapeutic [fused with Staphylococcus aureus enterotoxin E SEA/E120 superantigen (synthetic)]	Naptumomab estafenatox	ABR-217620, ANYARA, TTS CD3	Fab-G1-kappa [Mus musculus]	Renal cell carcinoma [226]	Phase III [NCT00420888]
				Nonsmall lung carcinoma [227]	Phase I [NCT00056537]
Diagnostic	Nofetumomab Merpentan	Carcinoma-Associated antigen	Fab fragment [Mus musculus]	Diagnostic imaging of small-cell lung cancer [228]	Phase M FDA approval 1996

Table 1. Cont.

Application [Radiolabeled/Conjugated/Fused]	International Nonproprietary Name	Common Name	Receptor Identification (Species)	Clinical Indication	Development Status (NCT Number)
Therapeutic	Onartuzumab	MetMAb, OA-5D5, OA5D5, PRO 143966	Fab-G1-kappa-[Fc-G1] [Humanized]	Metastatic Colorectal Cancers [229]	Phase II [NCT01418222]
				Solid tumors [230]	Phase III [NCT02488330]
Therapeutic [fused with TNF (tumor necrosis factor (TNF) superfamily member 2, TNFSF2, TNF-alpha, TNFA]	Onfekafusp alfa	L19TNF, L19TNF-alpha	[scFv-heavy-kappa - TNF (tumor necrosis factor (TNF) superfamily member 2, TNFSF2, TNF-alpha, TNFA)]-trimer [Homo sapiens]	Melanoma [231]	Phase II [NCT02076633]
				Solid tumors [232]	Phase I/II [NCT01253837]
Therapeutic [fused with Pseudomonas aeruginosa exotoxin A]	Oportuzumab monatox	VB4-845	scFv-kappa-heavy [Humanized]	Bladder Cancer [233]	Phase II [NCT00462488]
Therapeutic	Olrtertuzumab	TRU-016	VH-V-kappa-CH2 -CH3 [Humanized]	Chronic lymphocytic leukemia [234]	Phase I/II [NCT01188681]
				Non-Hodgkin's lymphoma [235]	Phase I [NCT00614042]
Therapeutic	Romilkimab	SAR156597, huTBTI3_2_1	[VH-H-Gamma4 VL-L-kappa]-dimer [Chimeric Humanized]	Idiopathic pulmonary fibrosis [236]	Phase II [NCT01529853]
Therapeutic	Solitomab	AMG 110, AMG-110, MT110	(scFv-kappa-heavy)-(scFv-heavy-kappa) [Mus musculus]	Systemic sclerosis [237]	Phase II [NCT02921971]
Therapeutic	Sonelokimab	M-1095, MSB-0010841	VH-VH'-VH, trivalent [Humanized Vicugna pacos (alpaca)]	Psoriasis [238]	Phase I [NCT02156466]
Therapeutic [fused with CD8A (COTM) -TNFRSF9 (CY1) - CD247 (CY2) (1:1)]	Tisagenlecleucel	Autologous T cells transduced with FMC63 scFv-8A-F9Z CAR (FMC63 scFv-CD8A-TNFRSF9-CD247 (CD3Z), CART19, CTL019, tisagenlecleucel-T)		Diffuse large B cell Lymphoma [239]	Phase I [NCT03630159]
				Acute lymphocytic leukemia [240]	Phase M FDA approval, 2018
Therapeutic	Vanucizumab	RG-7221, RG7221, RO5520985	IgG1-kappa-lambda with half-IG VL-CH1/VH-CK crossover [Humanized]	Solid tumors [241]	Phase I [NCT01688206]

Table 1. Cont.

Application [Radiolabeled/Conjugated/Fused]	International Nonproprietary Name	Common Name	Receptor Identification (Species)	Clinical Indication	Development Status (NCT Number)
Therapeutic	Vibecotamab	XmAb14045	half-IG G1-kappa/scFv-h-CH2-CH3 [Chimeric]	Acute Myelogenous Leukemia, B cell Acute Lymphoblastic Leukemia, Blastic Plasmacytoid Dendritic Cell Neoplasm, Chronic Myeloid Leukemia, Blast Crisis [242]	Phase I [NCT02730312]
Therapeutic	Vobarilizumab	(20A11-9mer-ALB11), ALX-0061	VH-VH' [Humanized]	Rheumatoid arthritis [243]	Phase II [NCT02518620]
				Systemic lupus erythematosus [244]	Phase II [NCT02437890]
Therapeutic	Zanidatamab	ZW-25, ZW25	[H-Gamma1_L-kappa]_scFv-VK-VH-h-CH2-CH3 [Humanized]	HER2+/HR+ Breast Cancer [245]	Phase II [NCT04222427]
				HER2-expressing Gastroesophageal Adenocarcinoma [246,247]	Phase II [NCT03929666]

4. Conclusions

The ever-increasing applications of antibody-based molecules as both therapeutic agents and key reagents for advanced diagnostic investigations have greatly expanded the demand of these crucial classes of molecules and the need for their production in high yield and purity. While the preparation of whole antibody molecules requires eukaryotic expression systems, antibody fragments like Fabs, scFvs and other similar surrogates that lack the glycosylation, can be conveniently prepared in *E. coli* backgrounds. The recent evolution of *E. coli* expression systems reinforces the use of this easy and cheap host-microorganism for an advisable production of antibody fragments in recombinant form. In Table 2, we report an updated list of antibody fragments described so far and the expression conditions utilized for their production, including expression localization (periplasmic, cytoplasmic), the type and format of antibody fragment, the vectors used, the inductor, the temperature and time of expression, the strain, the medium, the use of chaperones and the overall recovery. As explained in this review and reported in Table 2, during the last years, huge efforts have been done to adapt at best the *E. coli* machinery to the production of these "magic bullets" molecules, and a contribution has been also provided by structural biology and bioinformatics in addition to advanced molecular genetics, basic biology and chemical biology. Notable progress gas also emerged from the ever-increasing understanding of the unique structural features of the Ig-like domains as obtained by X-ray crystallography and accurate homology modeling studies. The structural knowledge of such basic units indeed provides a relevant contribution in the construct design for tuning the physicochemical and affinity properties and to improve the stability, the efficacy and the clinical potential of antibody-like molecules. Despite the high degree of similarity between the different components of this class of proteins and the growing availability of innovative strategies and robust tools, such as oxidizing mutant strains or plasmids for the overexpression of chaperones and foldases, and new growth media, it is evident that there is not a universal *E. coli*-based methodology for their efficient production, therefore, a trial and error optimization process is necessary for the determination of the successful experimental settings and to achieve scalability of antibody fragment expression processes at an industrial level.

Table 2. Summary of most relevant reported experimental settings for the production of Fab and scFv recombinant fragments in different *E. coli* compartments.

EXPRESSION	Ab-FRAGMENT	VECTOR	INDUCTOR	TEMP.	TIME	*E. coli* Strain	Medium	Chaperone	Recovery	Reference.
CYTOPLASMIC	Fab	pET23 modified	0.5 mM IPTG	30 °C	16 h	KEIO collection parental K12 *E. coli* strain [127]	Enpresso B	CyDisCo	3–50 mg/L	[54]
	scFv	pET23 modified	0.5 mM IPTG	30 °C	16 h	KEIO collection parental K12 *E. coli* strain [127]	Enpresso B	CyDisCo	4–271 mg/L	[54]
	scFv	pET22b	0.05 mM IPTG	30 °C	24 h	Shuffle	LB		147 mg/mL	[109]
	scFv	pET28b	1 mM IPTG	15 °C	48 h	Shuffle	TB	pG-KJE8 pG-Tf2	1–12.8 mg/ml	[102]
	Cyclic scFv	pET28b	1 mM IPTG	15 °C	48 h	Shuffle	TB	pET21-FKPB12 pG-KJE8	2.8 mg/mL	[36]
	Fab	pET28 modified	0.5 mM IPTG	30 °C	16 h	Shuffle	EnBase	SUMO fusion protein	12 mg/L	[87]
	Fab	pelB/pLAC	0.1 mM IPTG	30 °C	on	BL21	EnBase	pBAD/ DsbA 0.2% arabinose	30 mg/L	[88]
	Fab	pelB/pLKO4 β-lattamase	1 mM IPTG	26 °C	3 h	BL21	SB		10 mg/L	[60,62]
	Fab	Omp/pET22b	0.1 mM IPTG	25 °C	8 h	BL21(DE3)	LB	pKJE7 DnaK-dnaJ-grpE		[99]
PERIPLASMIC	Fab'	Omp/pK03 tac promotor pTTO vector	0.2 mM IPTG	30 °C	40 h	W3110 (ΔTsp, spr)	SM6G medium	DsbC	2.4 g/L Fermentation	[56]
	Fab	mal and pelB/pD881	50 mM L-rhamnose	30 °C	8 h	BL21(DE3)	Champion medium		25 mg/L	[96]
	Fab	phoA/STII	FRT-method	30 °C	12 h	W3110 (ilvG+/+ ΔphoA)	YS medium		332 mg/L Fermentation	[90]
	scFv	pRha67K/Omp	0.1 mM L-rhamnose	30 °C	16 h	W3110 (Δ rha Δlac)	LB		0.2 mg/mL	[68]

Table 2. Cont.

EXPRESSION	Ab-FRAGMENT	VECTOR	INDUCTOR	TEMP.	TIME	E. coli Strain	Medium	Chaperone	Recovery	Reference.
PERIPLASMIC?	scFv	pelB/pSAR2	15 mM L-rhamnose	25 °C	48 h	BL21(DE3)	TB		1.2 g/L	[71]
	scFv	pelB/pET22b	1 mM IPTG	25 °C	24 h	BL21(DE3)	LB	pKJE7 DnaK-dnaJ-grpE	65 ug/ml	[109]
	scFv	pelB/pET26b	0.2 mM IPTG	30 °C	4 h	BL21(DE3)	2xYT	DsbA and DsbC	33 mg/L	[170]
	scFv	pelB/pLBAD2				BL21	LB	DsbA	ND	[67]
	scFv	csA11 csB2 /pLBAD2 modified pelB sequence	0.02% arabinose	25 °C	26 h 30 h	BL21A	Lennox Broth		0.65 g/L Fermentation	[98]
	scFv	pelB/pET26 His-tag C terminal	0.1 mM IPTG 0.25% TRITON	25 °C	12 h	BL21(DE3)	M9-glucose medium		2.86 mg/L	[159]
EXTRACELLULAR	Fab	phoA/STII pRSFDuet modified	Starvation	20 °C	16 h	BL21(DE3)	LB and PLM medium		up to 10 mg/L	[150]

Author Contributions: A.S. and J.P.S. collected and analyzed the literature material. M.R. analyzed the literature material. A.S. drafted the manuscript. A.S. and M.R. edited the final manuscript. All authors have read and agreed to the published version of the manuscript.

Funding: Authors acknowledge the support from the "Research Project on CAR T cells for hematological malignancies and solid tumors" granted from Ministero della Salute. Support has been received also from Regione Campania for the projects: (i) Development of novel therapeutic approaches for treatment-resistant neoplastic diseases (SATIN)"; (ii) "Fighting Cancer resistance: Multidisciplinary integrated Platform for a technological Innovative Approach to Oncotherapies (Campania Oncotherapies)"; (iii) NANOCAN, NANOfotonica per la lotta al CANcro.

Acknowledgments: J.P.S. is supported by INCIPIT international PhD program cofounded by Marie Skolodowska-Curie Actions.

Conflicts of Interest: The authors declare no conflict of interests.

References

1. Bates, A.; Power, A.C. David vs. goliath: The structure, function, and clinical prospects of antibody fragments. *Antibodies* **2019**, *8*, 28. [CrossRef]
2. Kholodenko, I.V.; Kholodenko, R.V.; Manukyan, G.V.; Lupatov, A.Y.; Yarygin, K.N. Isolation of induced pluripotent cells from stromal liver cells of patients with alcoholic cirrhosis. *Bull. Exp. Biol. Med.* **2017**, *163*, 535–541. [CrossRef] [PubMed]
3. Sivaccumar, J.; Sandomenico, A.; Vitagliano, L.; Ruvo, M. Monoclonal antibodies: A prospective and retrospective view. *Curr. Med. Chem.* **2020**. [CrossRef] [PubMed]
4. Harmsen, M.M.; de Haard, H.J. Properties, production, and applications of camelid single-domain antibody fragments. *Appl. Microbiol Biotechnol.* **2007**, *77*, 13–22. [CrossRef] [PubMed]
5. English, H.; Hong, J.; Ho, M. Ancient species offers contemporary therapeutics: An update on shark VNAR single domain antibody sequences, phage libraries and potential clinical applications. *Antib. Ther.* **2020**, *3*, 1–9. [CrossRef] [PubMed]
6. Jovcevska, I.; Muyldermans, S. The therapeutic potential of nanobodies. *BioDrugs* **2020**, *34*, 11–26. [CrossRef]
7. de Marco, A. Recombinant expression of nanobodies and nanobody-derived immunoreagents. *Protein Expr. Purif.* **2020**, *172*, 105645. [CrossRef]
8. Cossins, A.J.; Harrison, S.; Popplewell, A.G.; Gore, M.G. Recombinant production of a VL single domain antibody in *Escherichia coli* and analysis of its interaction with peptostreptococcal protein L. *Protein Expr. Purif.* **2007**, *51*, 253–259. [CrossRef]
9. Mitchell, L.S.; Colwell, L.J. Comparative analysis of nanobody sequence and structure data. *Proteins* **2018**, *86*, 697–706. [CrossRef]
10. Uchanski, T.; Pardon, E.; Steyaert, J. Nanobodies to study protein conformational states. *Curr. Opin. Struct. Biol.* **2020**, *60*, 117–123. [CrossRef]
11. Barthelemy, P.A.; Raab, H.; Appleton, B.A.; Bond, C.J.; Wu, P.; Wiesmann, C.; Sidhu, S.S. Comprehensive analysis of the factors contributing to the stability and solubility of autonomous human VH domains. *J. Biol. Chem.* **2008**, *283*, 3639–3654. [CrossRef] [PubMed]
12. Muyldermans, S. Nanobodies: Natural single-domain antibodies. *Annu. Rev. Biochem.* **2013**, *82*, 775–797. [CrossRef] [PubMed]
13. Mitchell, L.S.; Colwell, L.J. Analysis of nanobody paratopes reveals greater diversity than classical antibodies. *Protein Eng. Des. Sel.* **2018**, *31*, 267–275. [CrossRef] [PubMed]
14. Zavrtanik, U.; Lukan, J.; Loris, R.; Lah, J.; Hadzi, S. Structural basis of epitope recognition by heavy-chain camelid antibodies. *J. Mol. Biol.* **2018**, *430*, 4369–4386. [CrossRef] [PubMed]
15. Konning, D.; Zielonka, S.; Grzeschik, J.; Empting, M.; Valldorf, B.; Krah, S.; Schroter, C.; Sellmann, C.; Hock, B.; Kolmar, H. Camelid and shark single domain antibodies: Structural features and therapeutic potential. *Curr. Opin. Struct. Biol.* **2017**, *45*, 10–16. [CrossRef]
16. Gu, X.; Jia, X.; Feng, J.; Shen, B.; Huang, Y.; Geng, S.; Sun, Y.; Wang, Y.; Li, Y.; Long, M. Molecular modeling and affinity determination of scFv antibody: Proper linker peptide enhances its activity. *Ann. Biomed. Eng.* **2010**, *38*, 537–549. [CrossRef]

17. Kortt, A.A.; Malby, R.L.; Caldwell, J.B.; Gruen, L.C.; Ivancic, N.; Lawrence, M.C.; Howlett, G.J.; Webster, R.G.; Hudson, P.J.; Colman, P.M. Recombinant anti-sialidase single-chain variable fragment antibody. Characterization, formation of dimer and higher-molecular-mass multimers and the solution of the crystal structure of the single-chain variable fragment/sialidase complex. *Eur. J. Biochem.* **1994**, *221*, 151–157. [CrossRef]
18. Iliades, P.; Kortt, A.A.; Hudson, P.J. Triabodies: Single chain Fv fragments without a linker form trivalent trimers. *FEBS Lett.* **1997**, *409*, 437–441. [CrossRef]
19. Le Gall, F.; Kipriyanov, S.M.; Moldenhauer, G.; Little, M. Di-, tri- and tetrameric single chain Fv antibody fragments against human CD19: Effect of valency on cell binding. *FEBS Lett.* **1999**, *453*, 164–168. [CrossRef]
20. Wang, S.; Zheng, C.; Liu, Y.; Zheng, H.; Wang, Z. Construction of multiform scFv antibodies using linker peptide. *J. Genet. Genom.* **2008**, *35*, 313–316. [CrossRef]
21. Worn, A.; Pluckthun, A. Stability engineering of antibody single-chain Fv fragments. *J. Mol. Biol.* **2001**, *305*, 989–1010. [CrossRef] [PubMed]
22. Sedykh, S.E.; Prinz, V.V.; Buneva, V.N.; Nevinsky, G.A. Bispecific antibodies: Design, therapy, perspectives. *Drug Des. Dev. Ther.* **2018**, *12*, 195–208. [CrossRef] [PubMed]
23. Huehls, A.M.; Coupet, T.A.; Sentman, C.L. Bispecific T-cell engagers for cancer immunotherapy. *Immunol. Cell Biol.* **2015**, *93*, 290–296. [CrossRef] [PubMed]
24. Slaney, C.Y.; Wang, P.; Darcy, P.K.; Kershaw, M.H. CARs versus BiTEs: A comparison between T cell-redirection strategies for cancer treatment. *Cancer Discov.* **2018**, *8*, 924–934. [CrossRef] [PubMed]
25. Alfthan, K.; Takkinen, K.; Sizmann, D.; Soderlund, H.; Teeri, T.T. Properties of a single-chain antibody containing different linker peptides. *Protein Eng.* **1995**, *8*, 725–731. [CrossRef]
26. Huston, J.S.; Levinson, D.; Mudgett-Hunter, M.; Tai, M.S.; Novotny, J.; Margolies, M.N.; Ridge, R.J.; Bruccoleri, R.E.; Haber, E.; Crea, R.; et al. Protein engineering of antibody binding sites: Recovery of specific activity in an anti-digoxin single-chain Fv analogue produced in *Escherichia coli*. *Proc. Natl. Acad. Sci. USA* **1988**, *85*, 5879–5883. [CrossRef]
27. Yusakul, G.; Sakamoto, S.; Pongkitwitoon, B.; Tanaka, H.; Morimoto, S. Effect of linker length between variable domains of single chain variable fragment antibody against daidzin on its reactivity. *Biosci. Biotechnol. Biochem.* **2016**, *80*, 1306–1312. [CrossRef] [PubMed]
28. Long, N.E.; Sullivan, B.J.; Ding, H.; Doll, S.; Ryan, M.A.; Hitchcock, C.L.; Martin, E.W., Jr.; Kumar, K.; Tweedle, M.F.; Magliery, T.J. Linker engineering in anti-TAG-72 antibody fragments optimizes biophysical properties, serum half-life, and high-specificity tumor imaging. *J. Biol. Chem.* **2018**, *293*, 9030–9040. [CrossRef]
29. Dudgeon, K.; Rouet, R.; Kokmeijer, I.; Schofield, P.; Stolp, J.; Langley, D.; Stock, D.; Christ, D. General strategy for the generation of human antibody variable domains with increased aggregation resistance. *Proc. Natl. Acad. Sci. USA* **2012**, *109*, 10879–10884. [CrossRef]
30. Dewi, K.S.; Retnoningrum, D.S.; Riani, C.; Fuad, A.M. Construction and periplasmic expression of the Anti-EGFRvIII ScFv antibody gene in *Escherichia coli*. *Sci. Pharm.* **2016**, *84*, 141–152. [CrossRef]
31. Hu, X.; O'Dwyer, R.; Wall, J.G. Cloning, expression and characterisation of a single-chain Fv antibody fragment against domoic acid in *Escherichia coli*. *J. Biotechnol.* **2005**, *120*, 38–45. [CrossRef] [PubMed]
32. Kim, Y.J.; Neelamegam, R.; Heo, M.A.; Edwardraja, S.; Paik, H.J.; Lee, S.G. Improving the productivity of single-chain Fv antibody against c-Met. by rearranging the order of its variable domains. *J. Microbiol. Biotechnol.* **2008**, *18*, 1186–1190. [PubMed]
33. Weatherill, E.E.; Cain, K.L.; Heywood, S.P.; Compson, J.E.; Heads, J.T.; Adams, R.; Humphreys, D.P. Towards a universal disulphide stabilised single chain Fv format: Importance of interchain disulphide bond location and vL-vH orientation. *Protein Eng. Des. Sel.* **2012**, *25*, 321–329. [CrossRef] [PubMed]
34. Fukuda, N.; Noi, K.; Weng, L.; Kobashigawa, Y.; Miyazaki, H.; Wakeyama, Y.; Takaki, M.; Nakahara, Y.; Tatsuno, Y.; Uchida-Kamekura, M.; et al. Production of single-chain fv antibodies specific for ga-pyridine, an advanced glycation end-product (age), with reduced inter.-domain motion. *Molecules* **2017**, *22*, 1695. [CrossRef]
35. Yamauchi, S.; Kobashigawa, Y.; Fukuda, N.; Teramoto, M.; Toyota, Y.; Liu, C.; Ikeguchi, Y.; Sato, T.; Sato, Y.; Kimura, H.; et al. Cyclization of single-chain Fv antibodies markedly suppressed their characteristic aggregation mediated by Inter.-Chain VH-VL interactions. *Molecules* **2019**, *24*, 2620. [CrossRef]
36. Liu, C.; Kobashigawa, Y.; Yamauchi, S.; Fukuda, N.; Sato, T.; Masuda, T.; Ohtsuki, S.; Morioka, H. Convenient method of producing cyclic single-chain Fv antibodies by split-intein-mediated protein ligation and chaperone co-expression. *J. Biochem.* **2020**. [CrossRef]

37. Rothlisberger, D.; Honegger, A.; Pluckthun, A. Domain interactions in the Fab fragment: A comparative evaluation of the single-chain Fv and Fab format engineered with variable domains of different stability. *J. Mol. Biol.* **2005**, *347*, 773–789. [CrossRef]
38. Humphreys, D.P.; Carrington, B.; Bowering, L.C.; Ganesh, R.; Sehdev, M.; Smith, B.J.; King, L.M.; Reeks, D.G.; Lawson, A.; Popplewell, A.G. A plasmid system for optimization of Fab' production in *Escherichia coli*: Importance of balance of heavy chain and light chain synthesis. *Protein Expr. Purif.* **2002**, *26*, 309–320. [CrossRef]
39. Reader, R.H.; Workman, R.G.; Maddison, B.C.; Gough, K.C. Advances in the production and batch reformatting of phage antibody libraries. *Mol. Biotechnol.* **2019**, *61*, 801–815. [CrossRef]
40. Sandborn, W.J.; Feagan, B.G.; Stoinov, S.; Honiball, P.J.; Rutgeerts, P.; Mason, D.; Bloomfield, R.; Schreiber, S.; Investigators, P.S. Certolizumab pegol for the treatment of Crohn's disease. *N. Engl. J. Med.* **2007**, *357*, 228–238. [CrossRef]
41. Jevsevar, S.; Kusterle, M.; Kenig, M. PEGylation of antibody fragments for half-life extension. *Methods Mol. Biol.* **2012**, *901*, 233–246. [PubMed]
42. Richards, D.A. Exploring alternative antibody scaffolds: Antibody fragments and antibody mimics for targeted drug delivery. *Drug Discov. Today Technol.* **2018**, *30*, 35–46. [CrossRef]
43. Rosano, G.L.; Morales, E.S.; Ceccarelli, E.A. New tools for recombinant protein production in *Escherichia coli*: A 5-year update. *Protein Sci.* **2019**, *28*, 1412–1422. [CrossRef] [PubMed]
44. Selas Castineiras, T.; Williams, S.G.; Hitchcock, A.G.; Smith, D.C. *E. coli* strain engineering for the production of advanced biopharmaceutical products. *FEMS Microbiol. Lett.* **2018**, *365*. [CrossRef] [PubMed]
45. Taylor, T.; Denson, J.P.; Esposito, D. Optimizing expression and solubility of proteins in *E. coli* using modified media and induction parameters. *Methods Mol. Biol.* **2017**, *1586*, 65–82.
46. Rosano, G.L.; Ceccarelli, E.A. Recombinant protein expression in *Escherichia coli*: Advances and challenges. *Front. Microbiol.* **2014**, *5*, 172. [CrossRef]
47. Studier, F.W. Stable expression clones and auto-induction for protein production in *E. coli*. *Methods Mol. Biol.* **2014**, *1091*, 17–32.
48. Wong, M.S.; Wu, S.; Causey, T.B.; Bennett, G.N.; San, K.Y. Reduction of acetate accumulation in *Escherichia coli* cultures for increased recombinant protein production. *Metab. Eng.* **2008**, *10*, 97–108. [CrossRef]
49. Kim, S.; Jeong, H.; Kim, E.Y.; Kim, J.F.; Lee, S.Y.; Yoon, S.H. Genomic and transcriptomic landscape of *Escherichia coli* BL21(DE3). *Nucleic Acids Res.* **2017**, *45*, 5285–5293. [CrossRef]
50. Lozano Terol, G.; Gallego-Jara, J.; Sola Martinez, R.A.; Canovas Diaz, M.; de Diego Puente, T. Engineering protein production by rationally choosing a carbon and nitrogen source using *E. coli* BL21 acetate metabolism knockout strains. *Microb. Cell Fact.* **2019**, *18*, 151. [CrossRef]
51. Lobstein, J.; Emrich, C.A.; Jeans, C.; Faulkner, M.; Riggs, P.; Berkmen, M. SHuffle, a novel *Escherichia coli* protein expression strain capable of correctly folding disulfide bonded proteins in its cytoplasm. *Microb. Cell Fact.* **2012**, *11*, 56. [CrossRef] [PubMed]
52. Wagner, S.; Klepsch, M.M.; Schlegel, S.; Appel, A.; Draheim, R.; Tarry, M.; Hogbom, M.; van Wijk, K.J.; Slotboom, D.J.; Persson, J.O.; et al. Tuning *Escherichia coli* for membrane protein overexpression. *Proc. Natl. Acad. Sci. USA* **2008**, *105*, 14371–14376. [CrossRef] [PubMed]
53. Mamat, U.; Wilke, K.; Bramhill, D.; Schromm, A.B.; Lindner, B.; Kohl, T.A.; Corchero, J.L.; Villaverde, A.; Schaffer, L.; Head, S.R.; et al. Detoxifying *Escherichia coli* for endotoxin-free production of recombinant proteins. *Microb. Cell Fact.* **2015**, *14*, 57. [CrossRef] [PubMed]
54. Gaciarz, A.; Veijola, J.; Uchida, Y.; Saaranen, M.J.; Wang, C.; Horkko, S.; Ruddock, L.W. Systematic screening of soluble expression of antibody fragments in the cytoplasm of *E. coli*. *Microb. Cell Fact.* **2016**, *15*, 22. [CrossRef] [PubMed]
55. Gaciarz, A.; Khatri, N.K.; Velez-Suberbie, M.L.; Saaranen, M.J.; Uchida, Y.; Keshavarz-Moore, E.; Ruddock, L.W. Efficient soluble expression of disulfide bonded proteins in the cytoplasm of *Escherichia coli* in fed-batch fermentations on chemically defined minimal media. *Microb. Cell Fact.* **2017**, *16*, 108. [CrossRef]
56. Ellis, M.; Patel, P.; Edon, M.; Ramage, W.; Dickinson, R.; Humphreys, D.P. Development of a high yielding *E. coli* periplasmic expression system for the production of humanized Fab' fragments. *Biotechnol. Prog.* **2017**, *33*, 212–220. [CrossRef]
57. Harding, C.M.; Feldman, M.F. Glycoengineering bioconjugate vaccines, therapeutics, and diagnostics in *E. coli*. *Glycobiology* **2019**, *29*, 519–529. [CrossRef]

58. Lizak, C.; Fan, Y.Y.; Weber, T.C.; Aebi, M. N-Linked glycosylation of antibody fragments in *Escherichia coli*. *Bioconjugate Chem.* **2011**, *22*, 488–496. [CrossRef]
59. Kightlinger, W.; Lin, L.; Rosztoczy, M.; Li, W.; DeLisa, M.P.; Mrksich, M.; Jewett, M.C. Design of glycosylation sites by rapid synthesis and analysis of glycosyltransferases. *Nat. Chem. Biol.* **2018**, *14*, 627–635. [CrossRef]
60. Kulmala, A.; Huovinen, T.; Lamminmaki, U. Effect of DNA sequence of Fab fragment on yield characteristics and cell growth of *E. coli*. *Sci. Rep.* **2017**, *7*, 3796. [CrossRef]
61. Angov, E.; Hillier, C.J.; Kincaid, R.L.; Lyon, J.A. Heterologous protein expression is enhanced by harmonizing the codon usage frequencies of the target gene with those of the expression host. *PLoS ONE* **2008**, *3*, e2189. [CrossRef]
62. Kulmala, A.; Huovinen, T.; Lamminmaki, U. Improvement of Fab expression by screening combinatorial synonymous signal sequence libraries. *Microb. Cell Fact.* **2019**, *18*, 157. [CrossRef] [PubMed]
63. Schmiedl, A.; Breitling, F.; Winter, C.H.; Queitsch, I.; Dubel, S. Effects of unpaired cysteines on yield, solubility and activity of different recombinant antibody constructs expressed in *E. coli*. *J. Immunol. Methods* **2000**, *242*, 101–114. [CrossRef]
64. Cerff, M.; Scholz, A.; Franzreb, M.; Batalha, I.L.; Roque, A.C.; Posten, C. In situ magnetic separation of antibody fragments from *Escherichia coli* in complex media. *BMC Biotechnol.* **2013**, *13*, 44. [CrossRef] [PubMed]
65. Guzman, L.M.; Belin, D.; Carson, M.J.; Beckwith, J. Tight regulation, modulation, and high-level expression by vectors containing the arabinose PBAD promoter. *J. Bacteriol.* **1995**, *177*, 4121–4130. [CrossRef] [PubMed]
66. Haldimann, A.; Daniels, L.L.; Wanner, B.L. Use of new methods for construction of tightly regulated arabinose and rhamnose promoter fusions in studies of the *Escherichia coli* phosphate regulon. *J. Bacteriol.* **1998**, *180*, 1277–1286. [CrossRef] [PubMed]
67. Kasli, I.M.; Thomas, O.R.T.; Overton, T.W. Use of a design of experiments approach to optimise production of a recombinant antibody fragment in the periplasm of *Escherichia coli*: Selection of signal peptide and optimal growth conditions. *AMB Express* **2019**, *9*, 5. [CrossRef] [PubMed]
68. Karyolaimos, A.; Ampah-Korsah, H.; Hillenaar, T.; Mestre Borras, A.; Dolata, K.M.; Sievers, S.; Riedel, K.; Daniels, R.; de Gier, J.W. Enhancing recombinant protein yields in the *E. coli* periplasm by combining signal. Peptide and production rate screening. *Front. Microbiol.* **2019**, *10*, 1511. [CrossRef]
69. Schlegel, S.; Rujas, E.; Ytterberg, A.J.; Zubarev, R.A.; Luirink, J.; de Gier, J.W. Optimizing heterologous protein production in the periplasm of *E. coli* by regulating gene expression levels. *Microb. Cell Fact.* **2013**, *12*, 24. [CrossRef]
70. Baumgarten, T.; Ytterberg, A.J.; Zubarev, R.A.; de Gier, J.W. Optimizing recombinant protein production in the *Escherichia coli* periplasm alleviates stress. *Appl. Environ. Microbiol.* **2018**, *84*. [CrossRef]
71. Petrus, M.L.C.; Kiefer, L.A.; Puri, P.; Heemskerk, E.; Seaman, M.S.; Barouch, D.H.; Arias, S.; van Wezel, G.P.; Havenga, M. A microbial expression system for high-level production of scFv HIV-neutralizing antibody fragments in *Escherichia coli*. *Appl. Microbiol. Biotechnol.* **2019**, *103*, 8875–8888. [CrossRef]
72. Choi, Y.J.; Morel, L.; Le Francois, T.; Bourque, D.; Bourget, L.; Groleau, D.; Massie, B.; Miguez, C.B. Novel, versatile, and tightly regulated expression system for *Escherichia coli* strains. *Appl. Environ. Microbiol.* **2010**, *76*, 5058–5066. [CrossRef]
73. Popov, M.; Petrov, S.; Nacheva, G.; Ivanov, I.; Reichl, U. Effects of a recombinant gene expression on ColE1-like plasmid segregation in *Escherichia coli*. *BMC Biotechnol.* **2011**, *11*, 18. [CrossRef]
74. Hausjell, J.; Kutscha, R.; Gesson, J.D.; Reinisch, D.; Spadiut, O. The effects of lactose induction on a plasmid-free, *E. coli* T7 expression system. *Bioengineering* **2020**, *7*, 8. [CrossRef]
75. Horga, L.G.; Halliwell, S.; Castineiras, T.S.; Wyre, C.; Matos, C.; Yovcheva, D.S.; Kent, R.; Morra, R.; Williams, S.G.; Smith, D.C.; et al. Tuning recombinant protein expression to match secretion capacity. *Microb. Cell Fact.* **2018**, *17*, 199. [CrossRef] [PubMed]
76. Ojima-Kato, T.; Morishita, S.; Uchida, Y.; Nagai, S.; Kojima, T.; Nakano, H. Rapid generation of monoclonal antibodies from single B cells by ecobody technology. *Antibodies* **2018**, *7*, 38. [CrossRef] [PubMed]
77. Upadhyay, A.K.; Murmu, A.; Singh, A.; Panda, A.K. Kinetics of inclusion body formation and its correlation with the characteristics of protein aggregates in *Escherichia coli*. *PLoS ONE* **2012**, *7*, e33951. [CrossRef] [PubMed]
78. Sarker, A.; Rathore, A.S.; Gupta, R.D. Evaluation of scFv protein recovery from *E. coli* by in vitro refolding and mild solubilization process. *Microb. Cell Fact.* **2019**, *18*, 5. [CrossRef]

79. Xu, L.; Song, X.; Jia, L. A camelid nanobody against EGFR was easily obtained through refolding of inclusion body expressed in *Escherichia coli*. *Biotechnol. Appl. Biochem.* **2017**, *64*, 895–901. [CrossRef]
80. Noguchi, T.; Nishida, Y.; Takizawa, K.; Cui, Y.; Tsutsumi, K.; Hamada, T.; Nishi, Y. Accurate quantitation for in vitro refolding of single domain antibody fragments expressed as inclusion bodies by referring the concomitant expression of a soluble form in the periplasms of *Escherichia coli*. *J. Immunol. Methods* **2017**, *442*, 1–11. [CrossRef]
81. Kaur, J.; Kumar, A.; Kaur, J. Strategies for optimization of heterologous protein expression in *E. coli*: Roadblocks and reinforcements. *Int. J. Biol. Macromol.* **2018**, *106*, 803–822. [CrossRef] [PubMed]
82. Gronemeyer, P.; Ditz, R.; Strube, J. Trends in Upstream and Downstream Process. Development for Antibody Manufacturing. *Bioengineering* **2014**, *1*, 188–212. [CrossRef] [PubMed]
83. Chong, L. *Molecular Cloning—A Laboratory Manual*, 3rd ed.; Science: Washington, DC, USA, 2001; Volume 292, p. 446.
84. Studier, F.W. Protein production by auto-induction in high density shaking cultures. *Protein Expr. Purif.* **2005**, *41*, 207–234. [CrossRef] [PubMed]
85. Krause, M.; Ukkonen, K.; Haataja, T.; Ruottinen, M.; Glumoff, T.; Neubauer, A.; Neubauer, P.; Vasala, A. A novel fed-batch based cultivation method provides high cell-density and improves yield of soluble recombinant proteins in shaken cultures. *Microb. Cell Fact.* **2010**, *9*, 11. [CrossRef]
86. Ukkonen, K.; Veijola, J.; Vasala, A.; Neubauer, P. Effect of culture medium, host strain and oxygen transfer on recombinant Fab antibody fragment yield and leakage to medium in shaken *E. coli* cultures. *Microb. Cell Fact.* **2013**, *12*, 73. [CrossRef]
87. Rezaie, F.; Davami, F.; Mansouri, K.; Agha Amiri, S.; Fazel, R.; Mahdian, R.; Davoudi, N.; Enayati, S.; Azizi, M.; Khalaj, V. Cytosolic expression of functional Fab fragments in *Escherichia coli* using a novel combination of dual SUMO expression cassette and EnBase((R)) cultivation mode. *J. Appl. Microbiol.* **2017**, *123*, 134–144. [CrossRef]
88. Rodriguez, C.; Nam, D.H.; Kruchowy, E.; Ge, X. Efficient antibody assembly in *E. coli* periplasm by disulfide bond. Folding factor Co-expression and culture optimization. *Appl. Biochem. Biotechnol.* **2017**, *183*, 520–529. [CrossRef] [PubMed]
89. Azarian, B.; Azimi, A.; Sepehri, M.; Samimi Fam, V.; Rezaie, F.; Talebkhan, Y.; Khalaj, V.; Davami, F. Proteomics investigation of molecular mechanisms affected by EnBase culture system in anti-VEGF fab fragment producing *E. coli* BL21 (DE3). *Prep. Biochem. Biotechnol.* **2019**, *49*, 48–57. [CrossRef]
90. Kim, S.J.; Ha, G.S.; Lee, G.; Lim, S.I.; Lee, C.M.; Yang, Y.H.; Lee, J.; Kim, J.E.; Lee, J.H.; Shin, Y.; et al. Enhanced expression of soluble antibody fragments by low-temperature and overdosing with a nitrogen source. *Enzyme Microb. Technol.* **2018**, *115*, 9–15. [CrossRef]
91. Dragosits, M.; Frascotti, G.; Bernard-Granger, L.; Vazquez, F.; Giuliani, M.; Baumann, K.; Rodriguez-Carmona, E.; Tokkanen, J.; Parrilli, E.; Wiebe, M.G.; et al. Influence of growth temperature on the production of antibody Fab fragments in different microbes: A host comparative analysis. *Biotechnol. Prog.* **2011**, *27*, 38–46. [CrossRef]
92. Rodriguez-Carmona, E.; Cano-Garrido, O.; Dragosits, M.; Maurer, M.; Mader, A.; Kunert, R.; Mattanovich, D.; Villaverde, A.; Vazquez, F. Recombinant Fab expression and secretion in *Escherichia coli* continuous culture at medium cell densities: Influence of temperature. *Process. Biochem.* **2012**, *47*, 446–452. [CrossRef]
93. Sevastsyanovich, Y.; Alfasi, S.; Overton, T.; Hall, R.; Jones, J.; Hewitt, C.; Cole, J. Exploitation of GFP fusion proteins and stress avoidance as a generic strategy for the production of high-quality recombinant proteins. *FEMS Microbiol. Lett.* **2009**, *299*, 86–94. [CrossRef] [PubMed]
94. Wyre, C.; Overton, T.W. Use of a stress-minimisation paradigm in high cell density fed-batch *Escherichia coli* fermentations to optimise recombinant protein production. *J. Ind. Microbiol. Biotechnol.* **2014**, *41*, 1391–1404. [CrossRef] [PubMed]
95. Rathore, A.S. Quality by design (QbD)-based process. development for purification of a biotherapeutic. *Trends Biotechnol.* **2016**, *34*, 358–370. [CrossRef] [PubMed]
96. Kumar, D.; Batra, J.; Komives, C.; Rathore, A.S. QbD based media development for the production of fab fragments in *E. coli*. *Bioengineering* **2019**, *6*, 29. [CrossRef]
97. Hsu, C.C.; Thomas, O.R.T.; Overton, T.W. Periplasmic expression in and release of Fab fragments from *Escherichia coli* using stress minimization. *J. Chem. Technol. Biotechnol.* **2016**, *91*, 815–822. [CrossRef]

98. Selas Castineiras, T.; Williams, S.G.; Hitchcock, A.; Cole, J.A.; Smith, D.C.; Overton, T.W. Development of a generic beta-lactamase screening system for improved signal peptides for periplasmic targeting of recombinant proteins in *Escherichia coli*. *Sci. Rep.* **2018**, *8*, 6986. [CrossRef]
99. Dariushnejad, H.; Farajnia, S.; Zarghami, N.; Aria, M.; Tanomand, A. Effect of DnaK/DnaJ/GrpE and DsbC Chaperons on Periplasmic Expression of Fab Antibody by *E. coli* SEC Pathway. *Int. J. Pept. Res. Ther.* **2019**, *25*, 67–74. [CrossRef]
100. Farajnia, S.; Ghorbanzadeh, V.; Dariushnejad, H. Effect of molecular chaperone on the soluble expression of recombinant fab fragment in *E. coli*. *Int. J. Pept. Res. Ther.* **2020**, *26*, 251–258. [CrossRef]
101. Yousefi, M.; Farajnia, S.; Mokhtarzadeh, A.; Akbari, B.; Ahdi Khosroshahi, S.; Mamipour, M.; Dariushnejad, H.; Ahmadzadeh, V. Soluble expression of humanized Anti-CD20 single chain antibody in *Escherichia coli* by cytoplasmic chaperones co-expression. *Avicenna J. Med. Biotechnol.* **2018**, *10*, 141–146.
102. Liu, C.; Kobashigawa, Y.; Yamauchi, S.; Toyota, Y.; Teramoto, M.; Ikeguchi, Y.; Fukuda, N.; Sato, T.; Sato, Y.; Kimura, H.; et al. Preparation of single-chain Fv antibodies in the cytoplasm of *Escherichia coli* by simplified and systematic chaperone optimization. *J. Biochem.* **2019**, *166*, 455–462. [CrossRef] [PubMed]
103. Mignon, C.; Mariano, N.; Stadthagen, G.; Lugari, A.; Lagoutte, P.; Donnat, S.; Chenavas, S.; Perot, C.; Sodoyer, R.; Werle, B. Codon harmonization—Going beyond the speed limit for protein expression. *FEBS Lett.* **2018**, *592*, 1554–1564. [CrossRef] [PubMed]
104. Fink, M.; Vazulka, S.; Egger, E.; Jarmer, J.; Grabherr, R.; Cserjan-Puschmann, M.; Striedner, G. Microbioreactor cultivations of fab-producing *Escherichia coli* reveal genome-integrated systems as suitable for prospective studies on direct fab expression effects. *Biotechnol. J.* **2019**, *14*, e1800637. [CrossRef] [PubMed]
105. Sharan, S.K.; Thomason, L.C.; Kuznetsov, S.G.; Court, D.L. Recombineering: A homologous recombination-based method of genetic engineering. *Nat. Protoc.* **2009**, *4*, 206–223. [CrossRef]
106. Dvorak, P.; Chrast, L.; Nikel, P.I.; Fedr, R.; Soucek, K.; Sedlackova, M.; Chaloupkova, R.; de Lorenzo, V.; Prokop, Z.; Damborsky, J. Exacerbation of substrate toxicity by IPTG in *Escherichia coli* BL21(DE3) carrying a synthetic metabolic pathway. *Microb. Cell Fact.* **2015**, *14*, 201. [CrossRef]
107. Huang, C.J.; Lin, H.; Yang, X. Industrial production of recombinant therapeutics in *Escherichia coli* and its recent advancements. *J. Ind. Microbiol. Biotechnol.* **2012**, *39*, 383–399. [CrossRef]
108. Meyer, Y.; Buchanan, B.B.; Vignols, F.; Reichheld, J.P. Thioredoxins and glutaredoxins: Unifying elements in redox biology. *Annu. Rev. Genet.* **2009**, *43*, 335–367. [CrossRef]
109. Ahmadzadeh, M.; Farshdari, F.; Nematollahi, L.; Behdani, M.; Mohit, E. Anti-HER2 scFv expression in *Escherichia coli* SHuffle((R))T7 express cells: Effects on solubility and biological activity. *Mol. Biotechnol.* **2020**, *62*, 18–30. [CrossRef]
110. Akbari, V.; Mir Mohammad Sadeghi, H.; Jafrian-Dehkordi, A.; Abedi, D.; Chou, C.P. Functional expression of a single-chain antibody fragment against human epidermal growth factor receptor 2 (HER2) in Escherichia coli. *J. Ind. Microbiol. Biotechnol.* **2014**, *41*, 947–956. [CrossRef]
111. Verdoliva, A.; Ruvo, M.; Cassani, G.; Fassina, G. Topological mimicry of cross-reacting enantiomeric peptide antigens. *J. Biol. Chem.* **1995**, *270*, 30422–30427. [CrossRef]
112. Russo, R.; Rega, C.; Caporale, A.; Tonon, G.; Scaramuzza, S.; Selis, F.; Ruvo, M.; Chambery, A. Ultra-performance liquid chromatography/multiple reaction monitoring mass spectrometry quantification of trastuzumab in human serum by selective monitoring of a specific peptide marker from the antibody complementarity-determining regions. *Rapid Commun. Mass Spectrom.* **2017**, *31*, 1184–1192. [CrossRef] [PubMed]
113. Levy, R.; Weiss, R.; Chen, G.; Iverson, B.L.; Georgiou, G. Production of correctly folded Fab antibody fragment in the cytoplasm of *Escherichia coli* trxB gor mutants via the coexpression of molecular chaperones. *Protein Expr. Purif.* **2001**, *23*, 338–347. [CrossRef] [PubMed]
114. Maeng, B.H.; Nam, D.H.; Kim, Y.H. Coexpression of molecular chaperones to enhance functional expression of anti-BNP scFv in the cytoplasm of *Escherichia coli* for the detection of B-type natriuretic peptide. *World J. Microbiol. Biotechnol.* **2011**, *27*, 1391–1398. [CrossRef] [PubMed]
115. Veisi, K.; Farajnia, S.; Zarghami, N.; Khoram Khorshid, H.R.; Samadi, N.; Ahdi Khosroshahi, S.; Zarei Jaliani, H. Chaperone-assisted soluble expression of a humanized Anti-EGFR ScFv antibody in *E. coli*. *Adv. Pharm. Bull.* **2015**, *5* (Suppl. S1), 621–627. [CrossRef]
116. Bukau, B.; Deuerling, E.; Pfund, C.; Craig, E.A. Getting newly synthesized proteins into shape. *Cell* **2000**, *101*, 119–122. [CrossRef]

117. de Marco, A.; Deuerling, E.; Mogk, A.; Tomoyasu, T.; Bukau, B. Chaperone-based procedure to increase yields of soluble recombinant proteins produced in *E. coli*. *BMC Biotechnol.* **2007**, *7*, 32. [CrossRef]
118. Sina, M.; Farajzadeh, D.; Dastmalchi, S. Effects of environmental factors on soluble expression of a humanized Anti-TNF-alpha scFv antibody in *Escherichia coli*. *Adv. Pharm. Bull.* **2015**, *5*, 455–461. [CrossRef]
119. Bach, H.; Mazor, Y.; Shaky, S.; Shoham-Lev, A.; Berdichevsky, Y.; Gutnick, D.L.; Benhar, I. *Escherichia coli* maltose-binding protein as a molecular chaperone for recombinant intracellular cytoplasmic single-chain antibodies. *J. Mol. Biol.* **2001**, *312*, 79–93. [CrossRef]
120. Yang, H.; Zhong, Y.; Wang, J.; Zhang, Q.; Li, X.; Ling, S.; Wang, S.; Wang, R. Screening of a ScFv antibody with high. affinity for application in human IFN-gamma immunoassay. *Front. Microbiol.* **2018**, *9*, 261. [CrossRef]
121. Ye, T.; Lin, Z.; Lei, H. High.-level expression and characterization of an anti-VEGF165 single-chain variable fragment (scFv) by small ubiquitin-related modifier fusion in *Escherichia coli*. *Appl. Microbiol. Biotechnol.* **2008**, *81*, 311–317. [CrossRef]
122. Sonoda, H.; Kumada, Y.; Katsuda, T.; Yamaji, H. Functional expression of single-chain Fv antibody in the cytoplasm of *Escherichia coli* by thioredoxin fusion and co-expression of molecular chaperones. *Protein Expr. Purif.* **2010**, *70*, 248–253. [CrossRef] [PubMed]
123. Esposito, D.; Chatterjee, D.K. Enhancement of soluble protein expression through the use of fusion tags. *Curr. Opin. Biotechnol.* **2006**, *17*, 353–358. [CrossRef] [PubMed]
124. Ojima-Kato, T.; Nagai, S.; Nakano, H. N-terminal SKIK peptide tag markedly improves expression of difficult-to-express proteins in *Escherichia coli* and Saccharomyces cerevisiae. *J. Biosci. Bioeng.* **2017**, *123*, 540–546. [CrossRef] [PubMed]
125. Ritthisan, P.; Ojima-Kato, T.; Damnjanovic, J.; Kojima, T.; Nakano, H. SKIK-zipbody-alkaline phosphatase, a novel antibody fusion protein expressed in *Escherichia coli* cytoplasm. *J. Biosci. Bioeng.* **2018**, *126*, 705–709. [CrossRef] [PubMed]
126. Ojima-Kato, T.; Fukui, K.; Yamamoto, H.; Hashimura, D.; Miyake, S.; Hirakawa, Y.; Yamasaki, T.; Kojima, T.; Nakano, H. 'Zipbody' leucine zipper-fused Fab in *E. coli* in vitro and in vivo expression systems. *Protein Eng. Des. Sel.* **2016**, *29*, 149–157. [CrossRef]
127. Baba, T.; Ara, T.; Hasegawa, M.; Takai, Y.; Okumura, Y.; Baba, M.; Datsenko, K.A.; Tomita, M.; Wanner, B.L.; Mori, H. Construction of *Escherichia coli* K-12 in-frame, single-gene knockout mutants: The Keio collection. *Mol. Syst. Biol.* **2006**, *2*, 2006 0008. [CrossRef]
128. Ren, G.; Ke, N.; Berkmen, M. Use of the SHuffle strains in production of proteins. *Curr. Protoc. Protein Sci.* **2016**, *85*, 5–26. [CrossRef]
129. Lagasse, H.A.; Alexaki, A.; Simhadri, V.L.; Katagiri, N.H.; Jankowski, W.; Sauna, Z.E.; Kimchi-Sarfaty, C. Recent advances in (therapeutic protein) drug development. *F1000 Res.* **2017**, *6*, 113. [CrossRef]
130. Choi, J.H.; Lee, S.Y. Secretory and extracellular production of recombinant proteins using *Escherichia coli*. *Appl. Microbiol. Biotechnol.* **2004**, *64*, 625–635. [CrossRef]
131. Mergulhao, F.J.; Summers, D.K.; Monteiro, G.A. Recombinant protein secretion in *Escherichia coli*. *Biotechnol. Adv.* **2005**, *23*, 177–202. [CrossRef]
132. Costa, T.R.; Felisberto-Rodrigues, C.; Meir, A.; Prevost, M.S.; Redzej, A.; Trokter, M.; Waksman, G. Secretion systems in Gram-negative bacteria: Structural and mechanistic insights. *Nat. Rev. Microbiol.* **2015**, *13*, 343–359. [CrossRef]
133. Tsirigotaki, A.; De Geyter, J.; Sostaric, N.; Economou, A.; Karamanou, S. Protein export through the bacterial Sec pathway. *Nat Rev Microbiol* **2017**, *15*, 21–36. [CrossRef]
134. Guerrero Montero, I.; Richards, K.L.; Jawara, C.; Browning, D.F.; Peswani, A.R.; Labrit, M.; Allen, M.; Aubry, C.; Dave, E.; Humphreys, D.P.; et al. *Escherichia coli* "TatExpress" strains export several g/L human growth hormone to the periplasm by the Tat pathway. *Biotechnol. Bioeng.* **2019**, *116*, 3282–3291. [CrossRef] [PubMed]
135. Messens, J.; Collet, J.F. Pathways of disulfide bond formation in *Escherichia coli*. *Int. J. Biochem. Cell Biol.* **2006**, *38*, 1050–1062. [CrossRef] [PubMed]
136. Shao, F.; Bader, M.W.; Jakob, U.; Bardwell, J.C. DsbG, a protein disulfide isomerase with chaperone activity. *J. Biol. Chem.* **2000**, *275*, 13349–13352. [CrossRef] [PubMed]
137. Saul, F.A.; Arie, J.P.; Vulliez-le Normand, B.; Kahn, R.; Betton, J.M.; Bentley, G.A. Structural and functional studies of FkpA from *Escherichia coli*, a cis/trans peptidyl-prolyl isomerase with chaperone activity. *J. Mol. Biol.* **2004**, *335*, 595–608. [CrossRef]

138. Schafer, U.; Beck, K.; Muller, M. Skp, a molecular chaperone of gram-negative bacteria, is required for the formation of soluble periplasmic intermediates of outer membrane proteins. *J. Biol. Chem.* **1999**, *274*, 24567–24574. [CrossRef]
139. Sklar, J.G.; Wu, T.; Kahne, D.; Silhavy, T.J. Defining the roles of the periplasmic chaperones SurA, Skp, and DegP in *Escherichia coli*. *Genes Dev.* **2007**, *21*, 2473–2484. [CrossRef]
140. Schlapschy, M.; Skerra, A. Periplasmic chaperones used to enhance functional secretion of proteins in *E. coli*. *Methods Mol. Biol.* **2011**, *705*, 211–224.
141. Wild, J.; Altman, E.; Yura, T.; Gross, C.A. DnaK and DnaJ heat shock proteins participate in protein export in *Escherichia coli*. *Genes Dev.* **1992**, *6*, 1165–1172. [CrossRef]
142. Bukau, B. Regulation of the *Escherichia coli* heat-shock response. *Mol. Microbiol.* **1993**, *9*, 671–680. [CrossRef]
143. Hews, C.L.; Cho, T.; Rowley, G.; Raivio, T.L. Maintaining integrity under stress: Envelope stress response regulation of pathogenesis in gram-negative bacteria. *Front. Cell. Infect. Microbiol.* **2019**, *9*, 313. [CrossRef] [PubMed]
144. Shokri, A.; Sanden, A.M.; Larsson, G. Growth rate-dependent changes in *Escherichia coli* membrane structure and protein leakage. *Appl. Microbiol. Biotechnol.* **2002**, *58*, 386–392. [PubMed]
145. Marschall, L.; Sagmeister, P.; Herwig, C. Tunable recombinant protein expression in *E. coli*: Promoter systems and genetic constraints. *Appl. Microbiol. Biotechnol.* **2017**, *101*, 501–512. [CrossRef]
146. Low, K.O.; Muhammad Mahadi, N.; Md Illias, R. Optimisation of signal peptide for recombinant protein secretion in bacterial hosts. *Appl. Microbiol. Biotechnol.* **2013**, *97*, 3811–3826. [CrossRef]
147. Freudl, R. Signal. peptides for recombinant protein secretion in bacterial expression systems. *Microb. Cell Fact.* **2018**, *17*, 52. [CrossRef]
148. Zhou, Y.; Lu, Z.; Wang, X.; Selvaraj, J.N.; Zhang, G. Genetic engineering modification and fermentation optimization for extracellular production of recombinant proteins using *Escherichia coli*. *Appl. Microbiol. Biotechnol.* **2018**, *102*, 1545–1556. [CrossRef] [PubMed]
149. Owji, H.; Nezafat, N.; Negahdaripour, M.; Hajiebrahimi, A.; Ghasemi, Y. A comprehensive review of signal peptides: Structure, roles, and applications. *Eur. J. Cell Biol.* **2018**, *97*, 422–441. [CrossRef]
150. Zalucki, Y.M.; Beacham, I.R.; Jennings, M.P. Biased codon usage in signal peptides: A role in protein export. *Trends Microbiol.* **2009**, *17*, 146–150. [CrossRef]
151. Zalucki, Y.M.; Beacham, I.R.; Jennings, M.P. Coupling between codon usage, translation and protein export in *Escherichia coli*. *Biotechnol. J.* **2011**, *6*, 660–667. [CrossRef]
152. Bentele, K.; Saffert, P.; Rauscher, R.; Ignatova, Z.; Bluthgen, N. Efficient translation initiation dictates codon usage at gene start. *Mol. Syst. Biol.* **2013**, *9*, 675. [CrossRef] [PubMed]
153. Hiller, K.; Grote, A.; Scheer, M.; Munch, R.; Jahn, D. PrediSi: Prediction of signal peptides and their cleavage positions. *Nucleic Acids Res.* **2004**, *32*, W375–W379. [CrossRef]
154. Almagro Armenteros, J.J.; Tsirigos, K.D.; Sonderby, C.K.; Petersen, T.N.; Winther, O.; Brunak, S.; von Heijne, G.; Nielsen, H. SignalP 5.0 improves signal peptide predictions using deep neural networks. *Nat. Biotechnol.* **2019**, *37*, 420–423. [CrossRef]
155. Orfanoudaki, G.; Markaki, M.; Chatzi, K.; Tsamardinos, I.; Economou, A. MatureP: Prediction of secreted proteins with exclusive information from their mature regions. *Sci. Rep.* **2017**, *7*, 3263. [CrossRef] [PubMed]
156. Thie, H.; Schirrmann, T.; Paschke, M.; Dubel, S.; Hust, M. SRP and Sec. pathway leader peptides for antibody phage display and antibody fragment production in *E. coli*. *New Biotechnol.* **2008**, *25*, 49–54. [CrossRef]
157. Lei, S.P.; Lin, H.C.; Wang, S.S.; Callaway, J.; Wilcox, G. Characterization of the Erwinia carotovora pelB gene and its product pectate lyase. *J. Bacteriol.* **1987**, *169*, 4379–4383. [CrossRef] [PubMed]
158. Demeu, L.M.K.; Soares, R.J.; Miranda, J.S.; Pacheco-Lugo, L.A.; Oliveira, K.G.; Cortez Plaza, C.A.; Billiald, P.; Ferreira de Moura, J.; Yoshida, N.; Alvarenga, L.M.; et al. Engineering a single-chain antibody against Trypanosoma cruzi metacyclic trypomastigotes to block cell invasion. *PLoS ONE* **2019**, *14*, e0223773. [CrossRef] [PubMed]
159. Na, K.I.; Kim, S.J.; Choi, D.S.; Min, W.K.; Kim, S.G.; Seo, J.H. Extracellular production of functional single-chain variable fragment against aflatoxin B1 using *Escherichia coli*. *Lett. Appl. Microbiol.* **2019**, *68*, 241–247. [CrossRef]
160. Luo, M.; Zhao, M.; Cagliero, C.; Jiang, H.; Xie, Y.; Zhu, J.; Yang, H.; Zhang, M.; Zheng, Y.; Yuan, Y.; et al. A general platform for efficient extracellular expression and purification of Fab from *Escherichia coli*. *Appl. Microbiol. Biotechnol.* **2019**, *103*, 3341–3353. [CrossRef]

161. Hjelm, A.; Karyolaimos, A.; Zhang, Z.; Rujas, E.; Vikstrom, D.; Slotboom, D.J.; de Gier, J.W. Tailoring *Escherichia coli* for the l-Rhamnose PBAD promoter-based production of membrane and secretory proteins. *ACS Synth. Biol.* **2017**, *6*, 985–994. [CrossRef]
162. Feige, M.J.; Hendershot, L.M.; Buchner, J. How antibodies fold. *Trends Biochem. Sci.* **2010**, *35*, 189–198. [CrossRef] [PubMed]
163. Johnson, G.; Wu, T.T. Kabat database and its applications: Future directions. *Nucleic Acids Res.* **2001**, *29*, 205–206. [CrossRef] [PubMed]
164. Ramm, K.; Gehrig, P.; Pluckthun, A. Removal of the conserved disulfide bridges from the scFv fragment of an antibody: Effects on folding kinetics and aggregation. *J. Mol. Biol.* **1999**, *290*, 535–546. [CrossRef] [PubMed]
165. Jager, M.; Pluckthun, A. The rate-limiting steps for the folding of an antibody scFv fragment. *FEBS Lett.* **1997**, *418*, 106–110. [CrossRef]
166. Bothmann, H.; Pluckthun, A. The periplasmic *Escherichia coli* peptidylprolyl cis, trans-isomerase FkpA. I. Increased functional expression of antibody fragments with and without cis-prolines. *J. Biol. Chem.* **2000**, *275*, 17100–17105. [CrossRef] [PubMed]
167. Sonoda, H.; Kumada, Y.; Katsuda, T.; Yamaji, H. Effects of cytoplasmic and periplasmic chaperones on secretory production of single-chain Fv antibody in *Escherichia coli*. *J. Biosci. Bioeng.* **2011**, *111*, 465–470. [CrossRef]
168. Ow, D.S.; Lim, D.Y.; Nissom, P.M.; Camattari, A.; Wong, V.V. Co-expression of Skp and FkpA chaperones improves cell viability and alters the global expression of stress response genes during scFvD1.3 production. *Microb. Cell Fact.* **2010**, *9*, 22. [CrossRef]
169. Levy, R.; Ahluwalia, K.; Bohmann, D.J.; Giang, H.M.; Schwimmer, L.J.; Issafras, H.; Reddy, N.B.; Chan, C.; Horwitz, A.H.; Takeuchi, T. Enhancement of antibody fragment secretion into the *Escherichia coli* periplasm by co-expression with the peptidyl prolyl isomerase, FkpA, in the cytoplasm. *J. Immunol. Methods* **2013**, *394*, 10–21. [CrossRef]
170. Sun, X.W.; Wang, X.H.; Yao, Y.B. Co-expression of Dsb proteins enables soluble expression of a single-chain variable fragment (scFv) against human type 1 insulin-like growth factor receptor (IGF-1R) in *E. coli*. *World J. Microbiol. Biotechnol.* **2014**, *30*, 3221–3227. [CrossRef]
171. Humphreys, D.P.; Chapman, A.P.; Reeks, D.G.; Lang, V.; Stephens, P.E. Formation of dimeric Fabs in *Escherichia coli*: Effect of hinge size and isotype, presence of interchain disulphide bond, Fab' expression levels, tail piece sequences and growth conditions. *J. Immunol. Methods* **1997**, *209*, 193–202. [CrossRef]
172. Wang, R.; Xiang, S.; Feng, Y.; Srinivas, S.; Zhang, Y.; Lin, M.; Wang, S. Engineering production of functional scFv antibody in *E. coli* by co-expressing the molecule chaperone Skp. *Front. Cell. Infect. Microbiol.* **2013**, *3*, 72. [CrossRef]
173. Su, L.; Xu, C.; Woodard, R.W.; Chen, J.; Wu, J. A novel strategy for enhancing extracellular secretion of recombinant proteins in *Escherichia coli*. *Appl. Microbiol. Biotechnol.* **2013**, *97*, 6705–6713. [CrossRef] [PubMed]
174. Bao, R.M.; Yang, H.M.; Yu, C.M.; Zhang, W.F.; Tang, J.B. An efficient protocol to enhance the extracellular production of recombinant protein from *Escherichia coli* by the synergistic effects of sucrose, glycine, and Triton X-100. *Protein Expr. Purif.* **2016**, *126*, 9–15. [CrossRef] [PubMed]
175. Yamanaka, H.; Kobayashi, H.; Takahashi, E.; Okamoto, K. MacAB is involved in the secretion of *Escherichia coli* heat-stable enterotoxin II. *J. Bacteriol.* **2008**, *190*, 7693–7698. [CrossRef] [PubMed]
176. Yamanaka, H.; Izawa, H.; Okamoto, K. Carboxy-terminal region involved in activity of *Escherichia coli* TolC. *J. Bacteriol.* **2001**, *183*, 6961–6964. [CrossRef]
177. Morra, R.; Shankar, J.; Robinson, C.J.; Halliwell, S.; Butler, L.; Upton, M.; Hay, S.; Micklefield, J.; Dixon, N. Dual transcriptional-translational cascade permits cellular level tuneable expression control. *Nucleic Acids Res.* **2016**, *44*, e21. [CrossRef] [PubMed]
178. Robinson, C.J.; Vincent, H.A.; Wu, M.C.; Lowe, P.T.; Dunstan, M.S.; Leys, D.; Micklefield, J. Modular riboswitch toolsets for synthetic genetic control in diverse bacterial species. *J. Am. Chem. Soc.* **2014**, *136*, 10615–10624. [CrossRef]
179. Ojima-Kato, T.; Nagai, S.; Nakano, H. Ecobody technology: Rapid monoclonal antibody screening method from single B cells using cell-free protein synthesis for antigen-binding fragment formation. *Sci. Rep.* **2017**, *7*, 13979. [CrossRef]

180. Jiang, X.; Suzuki, H.; Hanai, Y.; Wada, F.; Hitomi, K.; Yamane, T.; Nakano, H. A novel strategy for generation of monoclonal antibodies from single B cells using rt-PCR technique and in vitro expression. *Biotechnol. Prog.* **2006**, *22*, 979–988. [CrossRef]
181. Sabrina, Y.; Ali, M.; Nakano, H. In vitro generation of anti-hepatitis B monoclonal antibodies from a single plasma cell using single-cell RT-PCR and cell-free protein synthesis. *J. Biosci. Bioeng.* **2010**, *109*, 75–82. [CrossRef]
182. Ojima-Kato, T.; Hashimura, D.; Kojima, T.; Minabe, S.; Nakano, H. In vitro generation of rabbit anti-Listeria monocytogenes monoclonal antibody using single cell based RT-PCR linked cell-free expression systems. *J. Immunol. Methods* **2015**, *427*, 58–65. [CrossRef] [PubMed]
183. Sila-On, D.; Chertchinnapa, P.; Shinkai, Y.; Kojima, T.; Nakano, H. Development of a dual monoclonal antibody sandwich enzyme-linked immunosorbent assay for the detection of swine influenza virus using rabbit monoclonal antibody by Ecobody technology. *J. Biosci. Bioeng.* **2020**, *130*, 217–225. [CrossRef] [PubMed]
184. Zhao, X.; Ning, Q.; Mo, Z.; Tang, S. A promising cancer diagnosis and treatment strategy: Targeted cancer therapy and imaging based on antibody fragment. *Artif. Cells Nanomed. Biotechnol.* **2019**, *47*, 3621–3630. [CrossRef] [PubMed]
185. Dammes, N.; Peer, D. Monoclonal antibody-based molecular imaging strategies and theranostic opportunities. *Theranostics* **2020**, *10*, 938–955. [CrossRef] [PubMed]
186. Deonarain, M.P. Miniaturised 'antibody'-drug conjugates for solid tumours? *Drug Discov. Today Technol.* **2018**, *30*, 47–53. [CrossRef]
187. Martins, C.D.; Kramer-Marek, G.; Oyen, W.J.G. Radioimmunotherapy for delivery of cytotoxic radioisotopes: Current status and challenges. *Expert Opin. Drug Deliv.* **2018**, *15*, 185–196. [CrossRef]
188. Pietersz, G.A.; Wang, X.; Yap, M.L.; Lim, B.; Peter, K. Therapeutic targeting in nanomedicine: The future lies in recombinant antibodies. *Nanomedicine (Lond)* **2017**, *12*, 1873–1889. [CrossRef]
189. Falzone, L.; Salomone, S.; Libra, M. Evolution of cancer pharmacological treatments at the turn of the third millennium. *Front. Pharmacol.* **2018**, *9*, 1300. [CrossRef]
190. Fujiwara, K.; Masutani, M.; Tachibana, M.; Okada, N. Impact of scFv structure in chimeric antigen receptor on receptor expression efficiency and antigen recognition properties. *Biochem. Biophys. Res. Commun.* **2020**, *527*, 350–357. [CrossRef]
191. Thiele, H.; Schindler, K.; Friedenberger, J.; Eitel, I.; Furnau, G.; Grebe, E.; Erbs, S.; Linke, A.; Mobius-Winkler, S.; Kivelitz, D.; et al. Intracoronary compared with intravenous bolus abciximab application in patients with ST-elevation myocardial infarction undergoing primary percutaneous coronary intervention: The randomized Leipzig immediate percutaneous coronary intervention abciximab IV versus IC in ST-elevation myocardial infarction trial. *Circulation* **2008**, *118*, 49–57.
192. Azar, R.R.; McKay, R.G.; Thompson, P.D.; Hirst, J.A.; Mitchell, J.F.; Fram, D.B.; Waters, D.D.; Kiernan, F.J. Abciximab in primary coronary angioplasty for acute myocardial infarction improves short- and medium-term outcomes. *J. Am. Coll. Cardiol.* **1998**, *32*, 1996–2002. [CrossRef]
193. Randomised placebo-controlled trial of abciximab before and during coronary intervention in refractory unstable angina: The CAPTURE study. *Lancet* **1997**, *349*, 1429–1435. [CrossRef]
194. Kastrati, A.; Mehilli, J.; Neumann, F.J.; Dotzer, F.; ten Berg, J.; Bollwein, H.; Graf, I.; Ibrahim, M.; Pache, J.; Seyfarth, M.; et al. Abciximab in patients with acute coronary syndromes undergoing percutaneous coronary intervention after clopidogrel pretreatment: The ISAR-REACT 2 randomized trial. *JAMA* **2006**, *295*, 1531–1538. [CrossRef]
195. Burgess, G.; Boyce, M.; Jones, M.; Larsson, L.; Main, M.J.; Morgan, F.; Phillips, P.; Scrimgeour, A.; Strimenopoulou, F.; Vajjah, P.; et al. Randomized study of the safety and pharmacodynamics of inhaled interleukin-13 monoclonal antibody fragment VR942. *EBioMedicine* **2018**, *35*, 67–75. [CrossRef] [PubMed]
196. Ton, N.C.; Parker, G.J.; Jackson, A.; Mullamitha, S.; Buonaccorsi, G.A.; Roberts, C.; Watson, Y.; Davies, K.; Cheung, S.; Hope, L.; et al. Phase I evaluation of CDP791, a PEGylated di-Fab' conjugate that binds vascular endothelial growth factor receptor 2. *Clin. Cancer Res.* **2007**, *13*, 7113–7118. [CrossRef]
197. Bouchkouj, N.; Kasamon, Y.L.; de Claro, R.A.; George, B.; Lin, X.; Lee, S.; Blumenthal, G.M.; Bryan, W.; McKee, A.E.; Pazdur, R. FDA approval summary: Axicabtagene ciloleucel for relapsed or refractory large B-cell lymphoma. *Clin. Cancer Res.* **2019**, *25*, 1702–1708. [CrossRef]

198. Nastoupil, L.J.; Jain, M.D.; Feng, L.; Spiegel, J.Y.; Ghobadi, A.; Lin, Y.; Dahiya, S.; Lunning, M.; Lekakis, L.; Reagan, P.; et al. Standard-of-Care axicabtagene ciloleucel for relapsed or refractory large B-Cell lymphoma: Results from the US lymphoma CAR T consortium. *J. Clin. Oncol.* **2020**, JCO1902104. [CrossRef]
199. Neelapu, S.S.; Locke, F.L.; Bartlett, N.L.; Lekakis, L.J.; Miklos, D.B.; Jacobson, C.A.; Braunschweig, I.; Oluwole, O.O.; Siddiqi, T.; Lin, Y.; et al. Axicabtagene ciloleucel CAR T-Cell therapy in refractory large B-Cell lymphoma. *N. Engl. J. Med.* **2017**, *377*, 2531–2544. [CrossRef]
200. Rekers, N.H.; Zegers, C.M.; Germeraad, W.T.; Dubois, L.; Lambin, P. Long-lasting antitumor effects provided by radiotherapy combined with the immunocytokine L19-IL2. *Oncoimmunology* **2015**, *4*, e1021541. [CrossRef]
201. Weide, B.; Eigentler, T.; Catania, C.; Ascierto, P.A.; Cascinu, S.; Becker, J.C.; Hauschild, A.; Romanini, A.; Danielli, R.; Dummer, R.; et al. A phase II study of the L19IL2 immunocytokine in combination with dacarbazine in advanced metastatic melanoma patients. *Cancer Immunol. Immunother.* **2019**, *68*, 1547–1559. [CrossRef]
202. Coyle, L.; Morley, N.J.; Rambaldi, A.; Mason, K.D.; Verhoef, G.; Furness, C.; Zhang, A.; Jung, A.S.; Franklin, J.L. Open-label., phase 2 study of blinatumomab as second salvage therapy in adults with relapsed/refractory aggressive B-Cell Non-Hodgkin lymphoma. *Blood* **2018**, *132*. [CrossRef]
203. Viardot, A.; Goebeler, M.E.; Hess, G.; Neumann, S.; Pfreundschuh, M.; Adrian, N.; Zettl, F.; Libicher, M.; Sayehli, C.; Stieglmaier, J.; et al. Phase 2 study of the bispecific T-cell engager (BiTE) antibody blinatumomab in relapsed/refractory diffuse large B-cell lymphoma. *Blood* **2016**, *127*, 1410–1416. [CrossRef] [PubMed]
204. Jen, E.Y.; Xu, Q.; Schetter, A.; Przepiorka, D.; Shen, Y.L.; Roscoe, D.; Sridhara, R.; Deisseroth, A.; Philip, R.; Farrell, A.T.; et al. FDA approval: Blinatumomab for patients with B-cell precursor acute lymphoblastic leukemia in morphologic remission with minimal residual disease. *Clin. Cancer Res.* **2019**, *25*, 473–477. [CrossRef] [PubMed]
205. Dugel, P.U.; Koh, A.; Ogura, Y.; Jaffe, G.J.; Schmidt-Erfurth, U.; Brown, D.M.; Gomes, A.V.; Warburton, J.; Weichselberger, A.; Holz, F.G.; et al. HAWK and HARRIER: Phase 3, multicenter, randomized, double-masked trials of brolucizumab for neovascular age-related macular degeneration. *Ophthalmology* **2020**, *127*, 72–84. [CrossRef]
206. Duggan, S. Caplacizumab: First global approval. *Drugs* **2018**, *78*, 1639–1642. [CrossRef]
207. Gonzalez-Exposito, R.; Semiannikova, M.; Griffiths, B.; Khan, K.; Barber, L.J.; Woolston, A.; Spain, G.; von Loga, K.; Challoner, B.; Patel, R.; et al. CEA expression heterogeneity and plasticity confer resistance to the CEA-targeting bispecific immunotherapy antibody cibisatamab (CEA-TCB) in patient-derived colorectal cancer organoids. *J. Immunother. Cancer* **2019**, *7*, 101. [CrossRef]
208. Lang, L. FDA approves Cimzia to treat Crohn's disease. *Gastroenterology* **2008**, *134*, 1819. [CrossRef]
209. Gottlieb, A.B.; Blauvelt, A.; Thaci, D.; Leonardi, C.L.; Poulin, Y.; Drew, J.; Peterson, L.; Arendt, C.; Burge, D.; Reich, K. Certolizumab pegol for the treatment of chronic plaque psoriasis: Results through 48 weeks from 2 phase 3, multicenter, randomized, double-blinded, placebo-controlled studies (CIMPASI-1 and CIMPASI-2). *J. Am. Acad. Dermatol.* **2018**, *79*, 302–314 e6. [CrossRef]
210. Patel, A.M.; Moreland, L.W. Certolizumab pegol: A new biologic targeting rheumatoid arthritis. *Expert Rev. Clin. Immunol.* **2010**, *6*, 855–866. [CrossRef]
211. Bosch, P.C. Examination of the significant placebo effect in the treatment of interstitial cystitis/bladder pain syndrome. *Urology* **2014**, *84*, 321–326. [CrossRef]
212. Kishnani, P.; Lachmann, R.; Mozaffar, T.; Walters, C.; Case, L.; Appleby, M.; Libri, V.; Kak, M.; Wencel, M.; Landy, H. Safety and efficacy of VAL-1221, a novel fusion protein targeting cytoplasmic glycogen, in patients with late-onset Pompe disease. *Mol. Genet. Metab.* **2019**, *126*, S85–S86. [CrossRef]
213. Chamberlain, C.; Colman, P.J.; Ranger, A.M.; Burkly, L.C.; Johnston, G.I.; Otoul, C.; Stach, C.; Zamacona, M.; Dorner, T.; Urowitz, M.; et al. Repeated administration of dapirolizumab pegol in a randomised phase I study is well tolerated and accompanied by improvements in several composite measures of systemic lupus erythematosus disease activity and changes in whole blood transcriptomic profiles. *Ann. Rheum. Dis.* **2017**, *76*, 1837–1844. [CrossRef] [PubMed]
214. Tarsio, J.F.; Kelleher, P.J.; Tarsio, M.; Emery, J.M.; Lam, D.M.-K. Inhibition of cell proliferation on lens capsules by 4197X-ricin a immunoconjugate. *J. Cataract Refract. Surg.* **1997**, *23*, 260–266. [CrossRef]
215. Howard, J.F., Jr.; Bril, V.; Burns, T.M.; Mantegazza, R.; Bilinska, M.; Szczudlik, A.; Beydoun, S.; Garrido, F.; Piehl, F.; Rottoli, M.; et al. Randomized phase 2 study of FcRn antagonist efgartigimod in generalized myasthenia gravis. *Neurology* **2019**, *92*, e2661–e2673. [CrossRef] [PubMed]

216. Sahni, J.; Patel, S.S.; Dugel, P.U.; Khanani, A.M.; Jhaveri, C.D.; Wykoff, C.C.; Hershberger, V.S.; Pauly-Evers, M.; Sadikhov, S.; Szczesny, P.; et al. Simultaneous inhibition of angiopoietin-2 and vascular endothelial growth factor-A with faricimab in diabetic macular edema: BOULEVARD phase 2 randomized trial. *Ophthalmology* **2019**, *126*, 1155–1170. [CrossRef]
217. Lee, H.; Shields, A.F.; Siegel, B.A.; Miller, K.D.; Krop, I.; Ma, C.X.; LoRusso, P.M.; Munster, P.N.; Campbell, K.; Gaddy, D.F.; et al. (64)Cu-MM-302 positron emission tomography quantifies variability of enhanced permeability and retention of nanoparticles in relation to treatment response in patients with metastatic breast cancer. *Clin. Cancer Res.* **2017**, *23*, 4190–4202. [CrossRef]
218. Lebozec, K.; Jandrot-Perrus, M.; Avenard, G.; Favre-Bulle, O.; Billiald, P. Design, development and characterization of ACT017, a humanized Fab that blocks platelet's glycoprotein VI function without causing bleeding risks. *MAbs* **2017**, *9*, 945–958. [CrossRef]
219. Detalle, L.; Stohr, T.; Palomo, C.; Piedra, P.A.; Gilbert, B.E.; Mas, V.; Millar, A.; Power, U.F.; Stortelers, C.; Allosery, K.; et al. Generation and characterization of ALX-0171, a potent novel therapeutic nanobody for the treatment of respiratory syncytial virus infection. *Antimicrob. Agents Chemother.* **2016**, *60*, 6–13. [CrossRef]
220. Ali, S.O.; Yu, X.Q.; Robbie, G.J.; Wu, Y.; Shoemaker, K.; Yu, L.; DiGiandomenico, A.; Keller, A.E.; Anude, C.; Hernandez-Illas, M.; et al. Phase 1 study of MEDI3902, an investigational anti-Pseudomonas aeruginosa PcrV and Psl bispecific human monoclonal antibody, in healthy adults. *Clin. Microbiol. Infect.* **2019**, *25*, 629.e1–629.e6. [CrossRef]
221. Shi, R.; Takkar, N.; Murthy, B.; Mora, J.; Shevell, D.; Pupim, L.; Duchesne, D.; Throup, J.; Girgis, I.G. Pharmacokinetic and pharmacodynamic properties of lulizumab pegol, an Anti-CD28 antagonistic domain antibody, in normal healthy volunteers and patients with systemic lupus erythematosus. *J. Pharmacokinet. Pharmacodyn.* **2017**, *44*, S106.
222. Fleischmann, R.M.; Bliddal, H.; Blanco, F.J.; Schnitzer, T.J.; Peterfy, C.; Chen, S.; Wang, L.; Feng, S.; Conaghan, P.G.; Berenbaum, F.; et al. A Phase II trial of lutikizumab, an anti-interleukin-1alpha/beta dual variable domain immunoglobulin, in knee osteoarthritis patients with synovitis. *Arthritis Rheumatol.* **2019**, *71*, 1056–1069. [CrossRef] [PubMed]
223. Kreitman, R.J.; Pastan, I. Antibody fusion proteins: Anti-CD22 recombinant immunotoxin moxetumomab pasudotox. *Clin. Cancer Res.* **2011**, *17*, 6398–6405. [CrossRef] [PubMed]
224. Lin, A.Y.; Dinner, S.N. Moxetumomab pasudotox for hairy cell leukemia: Preclinical development to FDA approval. *Blood Adv.* **2019**, *3*, 2905–2910. [CrossRef] [PubMed]
225. Wayne, A.S.; Shah, N.N.; Bhojwani, D.; Silverman, L.B.; Whitlock, J.A.; Stetler-Stevenson, M.; Sun, W.; Liang, M.; Yang, J.; Kreitman, R.J.; et al. Phase 1 study of the anti-CD22 immunotoxin moxetumomab pasudotox for childhood acute lymphoblastic leukemia. *Blood* **2017**, *130*, 1620–1627. [CrossRef]
226. Elkord, E.; Burt, D.J.; Sundstedt, A.; Nordle, O.; Hedlund, G.; Hawkins, R.E. Immunological response and overall survival in a subset of advanced renal cell carcinoma patients from a randomized phase 2/3 study of naptumomab estafenatox plus IFN-alpha versus IFN-alpha. *Oncotarget* **2015**, *6*, 4428–4439. [CrossRef]
227. Borghaei, H.; Alpaugh, K.; Hedlund, G.; Forsberg, G.; Langer, C.; Rogatko, A.; Hawkins, R.; Dueland, S.; Lassen, U.; Cohen, R.B. Phase I dose escalation, pharmacokinetic and pharmacodynamic study of naptumomab estafenatox alone in patients with advanced cancer and with docetaxel in patients with advanced non-small-cell lung cancer. *J. Clin. Oncol.* **2009**, *27*, 4116–4123. [CrossRef]
228. Straka, M.R.; Joyce, J.M.; Myers, D.T. Tc-99m nofetumomab merpentan complements an equivocal bone scan for detecting skeletal metastatic disease from lung cancer. *Clin. Nucl. Med.* **2000**, *25*, 54–55. [CrossRef]
229. Bendell, J.C.; Hochster, H.; Hart, L.L.; Firdaus, I.; Mace, J.R.; McFarlane, J.J.; Kozloff, M.; Catenacci, D.; Hsu, J.J.; Hack, S.P.; et al. A Phase II randomized trial (GO27827) of first-line FOLFOX plus bevacizumab with or without the MET inhibitor onartuzumab in patients with metastatic colorectal cancer. *Oncologist* **2017**, *22*, 264–271. [CrossRef]
230. Morley, R.; Cardenas, A.; Hawkins, P.; Suzuki, Y.; Paton, V.; Phan, S.C.; Merchant, M.; Hsu, J.; Yu, W.; Xia, Q.; et al. Safety of onartuzumab in patients with solid tumors: Experience to date from the onartuzumab clinical trial program. *PLoS ONE* **2015**, *10*, e0139679. [CrossRef]
231. Danielli, R.; Patuzzo, R.; Di Giacomo, A.M.; Gallino, G.; Di Florio, A.; Cutala, O.; Lazzeri, A.; Fazio, C.; Giovannoni, L.; Ruffini, P.A.; et al. A phase II study of intratumoral application of L19IL21/L19TNF in melanoma patients in clinical stage III or stage IV M1a with presence of injectable cutaneous and/or subcutaneous lesions. *J. Clin. Oncol.* **2014**, *32*. [CrossRef]

232. Spitaleri, G.; Berardi, R.; Pierantoni, C.; De Pas, T.; Noberasco, C.; Libbra, C.; Gonzalez-Iglesias, R.; Giovannoni, L.; Tasciotti, A.; Neri, D.; et al. Phase I/II study of the tumour-targeting human monoclonal antibody-cytokine fusion protein L19-TNF in patients with advanced solid tumours. *J. Cancer Res. Clin. Oncol.* **2013**, *139*, 447–455. [CrossRef] [PubMed]
233. Kowalski, M.; Guindon, J.; Brazas, L.; Moore, C.; Entwistle, J.; Cizeau, J.; Jewett, M.A.; MacDonald, G.C. A phase II study of oportuzumab monatox: An immunotoxin therapy for patients with noninvasive urothelial carcinoma in situ previously treated with bacillus Calmette-Guerin. *J. Urol.* **2012**, *188*, 1712–1718. [CrossRef] [PubMed]
234. Robak, T.; Hellmann, A.; Kloczko, J.; Loscertales, J.; Lech-Maranda, E.; Pagel, J.M.; Mato, A.; Byrd, J.C.; Awan, F.T.; Hebart, H.; et al. Randomized phase 2 study of otlertuzumab and bendamustine versus bendamustine in patients with relapsed chronic lymphocytic leukaemia. *Br. J. Haematol.* **2017**, *176*, 618–628. [CrossRef]
235. Pagel, J.M.; Spurgeon, S.E.; Byrd, J.C.; Awan, F.T.; Flinn, I.W.; Lanasa, M.C.; Eisenfeld, A.J.; Stromatt, S.C.; Gopal, A.K. Otlertuzumab (TRU-016), an anti-CD37 monospecific ADAPTIR() therapeutic protein, for relapsed or refractory NHL patients. *Br. J. Haematol.* **2015**, *168*, 38–45. [CrossRef] [PubMed]
236. Raghu, G.; Richeldi, L.; Crestani, B.; Wung, P.; Bejuit, R.; Esperet, C.; Antoni, C.; Soubrane, C. SAR156597 in idiopathic pulmonary fibrosis: A phase 2 placebo-controlled study (DRI11772). *Eur. Respir. J.* **2018**, *52*. [CrossRef] [PubMed]
237. Khanna, D.; Tashkin, D.P.; Denton, C.P.; Lubell, M.W.; Vazquez-Mateo, C.; Wax, S. Ongoing clinical trials and treatment options for patients with systemic sclerosis-associated interstitial lung disease. *Rheumatology* **2019**, *58*, 567–579. [CrossRef] [PubMed]
238. Wasilewska, A.; Winiarska, M.; Olszewska, M.; Rudnicka, L. Interleukin-17 inhibitors. A new era in treatment of psoriasis and other skin diseases. *Postepy Dermatol. Alergol.* **2016**, *33*, 247–252. [CrossRef]
239. Schuster, S.J.; Bishop, M.R.; Tam, C.S.; Waller, E.K.; Borchmann, P.; McGuirk, J.P.; Jager, U.; Jaglowski, S.; Andreadis, C.; Westin, J.R.; et al. Tisagenlecleucel in adult relapsed or refractory diffuse large B-Cell lymphoma. *N. Engl. J. Med.* **2019**, *380*, 45–56. [CrossRef]
240. Prasad, V. Immunotherapy: Tisagenlecleucel—The first approved CAR-T-cell therapy: Implications for payers and policy makers. *Nat. Rev. Clin. Oncol.* **2018**, *15*, 11–12. [CrossRef]
241. Hidalgo, M.; Martinez-Garcia, M.; Le Tourneau, C.; Massard, C.; Garralda, E.; Boni, V.; Taus, A.; Albanell, J.; Sablin, M.P.; Alt, M.; et al. First-in-Human phase i study of single-agent vanucizumab, a first-in-class. bispecific anti-angiopoietin-2/anti-vegf-a antibody, in adult patients with advanced solid tumors. *Clin. Cancer Res.* **2018**, *24*, 1536–1545. [CrossRef]
242. Ravandi, F.; Bashey, A.; Foran, J.M.; Stock, W.; Mawad, R.; Blum, W.; Saville, M.W.; Johnson, C.M.; Vanasse, K.G.J.; Ly, T.; et al. Complete responses in relapsed/refractory Acute Myeloid Leukemia (AML) patients on a weekly dosing schedule of XmAb14045, a CD123 x CD3 T cell-engaging bispecific antibody: Initial results of a phase 1 study. *Blood* **2018**, *132*. [CrossRef]
243. Haddley, K. Vobarilizumab anti-interleukin-6 receptor subunit alpha (CD126; IL-6R) treatment of rheumatoid arthritis treatment of systemic lupus erythematosus. *Drugs Future* **2018**, *43*, 891–900. [CrossRef]
244. Haddley, K. Anifrolumab anti-interferon-alpha receptor 1(IFNAR1) monoclonal antibody treatment of systemic lupus erythematosus. *Drugs Future* **2018**, *43*, 471–481. [CrossRef]
245. Meric-Bernstam, F.; Beeram, M.; Blum, M.A.; Hausman, D.F.; Infante, J.R.; Patnaik, A.; Piha-Paul, S.A.; Rasco, D.W.; Rowse, G.; Thimmarayappa, J.; et al. Phase 1 dose escalation of ZW25, a HER2-targeted bispecific antibody, in patients (pts) with HER2-expressing cancers. *J. Clin. Oncol.* **2017**, *35*. [CrossRef]
246. Meric-Bernstam, F.; Chaves, J.; Oh, D.Y.; Lee, J.; Kang, Y.K.; Hamilton, E.; Mayordomo, J.; Cobleigh, M.; Vaklavas, C.; Elimova, E.; et al. Safety and efficacy of ZW25, a HER2-targeted bispecific antibody, in combination with chemotherapy in patients with locally advanced and/or metastatic HER2-expressing gastroesophageal cancer. *Mol. Cancer Ther.* **2019**, *18*. [CrossRef]
247. Meric-Bernstam, F.; Hanna, D.; Beeram, M.; Lee, K.W.; Kang, Y.K.; Chaves, J.; Lee, J.; Goodwin, R.; Vaklavas, C.; Oh, D.Y.; et al. Safety, anti-tumour activity, and biomarker results of the HER2-targeted bispecific antibody ZW25 in HER2-expressing solid tumours. *Ann. Oncol.* **2019**, *30*. [CrossRef]

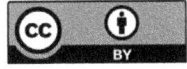 © 2020 by the authors. Licensee MDPI, Basel, Switzerland. This article is an open access article distributed under the terms and conditions of the Creative Commons Attribution (CC BY) license (http://creativecommons.org/licenses/by/4.0/).

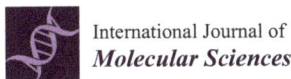 International Journal of
Molecular Sciences

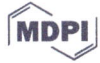

Review

Antibody-Drug Conjugates: The New Frontier of Chemotherapy

Sara Ponziani [1,†], Giulia Di Vittorio [2,†], Giuseppina Pitari [1], Anna Maria Cimini [1], Matteo Ardini [1], Roberta Gentile [2], Stefano Iacobelli [2], Gianluca Sala [2,3], Emily Capone [3], David J. Flavell [4], Rodolfo Ippoliti [1] and Francesco Giansanti [1,*]

1. Department of Life, Health and Environmental Sciences, University of L'Aquila, I-67100 L'Aquila, Italy; sara.ponziani@guest.univaq.it (S.P.); giuseppina.pitari@univaq.it (G.P.); annamaria.cimini@univaq.it (A.M.C.); matteo.ardini@univaq.it (M.A.); rodolfo.ippoliti@univaq.it (R.I.)
2. MediaPharma SrL, I-66013 Chieti, Italy; g.divittorio@mediapharma.it (G.D.V.); r.gentile@mediapharma.it (R.G.); s.iacobelli@mediapharma.it (S.I.); g.sala@unich.it (G.S.)
3. Department of Medical, Oral and Biotechnological Sciences, University of Chieti-Pescara, I-66100 Chieti, Italy; caponemily@gmail.com
4. The Simon Flavell Leukaemia Research Laboratory, Southampton General Hospital, Southampton SO16 6YD, UK; davidf@leukaemiabusters.org.uk
* Correspondence: francesco.giansanti@cc.univaq.it; Tel.: +39-0862433245; Fax: +39-0862423273
† These authors contributed equally to this work.

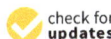

Received: 14 July 2020; Accepted: 30 July 2020; Published: 31 July 2020

Abstract: In recent years, antibody-drug conjugates (ADCs) have become promising antitumor agents to be used as one of the tools in personalized cancer medicine. ADCs are comprised of a drug with cytotoxic activity cross-linked to a monoclonal antibody, targeting antigens expressed at higher levels on tumor cells than on normal cells. By providing a selective targeting mechanism for cytotoxic drugs, ADCs improve the therapeutic index in clinical practice. In this review, the chemistry of ADC linker conjugation together with strategies adopted to improve antibody tolerability (by reducing antigenicity) are examined, with particular attention to ADCs approved by the regulatory agencies (the U.S. Food and Drug Administration (FDA) and the European Medicines Agency (EMA)) for treating cancer patients. Recent developments in engineering Immunoglobulin (Ig) genes and antibody humanization have greatly reduced some of the problems of the first generation of ADCs, beset by problems, such as random coupling of the payload and immunogenicity of the antibody. ADC development and clinical use is a fast, evolving area, and will likely prove an important modality for the treatment of cancer in the near future.

Keywords: Mabs; Antibody-Drug Conjugate; cancer therapy; drug targeting; payload; cross-linking

1. Introduction

The twentieth century has been characterized by basic and applied research leading to the discovery and use of an increasing number of cytotoxic chemotherapeutic compounds with the ability to rapidly kill dividing cancer cells in preference to non-dividing healthy cells. The well-known drawback of chemotherapy is due to the fact that these drugs, in addition to damaging cancer cells, also damage healthy tissues; thus, causing side effects, sometimes with serious consequences.

The challenge is, therefore, to search for drug delivery systems that achieve high cytotoxic efficacy against cancer cells, but with limited systemic toxicity. Antibody-drug conjugates (ADCs) offer the promise of achieving this objective and increase the therapeutic index significantly.

The approach to targeted chemotherapy comes from Paul Ehrlich's concept of the "magic bullet" formulated at the beginning of the twentieth century [1]. The principle of this concept, to avoid side effects, drugs must be guided and released into the tumor sites through association with ligands that are overexpressed or selectively expressed in the tumor. Ehrlich's proposal has been translated into practical applications for therapy due to the development of monoclonal antibodies in the mid-70s, combining the selectivity of recognition to the power of chemotherapeutic drugs [2]. To become a pharmacologically active drug, monoclonal antibodies can be linked to either a radioisotope (giving rise to Antibody radioimmunoconjugates, RAC), to a highly potent cytotoxic drug (antibody-drug conjugates, ADCs) or protein toxins (producing immunotoxins) [3,4].

The production of ADCs face several vital issues, such as the target cell selection, the nature of antigen, structure and stability of the antibody, the linker chemistry, and finally the cytotoxic payload.

One of the first problems encountered in the use of antibodies was the fact that murine antibodies are foreign proteins recognized as non-self by the human immune system that responds by producing human anti-mouse antibodies (HAMA). HAMAs can have toxic effects due to immune-complex formation in the patient and, thus, prevent further administration. With the technology of recombinant DNA, Phage display, and transgenic mice, it is now possible to create of completely human antibodies that are not immunogenic and greatly ameliorate such toxicities.

Chemotherapeutic drugs include antimetabolites (methotrexate, 6-mercaptopurine, 5-fluorouracile, cytarabine, gemcitabine, etc.), molecules interfering with microtubule polymerization (vinca alkaloids, taxanes), and molecules inducing damages on DNA (anthracyclines, nitrogen mustards). The most recent generation of chemotherapeutic molecules include both DNA damaging/alkylating agents (i.e., duocarmycin from Medarex/Bristol Mayer Squibb, Syntarge, calicheamicin from Wyeth/Pfizer, indolino-benzodiazepine from Immunogen), and molecules interfering with microtubule structure (i.e., maytansinoids, from immunogen, auristatin derivatives from Seattle Genetics). These compounds can kill cells with extremely high potency so that severe side effects greatly limit the administrable dose as a free drug. These compounds are therefore considered as ideal payload components of ADCs with high therapeutic index [5].

The conjugation strategy and chemistry chosen to represent a key factor for the success of ADCs, the homogeneity of ADC molecules being one of the main challenges in ADC design [2]. In deciding in which chemical conjugation process to use, it is necessary to develop a strategy that allows the reaction of those residues placed on the surface of the antibody through a chemical reactive group present on the linker. These strategies, depending on the type of residue (mainly amino groups of lysines or sulfhydryl groups of cysteines) that can lead to the production of mixed species whose Drug-Antibody Ratio (DARs) is variable. When the DAR is poorly controlled, this phenomenon can reduce the efficacy of the ADCs and furthermore increase aggregation possibility, the overall rate of clearance and release of the payload systemically at an early stage [6], although higher DAR values are beneficial for the overall potency. To improve the technology, focusing on obtaining homogeneous ADCs with a high therapeutic index, site-specific conjugation technologies have now been developed [7].

2. Basic Characteristics of the Conjugate

An ADC is composed of three different components (Figure 1): a monoclonal antibody, the payload, and the linker that joins the first two components. Different types of conjugation chemistry exist: as in the most common, linkage is obtained through lysine (ε-amine-group, -NH$_2$ in the deprotonated form) or cysteine (sulfhydryl-group, -SH). However, other conjugation strategies may also be pursued (see below). Whatever the conjugation strategy, it is vital that this does not affect the integrity and functionality of the antibody.

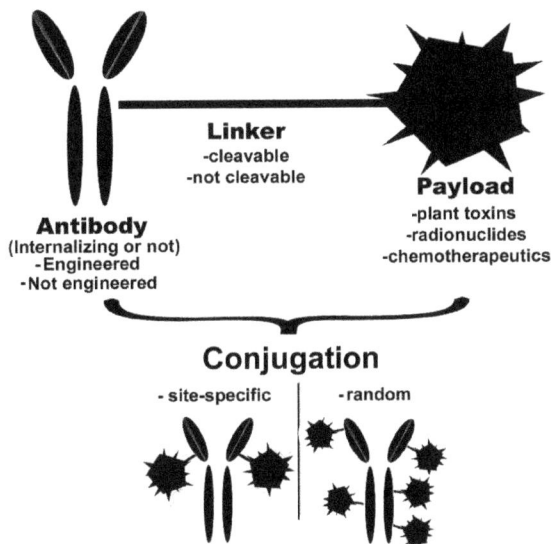

Figure 1. Schematic representation of various types of antibody-drug conjugates (ADCs) and their components.

2.1. Monoclonal Antibody

In the development of ADCs for cancer treatment, the choice of the antigen and, consequently, selection of the appropriate antibody plays a key role.

The antibody is chosen based on the molecular target recognition, with the highest affinity and selectivity for the target. Ideally, it should recognize an overexpressed target only at the tumor site to avoid delivering the pharmacological load inappropriately to non-target sites. For example, the (human epidermal growth factor receptor 2) (HER2) receptor is more than 100 times overexpressed in tumor tissues in comparison to the equivalent normal non-cancerous tissue [8].

The antigen against which the antibody is directed on the cancer cell should be present in high copy number ($>10^5$/cell.) [9]. So far, several antigens have been reported overexpressed in cancer tissues that can be exploited as targets for ADCs [10]. The antigen must be recognized and bound by the antibody with a reasonable affinty (Kd $\leq$ 10 nM) to ensure rapid uptake in the target cell [11].

In the first generation of ADCs, in many cases murine antibodies being recognized as foreign proteins generated a strong immune response with the production of anti-human antibodies that potentially reduced their therapeutic efficacy. This problem has been partially solved through the use of genetic engineering in second-generation ADCs, utilizing a mouse-human chimeric antibody format. The "humanized" chimeric antibody contains the mouse light and heavy chain variable regions that are linked to human constant regions. The chimeric ADCs showed promising results in cancer treatment but sometimes the problem of decreased efficiency and human anti-chimeric response were still present.

To overcome this problem, many efforts have been made to design a humanized monoclonal antibody, which contain only murine complementary determining regions (CDRs) regions combined with the human variable region [8] or fully human antibodies [12].

Usually, the antibodies used to construct ADCs are of the IgG1 class (Immunoglobulin G Subclass 1) (~150 kDa), but since antibodies in ADCs exploit the Fab region to recognize the antigen present at the end of light chains, only this region is essential to the antibody to carry out its function as a specific carrier. Therefore, in some cases, smaller antibody formats (i.e., antibody fragments that maintain the binding affinity for the receptor) have been used to create ADCs. These fragments can be obtained by IgG cleavage following papain digestion or recombinant production to produce Fabs and scFvs [13].

Selected antibodies and their derived ADCs can be directed against antigens that may or may not induce internalization through receptor-mediated endocytosis (RME), and by this criterion, ADCs can be classified as internalizing or non-internalizing.

2.1.1. Internalizing ADCs

Internalizing ADCs exploit RME to be internalized by target cells. In this case, the antibody performs a fundamental role as it favors the internalization of the target antigen receptor, which represents a crucial step for most ADCs to be effective. Although, as in the case of the anti-HER3 antibody EV20, the binding to the receptor and the internalization of receptor/antibody complex can alone induce cell death and inhibition of tumor growth [14–16].

Following internalization, the ADC can follow different endocytic routes that crucially may have profound effects on their cytotoxic efficacy. Clathrin-mediated and caveolae-mediated endocytosis (CME) in which the receptor mediates endocytosis and, alternatively, clathrin-caveolin-independent endocytosis, where the receptor does not mediate endocytosis [17]. The most common route to reach the cell cytoplasm, adopted by various ADCs, is CME, which is target antigen dependent. Molecules, such as epsin, dynamin, adaptor protein 2 (AP2), and phosphatidylinositol (4,5) bis-phosphate (PIP2) may increase accumulation of ADCs on the surface of cellular membrane [18] and assist the internalization of the ADC into the endo-lysosomal vesicle compartment.

Early endosomes form just below the membrane surface and usually endo-lysosomal vesicles containing ADCs progress to form late endosomes, whose lumens are acidic and may lead to the dissociation of antibodies from their receptors thus playing a vital role in recycling of antigen back to the membrane surface and subsequently lead to fusion of the late endosomal vesicle with lysosomes. The resulting pH decrease may also result in degradation of the ADC due to the numerous proteolytic enzymes present in the acidic lysosomal compartment with subsequent release of the drug payload. [19] (Figure 2).

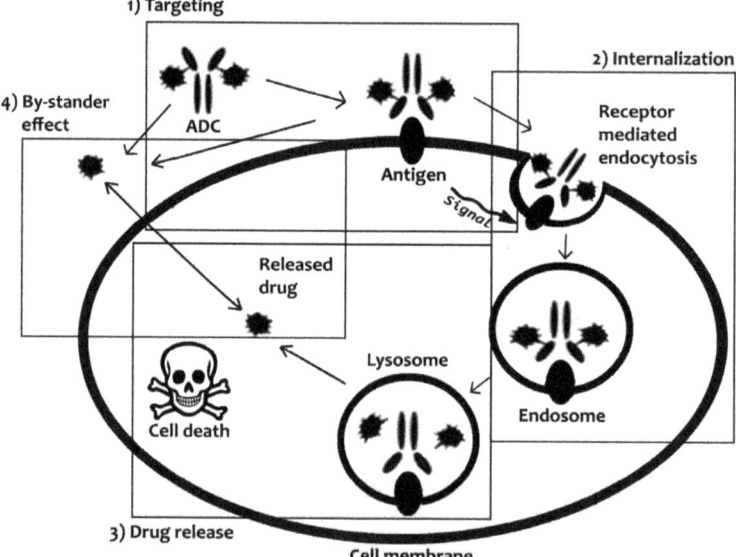

Figure 2. Schematic illustration of the mechanism of drug delivery and release mediated by ADCs.

Release of the drug within endolysosomal vesicles then results in the passive transport of drug payload into the cytosol where it can exert its pharmacological effect, killing the cancer cells via a molecule specific mechanism [20,21].

2.1.2. Non-Internalizing ADCs

The main pharmacological action of ADCs constructed with non-internalizing antibodies, relies on the cytotoxic payload exerting a bystander effect upon reaching the target tumor site. In this instance, once the ADC reaches the tumor site, proteolytic enzymes, or the reducing conditions in the tumor extracellular environment, act to liberate the drug payload, which facilitate the entry of drugs into the cells, by diffusion, pinocytosis, or other mechanisms. Once the released drugs start kill cancer cells, they release additional reducing agents or proteases, which in turn catalyze further release of drugs (Figure 2). This type of conjugates may also allow a by-stander effect on non-target cancer cells that are near the main target tumor mass, due to diffusion of the released drug into neighboring tumor cells of the drug [22].

It has been reported that an ADC directed against the alternatively spliced extracellular domain A of fibronectin induces a potent anticancer effect following the release of its payload after tumor cell death in the extracellular milieu. This allows the diffusion of the cytotoxic drug also into neighboring cells, and amplification of the process determined by a further release of reducing agents (e.g., cysteine, glutathione) [23].

2.2. Linkers

The linker component of the ADC, through which the covalent chemical bond between the drug and the antibody is created, should be chosen rationally, based on the mechanism of action of the antibody (whether internalizing or not) and limit potential chemical modifications to the drug in order to avoid loss of cytotoxicity. One of the main aims for the effective systemic delivery of an ADC is that the drug is released only at the target site; the linker, thus, must be stable enough in a biological environment (i.e., blood circulation) to avoid unwanted release of the pharmacological molecule.

There are two types of linkers available: cleavable and non-cleavable (Figure 3). The former can be used either in the design of either an internalizing or not internalizing ADC, because the release of the payload is required to take place in either the extracellular tumor environment, or within the lysosome or cytosol. This is possible because the extracellular environment of the tumor is highly reducing due to the presence of glutathione, which allows the release of payloads linked to the antibody via thiolic bonds. It also allows payload release via the degradation of peptide bonds in the presence of proteases such as Cathepsin B, whose overexpression in cancer drives its normal lysosomal localization towards extracellular secretion [24]. A cleavable linker, therefore, exploits differential conditions of reducing power or enzymatic degradation that can be present either outside or inside the target cell. Due to the chemical reactions needed to release the payload, the site of conjugation on the antibody is crucial to induce both stability in the plasma and availability to reduction or degradation on/into the target cell [25,26]. Non-cleavable linker-based ADC must, however, be internalizing, because to release their cytotoxic payload, the antibody component needs to be degraded by lysosomal or cytoplasmic proteases [27]. Furthermore, drugs linked to such linkers usually cannot exert a by-stander effect because upon degradation of the antibody by cellular proteases, they are released as fragments of antibody peptides that have a poor ability to permeate the cells. This type of non-cleavable linker has a higher efficiency for the treatment of tumors that express an antigen at high levels (to achieve a good clinical response and tumor regression, 99% of targeted cancer cells must be eliminated) or for hematological tumors [28,29].

A Disulfide linkers

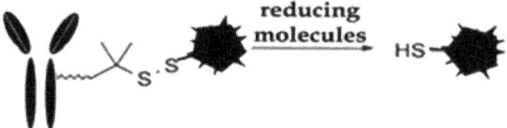

B Cathepsin B-responsive linker (Val-Cit)

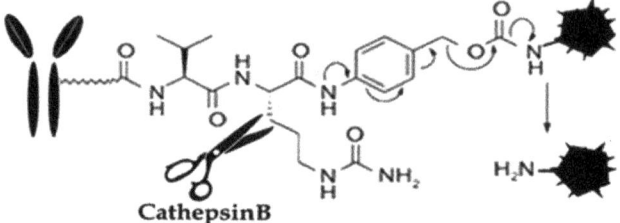

C Glycosidase-sensitive linker

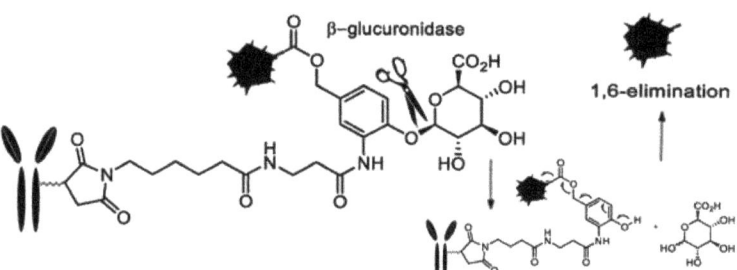

D Hydrazone linker

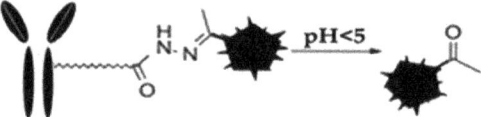

Figure 3. Available cleavable linkers in ADC (**A**) Disulfide linker, cleaved by reducing agents; (**B**) cathepsin B responsive linker, cleaved by Cathepsin B; (**C**) glycosidase-sensitive linker, cleaved by gluconidase; (**D**) hydrazone linker, cleaved by acidic environment.

2.2.1. Cleavable Linkers

Figure 3 above summarizes the most commonly used cleavable linkers that are described in detail in the sections that follow.

Disulfide Linkers

This type of linker is glutathione-sensitive. The disulfides are stable at physiological pH, in the systemic blood stream, but they are vulnerable to nucleophilic attack by thiols. Human serum albumin (HSA) represents the main thiol in plasma, being its concentration as high as >400 mM. Notwithstanding this high concentration, HSA fails to break the disulfide bond of ADC because its residue containing free thiol (Cys34) is found near a cleft in the molecule that is not significantly exposed to the solvent [30]. Conversely, disulfide-linked drugs resist reductive cleavage in the circulation because the glutathione (GSH) concentration in the blood (5 µmol/L) is lower than in the cytoplasm (1–10 mmol/L) allowing GSH thiol groups to be very effective in the cell cytoplasm also due to its well exposed position and its small size [31]. This difference in reductive potential between plasma and cytosol allows for the selective release of the intracellular payload of the ADCs. In addition, cancer cells cause oxidative stress that generates high GSH levels. Low glutathione levels in healthy tissues therefore discriminate release of the payload, also allowing the selective release of payload in close proximity to the tumor. ADCs with disulfide linkers are often associated with maytansinoid payloads, which were originally developed by Immunogen in 1992 [32]. To increase the stability of the bond, methyl groups may be added to surround disulfides in the linker structure [33], such as in the case of N-succinimidyl-4-(2-pyridyldithio)pentanoate (SPP) containing a single methyl, or N-succinimidyl-4-(2-pyridyldithio)butanoate (SPDB) containing two methyl groups.

Some ADC designs use a direct disulfide bond between the drug and the antibody. In this variety of ADC, the release of the drug is completely dependent on a strongly reducing tumor microenvironment [34]. Recently, ADCs with a direct disulfide bond between engineered cysteine residues and the thiols of maytansinoids payloads have been investigated [30]. By protecting disulfides reduction through antibody hindrance, these ADCs have good in vivo stability in mouse plasma. The results demonstrate that the DM3 payload is more stable than the DM1, given that only 10% of disulfide bonds are cleaved in plasma, a property that confers increased in vivo therapeutic activity in a murine model [35]. The structure of the whole antibody thus represents a protective environment significantly reducing the reductive release of the payload in the blood stream, but this in turn may limit the efficiency of release once at the tumor site. Other studies have shown that by creating an ADC using a small immunoprotein (SIP) antibody (small immunoprotein, comprised of an IgG, including variable regions from heavy and light chains linked through peptide plus additional C3 or C4 heavy chain proteins; see also below) and comparing the results with an analogous ADC constructed with intact IgG, the release of the drug by the ADC-SIP occurs faster. This is probably due to a more stable interchain disulfide bond in the SIP. However, by analyzing the stability of ADCs in mouse plasma, a half-life greater than 48 h with IgG and less than 3 h with SIP was determined. An analysis of the in vivo efficacy of the above compounds showed that the ADC-SIP experienced an accumulation and therefore a greater release than the IgG-ADC, despite there being a global accumulation of ADC-IgG after 24 h that was greater in the tumor than that observed for the ADC-SIP [23].

Cathepsin B-Sensitive Linker

The cysteine protease Cathepsin B is normally found inside late endosomes and lysosomal compartments in mammals. It is also implicated in tumor progression, being overexpressed by many cancers [36]. The carboxydipeptidase activity of Cathepsin B allows the splitting of a dipeptide linker that can bind a payload to the terminal C. This enzyme has various substrate target peptide sequences with Phe-Arg being the most common [36]. In addition, it also preferentially recognizes sequences such as valine-citrulline (Val-Cit) and phenylalanine-lysine (Phe-Lys) where the protease breaks a peptide bond on the C-terminal side of Val-Cit, Val-Ala, or Phe-Lys. Some studies have shown that a high pH basic environment increases the cleavage capacity [3] and that the hydrophobic residues Phe, Val, and Ala allow cleavage with cathepsin B that has the effect of increasing the stability in plasma. Sometimes, however, the payload can be too bulky in which case the use of a spacer that is stable and that does not alter the drugs chemistry, and functionality is necessary. One of the most used conjugation reagents is para-aminobenzyl carbamate (PABC) (Figure 4), that possesses a self-cleavage ability allowing it to release the unmodified payload [35]. For example, linkers containing Phe-Lys-PABC and Val-Cit-PABC, used for ADC with monomethyl-auristatin E (MMAE) payload, have a half-life in plasma for Phe-Lys-PABC of 12 h compared to 80 h for Val-Cit-PABC 80 h. This shorter half-life indicates that the linker with Phe-Lys-PABC is probably non-specific with the danger that it may exert off-target toxicity [37].

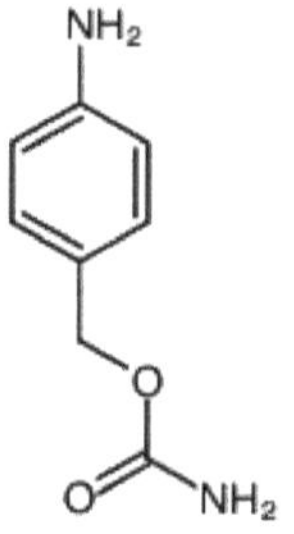

Figure 4. PABC, p-aminobenzyl carbamate, CAS#:918132-66-8.

To summarize, it has been shown that if these types of linker are coupled with paminobenzyloxycarbonyl (PABC) they work more efficiently as cleavable linkers (i.e., Val-Ala-PABC) for ADCs [38]. The PABC group acts as a spacer separating the toxic payload from Val-Cit sequence so that the active site of cathepsin B can gain better access to the cleavage sequence, thus, more effectively exploiting its protease activity, particularly if a large molecular sized payload is used. PABC is furthermore a self-immolate linker that, upon Cathepsin B cleavage, can undergo hydrolysis releasing the free drug to which it is attached (i.e., monomethyl-auristatin E (MMAE)) [39,40].

Hydrazone Linker

Hydrazone linkers or other similar molecules that are pH-dependent, have quite a stable structure at neutral pH (i.e., in the bloodstream at pH 7.4) and are hydrolyzed when they reach an acidic cellular compartment such as the lysosome (pH < 5) or late endosomes (pH 5.5–6.2). However, the degradation of this linker is not confined to the lysosome, but may, on occasion, also occur extracellularly. ADCs with a hydrazone linker hydrolyze only slowly under physiological conditions, with the slow release of the toxic payload [41]. A study with an antibody directed against mucin, conjugated via an acid-labile linker, showed good therapeutic effects in a preclinical pancreatic cancer model [42] where the tumor microenvironment is significantly more acidic than in normal tissues, due to the enhanced glycolysis taking place in the tumor with the consequent production of lactate to a level sufficient to induce extracellular cleavage of the linker. In mouse models, the slow release of the circulatory payload has produced promising results, but only in the presence of payloads with moderate cytotoxic activity. Payloads with higher cytotoxic activity, now widely used for the production of ADCs, demand the use linkers with higher stability to avoid the undesired release of the payload and resultant non-specific systemic toxicity [37].

Glycosidase-Sensitive Linkers

Glycosidases comprise hydrolytic lysosomal enzymes, such as β-glucuronidases that degrade β-glucuronic acid residues into polysaccharides. They are found in lysosomes and work under hydrophilic environments. β-glucuronidases, like cathepsin B, are also secreted in the necrotic areas of some tumors. They are also enzymatically active in the extracellular environment [43]. ADCs that contain β-glucuronic acid can reach a DAR = 8 without causing aggregation and without reducing the hydrophobicity of the ADC. Indeed, this type of linker greatly reduce plasma clearance of ADCs, thus increasing their efficacy in vivo [44]. It is also established that the use of Poly (Ethylene Glycol) PEG linkers increases the hydrophilicity of β-glucuronic acid and, thereby, increases the activity and efficiency of the ADC [30].

Another type of hydrolytic lysosomal enzyme, the β-galactosidases that degrade β-galactoside, are also overexpressed in some types of cancer [45]. An ADC based on trastuzumab linked to MMAE using a β-galactoside linker was shown to be more potent than an equivalent ADC based on a Val-Cit-PABC linker. This formulation of ADC-β-galactoside-DM1 has also been shown to be more efficient in vivo for the treatment of HER2+ breast tumors than the approved trastuzumab emtansine (T-DM1) [35].

2.2.2. Non-Cleavable Linkers

The most used non-cleavable linkers are alkylic and polymeric. For example, the MCC amine-to-sulfhydryl bifunctional cross-linker contains a cyclohexane ring structure that through steric hindrance protects the resulting thioether bond from hydrolysis [46]. The greatest advantage of non-cleavable versus cleavable linkers is their improved plasma stability; that results in reduced off-target toxicity in comparison to conjugates with cleavable linkers and thus provides greater stability and tolerability [47,48]. It is noteworthy that non-cleavable ADCs often have less activity against tumors due to the heterogeneity of target antigen expression where a bystander effect is an important contributor to therapeutic efficacy [49]. As described earlier, non-cleavable linkers require mAb degradation within the lysosome after ADC internalization to release the drug to the site of pharmacological activity in the cytosol. If the payload is linked to a charged amino acid such as lysine) with a Pi < 9.5, this will prevent escape of the drug by diffusion through the cell membrane and result in higher levels of drug-accumulation in the tumor cell which as a consequence should overcome the limitations of any bystander effect. In summary the major advantage of non-cleavable linkers is that they minimize drug release into the circulation thus limiting non-specific toxicity whilst maintaining, good in vivo stability [50].

Usually, non-cleavable linkers contain a thioether or maleimidocaproyl group. Examples of non-cleavable linker-based ADCs containing monomethyl auristatin F (MMAF), an anti-mitotic drug, where it was demonstrated that the drug is more potent if linked via a simple alkyl chain to the antibody. Conjugation effected with a non-reducible thioether linker demonstrated very good activity in both *in vitro* and in vivo [51].

2.3. Payloads

Currently, most ADCs are constructed with two main families of highly toxic compounds, acting either on microtubule or DNA structure. Among the first group, auristatins and maytansines payloads both act as tubulin inhibitors and have been widely used for construction of ADCs. Both molecules are potently cytotoxic against rapidly dividing cancer cells and have reduced toxicity to normal cells. Alternatively, calicheamicins and PBDs are DNA-damaging agents, inducing cell death by apoptotic mechanisms in all cells including cancer stem cells (CSCs), and for this reason, they do exert severe side effects. There is also a third category of drug that targets specific enzymes essential for cell survival. In general, the payloads suitable for an ADC must have: (a) good solubility in aqueous solutions allowing an easier conjugation to the antibody and ensuring enough solubility to ADC under physiological conditions; (b) a significantly higher cytotoxic activity (half maximal inhibitory concentration (IC_{50}) ranging from 0.01 to 0.1 nM) in comparison to clinically standard chemotherapeutic agents; (c) induce cancer cell death by apoptotic mechanisms; and (d) possess an appropriate functional group to facilitate conjugation to the antibody.

The most widely used commercialized drugs for ADC formulation comprise microtubule-targeting agents. The choice of tubulin inhibitors as payloads is appropriate since rapid cellular proliferation is one of the major discriminating features between cancerous and normal cells and antimitotic agents are in principle less toxic to the normal cells [52]. Vinca alkaloid, laulimalide, taxane, maytansine, and colchicine have all defined binding sites on microtubules. These molecules (Figure 5) can be grouped in two main categories depending on their mechanism of action: tubulin polymerization promoters (microtubule stabilizers) and tubulin polymerization inhibitors (microtubule destabilizers) [53]. In particular, microtubule stabilizers inhibit the formation of microtubules acting on the β-subunit of α-β tubulin dimers determining unregulated microtubule growth, as in case of Auristatin. In contrast, the mechanism of action of microtubule destabilizers is to block the polymerization of tubulin dimers by inhibiting the formation of mature microtubules, as is the case for maytansinoids (Figure 6).

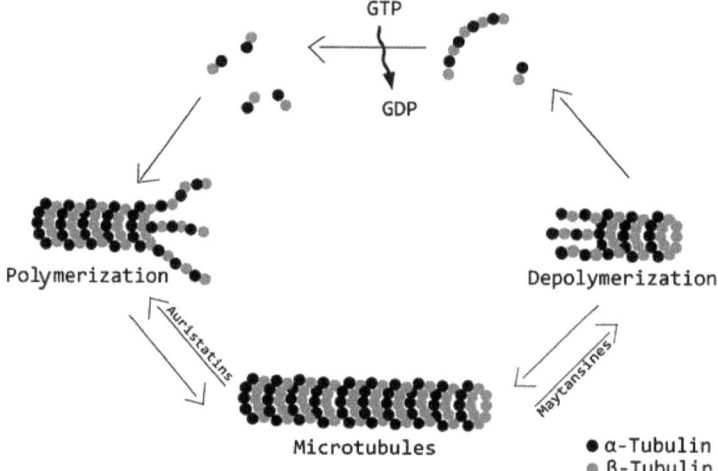

Figure 5. Mechanism of action of tubulin inhibitors payloads: polymerization promoters (microtubule stabilizers) and tubulin polymerization inhibitors (microtubule destabilizers). In the figure are two exemplifying drugs acting on microtubule formation: auristatins alters the formation of microtubules by binding on the β-subunit of α-β tubulin dimers; thus, producing uncontrolled growth of microtubules. Maytansines, on the contrary, stop tubulin dimers formation impairing the production of mature microtubules.

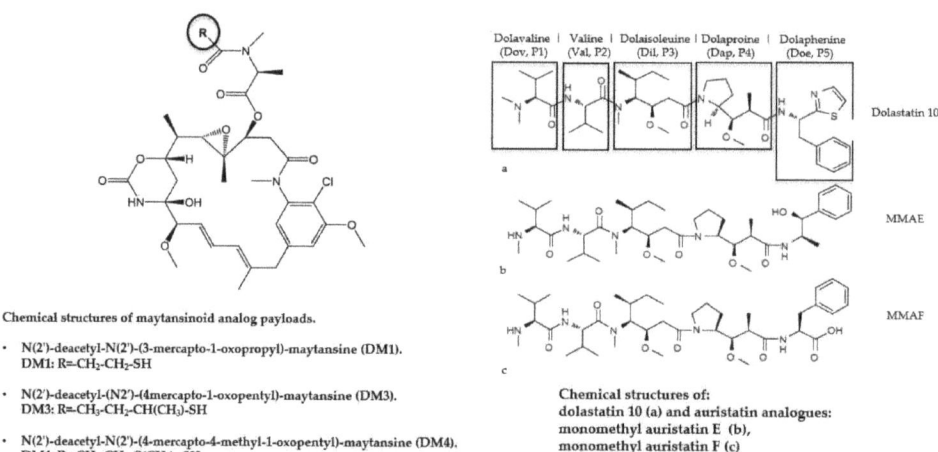

Figure 6. Classical microtubule-targeting agents: maytansinoids (**left**) and auristatin families (**right**).

Auristatin is a dolastatin synthetic analog. The original drug was isolated from *Dolabella auricularia* (sea hare) as dolastatin peptides, which successfully improved its water solubility to give auristatin [54]. Auristatins block tubulin assembly and induce cell cycle arrest in G2/M phase, causing cells to undergo apoptosis.

To prevent lysosomal payload degradation and to enhance drug efficacy two innovative auristatin derivatives (monomethyl auristatin E (MMAE) and monomethyl auristatin F (MMAF)) have been developed by Seattle Genetics. These two compounds are synthetic drugs derived by design from structure-activity relationship (SAR) analysis. These two new molecules are different due to a phenylalanine present at the C-terminus of MMAF that allows this latter compound to be more membrane impermeable. In contrast, MMAE can exit the cell and thus diffuse to nearby cells killing them through bystander effects [53].

Maytansinoids are derivatives of natural cytotoxic agents named maytansines, a family of toxins originally isolated from the cortex of *Maytenus serrata* possessing macrolide structure. Maytansine and maytansinoids alter microtubule polymerization thus inhibit the maturation of microtubules by binding to or in close proximity to the vinblastine-binding site on the β-subunit of tubulin. This consequently induces cell death through mitotic arrest [54].

ADCs that containing maytansinoid, are unfortunately substrates for multidrug resistance protein 1 (MDR1), a critical protein of the cell membrane that acts by actively pumping a wide variety of xenobiotics out of cells. To prevent this problem a series of hydrophilic linkers have been used in ADC chemistry. These linkers allow for an increased drug content (DAR) in ADCs s and subsequent increases in the amount of drug delivered to each target cell. The increased polarity introduced by such linkers allows the formation of maytansinoid metabolites that are poor substrates for efflux pumps thus overcoming MDR [55].

Maytansines are difficult to conjugate because they do not have reactive chemical groups. To overcome this problem, a series of derivatives containing SH groups have been created examples of which are, DM1 and DM4 that are substituted by methyl disulfide at the maytansine C3 N-acyl-N-methyl-L-alanyl ester side chain [56].

A third type of antimitotic payload includes tubulysins characterized by higher affinity of binding to the vinca domain of tubulin if compared with vinblastine. These agents exert a rapid disruption of the cytoskeleton and subsequent disassembly of the mitotic apparatus in proliferating cancer cells. This results in a block at G2/M of the cell cycle and subsequent apoptotic cell death [57] (Figure 7).

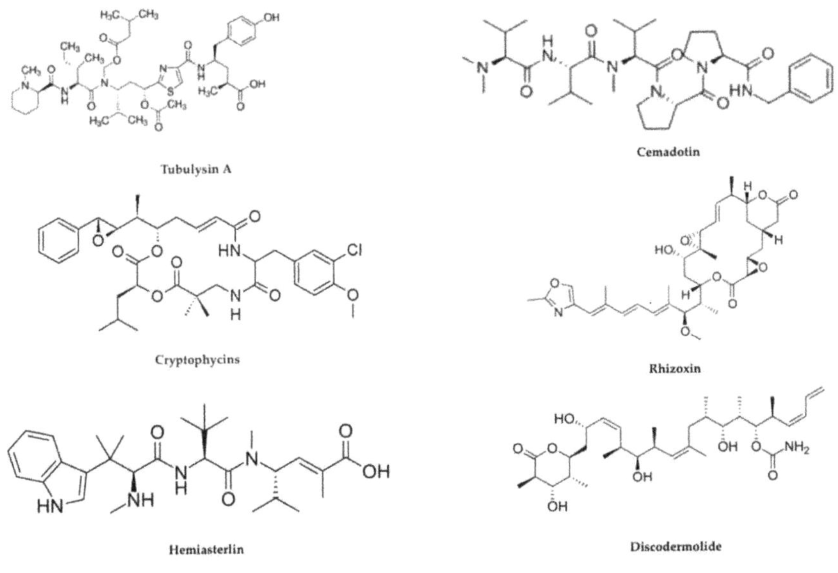

Figure 7. Other microtubule-targeting agents.

Tubulysins possess high degree of selective cytotoxicity against human cancer cells due to their rapid rate of division. Furthermore, they may also be effective against cancer cells overexpressing the P-glycoprotein or which possess mutations in tubulin gene. Tubulysins are comprised of a family with 14 different isoforms characterized by conserved core structure made of an L-isoleucine (Ile), a tubuvaline (Tuv), and an N-methylD-pipecolic acid (Mep) unit.

The first targeted drug (EC0305) based on tubulysin has been recently obtained by linking Tubulysin B to folic acid conjugate. Now several tubulysin D-based ADCs are under study [53].

To complete the family of drugs that bind to microtubules the following compounds are also worth mentioning:

Cryptophycins, a class of cytotoxins more potent than MMAE and DM1, isolated from *Nostoc cyanobacteria* induce tubulin depolymerization binding to microtubules. Cryptophycin-1 is the main component, acting on many solid tumors and additionally MDR cancer cells.

Hemiasterlin from marine sponges are naturally occurring tripeptides acting as potent inhibitors of cell growth. They bind to the tubulin vinca-site thus disrupting normal microtubule dynamics and consequently inhibiting tubulin polymerization. Taltobulin (HTI-286) is a fully synthetic analog of hemiasterlin and has been shown to be to be active against a variety of MDR cancer cell lines [53].

Cemadotin (LU103793) is a more hydrophilic synthetic pentapeptide analogous of dolastatin 15, possessing strong antiproliferative activity through inhibition of microtubule assembly and tubulin polymerization by binding at a novel site on tubulin. Cemadotin has been shown to be an effective payload for ADC construction [53].

Rhizoxin, a compound isolated from Rhizopus microspores (a fungus able to be infectious for humans causing mycosis) that binds to tubulin and causes inhibition of microtubule assembly [58].

Discodermolide is so far the most efficient natural promoter of tubulin assembly considered to be a very promising candidate for future ADC development [53].

There are furthermore other tubulin inhibitors that have been investigated for their possible use in ADC construction, such as taccalonolide A or B, taccalonolide AF or AJ, colchicine, epothilone A and B, taccalonolide AI-epoxide, CA-4, laulimalide, paclitaxel, and docetaxel, together with their synthetic analogous [53,59].

The second category of payload used for ADC construction is comprised of DNA-damaging drugs. This class of payload may be more effective than microtubule inhibitors with IC_{50} values in the picomolar, as opposed to the nanomolar range for microtubule inhibitors. This would make ADCs constructed with DNA damaging drug payloads more potent and therefore better suited for targeting antigens that are expressed at low levels on tumors. Furthermore, DNA-damaging drugs are fully capable of apoptotically killing non-dividing cells including cancer stem cells when used in combination with drugs that inhibit DNA repair and furthermore are capable of killing target cells at any point in the cell cycle [60].

There are at least four mechanisms of action exerted by DNA-damaging agents, which are as follows: (a) DNA double-strand breakage, (b) DNA alkylation, (c) DNA intercalation, and (d) DNA cross-linking. The most used DNA-damaging payloads are pyrrolobenzodiazepine, duocarmycins, doxorubicin, and calicheamicins [61] (Figure 8).

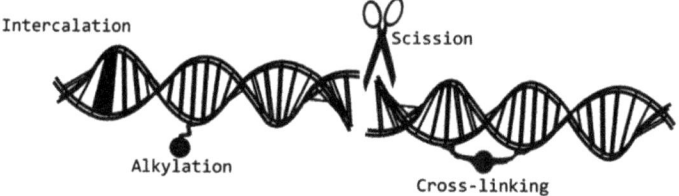

Figure 8. The four main mechanisms of action of DNA-damaging agents: DNA double-strand breakers, DNA alkylators, DNA intercalators, and DNA cross-linkers. DNA-damaging agents. These drugs can act at any phase of tumor cell life cycle.

Pyrrolobenzodiazepines (PBDs) were originally isolated from *Streptomyces* sp. and are natural products, possessing antibiotic and antitumor properties. PBD molecules bind in the minor groove of double- stranded DNAs to the C2-amino groups of guanine residues.

PBDs forms an adduct PBD/DNA in the minor groove of DNA, leading to decreased DNA repair and interfering with transcription factors binding to DNA, as well as to some enzyme functions including RNA polymerase and endonucleases.

Currently, additional to natural isolated monomeric forms of PBDs, synthetic PBD dimers are available, which in addition to forming monoadducts are also capable of forming intrastrand or interstrand DNA cross-links [62] (Figure 9).

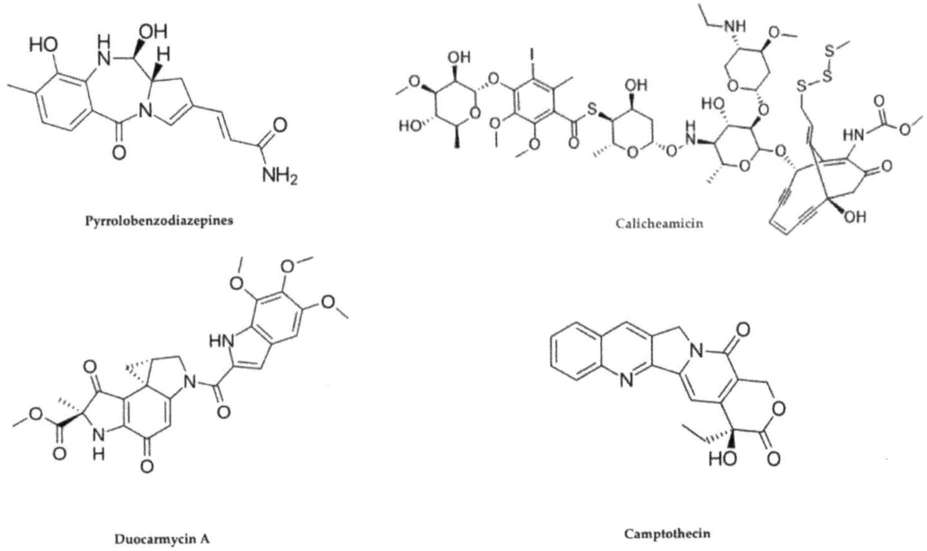

Figure 9. Examples of DNA-damaging drug payloads.

Duocarmycins, metabolites originally isolated from *Streptomyces* sp. are powerful cytotoxic substances because their mechanism of action involves alkylation of the DNA minor groove to form a stable adduct. Duocarmycins specifically bind to a sequence of five-base-pair rich in AT-rich where the central pyrroloindole may be easily accommodated. This results in irreversible DNA modification compromising its architecture that finally leads to DNA cleavage and apoptotic cell death. There are also synthetic analogs of duocarmycins available, such as adozelesin, bizelesin, and carzelesin.

Duocarmycins have impressively high cell cycle-independent cytotoxicity against a variety of proliferating cancer cells *in vitro* with IC_{50} values in the pM range [63].

The duocarmycin analogous DUBA (duocarmycin-hydroxybenzamide-azaindole), representing the duocarmycin final active drug metabolite, has been used to produce different new-generation ADCs that have been tested *in vitro* and in vivo to verify their therapeutic efficacy. An example is represented by SYD983, an anti-HER2 ADC, exerting clear anti-tumor activity in a mouse xenograft model (BT-474) and showing enough stability in human and macaque primate plasma [64].

The high toxicity of duocarmycins and their analogous makes them desirable candidates to maximize ADC cell-killing activity and also suggests that they may be effective agents to overcome multi drug resistant (MDR) tumor cells [65].

Calicheamicins (LL-E33288) are a class of antibiotics that were discovered in Texas following a search for novel fermentation-derived antitumor antibiotics that led to *Micromonospora echinospora*. These compounds are a class of enediyne-containing DNA-cleaving antitumor agent with a potency 4000–10,000 times greater than DNA intercalating drugs, such as Adriamycin and other similar.

The mechanism of action of calicheamicins after cell entry and nuclear diffusion is due to drug targeting and binding to the minor groove of DNA, causing double-strand breaks that induce apoptotic cell death [66].

Calicheamicins are extremely powerful drugs acting at sub-pM concentrations but also unfortunately exert significant non-specific toxicity, damaging the DNA of all cells. Their high toxicity means that they cannot be used directly as a single therapeutic agent in cancer treatment. Their inherent characteristics (i.e., high cytotoxicity, relatively small molecular size, mechanism of action) have however made calicheamicins useful payloads for the construction of ADCs [54].

Camptothecin (CPT) is a natural compound isolated from *Camptotheca acuminata* and is an inhibitor of the nuclear enzyme topoisomerase I. CPT molecules inhibit both DNA and RNA synthesis in mammalian cells, and have demonstrated to be strongly cytotoxic against a wide range of experimental tumors. Unfortunately, several clinical trials have shown considerable toxicity problems in patients due to their low solubility and resultant adverse side effects. To circumvent these limitations, camptothecin analogs topotecan (TPT) and irinotecan (camptothecin-11, CPT-11) that show improved water solubility have been approved by the FDA. These molecules were tested in clinical practice, and demonstrated significant antitumor activity and reduced toxicity [67].

SN-38 and DX-8951f are two additional CPT-analogs that have been used as ADC payloads. SN-38, an active CPT-11 metabolite that exploits inhibition of DNA topoisomerase to exert its anticancer activity [68].

In addition to all of the above-mentioned payloads, other molecules available also act as DNA-damaging agents for incorporation into newly emerging ADCs. Among these compounds, particular mention should be given to iSGD-1882 (DNA minor groove cross-linker derived from PBD dimers), centanamycin (binds to DNA and alkylates or intercalates into DNA), PNU-159682 (an anthracycline metabolite) [69], and uncialamycin (an enediyne natural product isolated from Streptomyces uncialis) [70], all active on different cancer cell lines, and finally indolinobenzodiazepine dimers (IGNs) bind to the DNA minor groove leading to DNA cross-linking [71].

Alternative Payloads

In addition to all the payloads discussed above, other molecules are available whose cytotoxicity is based on different mechanisms of action that include the direct induction of apoptosis, spliceosome, and RNA polymerase inhibition.

Bcl-2 family members, including Bcl-xL, are overexpressed in cancer and the BH3- binding domain on Bcl-xL has been targeted. Examples of such targeting agents comprise two anti-EGFR-Bcl-xL ADCs both of which possessed reasonable anti-tumor activity [72].

The spliceosome is an attractive target in cancer therapy, and thailanstatins have been shown to inhibit RNA splicing by the binding to different spliceosome subunits [61]. Thailanstatin A in fact was demonstrated to bind to the SF3b subunit of the spliceosome blocking RNA splicing and was used in the generation of an ADC (anti-Her2-thailanstatin). The Spliceostatins are potent spliceosome inhibitors of natural origin with interesting and potentially useful anticancer activities [61].

The final class of promising payloads are the transcription inhibitors targeting RNA polymerase II. Example of these compounds are the amatoxins, macrocyclic peptides produced by mushrooms of the genus Amanita, that are powerful and selective inhibitors of RNA polymerase II, thus resulting in the inhibition of protein synthesis [73].

β-amanitin has been covalently coupled to a MUC1-targeting mAb and this ADC has proven to be specifically cytotoxic against the human breast carcinoma cell lineT47D [74].

α-amanitin was efficiently targeted to cancer cells through an anti-HER2 mAb, with an IC_{50} value in the pM range. Moreover, α-amanitin has also been covalently linked to an EpCAM-targeting mAb, showing effective antiproliferative activity both *in vitro* and in vivo. An anti-PSMA-α-amanitin ADC has been recently observed to have in vivo antitumor activity when coupled using a stable and cleavable linker [56].

Amatoxins are highly water soluble, a property that facilitates the conjugation process and reduces ADC aggregation. Their low molecular weight, after release, allows for rapid kidney excretion in the urine. Amatoxins are also highly active against MDR cancer cells because they represent poor substrates for MDR mechanistic processes [71].

It should also be mentioned that payloads for conjugation to antibody can also include proteinaceous enzymes from plants (e.g., saporin, ricin A chain) [4,20] or bacterial toxins (PE, Pseudomonas exotoxin, DT, Diphtheria toxin) which induce cell death by irreversibly inhibiting protein synthesis catalytically [75,76]. Although this latter class of toxin molecule when conjugated to an antibody is commonly known as an immunotoxin, it is not considered a small molecule drug. The enzymatic nature of proteinaceous toxins as a payload represents added value since a single molecule may be sufficient to fatally intoxicate an individual cell. A variety of different linkers and payloads has been investigated over the years and because these are totally protein constructs, fully recombinant toxins are possible making this a promising production strategy [4].

The Figure 10 below summarizes all the payload categories discussed above in Section 2.3.

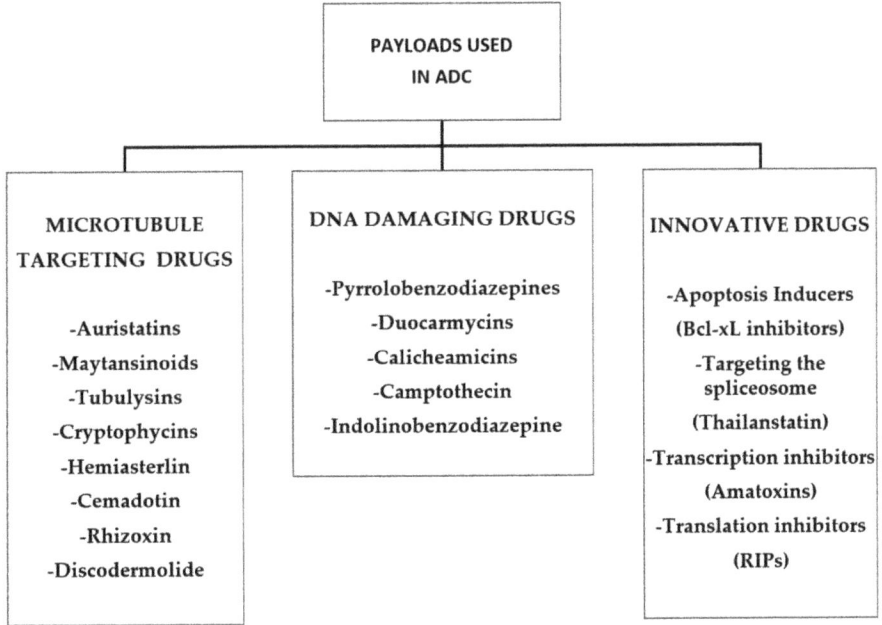

Figure 10. Summary diagram of the different classes of cytotoxic molecules used in ADC construction.

3. Conjugation Strategies

Most ADCs exploit the presence of lysine and cysteine residues within the polypeptide structure of the antibody as the point of conjugation. The average IgG_1 molecule for example, possesses approximately 90 lysine residues, but only 30 of these are accessible for conjugation, so theoretically the number of covalently coupled payloads could range from 1 to 30. Amide or amidine bond formation on the side chain of lysine is the most common reaction to effect covalent cross-linking of the antibody to the payload through exploitation of the reactive groups of linkers (i.e., *N*-hydroxysuccinimide esters, NHS; imidoesters) [77]. Figure 11 shows the main reactions used in the cross-linking procedures.

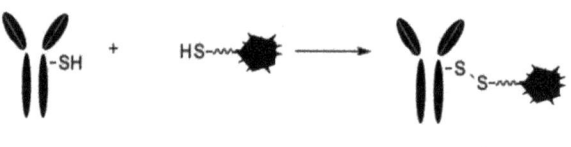

Figure 11. Main reactions used in the cross-linking procedures. (**A**) Lysine amide coupling, (**B**) Maleimide Alkylation, and (**C**) thiol-reactive conjugation.

The lysine-amide coupling conjugation is not site-specific and requires a pre-conjugation derivatization of the antibody and/or the payload in order for conjugation to proceed, very often using thiolic or citrulline-valine as linkers [77]. Alternatively, conjugation via cysteines requires that a partial reduction of the antibody is undertaken or a thiol-containing reagent (e.g., Trout's reagent) is used to introduce additional-SH groups available for the conjugation. This may cause destabilization of the whole IgG molecule and introduce structural heterogeneity into the final product. IgG$_1$ has four disulfide bridges, two that link the heavy to the light chains, and two in the hinge region, which bond together the two half-heavy chains of the whole antibody [78]. As one of the fundamental points of conjugation chemistry is the precise control of the drug Antibody Ratio (DAR), a recently used strategy is to achieve site-specific coupling of the payload by engineering the structure of the antibody. For example, the substitution of three cysteines in the hinge region with three serines yields an IgG molecule that fully retains its interactions between heavy and light chains [79]. Thus, through such modification of the cysteine residues, this leaves only two reactive cysteines, one on each chain, to yield an ADC product containing up to two molecules of drug per antibody. By refining the conjugation conditions, it is possible to obtain an extremely homogeneous product with the presence of the only conjugate with exactly two molecules of drug per antibody molecule (DAR 2) [23,34,79].

4. Site-Specific Enzymatic Conjugation

It is possible to use enzymatic methods to perform a site-specific controlled conjugation. This requires enzymes that react with the antibody and can induce a site- or amino acid sequence-specific modification. The most used enzymes are: sortase, transglutaminase, galactosyltransferase, and syaliltransferase. Sortase A from *Staphylococcus aureus* binds the LPXTG sequence and breaks the bond between glycine and threonine linking an oligoglycine (oligo-G) that can be used to bind the desired payload. A transglutaminase derived from *Streptomyces mobaraensis* catalyzes transpeptidation and recognizes an LLQG motif that has been inserted into a genetically engineered antibody, giving rise to a convenient site-specific ADC conjugation site. An application of a transglutaminase conjugation method gave rise to improvements in DAR for ADCs constructed with a branched linker that allowed for the loading of multiple payload molecules. Anami and coworkers developed an innovative conjugation method utilizing a branched linker on an anti-HER2 monoclonal antibody with MTGase, without a reduction in antibody binding affinity leading to the production of a homogeneous ADC molecular population with a remarkable increased DAR (up to 8) using monomethyl auristatin F as the payload [80].

The linkers used contain a lysine scaffold to generate a branch point and PEG spacers to increase ADC mobility. For MTGase-mediated antibody-linker conjugation, the presence of a primary amine is necessary as well as the presence of two reactive azide groups to link with the payloads [46]. Using MTGase this azide-linker can be bound to the glutamine residue Q295 in the IgG heavy chain. To generate an ADCs with DAR 2 the chosen payloads can be bound through azide-alkyne cyclization using a linear or branched linker to generate a DAR 4 ADC. This improved ADC showed increased *in vitro* cytotoxicity against HER2-expressing breast cancer cell lines compared to ADCs produced by more traditional methods [46].

An *N*-Glycan engineering strategy takes advantage of conserved Asn297 (N297) within the Fc domain in all IgG classes. In order to create a reactive aldehyde group on the *N*-glycan terminus it is possible to employ either β-1,4-galactosyltransferase (GalT) or α-2,6-sialyltransferase (SialT) enzymes to achieve this. The aldehyde groups enzymatically created are then used to conjugate amino-oxy-functionalized payloads [80]. Recently Bruins and coworkers used a mushroom tyrosinase to oxidize the exposed tyrosine residues on antibody to generate a 1,2-quinone, which can then be subjected to a nucleophilic reaction with thiols or amines from the side chains of amino acids such as cysteine, lysine, histidine, or any thus modified payload [81]. A further new recent strategy to improve ADC stability is site-specific conjugations using antibody engineered to incorporate non-natural amino acids (nnAA). The introduction of nnAA with orthogonal reactive functional groups (aldehyde, ketone, azido, or alkynyl tag) increases the homogeneity of ADCs and enables novel bioorthogonal chemistry that utilizes reactive groups that are different from the classical thiol or amine reactions. The most used nnAA or strategies are: seleno-cysteine, p-azidomethyl-L-phenylalanine (pAMF) p-acetyl phenylalanine (p-AcPhe), FGE (formylglycine generating enzyme) azide or alkynyl nnAA or glycan. To improve ADC stability, Transtuzumab was engineered to introduce p-AcPhe that could react through the carbonyl group (ketone) with a drug containing an alkoxy-amine to produce an oxime [82]. To achieve this, engineered new cell lines or cell free protein expression systems (OCFS: Open Cell Free Synthesis) were generated that possess the transcriptional machinery capable of inserting the a nnAA exactly where desired. In this system, the most important element needed for nnAA incorporation is a aminoacyl tRNA synthetase (aaRS) that charges a specific tRNA with the nnAA [83,84].

5. Approved ADCs and Future Perspectives

The ADC gemtuzumab ozogamicin, also known with the commercial name of Mylotarg® produced by Pfizer Inc., was the first ADC approved twenty years ago by the U.S. Food and Drug Administration (FDA). Mylotarg® was used to target the CD33 (Cluster of differentiation 33, sialic acid binding Ig-like lectin 3 (Siglec3)).

myeloid associated leukocyte differentiation antigen expressed by myeloid leukemia cells (CD33$^+$ AML). Currently, Mylotarg® is indicated for the treatment of patients diagnosed since at least two years with recurrent or refractory CD33$^+$ AML [85].

The Mylotarg® ADC was produced using a random conjugation technique with an amide bond interposed between the cleavable linker, hydrazone acetyl butyrate with the antibody attached to the calicheamicin payload via a lysine sidechain on the antibody [86]. The history of its approval has been complicated due to unexpected toxicities, in particular veno occlusive disease (VOD) in the liver in a significant proportion of patients. Myelotarg was initially approved by the FDA in the USA in 2000 but then voluntarily withdrawn from the market in 2011 following toxicity-related deaths and a lack of good clinical evidence showing its therapeutic benefits. Subsequently however, lower dose studies have demonstrated its safety and have clearly shown it to be of clinical benefit in a subset of AML patients [87].

In 2017, Myelotarg was once again approved by the FDA [88] and immediately following this approval another calicheamicin-based ADC using the same linker technology (linker-antibody bond and cytotoxin, bystander effect) inotuzumab ozogamicin (also known as Besponsa®) directed against the B-cell restricted differentiation antigen CD22 [89]. Besponsa®, was approved for use in the EU for the treatment of acute lymphoblastic leukemia currently under orphan drug status [90,91].

The second US, EU, and Japan approved ADC was brentuximab vedotin (Seattle Genetics, Inc. and Takeda Pharmaceutical Company Ltd.). The commercial name for this ADC is ADCETRIS® (Seattle Genetics Inc., n.d.) and is indicated for the treatment of Hodgkin's lymphoma targeting the Reed-Sternberg cell-associated antigen, CD30. This ADC was constructed using a protease-cleavable mc-VC-PABC linker and Monomethyl auristatin E (MMAE) as the cytotoxic drug payload [92]. The chemistry of linking method to provide a bystander effect is achieved through a dithiol bond via to a cysteine residue on the antibody. Adcetris® (brentuximab vedotin) has been approved by FDA in 2011 [93].

The final and most recent approved ADC at the time of writing is trastuzumab-emtansine (Roche Registration GmbH) sold under the commercial name Kadcyla®. The Trastuzumab (commercial name Herceptin) is a monoclonal antibody used as a naked antibody to treat HER2$^+$ breast cancer by targeting the antigen HER-2 (Human Epidermal growth factor Receptor) and triggering host-mediated antibody dependent cellular cytotoxicity (ADCC) while simultaneously downregulating EGFR-mediated growth signaling thereby inhibiting tumor growth [94]. The ADC Kadcyla® uses a maytansinoid derivative as the anti-neoplastic drug payload (DM-1) and a non-cleavable SMCC (amide antibody-linker) as linker. This ADC shows reduced bystander effect, strongest activity compared to Herceptin in certain conditions [86] and has been approved in the US, EU and Japan since 2013 [95–97].

Over the past two years, the FDA approved two new ADCs: Polivy® (Polatuzumab vedotin) and Lumoxiti® (Moxetumomab pasudotox). The Polivy® is a humanized monoclonal antibody, directed against CD79B (an antigen expressed by Large B-Cell lymphoma). Polivy is the first commercial therapeutic ADC produced using a site-specific covalent bond conjugated to the synthetic monomethyl auristatin E (MMAE) via engineered cysteines (THIOMABs) and using a protease-cleavable peptide linker to increase the plasma stability [98].

The Lumoxiti® is the first approved recombinant ADC. It is an innovative linkerless ADC is produced by genetic fusion between the Fv fragment of an anti-CD22 monoclonal with the 38 kDa fragment (PE38) of Pseudomonas exotoxin A [99].

We can underline that all the above-described approved ADCs (except the unique recombinant linkerless ADC Lumoxiti®) were developed using conventional random conjugation methods [100]. Table 1 reports shows all the approved and marketed ADCs.

Table 1. ADCs currently approved for clinical use.

Name	Antigen Target	Type of Cancer Target	Linker Type	Status
Mylotarg® (Gemtuzumab ozogamicin)	CD33	Myeloid leukemia B-cell lymphoma	Cleavable linker (hydrazone acetyl butyrate)	marketed
Besponsa® (Inotuzumab ozogamicin)	CD22	Lymphoblastic B leukemia	Cleavable linker (hydrazone acetyl butyrate)	marketed
Adcetris® (Brentuximab vedotin)	CD-30	Hodgkin's lymphoma	Protease-cleavable mc-VC PABC	marketed
Kadcyla® (Trastuzumab emtansine)	HER-2	HER2+ Breast cancer	Non cleavable thioether linker	marketed
Polivy® (Polatuzumab vedotin)	CD79B	Large B Cell lymphoma	Protease-cleavable	marketed
Lumoxiti® (Moxetumomab pasudotox)	CD22	Refractory hairy cell leukemia	Recombinant covalently fused (linkerless)	marketed

6. Future Perspectives

The approved ADCs are mostly indicated for the treatment of hematological malignancies and, with a few exceptions, their clinical activity has largely failed for solid tumors. The reasons for these failures may be attributed to the large molecular size of the ADC molecule that shows poor penetration into the tumor mass, thus resulting in poor in vivo efficacy [11]. For this reason, other forms of reduced sized antibodies such as single chain fragments of variable regions (scFv), i.e., v regions joined by a linker peptide, have been investigated, Also in the form of heterodimers of IgG and IgE, a small divalent immunoprotein (SIP, 75 kDa) or "minibody", a homodimer stabilized by a disulfide bond to its C-terminal [13]. The most explored antibody derivative variants are the dsFv and scFv. They are made of V_h and V_L domains linked through an interchain disulfide bond (dsFv) genetically engineered and linked covalently with a hydrophilic linker to form an scFv. Due to their modular nature, they can undergo multimerization into homo and hetero oligomers (diabody, triabody, tetrabody) strengthening antigen binding affinity and diversifying the different functionalities. The sdAbs (single domain antibodies) are smaller than scFvs, comprising 15-KDa V_h, V_l, or V_{hh} domains, also termed nanobodies, and containing the antigen domain in the terminal region of the hinge. Similarly, to scFv, these nanobodies can form homodimers increasing the binding affinity for the target antigen or formed into heterodimers with bispecific properties. Bispecific antibodies can interact simultaneously with two antigens on the same target cell, a property that potentially allows for an increase in the therapeutic window while decreasing the non-specific effects on non-target cells [101]. SIP antibodies have high affinity to their antigen and their turnover occurs in the liver. The technology for producing SIP antibodies was developed by Neri et al. [79] against fibronectin and other vascular antigens. These antigens, common in tumors, are stable and accessible. In addition, SIP have two C-terminal cysteines that allows a disulfide bridge with various payloads [102]. All these small fragments of antibodies as Fab, diabody and scFv, penetrate more rapidly into solid tumors but have a reduced serum half-life and undergo rapid renal elimination. This means that they are often eliminated before adequate absorption takes place at the tumor site.

Depending on the tumor under treatment, it is necessary to adequately choose and modify the Fc portion on the antibody to have the best possible response, especially to take advantage of the effect of the ADCC combined with other mechanisms of cell killing exerted via direct antibody-mediated cell signaling [2].

In addition to the above-mentioned ADCs, there are also other constructs and strategies to attack cancer cells that involve the conjugation of toxins or chemotherapeutic drugs to ligands or proteins that are overexpressed on the target cell. The most used ligands as carriers can be proteins or peptides. Another strategy is to use peptide-drug-conjugates that are made up of small, synthetic peptides [103–108]. These molecules appear to have an even faster penetration and elimination than the small antibody fragments we have described [102].

Nanomedicine is one of the formulation-based technologies to increase bioavailability of drugs. Nanotechnology can provide new treatment options for tumors due to the great potential for selective targeting and controlled drug release. Increasingly more attention is being paid to antibodies and their fragments as targeting ligands able to bind specific receptors that are overexpressed on tumor cells [109] for the delivery of nanoparticles.

Non-targeted nanoparticles such as liposomal-based preparations [110] polymeric [111] and metallic nanoparticles [112,113] are readily available for the conjugation with antibodies and drugs, potentially opening the possibility to develop theragnostic (therapeutics and diagnostics) agents. These formulations can reduce the toxicity profiles of the payloads and improve the therapeutic widow. One example is Doxil1, which has been on the market for 20 years as a liposomal preparation of doxorubicin, and is now being improved by PEGylation [114].

Antibody conjugate nanoparticles (ACNPs) are formed from a combination of ADC and nanotechnologies. ACNPs similarly to ADCs use antibodies to specifically target cancer cells for the delivery of encapsulated drugs.

Many ACNPs have been tested in clinical trials, but to date none has yet reached phase III trials [115].

In recent years, great progress has been made in developing effective nanoparticle-based drug targeting using conjugated antibodies. In addition, the use of antibody fragments combined with advances in molecular design are overcoming some of the problems associated with the large molecular size of unmodified antibodies [109].

With the adoption of strategies that improve the ability of ACNP to reach the tumor site to facilitate active targeting together with additional studies that are still needed to define and refine conjugation technology, size, shape and surface charge of nanoparticles will likely lead in the future to useful outcomes for these targeting reagents.

7. Conclusions

More than 80 ADCs are currently under investigation and are in various stages of clinical development for cancer treatment [116]. Current evidence indicates that the field of ADCs is a very promising one, even though in past years they have faced a number of clinical failures. Recent advances in technology now provide all of the necessary elements required for the facile production of humanized monoclonal antibodies, site-specific conjugation protocols, various potent cytotoxic payloads with different mechanisms of action, adaptable linker technologies, together with advanced analytic techniques [117]. With the availability of the new technologies and biomarker selection strategies, ADCs are set to represent an important contribution to the future of immuno-oncology.

Author Contributions: Conceptualization, F.G. and R.I.; Methodology, G.S. and S.I.; Software, S.P.; Validation, F.G., R.I.; Resources, S.P., R.G. and G.D.V.; Data Curation, S.P., G.P., E.C., M.A., R.G.; Writing-Original Draft Preparation, S.P., G.D.V., F.G., D.J.F. and R.I.; Writing-Review & Editing, A.M.C., G.S., S.I., D.J.F. and R.I.; Supervision, F.G., D.J.F. and R.I.; Project Administration, R.I., and S.I.; Funding Acquisition, R.I., G.S. and S.I. All authors have read and agreed to the published version of the manuscript.

Funding: F.G., A.M.C., R.I. are supported by University of L'Aquila, Fondi RIA di Ateneo. E.C. is recipient of an AIRC fellowship. G.S. is supported by AIRC (IG: 18467). S.P. program is funded by the Italian Ministry of Instruction, University, and Research under the national project PON ricerca e innovazione 2014–2020. M.A. supported by MIUR-Ministero dell'Istruzione, dell'Università e della Ricerca (Ministry of Education, University and Research) under national project PONRI 2014–2020 (N AIM1887574, CUP: E18H19000350007) co-funded by European Union through FSE and FESR.

Conflicts of Interest: G.S. and S.I. are shareholders of Mediapharma s.r.l. The other authors have no potential conflict of interest to report.

References

1. Strebhardt, K.; Ullrich, A. Paul Ehrlich's magic bullet concept: 100 years of progress. *Nat. Rev. Cancer* **2008**, *8*, 473–480. [CrossRef] [PubMed]
2. Hoffmann, R.M.; Coumbe, B.G.T.; Josephs, D.H.; Mele, S.; Ilieva, K.M.; Cheung, A.; Tutt, A.N.; Spicer, J.F.; Thurston, D.E.; Crescioli, S.; et al. Antibody structure and engineering considerations for the design and function of Antibody Drug Conjugates (ADCs). *OncoImmunology* **2018**, *7*, e1395127. [CrossRef] [PubMed]
3. Sochaj, A.M.; Świderska, K.W.; Otlewski, J. Current methods for the synthesis of homogeneous antibody-drug conjugates. *Biotechnol. Adv.* **2015**, *33*, 775–784. [CrossRef] [PubMed]
4. Giansanti, F.; Flavell, D.J.; Angelucci, F.; Fabbrini, M.S.; Ippoliti, R. Strategies to Improve the Clinical Utility of Saporin-Based Targeted Toxins. *Toxins (Basel)* **2018**, *10*, 82. [CrossRef] [PubMed]
5. Panowski, S.; Bhakta, S.; Raab, H.; Polakis, P.; Junutula, J.R. Site-specific antibody drug conjugates for cancer therapy. *mAbs* **2014**, *6*, 34–45. [CrossRef] [PubMed]
6. Singh, S.K.; Luisi, D.L.; Pak, R.H. Antibody-Drug Conjugates: Design, Formulation and Physicochemical Stability. *Pharm. Res.* **2015**, *32*, 3541–3571. [CrossRef]
7. Zhou, Q. Site-specific conjugation for ADC and beyond. *Biomedicines* **2017**, *5*, 64. [CrossRef]
8. Khongorzul, P.; Ling, C.J.; Khan, F.U.; Ihsan, A.U.; Zhang, J. Antibody-Drug Conjugates: A Comprehensive Review. *Mol. Cancer Res.* **2020**, *18*, 3–19. [CrossRef]
9. Chari, R.V.J.; Miller, M.L.; Widdison, W.C. Antibody-drug conjugates: An emerging concept in cancer therapy. *Angew. Chem. Int. Ed. Engl.* **2014**, *53*, 3796–3827. [CrossRef]
10. Weidle, U.H.; Maisel, D.; Klostermann, S.; Schiller, C.; Weiss, E.H. Intracellular proteins displayed on the surface of tumor cells as targets for therapeutic intervention with antibody-related agents. *Cancer Genom. Proteom.* **2011**, *8*, 49–63.
11. Gauzy-Lazo, L.; Sassoon, I.; Brun, M.P. Advances in Antibody-Drug Conjugate Design: Current Clinical Landscape and Future Innovations. *Slas Discov.* **2020**, *20*, 2472555220912955. [CrossRef] [PubMed]
12. Brüggemann, M.; Osborn, M.J.; Ma, B.; Hayre, J.; Avis, S.; Lundstrom, B.; Buelow, R. Human antibody production in transgenic animals. *Arch. Immunol. Exp. (Warsz)* **2015**, *63*, 101–108. [CrossRef] [PubMed]
13. Aguiar, S.; Dias, J.; Manuel, A.M.; Russo, R.; Gois, P.M.P.; da Silva, F.A.; Goncalves, J. Chimeric Small Antibody Fragments as Strategy to Deliver Therapeutic Payloads. *Adv. Protein Chem. Struct. Biol.* **2018**, 143–182. [CrossRef]
14. Sala, G.; Rapposelli, I.G.; Ghasemi, R.; Piccolo, E.; Traini, S.; Capone, E.; Rossi, C.; Pelliccia, A.; Di Risio, A.; D'Egidio, M.; et al. EV20, a NovelAnti-ErbB-3 Humanized Antibody, Promotes ErbB-3 Down-Regulation and Inhibits Tumor Growth In Vivo. *Transl. Oncol.* **2013**, *6*, 676–684. [CrossRef]
15. Prasetyanti, P.R.; Capone, E.; Barcaroli, D.; D'Agostino, D.; Volpe, S.; Benfante, A.; van Hooff, S.; Iacobelli, V.; Rossi, C.; Iacobelli, S.; et al. ErbB-3 activation by NRG-1β sustains growth and promotes vemurafenib resistance in BRAF-V600E colon cancer stem cells (CSCs). *Oncotarget* **2015**, *6*, 16902–16911. [CrossRef]
16. Ghasemi, R.; Rapposelli, I.G.; Capone, E.; Rossi, C.; Lattanzio, R.; Piantelli, M.; Sala, G.; Iacobelli, S. Dual targeting of ErbB-2/ErbB-3 results in enhanced antitumor activity in preclinical models of pancreatic cancer. *Oncogenesis* **2014**, *3*, e117. [CrossRef]
17. Conner, S.D.; Schmid, S.L. Regulated portals of entry into the cell. *Nature* **2003**, *422*, 37–44. [CrossRef]
18. Kalim, M.; Chen, J.; Wang, S.; Lin, C.; Ullah, S.; Liang, K.; Ding, Q.; Chen, S.; Zhan, J. Intracellular trafficking of new anticancer therapeutics: Antibody-drug conjugates. *Drug Des. Devel.* **2017**, *11*, 2265–2276. [CrossRef]
19. Rusten, T.E.; Vaccari, T.; Stenmark, H. Shaping development with ESCRTs. *Nat. Cell Biol.* **2011**, *14*, 38–45. [CrossRef]
20. Capone, E.; Giansanti, F.; Ponziani, S.; Lamolinara, A.; Iezzi, M.; Cimini, A.; Angelucci, F.; Sorda, R.; Laurenzi, V.; Natali, P.G.; et al. EV20-Sap, a novel anti-HER-3 antibody-drug conjugate, displays promising antitumor activity in melanoma. *Oncotarget* **2017**, *8*, 95412–95424. [CrossRef]
21. Capone, E.; Lamolinara, A.; D'Agostino, D.; Rossi, C.; De Laurenzi, V.; Iezzi, M.; Sala, G.; Iacobelli, S. EV20-mediated delivery of cytotoxic auristatin MMAF exhibits potent therapeutic efficacy in cutaneous melanoma. *J. Control Release* **2018**, *277*, 48–56. [CrossRef] [PubMed]
22. Staudacher, A.H.; Brown, M.P. Antibody drug conjugates and bystander killing: Is antigen-dependent internalisation required? *Br. J. Cancer* **2017**, *117*, 1736–1742. [CrossRef] [PubMed]

23. Dal Corso, A.; Gebleux, R.; Murer, P.; Soltermann, A.; Neri, V. A non-internalizing antibody-drug conjugate based on an anthracycline payload displays potent therapeutic activity in Vivo. *J. Control. Release* **2017**, *264*, 211–218. [CrossRef] [PubMed]
24. Mohamed, M.M.; Sloane, B.F. Cysteine cathepsins: Multifunctional enzymes in cancer. *Nat. Rev. Cancer* **2006**, *6*, 764–775. [CrossRef]
25. Lewis Phillips, G.D.; Li, G.; Dugger, D.L.; Crocker, L.M.; Parsons, K.L.; Mai, E.; Blättler, W.A.; Lambert, J.M.; Chari, R.V.; Lutz, R.J.; et al. Targeting HER2-positive breastcancer with trastuzumab-DM1, an antibody-cytotoxic drug conjugate. *Cancer Res.* **2008**, *68*, 9280–9290. [CrossRef]
26. Dorywalska, M.; Strop, P.; Melton-Witt, J.A.A.; Hasa-Moreno, A.; Farias, S.E.; Galindo Casas, M.; Delaria, K.; Lui, V.; Poulsen, K.; Loo, C.; et al. Effect of attachment site on stability of cleavable antibody drug conjugates. *Bioconjug. Chem.* **2015**, *26*, 650–659. [CrossRef]
27. Lu, J.; Jiang, F.; Lu, A.; Zhang, G. Linkers Having a Crucial Role in Antibody-Drug Conjugates. *Int. J. Mol. Sci.* **2016**, *17*, 561. [CrossRef]
28. Chari, R.V. Targeted cancer therapy: Conferring specificity to cytotoxic drugs. *Acc. Chem. Res.* **2008**, *41*, 98–107. [CrossRef]
29. Dorywalska, M.; Strop, P.; Melton-Witt, J.A.; Hasa-Moreno, A.; Farias, S.E.; Galindo Casas, M.; Delaria, K.; Lui, V.; Poulsen, K.; Sutton, J.; et al. Site-Dependent Degradation of a Non-Cleavable Auristatin-Based Linker-Payload in Rodent Plasma and Its Effect on ADC Efficacy. *PLoS ONE* **2015**, *10*, e0132282. [CrossRef]
30. Pillow, T.H.; Sadowsky, J.D.; Zhang, D.; Yu, S.F.; Del Rosario, G.; Xu, K.; He, J.; Bhakta, S.; Ohri, R.; Kozak, K.R.; et al. Decoupling stability and release in disulfide bonds with antibody-small molecule conjugates. *Chem. Sci.* **2017**, *8*, 366–370. [CrossRef]
31. Wu, B.; Zhang, G.; Shuang, S.; Choi, M.M. Biosensors for determination of glucose with glucose oxidase immobilized on an eggshell membrane. *Talanta* **2004**, *64*, 546–553. [CrossRef] [PubMed]
32. Chari, R.V.; Martell, B.A.; Gross, J.L.; Cook, S.B.; Shah, S.A.; Blättler, W.A.; McKenzie, S.J.; Goldmacher, V.S. Immunoconjugates containing novel maytansinoids: Promisinganticancer drugs. *Cancer Res.* **1992**, *52*, 127–131. [PubMed]
33. Saito, G.; Swanson, J.A.; Lee, K.D. Drug delivery strategy utilizing conjugation viareversible disulfide linkages: Role and site of cellular reducing activities. *Adv. Drug Deliv. Rev.* **2003**, *55*, 199–215. [CrossRef]
34. Giansanti, F.; Capone, E.; Ponziani, S.; Piccolo, E.; Gentile, R.; Lamolinara, A.; Di Campli, A.; Sallese, M.; Iacobelli, V.; Cimini, A.; et al. Secreted Gal-3BP is a novel promising target for non-internalizing Antibody-Drug Conjugates. *J. Control. Release* **2018**, *294*, 176–184. [CrossRef]
35. Bargh, J.; Isidro-Llobet, A.; Parker, J.; Spring, D. Cleavable linkers in antibody–drug conjugates. *Chem. Soc. Rev.* **2019**, *48*, 4361–4374. [CrossRef]
36. Dubowchik, G.M.; Mosure, K.; Knipe, J.O.; Firestone, R.A. Cathepsin B-sensitive dipeptide prodrugs. 2. Models of anticancer drugs paclitaxel (Taxol), mitomycin C and doxorubicin. *Bioorganic. Med. Chem. Lett.* **1998**, *8*, 3347–3352. [CrossRef]
37. Doronina, S.O.; Toki, B.E.; Torgov, M.Y.; Mendelsohn, B.A.; Cerveny, C.G.; Chace, D.F.; DeBlanc, R.L.; Gearing, R.P.; Bovee, T.D.; Siegall, C.B.; et al. Development of potent monoclonal antibody auristatin conjugates for cancer therapy. *Nat. Biotechnol.* **2003**, *21*, 778–784. [CrossRef]
38. Jain, N.; Smith, S.W.; Ghone, S.; Tomczuk, B. Current ADC Linker Chemistry. *Pharm. Res.* **2015**, *32*, 3526–3540. [CrossRef]
39. Dubowchik, G.M.; Firestone, R.A.; Padilla, L.; Willner, D.; Hofstead, S.J.; Mosure, K.; Knipe, J.O.; Lasch, S.J.; Trail, P.A. Cathepsin B-labile dipeptide linkers for lysosomal release of doxorubicin from internalizing immunoconjugates: Model studies of enzymatic drug release and antigen-specific in vitro anticancer activity. *Bioconjug. Chem.* **2002**, *13*, 855–869. [CrossRef]
40. Caculitan, N.G.; Dela, C.; Chuh, J.; Ma, Y.; Zhang, D.; Kozak, K.R.; Liu, Y.; Pillow, T.H.; Sadowsky, J.; Cheung, T.K.; et al. Cathepsin B Is Dispensable for Cellular Processing of Cathepsin B-Cleavable Antibody-Drug Conjugates. *Cancer Res.* **2017**, *77*, 7027–7037. [CrossRef]
41. Laguzza, B.C.; Nichols, C.L.; Briggs, S.L.; Cullinan, G.J.; Johnson, D.A.; Starling, J.J.; Baker, A.L.; Bumol, T.F.; Corvalan, J.R. New antitumor monoclonal antibody-vinca conjugates LY203725 and related compounds: Design, preparation, and representative in vivo activity. *J. Med. Chem.* **1989**, *32*, 548–555. [CrossRef] [PubMed]

42. Govindan, S.V.; Cardillo, T.M.; Sharkey, R.M.; Tat, F.; Gold, D.V.; Goldenberg, D.M. Milatuzumab-SN-38 conjugates for the treatment of CD74+ cancers. *Mol. Cancer* **2013**, *12*, 968–978. [CrossRef] [PubMed]
43. Tranoy-Opalinski, I.; Legigan, T.; Barat, R.; Clarhaut, J.; Thomas, M.; Renoux, B.; Papot, S. β-Glucuronidase-responsive prodrugs for selective cancer chemotherapy: An update. *Eur. J. Med. Chem.* **2014**, *74*, 302–313. [CrossRef] [PubMed]
44. Lyon, R.P.; Bovee, T.D.; Doronina, S.O.; Burke, P.J.; Hunter, J.H.; Neff-LaFord, H.D.; Jonas, M.; Anderson, M.E.; Setter, J.R.; Senter, P.D. Reducing hydrophobicity of homogeneous antibody-drug conjugates improves pharmacokinetics and therapeutic index. *Nat. Biotechnol.* **2015**, *33*, 733–735. [CrossRef]
45. Kolodych, S.; Michel, C.; Delacroix, S.; Koniev, O.; Ehkirch, A.; Eberova, J.; Cianférani, S.; Renoux, B.; Krezel, W.; Poinot, P.; et al. Development and evaluation of β-galactosidase-sensitive antibody-drug conjugates. *Eur. J. Med. Chem.* **2017**, *142*, 376–382. [CrossRef]
46. Lambert, J.M.; Chari, R.V. Ado-trastuzumab Emtansine (T-DM1): An antibody-drug conjugate (ADC) for HER2-positive breast cancer. *J. Med. Chem.* **2014**, *57*, 6949–6964. [CrossRef]
47. Kovtun, Y.V.; Audette, C.A.; Ye, Y.; Xie, H.; Ruberti, M.F.; Phinney, S.J.; Leece, B.A.; Chittenden, T.; Blättler, W.A.; Goldmacher, V.S. Antibody-drug conjugates designed toeradicate tumors with homogeneous and heterogeneous expression of the targetantigen. *Cancer Res.* **2006**, *66*, 3214–3221. [CrossRef]
48. Oflazoglu, E.; Stone, I.J.; Gordon, K.; Wood, C.G.; Repasky, E.A.; Grewal, I.S.; Law, C.L.; Gerber, H.P. Potent anticarcinoma activity of the humanized anti-CD70 antibody h1F6 conjugated to the tubulin inhibitor auristatin via an uncleavable linker. *Clin. Cancer Res.* **2008**, *14*, 6171–6180. [CrossRef]
49. Polson, A.G.; Calemine-Fenaux, J.; Chan, P.; Chang, W.; Christensen, E.; Clark, S.; de Sauvage, F.J.; Eaton, D.; Elkins, K.; Elliott, J.M.; et al. Antibody-drug conjugates for the treatment of non-Hodgkin's lymphoma: Target and linker-drug selection. *Cancer Res.* **2009**, *69*, 2358–2364. [CrossRef]
50. Sau, S.; Alsaab, H.O.; Kashaw, S.K.; Tatiparti, K.; Iyer, A.K. Advances in antibody-drugconjugates: A new era of targeted cancer therapy. *Drug Discov. Today* **2017**, *22*, 1547–1556. [CrossRef]
51. Doronina, S.O.; Mendelsohn, B.A.; Bovee, T.D.; Cerveny, C.G.; Alley, S.C.; Meyer, D.L.; Oflazoglu, E.; Toki, B.E.; Sanderson, R.J.; Zabinski, R.F.; et al. Enhanced activity of monomethylauristatin F through monoclonal antibody delivery: Effects of linker technology on efficacy and toxicity. *Bioconjug. Chem.* **2006**, *17*, 114–124. [CrossRef]
52. Lencer, W.I.; Blumberg, R.S. A passionate kiss, then run: Exocytosis and recycling of IgG by FcRn. *Trends Cell Biol.* **2005**, *15*, 5–9. [CrossRef]
53. Chen, H.; Lin, Z.; Arnst, K.E.; Miller, D.D.; Li, W. Tubulin inhibitor-based antibody-drug conjugates for cancer therapy. *Molecules* **2017**, *22*, 1281. [CrossRef]
54. Anderl, J.; Faulstich, H.; Hechler, T.; Kulke, M. Antibody–Drug Conjugate Payloads. *Methods Mol. Biol.* **2013**, *1045*, 51–70. [CrossRef]
55. Zakacs, G.; Paterson, J.K.; Ludwig, J.A.; Booth-Genthe, C.; Gottesman, M.M. Targeting multidrug resistance in cancer. *Nat. Rev. Drug Discov.* **2006**, *5*, 219–234. [CrossRef] [PubMed]
56. Leung, D.; Wurst, J.M.; Liu, T.; Martinez, R.M.; Datta-Mannan, A.; Feng, Y. Antibody Conjugates-Recent Advances and Future Innovations. *Antibodies (Basel)* **2020**, *9*, 2. [CrossRef] [PubMed]
57. Kaur, G.; Hollingshead, M.; Holbeck, S.; Schauer-Vukasinovic, V.; Camalier, R.F.; Domling, A.; Agarwal, S. Biological evaluation of tubulysin A: A potential anticancer and antiangiogenic natural product. *Biochem. J.* **2006**, *396*, 235–242. [CrossRef] [PubMed]
58. Prota, A.E.; Bargsten, K.; Diaz, J.F.; Marsh, M.; Cuevas, C.; Liniger, M.; Steinmetz, M.O. A new tubulin-binding site and pharmacophore for microtubule destabilizing anticancer drugs. *Proc. Natl. Acad. Sci. USA* **2014**, *111*, 13817–13821. [CrossRef] [PubMed]
59. Dumontet, C.; Jordan, M.A. Microtubule-binding agents: A dynamic field of cancer therapeutics. *Nat. Rev. Drug Discov.* **2010**, *99*, 790–803. [CrossRef]
60. Kastenhuber, E.R.; Lowe, S.W. Putting p53 in Context. *Cell* **2017**, *170*, 1062–1078. [CrossRef]
61. Yaghoubi, S.; Karimi, M.H.; Lotfinia, M.; Gharibi, T.; Mahi-Birjand, M.; Kavi, E.; Hosseini, F.; Sineh Sepehr, K.; Khatami, M.; Bagheri, N.; et al. Potential drugs used in the antibody-drug conjugate (ADC) architecture for cancer therapy. *J. Cell. Physiol.* **2020**, *235*, 31–64. [CrossRef]
62. Antonow, D.; Thurston, D.E. Synthesis of DNA-interactive pyrrolo[2,1-c][1,4]benzodiazepines (PBDs). *Chem. Rev.* **2011**, *111*, 2815–2864. [CrossRef]

63. Tietze, L.F.; Schmuck, K. Prodrugs for targeted tumor therapies: Recent developments in ADEPT, GDEPT and PMT. *Curr. Pharm. Des.* **2011**, *17*, 3527–3547. [CrossRef]
64. Dokter, W.; Ubink, R.; van der Lee, M.; van der Vleuten, M.; van Achterberg, T.; Jacobs, D.; Loosveld, E.; van den Dobbelsteen, D.; Egging, D.; Mattaar, E.; et al. Preclinical profile of theHER2-targeting ADC SYD983/SYD985: Introduction of a new duocarmycin-basedlinker-drug platform. *Mol. Cancer* **2014**, *13*, 2618–2629. [CrossRef]
65. Rinnerthaler, G.; Gampenrieder, S.P.; Greil, R. HER2 Directed Antibody-Drug-Conjugates beyond T-DM1 in Breast Cancer. *Int. J. Mol. Sci.* **2019**, *20*, 1115. [CrossRef]
66. Gebleux, R.; Casi, G. Antibody-drug conjugates: Current status and future perspectives. *Pharm. Ther.* **2016**, *167*, 48–59. [CrossRef]
67. Adams, D.J.; Dewhirst, M.W.; Flowers, J.L.; Gamcsik, M.P.; Colvin, O.M.; Manikumar, G.; Wani, M.C.; Wall, M.E. Camptothecin analogues with enhanced antitumor activity at acidic pH. *Cancer Chemother. Pharm.* **2000**, *46*, 263–271. [CrossRef]
68. Starodub, A.N.; Ocean, A.J.; Shah, M.A.; Guarino, M.J.; Picozzi, V.J.; Vahdat, L.T.; Thomas, S.S.; Govindan, S.V.; Maliakal, P.P.; Wegener, W.A. First-in-human trial of a novel anti-trop-2 antibody-SN-38 conjugate, sacituzumab govitecan, for the treatment of diverse metastatic solid tumors. *Clin. Cancer Res.* **2015**, *21*, 3870–3878. [CrossRef]
69. Yu, Q.; Ding, J. Precision cancer medicine: Where to target? *Acta Pharmacol. Sin.* **2015**, *36*, 1161–1162. [CrossRef]
70. Chowdari, N.S.; Pan, C.; Rao, C.; Langley, D.R.; Sivaprakasam, P.; Sufi, B.; Derwin, D.; Wang, Y.; Kwok, E.; Passmore, D.; et al. Uncialamycin as a novel payload for antibody drug conjugate (ADC) based targeted cancer therapy. *Bioorganic. Med. Chem. Lett.* **2019**, *29*, 466–470. [CrossRef]
71. Kim, E.G.; Kim, K.M. Strategies and advancement in antibody- drug conjugate optimization for targeted cancer therapeutics. *Biomol. Ther. (Seoul)* **2015**, *23*, 493–509. [CrossRef]
72. Hennessy, E.J. Selective inhibitors of Bcl-2 and Bcl-xL: Balancing antitumor activity with on-target toxicity. *Bioorganic. Med. Chem. Lett.* **2016**, *26*, 2105–2114. [CrossRef] [PubMed]
73. Hallen, H.E.; Luo, H.; Scott-Craig, J.S.; Walton, J.D. Gene family encoding the major toxins of lethal Amanita mushrooms. *Proc. Natl. Acad. Sci. USA* **2007**, *104*, 19097–19101. [CrossRef] [PubMed]
74. Danielczyk, A.; Stahn, R.; Faulstich, D.; Löffler, A.; Märten, A.; Karsten, U.; Goletz, S. PankoMab: A potent new generation anti-tumour MUC1 antibody. *Cancer Immunol. Immunother. CII* **2006**, *55*, 1337–1347. [CrossRef] [PubMed]
75. Kaplan, G.; Mazor, R.; Lee, F.; Jang, Y.; Leshem, Y.; Pastan, I. Improving the In Vivo Efficacy of an Anti-Tac (CD25) Immunotoxin by Pseudomonas Exotoxin A Domain II Engineering. *Mol. Cancer Ther.* **2018**, *17*, 1486–1493. [CrossRef]
76. Kaplan, G.; Lee, F.; Onda, M.; Kolyvas, E.; Bhardwaj, G.; Baker, D.; Pastan, I. Protection of the Furin Cleavage Site in Low-Toxicity Immunotoxins Based on Pseudomonas Exotoxin A. *Toxins* **2016**, *8*, 217. [CrossRef] [PubMed]
77. Tsuchikama, K.; An, Z. Antibody-drug conjugates: Recent advances in conjugation and linker chemistries. *Protein Cell* **2018**, *9*, 33–46. [CrossRef]
78. Liu, H.; May, K. Disulfide bond structures of IgG molecules: Structural variations, chemical modifications and possible impacts to stability and biological function. *mABs* **2012**, *4*, 17–23. [CrossRef]
79. Gébleux, R.; Wulhfard, S.; Casi, G.; Neri, D. Antibody Format and Drug Release RateDetermine the Therapeutic Activity of Noninternalizing Antibody-Drug Conjugates. *Mol. Cancer Ther.* **2015**, *14*, 2606–2612. [CrossRef]
80. Anami, Y.; Xiong, W.; Gui, X.; Deng, M.; Zhang, C.C.; Zhang, N.; An, Z.; Tsuchikama, K. Enzymatic conjugation using branched linkers for constructing homogeneous antibody-drug conjugates with high potency. *Org. Biomol. Chem.* **2017**, *15*, 5635–5642. [CrossRef]
81. Bruins, J.J.; Westphal, A.H.; Albada, B.; Wagner, K.; Bartels, L.; Spits, H.; van Berkel, W.J.H.; van Delft, F.L. Inducible, Site-Specific Protein Labeling by Tyrosine Oxidation-Strain-Promoted (4 + 2) Cycloaddition. *Bioconjug. Chem.* **2017**, *28*, 1189–1193. [CrossRef]
82. Axup, J.Y.; Bajjuri, K.M.; Ritland, M.; Hutchins, B.M.; Kim, C.H.; Kazane, S.A. Synthesis of site-specific antibody-drug conjugates using unnatural amino acids. *Proc. Natl. Acad. Sci. USA* **2012**, *109*, 16101–16106. [CrossRef] [PubMed]

83. Tian, F.; Lu, Y.; Manibusan, A.; Sellers, A.; Tran, H.; Sun, Y.; Phuong, T.; Barnett, R.; Hehli, B. A general approach to site-specific antibody drug conjugates. *Proc. Natl. Acad. Sci. USA* **2014**, *111*, 1766–1771. [CrossRef] [PubMed]
84. Zimmerman, E.S.; Heibeck, T.H.; Gill, A.; Li, X.; Murray, C.J.; Madlansacay, M.R.; Tran, C.; Uter, N.T.; Yin, G.; Rivers, P.J.; et al. Production of site-specific antibody-drug conjugates using optimized non-natural amino acids in a cell-free expression system. *Bioconjug. Chem.* **2014**, *25*, 351–361. [CrossRef]
85. Norsworthy, K.J.; Ko, C.W.; Lee, J.E.; Liu, J.; John, C.S.; Przepiorka, D.; Farrell, A.T.; Pazdur, R. FDA Approval Summary: Mylotarg for Treatment of Patients with Relapsed orRefractory CD33-Positive Acute Myeloid Leukemia. *Oncologist* **2018**, *23*, 1103–1108. [CrossRef] [PubMed]
86. Ricart, A.D. Antibody-drug conjugates of calicheamicin derivative: Gemtuzumab ozogamicin and inotuzumab ozogamicin. *Clin. Cancer Res.* **2011**, *17*, 6417–6427. [CrossRef] [PubMed]
87. Tanimoto, T.; Tsubokura, M.; Mori, J.; Pietrek, M.; Ono, S.; Kami, M. Differences in drugapproval processes of 3 regulatory agencies: A case study of gemtuzumabozogamicin. *Invest. New Drugs* **2013**, *31*, 473–478. [CrossRef]
88. FDA. FDA Approves Mylotarg for Treatment of Acute Myeloid leukemia [WWW]. 2017. Available online: https://www.fda.gov/newsevents/newsroom/pressannouncements/ucm574507.htm (accessed on 1 September 2017).
89. FDA. FDA Approves New Treatment for Adults with Relapsed or Refractory Acute Lymphoblastic Leukemia [WWW]. 2017. Available online: https://www.fda.gov/newsevents/newsroom/pressannouncements/ucm572131.htm (accessed on 17 August 2017).
90. EMA Besponsa. Inotuzumab ozogamicin [WWW]. 2017. Available online: http://www.ema.europa.eu/ema/index.jsp?curl=pages/medicines/human/medicines/004119/human_med_002109.jsp&mid=WC0b01ac058001d124 (accessed on 28 June 2017).
91. Lamb, Y.N. Inotuzumab Ozogamicin: First Global Approval. *Drugs* **2017**, *77*, 1603–1610. [CrossRef]
92. Moek, K.L.; de Groot, D.J.A.; de Vries, E.G.E.; Fehrmann, R.S.N. The antibody-drug conjugate target landscape across a broad range of tumour types. *Ann. Oncol.* **2017**, *28*, 3083–3091. [CrossRef]
93. Dan, N.; Setua, S.; Kashyap, V.K.; Khan, S.; Jaggi, M.; Yallapu, M.M.; Chauhan, S.C. Antibody-Drug Conjugates for Cancer Therapy: Chemistry to Clinical Implications. *Pharmaceuticals (Basel)* **2018**, *11*, 32. [CrossRef]
94. EMA Herceptin. Trastuzumab [WWW]. 2018. Available online: http://www.ema.europa.eu/ema/index.jsp?curl=pages/medicines/human/medicines/000278/human_med_000818.jsp&mid=WC0b01ac058001d124 (accessed on 14 May 2018).
95. EMA Kadcyla. Trastuzumab Emtansine [WWW]. 2018. Available online: http://www.ema.europa.eu/ema/index.jsp?curl=pages/medicines/human/medicines/002389/human_med_001712.jsp&mid=WC0b01ac058001d124 (accessed on 14 May 2018).
96. FDA Drug Approval Package. Kadcyla (Ado-Trastuzumab Emtansine) Injection [WWW]. 2013. Available online: https://www.accessdata.fda.gov/drugsatfda_docs/nda/2013/125427Orig1s000TOC.cfm (accessed on 18 May 2018).
97. PMDA Trastuzumab emtansine. Review Report [WWW]. 2013. Available online: http://www.pmda.go.jp/files/000153735.pdf (accessed on 14 May 2018).
98. Deeks, E.D. Polatuzumab Vedotin: First Global Approval. *Drugs* **2019**, *79*, 1467–1475. [CrossRef]
99. Dhillon, S. Moxetumomab Pasudotox: First Global Approval. *Drugs* **2018**, *78*, 1763–1767. [CrossRef] [PubMed]
100. Yoder, N.C.; Bai, C.; Tavares, D.; Widdison, W.C.; Whiteman, K.R.; Wilhelm, A.; Wilhelm, S.D.; McShea, M.A.; Maloney, E.K.; Ab, O.; et al. A Case Study Comparing Heterogeneous Lysine- and Site-Specific Cysteine-Conjugated Maytansinoid Antibody-Drug Conjugates (ADCs) Illustrates the Benefits of Lysine Conjugation. *Mol. Pharm.* **2019**, *16*, 3926–3937. [CrossRef] [PubMed]
101. Goulet, D.R.; Atkins, W.M. Considerations for the Design of Antibody-Based Therapeutics. *J. Pharm. Sci.* **2020**, *109*, 74–103. [CrossRef] [PubMed]
102. Deonarain, M.P. Miniaturised 'antibody'-drug conjugates for solid tumours? *Drug Discov. Today Technol.* **2018**, *30*, 47–53. [CrossRef]

103. Cimini, A.; Mei, S.; Benedetti, E.; Laurenti, G.; Koutris, I.; Cinque, B.; Cifone, M.G.; Galzio, R.; Pitari, G.; Di Leandro, L.; et al. Distinct cellular responses induced by saporin and a transferrin-saporinconjugate in two different human glioblastoma cell lines. *J. Cell Physiol.* **2012**, *227*, 939–951. [CrossRef]
104. Della Cristina, P.; Castagna, M.; Lombardi, A.; Barison, E.; Tagliabue, G.; Ceriotti, A.; Koutris, I.; Di Leandro, L.; Giansanti, F.; Vago, R.; et al. Systematic comparison of single-chain Fvantibody-fusion toxin constructs containing Pseudomonas Exotoxin A or saporinproduced in different microbial expression systems. *Microb. Cell Fact.* **2015**, *14*, 19. [CrossRef]
105. Giansanti, F.; Di Leandro, L.; Koutris, I.; Pitari, G.; Fabbrini, M.S.; Lombardi, A.; Flavell, D.J.; Flavell, S.U.; Gianni, S.; Ippoliti, R. Engineering a switchable toxin: Thepotential use of PDZ domains in the expression, targeting and activation ofmodified saporin variants. *Protein Eng. Des. Sel.* **2010**, *23*, 61–68. [CrossRef]
106. Giansanti, F.; Sabatini, D.; Pennacchio, M.R.; Scotti, S.; Angelucci, F.; Dhez, A.C.; Antonosante, A.; Cimini, A.; Giordano, A.; Ippoliti, R. PDZ Domain in the Engineeringand Production of a Saporin Chimeric Toxin as a Tool for targeting Cancer Cells. *J. Cell Biochem.* **2015**, *116*, 1256–1266. [CrossRef]
107. Provenzano, E.A.; Posteri, R.; Giansanti, F.; Angelucci, F.; Flavell, S.U.; Flavell, D.J.; Fabbrini, M.S.; Porro, D.; Ippoliti, R.; Ceriotti, A.; et al. Optimization of construct design and fermentation strategy for the production ofbioactive ATF-SAP, a saporin based anti-tumoral uPAR-targeted chimera. *Microbcell Fact.* **2016**, *15*, 194. [CrossRef]
108. Dhez, A.C.; Benedetti, E.; Antonosante, A.; Panella, G.; Ranieri, B.; Florio, T.M.; Cristiano, L.; Angelucci, F.; Giansanti, F.; Di Leandro, L.; et al. Targeted therapy of human glioblastoma via delivery of a toxinthrough a peptide directed to cell surface nucleolin. *J. Cell Physiol.* **2018**, *233*, 4091–4105. [CrossRef]
109. Marques, A.C.; Costa, P.J.; Velho, S.; Amaral, M.H. Functionalizing nanoparticles with cancer-targeting antibodies: A comparison of strategies. *J. Control. Release* **2020**, *320*, 180–200. [CrossRef] [PubMed]
110. El Maghraby, G.M.; Arafa, M.F. Liposomes for enhanced cellular uptake of anticancer agents. *Curr. Drug Deliv.* **2020**. [CrossRef] [PubMed]
111. Sun, H.; Erdman, W.; Yuan, Y.; Mohamed, M.A.; Xie, R.; Gong, S.; Cheng, C. Crosslinked polymer nanocapsules for therapeutic, diagnostic, and theranostic applications. *Wiley Interdiscip. Rev. Nanomed. Nanobiotechnol.* **2020**, e1653. [CrossRef] [PubMed]
112. Jindal, M.; Nagpal, M.; Singh, M.; Aggarwal, G.; Dhingra, G.A. Gold Nanoparticles- Boon in Cancer Theranostics. *Curr. Pharm. Des.* **2020**. [CrossRef]
113. Ardini, M.; Huang, J.; Sánchez, C.S.; Mousavi, M.Z.; Caprettini, V.; Maccaferri, N.; Melle, G.; Bruno, G.; Pasquale, L.; Garoli, D.; et al. Live Intracellular Biorthogonal Imaging by Surface Enhanced Raman Spectroscopy using Alkyne-Silver Nanoparticles Clusters. *Sci. Rep.* **2018**, *8*, 1265.
114. Wang, H.; Zheng, M.; Gao, J.; Wang, J.; Zhang, Q.; Fawcett, J.P.; He, Y.; Gu, J. Uptake and release profiles of PEGylated liposomal doxorubicin nanoparticles: A comprehensive picture based on separate determination of encapsulated and total drug concentrations in tissues of tumor-bearing mice. *Talanta* **2020**, *208*, 120358. [CrossRef]
115. Johnston, M.C.; Scott, C.J. Antibody conjugated nanoparticles as a novel form of antibody drug conjugate chemotherapy. *Drug Discov. Today Technol.* **2018**, *30*, 63–69. [CrossRef]
116. Coats, S.; Williams, M.; Kebble, B.; Dixit, R.; Tseng, L.; Yao, N.S.; Tice, D.A.; Soria, J.C. Antibody-Drug Conjugates: Future Directions in Clinical and Translational Strategies to Improve the Therapeutic Index. *Clin. Cancer Res.* **2019**, *12*. [CrossRef]
117. Drake, P.M.; Rabuka, D. Recent Developments in ADC Technology: Preclinical Studies Signal Future Clinical Trends. *Bio. Drugs* **2017**, *31*, 521–531. [CrossRef]

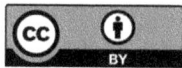 © 2020 by the authors. Licensee MDPI, Basel, Switzerland. This article is an open access article distributed under the terms and conditions of the Creative Commons Attribution (CC BY) license (http://creativecommons.org/licenses/by/4.0/).

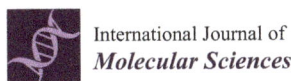

Review

B-Cell Maturation Antigen (BCMA) as a Target for New Drug Development in Relapsed and/or Refractory Multiple Myeloma

Hanley N. Abramson

Department of Pharmaceutical Sciences, Wayne State University, Detroit, MI 48202, USA; ac2531@wayne.edu

Received: 2 July 2020; Accepted: 20 July 2020; Published: 22 July 2020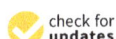

Abstract: During the past two decades there has been a major shift in the choice of agents to treat multiple myeloma, whether newly diagnosed or in the relapsed/refractory stage. The introduction of new drug classes, such as proteasome inhibitors, immunomodulators, and anti-CD38 and anti-SLAMF7 monoclonal antibodies, coupled with autologous stem cell transplantation, has approximately doubled the disease's five-year survival rate. However, this positive news is tempered by the realization that these measures are not curative and patients eventually relapse and/or become resistant to the drug's effects. Thus, there is a need to discover newer myeloma-driving molecular markers and develop innovative drugs designed to precisely regulate the actions of such putative targets. B cell maturation antigen (BCMA), which is found almost exclusively on the surfaces of malignant plasma cells to the exclusion of other cell types, including their normal counterparts, has emerged as a specific target of interest in this regard. Immunotherapeutic agents have been at the forefront of research designed to block BCMA activity. These agents encompass monoclonal antibodies, such as the drug conjugate belantamab mafodotin; bispecific T-cell engager strategies exemplified by AMG 420; and chimeric antigen receptor (CAR) T-cell therapeutics that include idecabtagene vicleucel (bb2121) and JNJ-68284528.

Keywords: myeloma; BCMA; bispecific T-cell engager; antibody-drug conjugates; chimeric antigen receptor T-cells; belantamab mafodotin; idecabtagene vicleucel; JNJ-68284528

1. Introduction

Multiple myeloma (MM) is a hematological cancer characterized by clonal plasma cell proliferation in the bone marrow along with high levels of monoclonal immunoglobulins in the blood and/or urine. Ranking behind non-Hodgkin's lymphoma, MM is the second most common blood cancer and the 14th most prevalent cancer overall. It is estimated that in 2020 a total of 32,270 (54.3% male) new cases of the disease will be diagnosed and be responsible for 12,830 deaths in the U.S. [1]. Active MM, which is accompanied by a tetrad of symptoms, generally abbreviated CRAB—hypercalcemia, renal insufficiency, anemia, and bone lesions—often is preceded by an asymptomatic phase known as monoclonal gammopathy of undetermined significance (MGUS). Progression from MGUS to MM, which carries a risk of about 1% per year [2], may also include another asymptomatic state known as smoldering myeloma [3]. The most recent pertinent guidelines for the diagnosis and treatment of MM have been issued by the National Comprehensive Cancer Network (NCCN) [4].

The therapy of MM has seen remarkable progress over the past half century. Beginning in the mid-1960s and continuing for more than three decades, alkylating agents, principally melphalan and cyclophosphamide, often accompanied by corticosteroids, were considered standard therapy for the disease. Starting in the 1990s, treatment protocols for the disease were augmented by autologous stem cell transplantation (ASCT). This established paradigm shifted dramatically starting in the late 1990s with the discovery of thalidomide's immunomodulatory actions that conferred remarkable anti-myeloma properties on this formerly ignominious agent. This was followed by the mechanistically related lenalidomide in 2005 and later (2013) pomalidomide. Furthermore, the discovery of the anti-myeloma activity of the proteasome inhibitor bortezomib in 2003, subsequently followed by carfilzomib and ixazomib, provided substantive additions to the armamentarium available to fight the disease. In 2015, in another remarkable turn of events, the Food and Drug Administration (FDA) approved two monoclonal antibodies (mAbs)—daratumumab and elotuzumab—for treating MM. Both target glycoproteins found on the surface of MM cells, CD38 and SLAMF7, respectively. Another anti-CD38 mAb, isatuximab-irfc, was approved by the FDA in 2020. Rounding out the currently FDA-approved treatment modalities for MM are the pan-histone deacetylase inhibitor panobinostat (2015) and the nuclear export inhibitor selinexor (2019). The success of these therapeutic advances over the past four decades is attested to by the more than doubling of the disease's five-year survival rate, from 24.5% in 1975–77 to 55.1% in 2010–2016 [5]. Nevertheless, MM remains largely incurable and relapse and refractoriness to treatment continue as major problems [4], spurring the search for newer molecular targets and discovery of drugs exquisitely designed to modulate the actions of these targets.

2. The BAFF/APRIL/BCMA Axis

B-cell activating factor (BAFF; BLyS; TALL-1) and APRIL (a proliferation-inducing ligand) are two homologous members of the tumor necrosis factor (TNF) superfamily [6,7] that have received much recent attention for their roles in the pathology of lupus erythematosus, rheumatoid arthritis, and other autoimmune diseases [8,9]. There also is evidence that the production of both of these cytokines in the bone marrow microenvironment plays a key role in the viability and proliferation of myeloma cells [10]. Moreover, MM disease progression and prognosis have been linked with BAFF and APRIL serum levels [11]. Both BAFF and APRIL serve as ligands for two TNF receptor family members located on the myeloma cell surface—transmembrane activator and calcium modulator and cyclophilin ligand interactor (TACI) and B-cell maturation antigen (BCMA). In addition, BAFF binds to a third myeloma cell receptor, BAFF-R (Figure 1).

Two inhibitors of both BAFF and APRIL, atacicept and tabalumab, each have been studied in several immune-related conditions, including MM, but have failed to exhibit substantial efficacy in any trials [12,13]. Moreover, BION-1301, a humanized anti-APRIL antibody, that had been considered a possibility for clinical development in MM has been dropped from further consideration in myeloma due to failure to achieve objective responses in a phase I study (NCT03340883) [14].

However, the bulk of attention on the BAFF/APRIL/BCMA axis in MM has been focused on BCMA as a major target of interest, particularly in three immunotherapy fronts: as a mAb (both naked and drug-conjugated); as a component of the bispecific T-cell engager (BiTE) strategy; and in conjunction with chimeric antigen receptor (CAR) T-cell therapy.

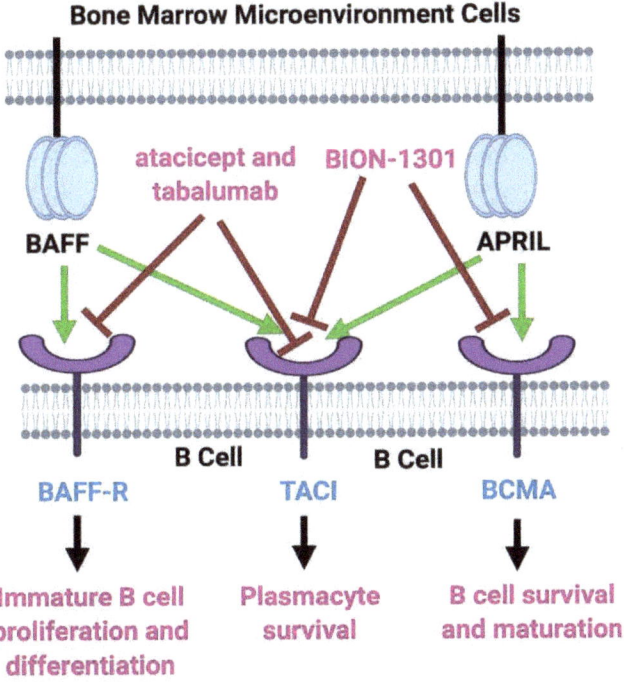

Figure 1. BAFF/APRIL/BCMA Axis. Tumor necrosis factor (TNF) family members BAFF (B-cell activating factor) and APRIL (a proliferation-inducing ligand) are cytokines secreted in the bone marrow microenvironment that play key roles in B cell development, as well as in supporting the viability and proliferation of plasma cells in multiple myeloma. Both BAFF and APRIL serve as ligands for two receptors on the myeloma cell surface—transmembrane activator and calcium modulator and cyclophilin ligand interactor (TACI) and B-cell maturation antigen (BCMA). BAFF also binds to BAFF-R, another myeloma cell receptor. The receptor blockers shown, atacicept, tabalumab, and BION-1301, have been studied in MM patients but have failed to provide evidence of efficacy. On the other hand, inhibitors of BCMA have demonstrated great potential in the therapy of MM. Created with BioRender.com.

3. BCMA

BCMA (CD269; TNFRSF17), also a member of the TNF receptor superfamily, was first identified in the early 1990s [15–18]. Expression of this 184-amino acid glycoprotein plays a major role in B-cell maturation and differentiation into plasma cells [19]. Structurally, BCMA is comprised of three major domains: extracellular (amino acids 1–54, linked by disulfide bonds at positions 8–21, 24–37, and 28–41), transmembrane (amino acids 55–77), and cytoplasmic (amino acids 78–184). In normal human tissues, both BCMA protein and mRNA are found almost exclusively on plasma cells and are selectively overexpressed during plasmacyte malignant transformation, promoting tumor cell growth, survival, and drug resistance, primarily through activation of the NFκB, AKT, phosphoinositide 3-kinase (PI3K), STAT3, and MAPK intracellular signal transduction cascades [20–24]. This consistent elevation and virtually sole confinement of BCMA on the surface of MM cells from both cell lines and patient samples has made BCMA a compelling target for drug discovery and development in MM [25,26]. In addition, several studies have provided substantial evidence pointing to the value of using membrane bound BCMA measurements not only as a biomarker for MM diagnosis and prognosis, but also as a possible predictor of response to treatment [27]. Moreover, the finding that BCMA is expressed at similar levels during the various stages of MM, from previously untreated to relapse, suggests that BCMA may be a valid therapeutic target throughout the course of the disease [28].

Blood levels of a soluble form of BCMA (sBCMA), the result of the shedding of BCMA from the plasma cell surface due to cleavage by γ-secretase [29], have been shown to be elevated in MM patients and are linked to inferior clinical outcomes [30]. sBCMA, which is comprised of the extracellular domain plus a portion of the transmembrane domain of BCMA [29], not only lowers the density of the target antigen but also provides a soluble decoy capable of limiting the efficacy of anti-BCMA agents currently under development. This potential hurdle has stimulated the search for γ-secretase inhibitors, which already have attained a prominent role in the quest for drugs to treat Alzheimer's disease and a number of Notch-overexpressing cancers [31,32], as well as to enhance outcomes in BCMA-directed therapies [33,34].

4. Anti-BCMA Monoclonal Antibodies

A core feature of IgG antibodies is the presence of an abundance of fucosyl groups in the N-linked biantennary complex oligosaccharides found in the Fc region [35]. Removal of these groups has become a well-established strategy for enhancing antibody-dependent cellular cytotoxicity (ADCC) through binding to FcγIIIa receptors on natural killer (NK) cells [36,37]. Two such afucosylated anti-BCMA antibodies are described below: the antibody-drug conjugate (ADC) belantamab mafodotin and the naked antibody SEA-BCMA.

Belantamab mafodotin (GSK2857916) is an ADC, in which the antibody is coupled to the microtubule inhibitor monomethylauristatin F (MMAF) through a protease-resistant maleimidocaproyl linker [38]. Binding to the BCMA receptor disrupts BAFF and APRIL signaling to induce ADCC, while the conjugated component produces myeloma cell arrest at the G2/M checkpoint [39]. This immunoconjugate continues to be studied in relapsed and/or refractory MM (RRMM) patients in the DREAMM series of trials (see Table 1). The phase II DREAMM-2 study (NCT03525678) showed that this agent, which has been granted breakthrough therapy and priority review status for RRMM by the FDA, as well as PRIME designation from the European Medicines Agency, has an acceptable safety profile with corneal problems, thrombocytopenia, and anemia, attributed to the MMAF payload, cited as the most commonly observed adverse events. However, the objective response rate (ORR) was only 31% in the DREAMM-2 trial [40] compared to the results of an earlier exploratory study (NCT02064387, DREAMM-1) in which an ORR of 60% was found [41]. Recruitment is currently ongoing for a phase II trial (DREAMM-5; NCT04126200) [42] that includes, along with belantamab mafodotin, two T-cell co-stimulatory agonistic mAbs, GSK3174998 and GSK3359609, which target OX40 [43] and inducible co-stimulator (ICOS) [44,45], respectively. Additionally included in the DREAM-5 trial is a study of the γ-secretase inhibitor nirogacestat (PF-03084014), which blocks the shedding of BCMA from the plasma membrane surface, an approach that has been shown, as stated earlier, to improve effectiveness of anti-BCMA therapy [29]. The conjugate also is under investigation in combination with lenalidomide and bortezomib in a phase II study (NCT03544281; DREAMM-6) [46]. Finally, two phase III studies of belantamab mafodotin recently have been launched: one in combination with pomalidomide (NCT04162210; DREAMM-3) and the other with daratumumab plus bortezomib (NCT04246047; DREAMM-7).

Table 1. Active trials of anti- B cell maturation antigen (BCMA) monoclonal antibodies and their drug conjugates in relapsed/refractory multiple myeloma (RRMM).

Trial ID [References]	Treatment	Phase	Enrollment	Trial Title
NCT02064387 [41]	Belantamab mafodotin (GSK2857916)	I	79	A Phase I Open-label, Dose Escalation Study to Investigate the Safety, Pharmacokinetics, Pharmacodynamics, Immunogenicity and Clinical Activity of the Antibody Drug Conjugate GSK2857916 in Subjects With Relapsed/Refractory Multiple Myeloma and Other Advanced Hematologic Malignancies Expressing BCMA (DREAMM 1)
NCT03525678 [40]	Belantamab mafodotin (GSK2857916)	II	221	A Phase II, Open Label, Randomized, Two-Arm Study to Investigate the Efficacy and Safety of Two Doses of the Antibody Drug Conjugate GSK2857916 in Participants With Multiple Myeloma Who Had 3 or More Prior Lines of Treatment, Are Refractory to a Proteasome Inhibitor and an Immunomodulatory Agent and Have Failed an Anti-CD38 Antibody (DREAMM 2)
NCT04162210	Belantamab mafodotin (GSK2857916) + Pom + low dose Dex	III	380	A Phase III, Open-Label, Randomized Study to Evaluate the Efficacy and Safety of Single Agent Belantamab Mafodotin Compared to Pomalidomide Plus Low dose Dexamethasone (Pom/Dex) in Participants with Relapsed/Refractory Multiple Myeloma (RRMM) (DREAMM 3)
NCT03848845	Belantamab mafodotin (GSK2857916) + Pemb	II	40	A Phase I/II Single Arm Open-Label Study to Explore Safety and Clinical Activity of GSK2857916 Administered in Combination With Pembrolizumab in Subjects With Relapsed/Refractory Multiple Myeloma—DREAMM 4
NCT04126200 [42]	Belantamab mafodotin (GSK2857916) + GSK3174998 + GSK3359609 + Nirogacestat	II	464	A Phase I/II, Randomized, Open-label Platform Study Utilizing a Master Protocol to Study Belantamab Mafodotin (GSK2857916) as Monotherapy and in Combination With Anti-Cancer Treatments in Participants with Relapsed/ Refractory Multiple Myeloma (RRMM)—DREAMM 5
NCT03544281 [46]	Belantamab mafodotin (GSK2857916) + Len + Dex + Bort	II	123	A Phase I/II, Open-label, Dose Escalation and Expansion Study to Evaluate Safety, Tolerability, and Clinical Activity of the Antibody-Drug Conjugate GSK2857916 Administered in Combination With Lenalidomide Plus Dexamethasone (Arm A), or Bortezomib Plus Dexamethasone (Arm B) in Participants With Relapsed / Refractory Multiple Myeloma—DREAMM 6
NCT04246047	Belantamab mafodotin (GSK2857916) + Dara + Bort + Dex	III	478	A Multicenter, Open-Label, Randomized Phase III Study to Evaluate the Efficacy and Safety of the Combination of Belantamab Mafodotin, Bortezomib, and Dexamethasone (B-Vd) Compared With the Combination of Daratumumab, Bortezomib and Dexamethasone (D-Vd) in Participants With Relapsed/Refractory Multiple Myeloma—DREAMM 7

Table 1. Cont.

Trial ID [References]	Treatment	Phase	Enrollment	Trial Title
NCT03582033	SEA-BCMA + Dex	I	185	A Phase 1 Study of SEA-BCMA in Patients with Relapsed or Refractory Multiple Myeloma
NCT03489525 [47,48]	MEDI2228	I	106	A Phase 1, Open-label Study to Evaluate the Safety, Pharmacokinetics, Immunogenicity, and Preliminary Efficacy of MEDI2228 in Subjects with Relapsed/Refractory Multiple Myeloma
NCT04036461	CC-99712	I	120	A Phase 1, Multicenter, Open-label, Dose Finding Study of CC-99712, a BCMA Antibody-Drug Conjugate, in Subjects with Relapsed and Refractory Multiple Myeloma

Abbreviations: Bort = bortezomib; Dara = daratumumab; Dex = dexamethasone; Len = lenalidomide; Pemb = pembrolizumab; Pom = pomalidomide.

Another afucosylated IgG1 mAb is the humanized antibody from Seattle Genetics known as SEA-BCMA, which has shown promising anti-myeloma activity in pre-clinical models [49] and is the subject of an ongoing phase I study in RRMM (NCT03582033) for which patients currently are being recruited. However, a myeloma-based clinical trial (NCT03266692) of SEA-BCMA in combination with the antibody-coupled T-cell receptor ACTR087 was terminated by the sponsor, following reports of serious adverse effects in an FDA-halted trial that employed ACTR087 and rituximab in a B-cell lymphoma study (NCT02776813) [50].

MEDI2228 is a fully human antibody conjugated to a dimeric minor-groove binding pyrrolobenzodiazepine payload (tesirine) via a protease-cleavable dipeptide (valine-alanine) linker [51]. The conjugate is rapidly internalized and trafficked to the lysosome where the warhead is released leading to DNA damage and subsequent apoptosis. Preclinical studies in mice demonstrated the strong anti-myeloma effects of MEDI2228 even in the presence of clinically significant levels of sBCMA [47,48]. A phase I clinical trial (NCT03489525) has been initiated to determine appropriate dosing of MEDI2228 in RRMM patients, although no data have been reported thus far. CC-99712 is another ADC (composition not available) that recently entered a clinical trial (NCT04036461) for RRMM but results have yet to be described.

5. T-Cell-Engaging Bispecific Antibodies

In recent years, T-cell-based antibody therapeutics have assumed an important role in the fight against a number of cancers, including MM. Two main areas of research have dominated this arena: T-cell-engaging bispecific antibodies (T-BsAbs) and chimeric antigen receptor (CAR) T-cell therapies. Based on a concept originally advanced by Nisonoff in the early 1960s [52], T-BsAbs are predicated on the design of a dual-targeting antibody constructed so as to enable one arm initially to bind to the CD3 co-receptor complex on T-cells, while the other arm subsequently is directed to tumor cells via a tumor-associated antigen. The numerous variations on this basic strategy that facilitates recruitment of cytotoxic T-cells to tumor cells in order to effect lysis of the latter recently have been the subject of several extensive reviews [53–58]. The cytotoxicity induced by the immunological synapse thus created is due to T-cell release of two cytolytic-initiating proteins—perforin, which produces transmembrane pores in the tumor cell and granzyme B, which navigates through the created pores to initiate apoptosis in the tumor cells [59–62]. The strategy differs substantially from regular T-cell mediated cytotoxicity in a number of respects. For example, the need for antibody-presenting cells is circumvented, the formation of a major histocompatibility complex (MHC)/antigen complex is not required, and co-stimulatory molecules are not involved. Moreover, such constructs enable "off-the-shelf" use by obviating any requirement for ex vivo T-cell manipulation. Additionally, such constructs produce a polyclonal expansion of T memory cells as a result of persistent T-cell activation. The density of the tumor antigen, as well as the relative binding affinities of each arm for their respective targets and biodistribution, are among the key characteristics of T-BsAbs that impact each construct's therapeutically relevant properties and which may be fine-tuned to optimize activity [63–66]. Table 2 lists the currently active clinical trials that include T-cell engaging bispecific antibodies for the treatment of RRMM.

Table 2. Active trials of T-cell-engaging bispecific antibodies in RRMM.

Trial ID [References]	Treatment	Phase	Enrollment	Trial Title
NCT02514239 [67]	AMG 420 (BI 836909)	I	43	An Open Label, Phase I, Dose Escalation Study to Characterize the Safety, Tolerability, Pharmacokinetics, and Pharmacodynamics of Intravenous Doses of BI 836909 in Relapsed and/or Refractory Multiple Myeloma Patients
NCT03287908 [68]	AMG 701	I/II	270	A Phase 1/2 Open-label Study Evaluating the Safety, Tolerability, Pharmacokinetics, Pharmacodynamics, and Efficacy of AMG 701 in Subjects with Multiple Myeloma (ParadigMM-1B)
NCT03761108 [69]	REGN5458	I/II	74	Phase 1/2 FIH Study of REGN5458 (Anti-BCMA x Anti-CD3 Bispecific Antibody) in Patients with Relapsed or Refractory Multiple Myeloma
NCT04083534	REGN5459	I/II	56	Phase 1/2 FIH Study of REGN5459 (Anti-BCMA x Anti-CD3 Bispecific Antibody) in Patients with Relapsed or Refractory Multiple Myeloma
NCT03145181 [70]	Teclistamab (JNJ-64007957)	I	160	A Phase 1, First-in-Human, Open-Label, Dose Escalation Study of JNJ-64007957, a Humanized BCMA x CD3 DuoBody® Antibody in Subjects with Relapsed or Refractory Multiple Myeloma
NCT04108195	Daratumumab + Talquetamab + Teclistamab (JNJ-64007957)	I	100	A Phase 1b Study of Subcutaneous Daratumumab Regimens in Combination With Bispecific T Cell Redirection Antibodies for the Treatment of Subjects with Multiple Myeloma
NCT03269136 [71–73]	PF-06863135	I	80	A Phase I, Open Label Study to Evaluate the Safety, Pharmacokinetic, Pharmacodynamic and Clinical Activity of Pf-06863135, a B-Cell Maturation Antigen (BCMA)-CD3 Bispecific Antibody, In Patients with Relapsed/Refractory Advanced Multiple Myeloma (MM)
NCT03486067 [74]	CC-93269	I	120	A Phase 1, Open-label, Dose Finding Study of CC-93269, a BCMA X CD3 T Cell Engaging Antibody, in Subjects with Relapsed and Refractory Multiple Myeloma.
NCT03933735 [75,76]	TNB-383B	I	72	A Multicenter, Phase 1, Open-label, Dose-escalation and Expansion Study of TNB-383B, a Bispecific Antibody Targeting BCMA in Subjects with Relapsed or Refractory Multiple Myeloma
NCT04184050 [77]	HPN217	I/II	70	A Phase 1/2 Open-label, Multicenter, Dose Escalation and Dose Expansion Study of the Safety, Tolerability, and Pharmacokinetics of HPN217 in Patients With Relapsed/Refractory Multiple Myeloma

Bi-specific T-cell engagers (BiTEs®), developed by Micromet in collaboration with Amgen, represent one type of T-BsAB in which the cross-link is provided by tandem single-chain variable fragments (scFvs) [63,78]. This innovative approach to cancer immunotherapy has borne fruit in the form of the CD3-CD19 cross-linking construct blinatumomab (Blincyto®) that was granted accelerated FDA approval in 2014 for use in Philadelphia chromosome-negative B-cell precursor acute lymphocytic leukemia (B-cell ALL), an indication that since has been expanded to include B-ALL patients with minimal residual disease (MRD) [79,80]. Blinatumomab, combined with ASCT, has been the subject of one RRMM-based trial (NCT03173430), which recently was terminated due to "slow patient accrual". However, the bulk of myeloma-related work using BiTEs has been based on recombinant antibodies to two different epitopes designed to cross-link the CD3ζ chains on the surface of tumor-specific T-cells and the targeted myeloma-BCMA.

Two of the most important and frequently encountered adverse effects that accompany T-cell activating immunotherapies, including those based on T-BsAbs and CAR T-cell formats, are the cytokine release syndrome (CRS; cytokine storm) and neurotoxicity (CAR T-cell-related encephalopathy syndrome; CRES), both of which may be life-threatening [81–83]. Almost without exception, CRS is seen in varying degrees of severity in a percentage of participants in every trial of the immunotherapeutic agents described in this and the following section. For example, in an analysis of 15 trials of anti-CD19 or anti-BCMA CAR T-cell constructs, of a total of 977 patients, 62.3% (range: 11% to 100%) experienced some degree of CRS with 18.4% (range 0.8% to 46%) in grades 3 or 4 [82]. Comparisons such as this highlight the problem of assessing the risk of developing CRS and its severity with any specific immunotherapeutic regimen, being subject to influences such as the type of malignancy under study, the structure and target of the immunotherapeutic product involved, and the grading scales used [84].

In its most serious form, the syndrome, which also has been implicated as a serious contributor to the lethal effects of COVID-19 infections [85,86], bears resemblance to a severe inflammatory response. As the name implies, the syndrome has been attributed to the expression and release of various cytokines, most notably IL-6, TNF-α, and IFN-γ [87]. Management of CRS includes corticosteroid infusions and the IL-6 receptor antagonist tocilizumab, which has been approved for the treatment of CAR T-cell associated CRS [88,89]. However, there have been no randomized controlled studies comparing the efficacy of corticosteroids and tocilizumab in the management of CRS. The pathophysiology and management of CRES, which generally occurs within the first two weeks of therapy, have been reviewed by Neelapu [88]. As noted for a few of the products described in subsequent discussions, in some cases the CAR T-cells have been designed to contain a safety switch consisting of a transduced receptor, like CD20 or non-functional truncated epidermal growth factor receptor (EGFR), that can be switched "off" through administration of an antagonist—in these cases, rituximab or cetuximab, respectively—to curtail CAR T-cell toxicity through ADCC and complement dependent cytotoxicity (CDC) [90,91]. Another type of safety switch is based on the dimerization of caspase-9 to activate apoptosis upon exposure to a synthetic dimerizing drug, such as remiducid [92–95].

AMG 420 (BI-836909), which has been granted fast-track status by the FDA, has shown favorable results in a trial (NCT02514239) of 42 RRMM patients with an overall ORR of 31%, including 70% (7/10) in patients receiving the maximum tolerated dose of 400 g/day. The most serious treatment-related adverse events noted in this study were infections and polyneuropathy. CRS, mostly grade 1, was observed in 38% of patients [67]. AMG 701, whose Fc domain has been engineered to produce a longer serum half-life compared to AMG 420, is currently the subject of a phase I trial (NCT03287908) as monotherapy for RRMM. A preclinical study [68] suggests that a follow-up trial of AMG 701 combined with an immunomodulator may be warranted. REGN5458 (NCT03761108) and REGN5459 (NCT04083534) are two BCMAxCD3 bispecific antibodies developed by Regeneron in partnership with Sanofi. Both are in phase I trials in RRMM patients, although to date preliminary data have been reported only for the former study [69].

Another BCMAxCD3 bispecific antibody teclistamab (JNJ-64007957) has been shown to be well-tolerated in a monkey model [70] and has been included in two clinical trials in RRMM—a phase I dose-escalation study (NCT03145181) and a phase I trial in combination with subcutaneous daratumumab (NCT04108195) plus the CD3xGPRC5D bispecific construct talquetamab. PF-06863135 (PF-3135), a BCMA-CD3 formatted BiTE derived from hinge-mutation engineering of an IgG2a backbone, is presently in a phase I trial (NCT03269136) for RRMM [71–73]. Another humanized IgG T-cell engager under clinical scrutiny is CC-93269 (NCT03486067), whose two arms bind in a 2 + 1 format—bivalently to BCMA and monovalently to CD3ε [74].

TNB-383B, under development by Tenebio in collaboration with Abbvie, differs from the other T-BsAbs currently being tested for anti-myeloma activity in that its structure consists of a single immunoglobulin light chain domain in addition to two variable heavy chains. The resulting BCMAxCD3 bispecific format possesses strong T-cell activation kinetics and a low-affinity anti-CD3 arm, resulting in reduced levels of cytokine release while retaining high cytotoxic activity, as demonstrated by studies conducted in vitro and in a mouse xenograft model [75]. TNB-383B, which was granted orphan drug status by the FDA in November 2019, currently is the subject of a phase I trial (NCT03933735) in RRMM [76]. There are a number of other bispecific antibodies that have shown promise for RRMM in preclinical studies. These include TNB-381M [96], FPA-151 [96], EM801 [28], and AP163 [97].

HPN217 provides an example of a tri-specific antibody format. Developed by Harpoon Therapeutics and the subject of a phase I/II trial for RRMM (NCT04184050), HPN217 is comprised of three binding domains in a single chain—an N-terminal BCMA-binding component, a C-terminal single-chain CD3ε TCR-binding portion; and a central domain that binds to human serum albumin. This product's extended half-life, compared to bispecific formats, has been attributed to its smaller size and flexibility [77].

In addition to BCMAxCD3-based bispecific antibody formats, efforts have been made to develop BCMA-targeted constructs that bind to receptors on NK cells, which, like cytotoxic T-cells, mediate cytotoxicity through release of granzyme and perforin, as well as expression of various apoptosis-inducing ligands [98]. One such construct is a tri-specific product that binds CD16A on NK cells to both BCMA and CD200 on myeloma cells [26,99]. Another is Compass Therapeutics' CTX-4419, which binds myeloma cell BCMA to both CD16A and p30 on NK cells and has shown some initial promise in preclinical work. Interestingly, NK CD16A engagement is not required for the tumor cell-killing properties of this product [100]. Similar properties have been reported for the related NK cell-engaging multispecific antibodies CTX-8573 [101] and AFM26 [102].

6. Chimeric Antigen Receptor (CAR) T-Cells

6.1. Autologous CAR T-Cell Therapy

Chimeric antigen receptor (CAR) T-cell therapy has emerged in recent years to a position of prominence in the immunotherapy of cancer [103,104]. This form of adoptive cell transfer (ACT) is designed to convert patient-derived cytotoxic T-cells into specific killers of cancer cells through the use of recombinant DNA techniques by which a viral vector is constructed to express a chimeric receptor against an antigen found on cancer cells. The engineered T-cells are then reinfused into the patient with the intent of lethally attaching to the targeted malignant cells. The technique has been used with success in certain hematological cancers, particularly B-cell malignancies, although solid tumors remain a substantial challenge [105].

The first CAR T-cell products, approved by the FDA in 2017, were tisagenlecleucel (CTL019; Kymriah®) and axicabtagene ciloleucel (axi-cel; Yescart®), scFv constructs directed against the CD19 antigen, which is uniformly expressed on the surface of malignant B lymphocytes. The former was approved for B-cell acute lymphoblastic leukemia and the latter for diffuse large B-cell lymphoma. The two products differ in a number of respects, such as in the co-stimulatory domain engineered into its chimeric receptor: 4-1BB (CD137; to enhance memory persistence) in tisagenlecleucel and CD28 (to afford greater peak expansion) in axi-cel. In addition, tisagenlecleucel uses a lentiviral vector in the manufacturing process while axi-cel is retroviral-based [106–111].

Although ORRs in the range of 80% or higher have been observed in trials of CAR T-cells targeting CD19, durable remissions have been much more difficult to realize [112–115]. However, numerous studies have demonstrated the benefits of pre-ACT lymphodepletion, usually consisting of fludarabine and cyclophosphamide, in several CAR T-cell-based trials in terms of improved T-cell peak expansion and persistence and clinical outcomes [116]. While lymphodepletion, first shown to be efficacious in malignant melanoma patients [117,118], provides transient tumor control while creating space for CAR T-cell expansion in the bone marrow, the mechanism underlying the improved efficacy putatively attributed to lymphodepletion is not known. Among the proposals advanced to explain the effect are enhanced levels of monocyte chemoattract protein-1 (MCP-1) [119]; elimination of sinks for homeostatic cytokines, such as interleukin-2 (IL-2), IL-7, and IL-15 [120]; and downregulation of indoleamine 2,3-dioxygenase in tumor cells [121].

Whereas CD19 has proven to be a very fruitful target for B-cell malignancies, this has not been the case when applied to MM. As a rule, CD19 is not typically expressed on malignant plasma cells, although it is present on their normal counterparts [122,123]. On the other hand, CD19 has been found to be highly expressed by plasma cells in the bone marrow of MGUS patients, leading to speculation that such cells might be myeloma stem cells [124,125]. However, a trial (NCT02135406) of tisagenlecleucel combined with ASCT produced only a poor clinical benefit in ten MM subjects [126]. Meanwhile, emphasis has shifted to BCMA as a major focus of myeloma-based studies applying the principles of CAR T-cell technology [127,128]. Several of these products, based on the BCMA target, are described below. Table 3 lists the currently active clinical trials that include anti-BCMA directed CAR T-cell constructs.

Table 3. Active trials of BCMA-targeted chimeric antigen receptor T-Cells in RRMM.

Trial ID [References]	Treatment	Phase	Enrollment	Trial Title
NCT02215967 [129]	Anti-BCMA-CAR T cells + Ctx + Flu	I	30	A Phase I Clinical Trial of T-Cells Targeting B-Cell Maturation Antigen for Previously Treated Multiple Myeloma
NCT03502577 [34]	Anti-BCMA-CAR T cells + Ctx + Flu + LY3039478 (gamma-secretase inhibitor)	I	18	A Phase I Study of B-Cell Maturation Antigen (BCMA)-Specific Chimeric Antigen Receptor T Cells in Combination With JSMD194, a Small Molecule Inhibitor of Gamma Secretase, in Patients With Relapsed or Persistent Multiple Myeloma
NCT02658929 [130]	bb2121	I	67	A Phase 1 Study of bb2121 in BCMA-Expressing Multiple Myeloma (CRB-401)
NCT03361748 [131]	Idecabtagene vicleucel (bb2121)	II	149	A Phase 2, Multicenter Study to Determine the Efficacy and Safety of bb2121 in Subjects with Relapsed and Refractory Multiple Myeloma (KarMMa-1)
NCT03601078 [132]	Idecabtagene vicleucel (bb2121)	II	181	A Phase 2, Multicohort, Open-label, Multicenter Study to Evaluate the Efficacy and Safety of bb2121 in Subjects With Relapsed and Refractory Multiple Myeloma and in Subjects with Clinical High-Risk Multiple Myeloma (KarMMa-2)
NCT03651128	Idecabtagene vicleucel (bb2121) + standard MM regimens	III	381	A Phase 3, Multicenter, Randomized, Open-label Study to Compare the Efficacy and Safety of bb2121 Versus Standard Regimens in Subjects with Relapsed and Refractory Multiple Myeloma (RRMM) (KarMMa-3)

Table 3. Cont.

Trial ID [References]	Treatment	Phase	Enrollment	Trial Title
NCT04196491	Idecabtagene vicleucel (bb2121) + Carf + Ctx + Flu + Len	I	60	A Phase 1, Open-label, Multicenter Study to Evaluate the Safety of bb2121 in Subjects with High Risk, Newly Diagnosed Multiple Myeloma (KarMMa-4)
NCT02786511	Idecabtagene vicleucel (bb2121)	–	50	Longterm Follow-up of Subjects Treated With bb2121
NCT03274219 [133]	bb21217	I	74	A Phase 1 Study of bb21217, an Anti-BCMA CAR T Cell Drug Product, in Relapsed and/or Refractory Multiple Myelom
NCT03090659 [134–136]	JNJ-68284528 (LCAR-B38M)	I/II	100	A Clinical Study of Legend Biotech BCMA-chimeric Antigen Receptor Technology in Treating Relapsed/Refractory (R/R) Multiple Myeloma Patients (LEGEND-2)
NCT03548207 [137]	JNJ-68284528 (LCAR-B38M)	I/II	118	A Phase 1b-2, Open-Label Study of JNJ-68284528, A Chimeric Antigen Receptor T-Cell (CAR-T) Therapy Directed Against BCMA in Subjects with Relapsed or Refractory Multiple Myeloma (CARTITUDE-1)
NCT04133636	JNJ-68284528 (LCAR-B38M) + Len	II	80	A Phase 2, Multicohort Open-Label Study of JNJ-68284528, a Chimeric Antigen Receptor T Cell (CAR-T) Therapy Directed Against BCMA in Subjects with Multiple Myeloma (CARTITUDE-2)
NCT04181827	JNJ-68284528 (LCAR-B38M) + Pom + Bort + Dex + Dara	III	400	A Phase 3 Randomized Study Comparing JNJ-68284528, a Chimeric Antigen Receptor T Cell (CAR-T) Therapy Directed Against BCMA, Versus Pomalidomide, Bortezomib and Dexamethasone (PVd) or Daratumumab, Pomalidomide and Dexamethasone (DPd) in Subjects with Relapsed and Lenalidomide-Refractory Multiple Myeloma (CARTITUDE-4)
NCT03288493 [138]	P-BCMA-101 + Rimiducid	I/II	220	Open-Label, Multicenter, Phase 1 Study to Assess the Safety of P BCMA-101 in Subjects with Relapsed / Refractory Multiple Myeloma (MM) Followed by a Phase 2 Assessment of Response and Safety (PRIME)
NCT03741127 [139]	P-BCMA-101 + Rimiducid	I	100	Open Label, Multicenter, Long-Term Follow-Up Study for Subjects Treated With P-BCMA-101
NCT03070327 [55,140]	MCARH171 + Ctx + Len	I	20	A Phase I Trial of B-cell Maturation Antigen (BCMA) Targeted EGFRt/BCMA-41BBz Chimeric Antigen Receptor (CAR) Modified T Cells With or Without Lenalidomide for the Treatment of Multiple Myeloma (MM)
NCT03338972 [55,141]	FCARH143 + Ctx + Flu	I	25	A Phase I Study of Adoptive Immunotherapy for Advanced B-Cell Maturation Antigen (BCMA)+ Multiple Myeloma With Autologous CD4+ and CD8+ T Cells Engineered to Express a BCMA-Specific Chimeric Antigen Receptor

Table 3. Cont.

Trial ID [References]	Treatment	Phase	Enrollment	Trial Title
NCT03430011 [55,142]	JCARH125	I/II	245	An Open-Label Phase 1/2 Study of JCARH125, BCMA-targeted Chimeric Antigen Receptor (CAR) T Cells, in Subjects With Relapsed or Refractory Multiple Myeloma
NCT03975907 [143]	CT053	I/II	62	An Open Label, Phase I/II Clinical Trial to Evaluate the Safety and Efficacy of Fully Human Anti-BCMA Chimeric Antibody Receptor Autologous T Cell (CAR T Infusion in Patients With Relapsed and/or Refractory Multiple Myeloma
NCT03915184 [143]	CT053	I	70	Open Label, Multi-center, Phase 1b/2 Clinical Trial to Evaluate the Safety and Efficacy of Autologous CAR BCMA T Cells (CT053) in Patients With Relapsed and/or Refractory Multiple Myeloma
NCT04155749	CART-ddBCMA	I	12	Master Protocol for the Phase 1 Study of Cell Therapies for the Treatment of Patients With Relapsed Refractory Multiple Myeloma, Including Long-term Safety Follow-up
NCT03448978 [144]	Descartes-08 + Ctx + Flu	I/II	30	Combined Phase I-Phase II Study of Autologous CD8+ T-cells Transiently Expressing a Chimeric Antigen Receptor Directed to B-Cell Maturation Antigen in Patients With Multiple Myeloma
NCT02546167 [145–147]	CART-BCMA	I	25	Pilot Study Of Redirected Autologous T Cells Engineered To Contain an Anti-BCMA scFv Coupled To TCRζ And 4-1BB Signaling Domains in Patients With Relapsed and/or Refractory Multiple Myeloma
NCT03455972 [148]	CART-anti-CD19/BCMAI	I	15	Study of T Cells Targeting CD19/BCMA (CART-19/BCMA) for High Risk Multiple Myeloma Followed With Auto-HSCT
NCT03196414 [149]	CART-anti-CD19/BCMAI	I	10	Study of T Cells Targeting CD138/BCMA/CD19/More Antigens (CART-138/BCMA/19/More) for Chemotherapy Refractory and Relapsed Multiple Myeloma
NCT03549442 [150]	BCMA CART + huCART19	I	39	Phase 1 Study of CART-BCMA With or Without huCART19 as Consolidation of Standard First or Second-Line Therapy for High-Risk Multiple Myeloma
NCT03706547 [150]	Anti-CD19/BCMA CAR-T cells	I	20	Clinical Study of Anti-CD19/BCMA Bispecific Chimeric Antigen Receptors (CARs) T Cell Therapy for Relapsed and Refractory Multiple Myeloma
NCT03767725 [150]	Anti-BCMA or/and Anti-CD19 CAR Autologous T Cells	I	10	Phase I Trial Study of Anti-BCMA (B-cell Maturation Antigen) or/and Anti-CD19 Chimeric Antigen Receptor T Cells (CART Cell) Treatment for the Patient of Relapsed Multiple Myeloma
NCT03602612 [151]	Anti-BCMA CAR T cells + Ctx + Flu	I	42	A Phase I Clinical Trial of T Cells Expressing a Novel Fully-human Anti-BCMA CAR for Treating Multiple Myeloma

Table 3. Cont.

Trial ID [References]	Treatment	Phase	Enrollment	Trial Title
NCT04093596 [152–154]	ALLO-715 + ALLO-647 + Ctx + Flu	I	90	A Single-Arm, Open-Label, Phase 1 Study of the Safety, Efficacy, and Cellular Kinetics/ Pharmacodynamics of ALLO-715 to Evaluate an Anti-BCMA Allogeneic CAR T Cell Therapy in Subjects With Relapsed/Refractory Multiple Myeloma (UNIVERSAL)
NCT04171843 [155]	PBCAR269A + Ctx + Flu	I/II	48	A Phase 1/2a, Open-label, Dose-escalation, Dose-expansion Study to Evaluate the Safety and Clinical Activity of PBCAR269A in Study Participants With Relapsed/Refractory Multiple Myeloma

Abbreviations: Bort = bortezomib; Carf = carfilzomib; Ctx = cyclophosphamide; Dara = daratumumab; Dex = dexamethasone; Flu = fludarabine; Len = lenalidomide; Pom = pomalidomide.

The first in-human study (NCT02215967) of an anti-BCMA CAR T-cell preparation in RRMM was conducted using a lentivirus engineered construct comprised of an anti-BCMA scFv, linked in tandem to a CD8 hinge, a transmembrane region, a co-stimulatory domain (CD28), and CD3ζ as the T-cell activator [156] (Figure 2). An ORR of 81% and a median progression-free survival (PFS) of 31 weeks was reported for 16 patients who received a dose of 9×10^6 T-cells per kg, the highest dose used in the trial. The subjects in this study previously had undergone a median of 9.5 lines of therapy for MM [129].

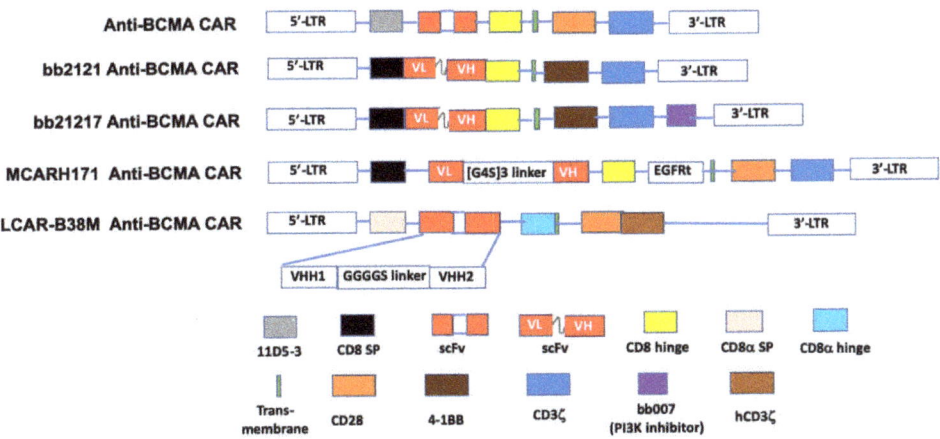

Figure 2. The schematic diagram of representative structures of BCMA-targeted chimeric antigen receptors (CAR). The BCMA CARs contain a single-chain of BCMA antibody variable fragment (ScFv), a transmembrane domain, a hinge region, a co-stimulation domain (4-1BB, CD28 or OX40), and a CD3ζ domain. Additional sequences (such as PI3K inhibitor) are added to enhance identification of CAR+ T cells. LCAR-B38M CAR contains two epitopes of BCMA scFv, VHH1 and VHH2. PI3K: phosphoinositol 3-kinase. Adapted from Lin et al. [156] with permission through Copyright Clearance Center, Inc.

Idecabtagene vicleucel (bb2121; Ide-cel) is an anti-BCMA scFv fused to the CD137 (4-1BB) co-stimulatory and CD3ζ signaling domains [157]. Following its designation by the FDA as a breakthrough therapy in 2017, bb2121 has been included in a series of phased trials designated KarMMa-1 through KarMMa-4 (NCT03361748 [131], NCT03601078, NCT03651128, and NCT04196491, respectively). Data on the first 33 RR myeloma patients (NCT02658929) [130] in the KarMMa-1 study revealed an ORR of 85%, including 15 patients with complete responses, although six of these subsequently relapsed. The median PFS in this study was 11.8 months. Moreover, 100% (16/16) of evaluable responders in this study with a partial response or better exhibited MRD negativity. Both grade 3 or 4 hematologic (primarily neutropenia) and neurotoxic (42%, all but one of grade 1 or 2) adverse effects were reported. CRS was noted in 76% of the patients. A press release from BMS and bluebird bio, the drug's sponsors [132], reported data on the KarMMa-2 trial that included 128 evaluable RRMM patients, who were administered either 150, 300, or 450×10^6 CAR T-cells. A median PFS of 8.6 months was found and the toxicity profile was similar to that reported in the earlier phase. Based on these data, a Biologic License Application was submitted to the FDA in early 2020 [158].

A next-generation construct is bb21217, which employs the same lentiviral design as bb2121 but to which an extra PI3K inhibitor domain (bb007) has been added during ex vivo culturing. This production modification has been shown to significantly enhance CAR T-cell-based immunotherapy by enriching the final product's population of memory-like T-cells, thereby augmenting T-cell durability and potency [159]. Currently, bb21217 is the subject of a phase I dose-escalation trial (NCT03274219) in RRMM patients. Adverse event data have been reported for 22 patients thus far in this trial—13 developed CRS while 5 experienced neurotoxicity and both toxicities were reported resolved. Clinical responses were observed in 15 of 18 evaluable patients, although 6 subsequently experienced relapse. Persistence of CAR T-cells was detected in six of the eight patients evaluated at six months, while two patients had detectable levels after 18 months [133].

JNJ-68284528 (LCAR-B38M; JNJ-4528) is unique among BCMA-targeted T-cell therapies in that it is directed against two BCMA epitopes (VH1 and VH2) to confer improved affinity for BCMA-expressing cells. Data on 57 patients, who had received an average of three prior therapies, in the phase I LEGEND-2 trial (NCT03090659) of JNJ-68284528 showed an ORR of 88% and PFS of 15 months. CRS, mostly grades 1 or 2, was seen in 83% of subjects [134–136]. Reported results from 21 evaluable RRMM patients in the CARTITUDE-1 phase Ib/II trial (NCT03548207) [137] were similar (91% ORR, no PFS given, CRS 88%) to those seen in the LEGEND-2 study. In 2019, as a result of these two trials the EMA accorded JNJ-68284528 PRIME status and the FDA provided this agent with the Breakthrough Therapy Designation. CARTITUDE-2 (NCT04133636) and CARTITUDE-4 (NCT04181827) are additional trials that have been initiated to further study the efficacy of JNJ-68284528 in RRMM patients. Significantly, the latter is a phase III investigation aimed at comparing this CAR-T product with standard triplet therapy.

P-BCMA-101, which received FDA Orphan Drug status in 2019, is a fully humanized anti-BCMA CAR T-cell product, in which a CD3ζ/4-1BB signaling domain is fused to a non-immunoglobulin Centyrin® scaffold. In comparison, such constructs are smaller than those patterned on immunoglobulins, have higher binding affinities, improved stability, reduced immunogenicity, and lower production cost. These qualities are attributed to use of transposon (piggy-BAC®)-based technology, instead of a viral vector, in the manufacturing process [160]. Moreover, pre-clinical work showed that the process yields a preponderance of T stem cell memory cells (T_{scm}), which offers a potential for therapeutic longevity [161]. A phase I trial (NCT03288493; PRIME) of P-BCMA-101, in 12 heavily pretreated RRMM patients, showed an ORR of 83% in 6 who were evaluated, 1 of whom experienced grade 2 CRS, although additional data more fully supporting the efficacy and safety of this agent have yet to appear [138]. However, according to the drug's sponsor (Poseida Therapeutics), a 15 year follow-up study has been designed and implemented to explore these issues in depth (NCT03741127) [139]. These latter two trials of P-BCMA-101 also are noteworthy for their inclusion of remiducid as a safety switch apoptosis activator, acting through induction of caspase-9 [92–95].

JCARH125 and FCARH143 are two fully human svFv bicistronic constructs incorporating the 4-1BB co-stimulatory domain [162]. Both CARs use a lentiviral vector but differ in the method of production. Related to these is MCARH171, a gamma-retroviral engineered product that features a truncated EGFR safety system that can be activated by cetuximab when warranted to mitigate CAR T-cell toxicity [163]. Active clinical trials of these three CAR T-cell products are included in Table 3.

CT053 and CT103A are lentivirus vector-based BCMA-targeted CAR T-cell constructs containing a fully human scFv, a CD8α hinge, as well as transmembrane, 4-1BB co-stimulatory, and CD3ζ activation domains, currently under development by CARSgen Therapeutics. The FDA has granted CT053 the Regenerative Medicine Advanced Therapy (RMAT) designation, based on the initial results of ongoing trials in China (NCT03975907) and the US (NCT03915184) in RRMM patients who previously had been treated with a median of four prior regimens [143,164]. CT103A is being studied in China for RRMM (Chinese Clinical Trial Register ChiCTR1800018137). An ORR of 100% was reported for the first 16 patients who received CT103A in a phase I trial [165].

Among other BCMA-targeted CAR T-cell platforms that recently have entered trials for RRMM are Arcelix's CART-ddBCMA in which the scFv binding domain is replaced by a proprietary soluble protein antigen-receptor X-linker (sparX) (NCT04155749; 15 year study); Descartes-08, a CD8$^+$ T-cell preparation whose co-stimulatory domain remains undisclosed (NCT03448978) [144]; and another CD3-4-1BB product referred to only as CART-BCMA (NCT02546167) [145–147].

Both CD19- and BCMA-targeted CAR T-cells have been used in combination in a few trials [150]; for example, NCT03455972 (newly diagnosed MM) [148] and NCT03196414 [149] (RRMM). Three additional trials that use variations on this combination protocol are NCT03549442, NCT03706547, and NCT03767725, although no results have yet been reported for these studies.

A significant departure from the standard scFv design pattern is seen in a BCMA-targeting CAR, designated as FHVH-BCMA-T (FHVH33-CD8BBZ), which contains a fully human heavy-chain-only binding domain (FHVH33). The construct, by eliminating linker-connected light chains, was predicted to reduce the risk of recipient immune responses [166]. The initial results of a trial (NCT03602612) of the drug in 12 patients who had previously received a median of 6 lines of anti-myeloma therapy, showed objective responses in 10 subjects. Although 11 of the 12 patients developed CRS, only 1 was considered grade 3 and that was resolved by tocilizumab [151].

6.2. Allogeneic CAR T-Cell Therapy

The generation of short-lived responses, coupled with high risk of CRS and other dose-limiting adverse effects, remains one of the drawbacks of autologously administered BCMA-targeted CAR T-cells in MM. In efforts to mitigate these issues, some CAR T-cell originators have turned their attention toward the potential development of "off-the-shelf" allogeneic products that use T-cells derived from healthy donors. One such example is ALLO-715 whose production process uses the proprietary Transcription Activator-like Effector Nuclease (TALEN^{TM}) in a site-specific BCMA gene-editing technique designed to limit T-cell receptor-mediated immune responses in the final product [152–154,167]. Following promising pre-clinical results in a murine model, ALLO-715 was advanced to a phase I trial (NCT04093596) for which patient recruitment has been initiated. ALLO-715 is noteworthy for its incorporation of a CD20-based mimotope as a rituximab-enabled safety switch, activation of which may be employed to specifically and efficiently eliminate CAR T-cells through ADCC and complement dependent cytotoxicity (CDC) [91,168] where required to relieve toxicity. This is the first anti-BCMA CAR T-cell product utilizing a CD20-based approach for this purpose. This trial also is noteworthy for its use of an anti-CD52 antibody, ALLO-647, as a selective lymphodepletion agent.

Another allogeneic BCMA-targeted CAR T-cell candidate under development for RRMM is PBCAR269A, a product of Precision BioSciences' proprietary ARCUS® nuclease gene-editing platform, which is predicated on the homing endonuclease I-CreI scaffold [155,169]. In 2020, PBCAR269A was advanced to a myeloma-based phase I trial (NCT04171843) based on data presented recently on two other products in the company's allogeneic CAR T-cell portfolio on other cancers: PBCAR0191 (NCT03666000) and PBCAR20A (NCT04030195), which target CD19 and CD20, respectively.

Finally, encouraging preclinical data recently have appeared that portends the possibility of engineering CARs that employ T-cell alternatives, such as NK cells [170,171], to generate novel systems targeting BCMA for future allogeneic product development in the quest for innovative anti-myeloma treatments.

7. Summary and Future Prospects

The armamentarium of available treatment modalities for MM, formerly restricted to alkylating agents and corticosteroids, has changed dramatically in the past two decades with the introduction of agents working by novel mechanisms, such as proteasome inhibition, immunomodulation, and CD38 blockade. The collective effect has been a remarkable improvement in the disease's five-year survival rate. However, this success is tempered by the almost invariable relapse and refractoriness to treatment that eventually emerge. This has spurred an ongoing quest for innovative targets subject to control through new drug discovery efforts, especially in the relapsed/refractory setting. One such target is BCMA, whose virtually exclusive confinement to malignant plasma cells has attracted much attention as an immunotherapeutic point of attack in myeloma-based new drug development. In this there is some reason for optimism.

In support of that positive outlook is the BCMA-targeting ADC belantamab mafodotin (GSK2857916), the subject of two recently launched phase III trials wherein the drug is combined with either pomalidomide or daratumumab plus bortezomib. The results of these and other future trials will help determine the eventual role of ADCs in myeloma-based therapeutics. In addition to its comparative simplicity of manufacture and consequential cost-savings benefit, a significant advantage of this ADC over other BCMA-targeted immunotherapies is that it carries virtually no risk of potentially lethal CRS.

Although several T-cell engaging bispecific antibodies targeting BCMA have been developed for treating MM, to date none has been included in myeloma studies beyond early phase trials. The most advanced member of this group, the BiTE construct AMG 420, has shown some encouraging efficacy but suffers from the requirement for continuous intravenous infusion although intermittent dosing is being investigated [67]. The related BiTE product, AMG 701, with its extended half-life and potential for once-weekly dosing may offer a more suitable alternative for future large-scale development in this drug class [68]. Several additional T-cell engaging products with similarly favorable pharmacokinetics recently have entered RRMM trials.

Most of the current interest in the prospects for immunotherapy in RRMM lies in CAR T-cell technology. Since the successful 2017 introduction of two CD19-targeting CAR T-cell products for certain B-cell leukemias and lymphomas (tisagenlecleucel and axicabtagene ciloleucel), there has been a flurry of activity geared toward the development of similar type constructs targeting BCMA. At this point, the two leading candidates appear to be Idecabtagene vicleucel (bb2121) and JNJ-68284528 (LCAR-B38M), both of which are in phase III trials. In the meantime, a number of products in this class continue to enter the pipeline each year and the flow shows no sign of abating. As the field continues to mature and engineering and manufacturing technologies evolve toward optimization and planning for future trials of these products moves forward, serious challenges need to be addressed if CAR T-cell technology is to take its place in the spectrum of accepted regimens available to treat MM, not only in the relapsed/refractory stage but perhaps eventually in earlier lines of therapy for the disease. Investigations aimed at informing dose levels compatible with maximizing response depth and durability while reducing adverse effects, especially CRS, continue apace. In addition, studies of additional efficacy determinants, such as kill-switch design and employment and the role, mode, and mechanism of lymphodepletion, will continue to determine the utility of CAR T-cell therapeutics in RRMM going forward. In the background looms the question of how the process can be made applicable to allogeneic products that offer off-the-shelf advantages, even as a few attempts to develop such products have begun to appear on the scene. The challenges ahead are formidable but the current level of activity in the myeloma-based CAR T-cell therapeutics arena augurs well for a promising future in which BCMA will continue to play a major role as a highly attractive target for conceptualizing new drug design and development, as well as a potential cure for this unrelenting disease.

Funding: This research received no external funding.

Conflicts of Interest: The author declares no conflict of interest.

References

1. Siegel, R.L.; Miller, K.D.; Jemal, A. Cancer statistics, 2020. *CA Cancer J. Clin.* **2020**, *70*, 7–30. [CrossRef] [PubMed]
2. Kyle, R.A.; Therneau, T.M.; Rajkumar, S.V.; Offord, J.R.; Larson, D.R.; Plevak, M.F.; Melton, L.J., 3rd. A long-term study of prognosis in monoclonal gammopathy of undetermined significance. *N. Engl. J. Med.* **2002**, *346*, 564–569. [CrossRef] [PubMed]
3. Kyle, R.A.; Remstein, E.D.; Therneau, T.M.; Dispenzieri, A.; Kurtin, P.J.; Hodnefield, J.M.; Larson, D.R.; Plevak, M.F.; Jelinek, D.F.; Fonseca, R.; et al. Clinical course and prognosis of smoldering (asymptomatic) multiple myeloma. *N. Engl. J. Med.* **2007**, *356*, 2582–2590. [CrossRef] [PubMed]
4. Kumar, S.K.; Callander, N.S.; Hillengass, J.; Liedtke, M.; Baljevic, M.; Campagnaro, E.; Castillo, J.J.; Chandler, J.C.; Cornell, R.F.; Costello, C.; et al. NCCN guidelines insights: Multiple myeloma, version 1.2020. *J. Natl. Compr. Cancer Netw.* **2019**, *17*, 1154–1165. [CrossRef] [PubMed]
5. *SEER Cancer Statistics Review (CSR) 1975–2017: Myeloma*; National Cancer Institute: Bethesda, MD, USA, 2020.
6. So, T.; Ishii, N. The TNF-TNFR family of co-signal molecules. *Adv. Exp. Med. Biol.* **2019**, *1189*, 53–84.
7. Moore, P.A.; Belvedere, O.; Orr, A.; Pieri, K.; LaFleur, D.W.; Feng, P.; Soppet, D.; Charters, M.; Gentz, R.; Parmelee, D.; et al. BLyS: Member of the tumor necrosis factor family and B lymphocyte stimulator. *Science* **1999**, *285*, 260–263. [CrossRef]
8. Shabgah, A.G.; Shariati-Sarabi, Z.; Tavakkol-Afshari, J.; Mohammadi, M. The role of BAFF and APRIL in rheumatoid arthritis. *J. Cell. Physiol.* **2019**, *234*, 17050–17063. [CrossRef]
9. Baert, L.; Manfroi, B.; Casez, O.; Sturm, N.; Huard, B. The role of APRIL—A proliferation inducing ligand—In autoimmune diseases and expectations from its targeting. *J. Autoimmun.* **2018**, *95*, 179–190. [CrossRef]
10. Pan, J.; Sun, Y.; Zhang, N.; Li, J.; Ta, F.; Wei, W.; Yu, S.; Ai, L. Characteristics of BAFF and APRIL factor expression in multiple myeloma and clinical significance. *Oncol. Lett.* **2017**, *14*, 2657–2662. [CrossRef]
11. Hengeveld, P.J.; Kersten, M.J. B-cell activating factor in the pathophysiology of multiple myeloma: A target for therapy? *Blood Cancer J.* **2015**, *5*, e282. [CrossRef]
12. Raje, N.S.; Moreau, P.; Terpos, E.; Benboubker, L.; Grzasko, N.; Holstein, S.A.; Oriol, A.; Huang, S.Y.; Beksac, M.; Kuliczkowski, K.; et al. Phase 2 study of tabalumab, a human anti-B-cell activating factor antibody, with bortezomib and dexamethasone in patients with previously treated multiple myeloma. *Br. J. Haematol.* **2017**, *176*, 783–795. [CrossRef]
13. Rossi, J.F.; Moreaux, J.; Hose, D.; Requirand, G.; Rose, M.; Rouille, V.; Nestorov, I.; Mordenti, G.; Goldschmidt, H.; Ythier, A.; et al. Atacicept in relapsed/refractory multiple myeloma or active Waldenstrom's macroglobulinemia: A phase I study. *Br. J. Cancer* **2009**, *101*, 1051–1058. [CrossRef] [PubMed]
14. Bensinger, W.; Raptis, A.; Berenson, J.; Spira, A.; Nooka, A.; Chaudhry, M.; van Zandvoort, P.; Nair, N.; Lo, J.; Elassaiss-Schaap, J.; et al. Phase 1 study of safety and tolerability of BION-1301 in patients with relapsed or refractory multiple myeloma. *J. Clin. Oncol.* **2019**, *37*, 8012. [CrossRef]
15. Laabi, Y.; Gras, M.P.; Brouet, J.C.; Berger, R.; Larsen, C.J.; Tsapis, A. The BCMA gene, preferentially expressed during B lymphoid maturation, is bidirectionally transcribed. *Nucleic Acids Res.* **1994**, *22*, 1147–1154. [CrossRef] [PubMed]
16. Kozlow, E.J.; Wilson, G.L.; Fox, C.H.; Kehrl, J.H. Subtractive cDNA cloning of a novel member of the Ig gene superfamily expressed at high levels in activated B lymphocytes. *Blood* **1993**, *81*, 454–461. [CrossRef] [PubMed]
17. Zhou, L.J.; Schwarting, R.; Smith, H.M.; Tedder, T.F. A novel cell-surface molecule expressed by human interdigitating reticulum cells, Langerhans cells, and activated lymphocytes is a new member of the Ig superfamily. *J. Immunol.* **1992**, *149*, 735–742.
18. Laabi, Y.; Gras, M.P.; Carbonnel, F.; Brouet, J.C.; Berger, R.; Larsen, C.J.; Tsapis, A. A new gene, BCM, on chromosome 16 is fused to the interleukin 2 gene by a t(4;16)(q26;p13) translocation in a malignant T cell lymphoma. *EMBO J.* **1992**, *11*, 3897–3904. [CrossRef]
19. O'Connor, B.P.; Raman, V.S.; Erickson, L.D.; Cook, W.J.; Weaver, L.K.; Ahonen, C.; Lin, L.L.; Mantchev, G.T.; Bram, R.J.; Noelle, R.J. BCMA is essential for the survival of long-lived bone marrow plasma cells. *J. Exp. Med.* **2004**, *199*, 91–98. [CrossRef]

20. Shen, X.; Guo, Y.; Qi, J.; Shi, W.; Wu, X.; Ju, S. Binding of B-cell maturation antigen to B-cell activating factor induces survival of multiple myeloma cells by activating Akt and JNK signaling pathways. *Cell Biochem. Funct.* **2016**, *34*, 104–110. [CrossRef]
21. Demchenko, Y.N.; Kuehl, W.M. A critical role for the NFkB pathway in multiple myeloma. *Oncotarget* **2010**, *1*, 59–68. [CrossRef]
22. Chatterjee, M.; Jain, S.; Stuhmer, T.; Andrulis, M.; Ungethum, U.; Kuban, R.J.; Lorentz, H.; Bommert, K.; Topp, M.; Kramer, D.; et al. STAT3 and MAPK signaling maintain overexpression of heat shock proteins 90 alpha and beta in multiple myeloma cells, which critically contribute to tumor-cell survival. *Blood* **2007**, *109*, 720–728. [CrossRef]
23. Lentzsch, S.; Chatterjee, M.; Gries, M.; Bommert, K.; Gollasch, H.; Dorken, B.; Bargou, R.C. PI3-K/AKT/FKHR and MAPK signaling cascades are redundantly stimulated by a variety of cytokines and contribute independently to proliferation and survival of multiple myeloma cells. *Leukemia* **2004**, *18*, 1883–1890. [CrossRef] [PubMed]
24. Chatterjee, M.; Stuhmer, T.; Herrmann, P.; Bommert, K.; Dorken, B.; Bargou, R.C. Combined disruption of both the MEK/ERK and the IL-6R/STAT3 pathways is required to induce apoptosis of multiple myeloma cells in the presence of bone marrow stromal cells. *Blood* **2004**, *104*, 3712–3721. [CrossRef] [PubMed]
25. Carpenter, R.O.; Evbuomwan, M.O.; Pittaluga, S.; Rose, J.J.; Raffeld, M.; Yang, S.; Gress, R.E.; Hakim, F.T.; Kochenderfer, J.N. B-cell maturation antigen is a promising target for adoptive T-cell therapy of multiple myeloma. *Clin. Cancer Res.* **2013**, *19*, 2048–2060. [CrossRef] [PubMed]
26. Cho, S.F.; Anderson, K.C.; Tai, Y.T. Targeting B cell maturation antigen (BCMA) in multiple myeloma: Potential uses of BCMA-based immunotherapy. *Front. Immunol.* **2018**, *9*, 1821. [CrossRef] [PubMed]
27. Shah, N.; Chari, A.; Scott, E.; Mezzi, K.; Usmani, S.Z. B-cell maturation antigen (BCMA) in multiple myeloma: Rationale for targeting and current therapeutic approaches. *Leukemia* **2020**, *34*, 985–1005. [CrossRef] [PubMed]
28. Seckinger, A.; Delgado, J.A.; Moser, S.; Moreno, L.; Neuber, B.; Grab, A.; Lipp, S.; Merino, J.; Prosper, F.; Emde, M.; et al. Target expression, generation, preclinical activity, and pharmacokinetics of the BCMA-T cell bispecific antibody EM801 for multiple myeloma treatment. *Cancer Cell* **2017**, *31*, 396–410. [CrossRef]
29. Laurent, S.A.; Hoffmann, F.S.; Kuhn, P.H.; Cheng, Q.; Chu, Y.; Schmidt-Supprian, M.; Hauck, S.M.; Schuh, E.; Krumbholz, M.; Rubsamen, H.; et al. Gamma-secretase directly sheds the survival receptor BCMA from plasma cells. *Nat. Commun.* **2015**, *6*, 7333. [CrossRef]
30. Sanchez, E.; Li, M.; Kitto, A.; Li, J.; Wang, C.S.; Kirk, D.T.; Yellin, O.; Nichols, C.M.; Dreyer, M.P.; Ahles, C.P.; et al. Serum B-cell maturation antigen is elevated in multiple myeloma and correlates with disease status and survival. *Br. J. Haematol.* **2012**, *158*, 727–738. [CrossRef]
31. Golde, T.E.; Koo, E.H.; Felsenstein, K.M.; Osborne, B.A.; Miele, L. Gamma-secretase inhibitors and modulators. *Biochim. Biophys. Acta* **2013**, *1828*, 2898–2907. [CrossRef]
32. Yuan, X.; Wu, H.; Xu, H.; Xiong, H.; Chu, Q.; Yu, S.; Wu, G.S.; Wu, K. Notch signaling: An emerging therapeutic target for cancer treatment. *Cancer Lett.* **2015**, *369*, 20–27. [CrossRef]
33. Sanchez, E.; Gillespie, A.; Tang, G.; Ferros, M.; Harutyunyan, N.M.; Vardanyan, S.; Gottlieb, J.; Li, M.; Wang, C.S.; Chen, H.; et al. Soluble B-cell maturation antigen mediates tumor-induced immune deficiency in multiple myeloma. *Clin. Cancer Res.* **2016**, *22*, 3383–3397. [CrossRef] [PubMed]
34. Pont, M.J.; Hill, T.; Cole, G.O.; Abbott, J.J.; Kelliher, J.; Salter, A.I.; Hudecek, M.; Comstock, M.L.; Rajan, A.; Patel, B.K.R.; et al. Gamma-secretase inhibition increases efficacy of BCMA-specific chimeric antigen receptor T cells in multiple myeloma. *Blood* **2019**, *134*, 1585–1597. [CrossRef] [PubMed]
35. Zauner, G.; Selman, M.H.; Bondt, A.; Rombouts, Y.; Blank, D.; Deelder, A.M.; Wuhrer, M. Glycoproteomic analysis of antibodies. *Mol. Cell. Proteom.* **2013**, *12*, 856–865. [CrossRef] [PubMed]
36. Satoh, M.; Iida, S.; Shitara, K. Non-fucosylated therapeutic antibodies as next-generation therapeutic antibodies. *Expert Opin. Biol. Ther.* **2006**, *6*, 1161–1173. [CrossRef]
37. Mori, K.; Iida, S.; Yamane-Ohnuki, N.; Kanda, Y.; Kuni-Kamochi, R.; Nakano, R.; Imai-Nishiya, H.; Okazaki, A.; Shinkawa, T.; Natsume, A.; et al. Non-fucosylated therapeutic antibodies: The next generation of therapeutic antibodies. *Cytotechnology* **2007**, *55*, 109–114. [CrossRef]
38. Tai, Y.T.; Anderson, K.C. Targeting B-cell maturation antigen in multiple myeloma. *Immunotherapy* **2015**, *7*, 1187–1199. [CrossRef] [PubMed]

39. Tai, Y.T.; Mayes, P.A.; Acharya, C.; Zhong, M.Y.; Cea, M.; Cagnetta, A.; Craigen, J.; Yates, J.; Gliddon, L.; Fieles, W.; et al. Novel afucosylated anti-B cell maturation antigen-monomethyl auristatin F antibody-drug conjugate (GSK2857916) induces potent and selective anti-multiple myeloma activity. *Blood* **2014**, *123*, 3128–3138. [CrossRef]
40. Lonial, S.; Lee, H.C.; Badros, A.; Trudel, S.; Nooka, A.K.; Chari, A.; Abdallah, A.O.; Callander, N.; Lendvai, N.; Sborov, D.; et al. Belantamab mafodotin for relapsed or refractory multiple myeloma (DREAMM-2): A two-arm, randomised, open-label, phase 2 study. *Lancet Oncol.* **2019**, *21*, 207–221. [CrossRef]
41. Trudel, S.; Lendvai, N.; Popat, R.; Voorhees, P.M.; Reeves, B.; Libby III, E.N.; Richardson, P.G.; Anderson, L.; Sutherland, H.; Yong, K.; et al. Deep and durable responses in patients (pts) with relapsed/refractory multiple myeloma (MM) treated with monotherapy GSK2857916, an antibody drug conjugate against B-cell maturation antigen (BCMA): Preliminary results from part 2 of study BMA117159. *Blood* **2017**, *130*, 741.
42. Richardson, P.G.; Biswas, S.; Holkova, B.; Jackson, N.; Netherway, T.; Bao, W.; Ferron-Brady, G.; Yeakey, A.; Shelton, C.; Montes De Oca, R.; et al. Dreamm-5: Platform trial evaluating belantamab mafodotin (a BCMA-directed immuno-conjugate) in combination with novel agents in relapsed or refractory multiple myeloma (RRMM). *Blood* **2019**, *134*, 1857. [CrossRef]
43. Infante, J.R.; Ahlers, C.M.; Hodi, F.S.; Postel-Vinay, S.; Schellens, J.H.M.; Heymach, J.; Autio, K.A.; Barnette, M.S.; Struemper, H.; Watmuff, M.; et al. ENGAGE-1: A first in human study of the OX40 agonist GSK3174998 alone and in combination with pembrolizumab in patients with advanced solid tumors. *J. Clin. Oncol.* **2016**, *34*, TPS3107. [CrossRef]
44. Angevin, E.; Barnette, M.S.; Bauer, T.M.; Cho, D.C.; Ellis, C.E.; Gan, H.K.; Hansen, A.R.; Hoos, A.; Jewell, R.C.; Katz, J.; et al. INDUCE-1: A phase I open-label study of GSK3359609, an ICOS agonist antibody, administered alone and in combination with pembrolizumab in patients with advanced solid tumors. *J. Clin. Oncol.* **2017**, *35*, TPS3113. [CrossRef]
45. Han, X.; Vesely, M.D. Stimulating T cells against cancer with agonist immunostimulatory monoclonal antibodies. *Int. Rev. Cell Mol. Biol.* **2019**, *342*, 1–25. [PubMed]
46. Nooka, A.K.; Stockerl-Goldstein, K.; Quach, H.; Forbes, A.; Mateos, M.V.; Khot, A.; Tan, A.; Abonour, R.; Chopra, B.; Rogers, R.; et al. DREAMM-6: Safety and tolerability of belantamab mafodotin in combination with bortezomib/dexamethasone in relapsed/refractory multiple myeloma (RRMM). *J. Clin. Oncol.* **2020**, *38*, 8502. [CrossRef]
47. Kinneer, K.; Flynn, M.; Thomas, S.B.; Meekin, J.; Varkey, R.; Xiao, X.; Zhong, H.; Breen, S.; Hynes, P.G.; Fleming, R.; et al. Preclinical assessment of an antibody-PBD conjugate that targets BCMA on multiple myeloma and myeloma progenitor cells. *Leukemia* **2019**, *33*, 766–771. [CrossRef]
48. Kinneer, K.; Meekin, J.; Varkey, R.; Xiao, X.; Zhong, H.; Breen, S.; Hurt, E.; Thomas, S.; Flynn, M.; Hynes, P.; et al. Preclinical evaluation of MEDI2228, a BCMA-targeting pyrrolobenzodiazepine-linked antibody drug conjugate for the treatment of multiple myeloma. *Blood* **2017**, *130*, 3153.
49. Van Epps, H.; Anderson, M.; Yu, C.; Klussman, K.; Westendorf, L.; Carosino, C.; Manlove, L.; Cochran, J.; Neale, J.; Benjamin, D.; et al. SEA-BCMA: A highly active enhanced antibody for multiple myeloma. *Cancer Res.* **2018**, *78*, 3833.
50. Nikitorowicz-Buniak, J. FDA Safety Concerns Halt ACTR087 B Cell Non-Hodgkin Lymphoma Clinical Trial. Available online: https://lymphomahub.com/medical-information/fda-safety-concerns-halt-actr087-b-cell-non-hodgkin-lymphoma-clinical-trial (accessed on 11 June 2020).
51. Tiberghien, A.C.; Levy, J.N.; Masterson, L.A.; Patel, N.V.; Adams, L.R.; Corbett, S.; Williams, D.G.; Hartley, J.A.; Howard, P.W. Design and synthesis of tesirine, a clinical antibody-drug conjugate pyrrolobenzodiazepine dimer payload. *ACS Med. Chem. Lett.* **2016**, *7*, 983–987. [CrossRef]
52. Nisonoff, A.; Rivers, M.M. Recombination of a mixture of univalent antibody fragments of different specificity. *Arch. Biochem. Biophys.* **1961**, *93*, 460–462. [CrossRef]
53. Tai, Y.T.; Anderson, K.C. B cell maturation antigen (BCMA)-based immunotherapy for multiple myeloma. *Expert Opin. Biol. Ther.* **2019**, *19*, 1143–1156. [CrossRef] [PubMed]
54. Wang, Q.; Chen, Y.; Park, J.; Liu, X.; Hu, Y.; Wang, T.; McFarland, K.; Betenbaugh, M.J. Design and production of bispecific antibodies. *Antibodies (Basel, Switzerland)* **2019**, *8*, 43. [CrossRef] [PubMed]
55. Cohen, A.D.; Raje, N.; Fowler, J.A.; Mezzi, K.; Scott, E.C.; Dhodapkar, M.V. How to train your T cells: Overcoming immune dysfunction in multiple myeloma. *Clin. Cancer Res.* **2020**, *26*, 1541–1554. [CrossRef] [PubMed]

56. Suurs, F.V.; Lub-de Hooge, M.N.; de Vries, E.G.E.; de Groot, D.J.A. A review of bispecific antibodies and antibody constructs in oncology and clinical challenges. *Pharmacol. Ther.* **2019**, *201*, 103–119. [CrossRef]
57. Ahamadi-Fesharaki, R.; Fateh, A.; Vaziri, F.; Solgi, G.; Siadat, S.D.; Mahboudi, F.; Rahimi-Jamnani, F. Single-chain variable fragment-based bispecific antibodies: Hitting two targets with one sophisticated arrow. *Mol. Ther. Oncolytics* **2019**, *14*, 38–56. [CrossRef]
58. Wu, Z.; Cheung, N.V. T cell engaging bispecific antibody (T-BsAb): From technology to therapeutics. *Pharmacol. Ther.* **2018**, *182*, 161–175. [CrossRef]
59. Viardot, A.; Bargou, R. Bispecific antibodies in haematological malignancies. *Cancer Treat. Rev.* **2018**, *65*, 87–95. [CrossRef]
60. Offner, S.; Hofmeister, R.; Romaniuk, A.; Kufer, P.; Baeuerle, P.A. Induction of regular cytolytic T cell synapses by bispecific single-chain antibody constructs on MHC class I-negative tumor cells. *Mol. Immunol.* **2006**, *43*, 763–771. [CrossRef]
61. Haas, C.; Krinner, E.; Brischwein, K.; Hoffmann, P.; Lutterbuse, R.; Schlereth, B.; Kufer, P.; Baeuerle, P.A. Mode of cytotoxic action of T cell-engaging BiTE antibody MT110. *Immunobiology* **2009**, *214*, 441–453. [CrossRef]
62. Thiery, J.; Keefe, D.; Boulant, S.; Boucrot, E.; Walch, M.; Martinvalet, D.; Goping, I.S.; Bleackley, R.C.; Kirchhausen, T.; Lieberman, J. Perforin pores in the endosomal membrane trigger the release of endocytosed granzyme B into the cytosol of target cells. *Nat. Immunol.* **2011**, *12*, 770–777. [CrossRef]
63. Baeuerle, P.A.; Reinhardt, C. Bispecific T-cell engaging antibodies for cancer therapy. *Cancer Res.* **2009**, *69*, 4941–4944. [CrossRef] [PubMed]
64. Mazor, Y.; Sachsenmeier, K.F.; Yang, C.; Hansen, A.; Filderman, J.; Mulgrew, K.; Wu, H.; Dall'Acqua, W.F. Enhanced tumor-targeting selectivity by modulating bispecific antibody binding affinity and format valence. *Sci. Rep.* **2017**, *7*, 40098. [CrossRef] [PubMed]
65. Velders, M.P.; van Rhijn, C.M.; Oskam, E.; Fleuren, G.J.; Warnaar, S.O.; Litvinov, S.V. The impact of antigen density and antibody affinity on antibody-dependent cellular cytotoxicity: Relevance for immunotherapy of carcinomas. *Br. J. Cancer* **1998**, *78*, 478–483. [CrossRef]
66. Mandikian, D.; Takahashi, N.; Lo, A.A.; Li, J.; Eastham-Anderson, J.; Slaga, D.; Ho, J.; Hristopoulos, M.; Clark, R.; Totpal, K.; et al. Relative target affinities of T-cell-dependent bispecific antibodies determine biodistribution in a solid tumor mouse model. *Mol. Cancer Ther.* **2018**, *17*, 776–785. [CrossRef] [PubMed]
67. Topp, M.S.; Duell, J.; Zugmaier, G.; Attal, M.; Moreau, P.; Langer, C.; Krönke, J.; Facon, T.; Salnikov, A.V.; Lesley, R.; et al. Anti-B-cell maturation antigen BiTE molecule AMG 420 induces responses in multiple myeloma. *J. Clin. Oncol.* **2020**, *38*, 775–783. [CrossRef] [PubMed]
68. Cho, S.-F.; Lin, L.; Xing, L.; Wen, K.; Yu, T.; Wahl, J.; Matthes, K.; Munshi, N.; Anderson, K.C.; Arvedson, T.; et al. AMG 701, a half-life extended anti-BCMA BiTE®, potently induces T cell-redirected lysis of human multiple myeloma cells and can be combined with IMiDs to overcome the immunosuppressive bone marrow microenvironment. *Clin. Lymphoma Myeloma Leuk.* **2019**, *19*, e54. [CrossRef]
69. Cooper, D.; Madduri, D.; Lentzsch, S.; Jagannath, S.; Li, J.; Boyapati, A.; Adriaens, L.; Chokshi, D.; Zhu, M.; Lowy, I.; et al. Safety and preliminary clinical activity of REGN5458, an anti-BCMA x anti-CD3 bispecific antibody, in patients with relapsed/refractory multiple myeloma. *Blood* **2019**, *134*, 3176. [CrossRef]
70. Girgis, S.; Shetty, S.; Jiao, T.; Amuzie, C.; Weinstock, D.; Watson, R.G.; Ford, J.; Pillarisetti, K.; Baldwin, E.; Bellew, K. Exploratory pharmacokinetic/pharmacodynamic and tolerability study of BCMAxCD3 in cynomolgus monkeys. *Blood* **2016**, *128*, 5668. [CrossRef]
71. Suzuki, S.; Annaka, H.; Konno, S.; Kumagai, I.; Asano, R. Engineering the hinge region of human IgG1 Fc-fused bispecific antibodies to improve fragmentation resistance. *Sci. Rep.* **2018**, *8*, 17253. [CrossRef]
72. Lesokhin, A.M.; Raje, N.; Gasparetto, C.J.; Walker, J.; Krupka, H.I.; Joh, T.; Taylor, C.T.; Jakubowiak, A.J. A phase I, open-label study to evaluate the safety, pharmacokinetic, pharmacodynamic, and clinical activity of PF-06863135, a B-cell maturation antigen/CD3 bispecific antibody, in patients with relapsed/refractory advanced multiple myeloma. *Blood* **2018**, *132*, 3229. [CrossRef]
73. Raje, N.S.; Jakubowiak, A.; Gasparetto, C.; Cornell, R.F.; Krupka, H.I.; Navarro, D.; Forgie, A.J.; Udata, C.; Basu, C.; Chou, J.; et al. Safety, clinical activity, pharmacokinetics, and pharmacodynamics from a phase I study of PF-06863135, a B-cell maturation antigen (BCMA)–CD3 bispecific antibody, in patients with relapsed/refractory multiple myeloma (RRMM). *Blood* **2019**, *128*, 1869. [CrossRef]

74. Costa, L.J.; Wong, S.W.; Bermúdez, A.; de la Rubia, J.; Mateos, M.-V.; Ocio, E.M.; Rodríguez-Otero, P.; San-Miguel, J.; Li, S.; Sarmiento, R.; et al. First clinical study of the B-cell maturation antigen (BCMA) 2+1 T cell engager (TCE) CC-93269 in patients (pts) with relapsed/refractory multiple myeloma (RRMM): Interim results of a phase 1 multicenter trial. *Blood* **2019**, *134*, 143. [CrossRef]
75. Trinklein, N.D.; Pham, D.; Schellenberger, U.; Buelow, B.; Boudreau, A.; Choudhry, P.; Clarke, S.C.; Dang, K.; Harris, K.E.; Iyer, S.; et al. Efficient tumor killing and minimal cytokine release with novel T-cell agonist bispecific antibodies. *mAbs* **2019**, *11*, 639–652. [CrossRef] [PubMed]
76. Buelow, B.; D'Souza, A.; Rodriguez, C.; Vij, R.; Nath, R.; Snyder, M.; Pham, D.; Patel, A.; Iyer, S. A multicenter, phase 1, open-label, dose-escalation and expansion study of TNB-383B, a bispecific antibody targeting BCMA in subjects with relapsed or refractory multiple myeloma. *Blood* **2019**, *134*, 1874. [CrossRef]
77. Law, C.L.; Aaron, W.; Austin, R.; Barath, M.; Callihan, E.; Evans, T.; Gamez Guerrero, M.; Hemmati, G.; Jones, A.; Kwant, K.; et al. Preclinical and nonclinical characterization of HPN217: A tri-Specific T cell activating construct (TriTAC) targeting B cell maturation antigen (BCMA) for the treatment of multiple myeloma. *Blood* **2018**, *132*, 3225. [CrossRef]
78. Dahlen, E.; Veitonmaki, N.; Norlen, P. Bispecific antibodies in cancer immunotherapy. *Ther. Adv. Vaccines Immunother.* **2018**, *6*, 3–17. [CrossRef]
79. Sanford, M. Blinatumomab: First global approval. *Drugs* **2015**, *75*, 321–327. [CrossRef]
80. Jen, E.Y.; Xu, Q.; Schetter, A.; Przepiorka, D.; Shen, Y.L.; Roscoe, D.; Sridhara, R.; Deisseroth, A.; Philip, R.; Farrell, A.T.; et al. FDA approval: Blinatumomab for patients with B-cell precursor acute lymphoblastic leukemia in morphologic remission with minimal residual disease. *Clin. Cancer Res.* **2019**, *25*, 473–477. [CrossRef]
81. Strohl, W.R.; Naso, M. Bispecific T-cell redirection versus chimeric antigen receptor (CAR)-T cells as approaches to kill cancer cells. *Antibodies (Basel, Switzerland)* **2019**, *8*, 41. [CrossRef]
82. Shimabukuro-Vornhagen, A.; Godel, P.; Subklewe, M.; Stemmler, H.J.; Schlosser, H.A.; Schlaak, M.; Kochanek, M.; Boll, B.; von Bergwelt-Baildon, M.S. Cytokine release syndrome. *J. Immunother. Cancer* **2018**, *6*, 56. [CrossRef]
83. Kennedy, L.B.; Salama, A.K.S. A review of cancer immunotherapy toxicity. *CA Cancer J. Clin.* **2020**, *70*, 86–104. [CrossRef]
84. Brudno, J.N.; Kochenderfer, J.N. Recent advances in CAR T-cell toxicity: Mechanisms, manifestations and management. *Blood Rev.* **2019**, *34*, 45–55. [CrossRef] [PubMed]
85. Mehta, P.; McAuley, D.F.; Brown, M.; Sanchez, E.; Tattersall, R.S.; Manson, J.J. COVID-19: Consider cytokine storm syndromes and immunosuppression. *Lancet* **2020**, *395*, 1033–1034. [CrossRef]
86. Soy, M.; Keser, G.; Atagündüz, P.; Tabak, F.; Atagündüz, I.; Kayhan, S. Cytokine storm in COVID-19: Pathogenesis and overview of anti-inflammatory agents used in treatment. *Clin. Rheumatol.* **2020**, *39*, 2085–2094. [CrossRef] [PubMed]
87. Brudno, J.N.; Kochenderfer, J.N. Toxicities of chimeric antigen receptor T cells: Recognition and management. *Blood* **2016**, *127*, 3321–3330. [CrossRef] [PubMed]
88. Neelapu, S.S.; Tummala, S.; Kebriaei, P.; Wierda, W.; Gutierrez, C.; Locke, F.L.; Komanduri, K.V.; Lin, Y.; Jain, N.; Daver, N.; et al. Chimeric antigen receptor T-cell therapy—Assessment and management of toxicities. *Nat. Rev. Clin. Oncol.* **2018**, *15*, 47–62. [CrossRef]
89. Le, R.Q.; Li, L.; Yuan, W.; Shord, S.S.; Nie, L.; Habtemariam, B.A.; Przepiorka, D.; Farrell, A.T.; Pazdur, R. FDA approval summary: Tocilizumab for treatment of chimeric antigen receptor T cell-induced severe or life-threatening cytokine release syndrome. *Oncologist* **2018**, *23*, 943–947. [CrossRef]
90. Yu, S.; Yi, M.; Qin, S.; Wu, K. Next generation chimeric antigen receptor T cells: Safety strategies to overcome toxicity. *Mol. Cancer* **2019**, *18*, 125. [CrossRef]
91. Griffioen, M.; van Egmond, E.H.; Kester, M.G.; Willemze, R.; Falkenburg, J.H.; Heemskerk, M.H. Retroviral transfer of human CD20 as a suicide gene for adoptive T-cell therapy. *Haematologica* **2009**, *94*, 1316–1320. [CrossRef]
92. Diaconu, I.; Ballard, B.; Zhang, M.; Chen, Y.; West, J.; Dotti, G.; Savoldo, B. Inducible caspase-9 selectively modulates the toxicities of CD19-specific chimeric antigen receptor-modified T cells. *Mol. Ther.* **2017**, *25*, 580–592. [CrossRef]

93. Straathof, K.C.; Pulè, M.A.; Yotnda, P.; Dotti, G.; Vanin, E.F.; Brenner, M.K.; Heslop, H.E.; Spencer, D.M.; Rooney, C.M. An inducible caspase 9 safety switch for T-cell therapy. *Blood* **2005**, *105*, 4247–4254. [CrossRef] [PubMed]
94. Di Stasi, A.; Tey, S.K.; Dotti, G.; Fujita, Y.; Kennedy-Nasser, A.; Martinez, C.; Straathof, K.; Liu, E.; Durett, A.G.; Grilley, B.; et al. Inducible apoptosis as a safety switch for adoptive cell therapy. *N. Engl. J. Med.* **2011**, *365*, 1673–1683. [CrossRef] [PubMed]
95. Gargett, T.; Brown, M.P. The inducible caspase-9 suicide gene system as a "safety switch" to limit on-target, off-tumor toxicities of chimeric antigen receptor T cells. *Front. Pharmacol.* **2014**, *5*, 235. [CrossRef] [PubMed]
96. Nie, S.; Wang, Z.; Moscoso-Castro, M.; D'Souza, P.; Lei, C.; Xu, J.; Gu, J. Biology drives the discovery of bispecific antibodies as innovative therapeutics. *Antib. Ther.* **2020**, *3*, 18–62. [CrossRef]
97. Li, Z.; Li, Q.; Zhang, G.; Ma, X.; Hu, X.; Ouyang, K.; Li, B.; Liu, Z. A novel bispecific BCMAxCD3 T cell-engaging antibody that treat multiple myeloma (MM) with minimal cytokine secretion. *Ann. Oncol.* **2019**, *30*, V808. [CrossRef]
98. Smyth, M.J.; Cretney, E.; Kelly, J.M.; Westwood, J.A.; Street, S.E.; Yagita, H.; Takeda, K.; van Dommelen, S.L.; Degli-Esposti, M.A.; Hayakawa, Y. Activation of NK cell cytotoxicity. *Mol. Immunol.* **2005**, *42*, 501–510. [CrossRef]
99. Gantke, T.; Weichel, M.; Reusch, U.; Ellwanger, K.; Fucek, I.; Griep, R.; Molkenthin, V.; Kashala, O.; Treder, M. Trispecific antibodies for selective CD16A-directed NK-cell engagement in multiple myeloma. *Blood* **2016**, *128*, 4513. [CrossRef]
100. Draghi, M.; Schafer, J.L.; Nelson, A.; Frye, Z.; Oliphant, A.; Haserlat, S.; Lajoie, J.; Rogers, K.; Villinger, F.; Schmidt, M.; et al. Preclinical development of a first-in-class NKp30xBCMA NK cell engager for the treatment of multiple myeloma. *Cancer Res.* **2019**, *79*, 4972.
101. Watkins-Yoon, J.; Guzman, W.; Oliphant, A.; Haserlat, S.; Leung, A.; Chottin, C.; Ophir, M.; Vekeria, J.; Nelson, A.P.; Frye, Z.; et al. CTX-8573, an innate-cell engager targeting BCMA, is a highly potent multispecific antibody for the treatment of multiple myeloma. *Blood* **2019**, *134*, 3182. [CrossRef]
102. Ross, T.; Reusch, U.; Wingert, S.; Haneke, T.; Klausz, K.; Otte, A.K.; Schub, N.; Knackmuss, S.; Müller, T.; Ellwanger, K.; et al. Preclinical characterization of AFM26, a novel B cell maturation antigen (BCMA)-directed tetravalent bispecific antibody for high affinity retargeting of NK cells against myeloma. *J. Clin. Oncol.* **2018**, *35*, 1927. [CrossRef]
103. Roex, G.; Feys, T.; Beguin, Y.; Kerre, T.; Poire, X.; Lewalle, P.; Vandenberghe, P.; Bron, D.; Anguille, S. Chimeric antigen receptor-T-cell therapy for B-cell hematological malignancies: An update of the pivotal clinical trial data. *Pharmaceutics* **2020**, *12*, 194. [CrossRef] [PubMed]
104. Rosenbaum, L. Tragedy, perseverance, and chance—The story of CAR-T therapy. *N. Engl. J. Med.* **2017**, *377*, 1313–1315. [CrossRef]
105. Ruella, M.; June, C.H. Chimeric antigen receptor T cells for B cell neoplasms: Choose the right CAR for you. *Curr. Hematol. Malig. Rep.* **2016**, *11*, 368–384. [CrossRef] [PubMed]
106. Radic, M. Armed and accurate: Engineering cytotoxic T cells for eradication of leukemia. *BMC Biotechnol.* **2012**, *12*, 6. [CrossRef] [PubMed]
107. Wall, D.A.; Krueger, J. Chimeric antigen receptor T cell therapy comes to clinical practice. *Curr. Oncol.* **2020**, *27* (Suppl. 2), S115–S123. [CrossRef] [PubMed]
108. Badar, T.; Shah, N.N. Chimeric antigen receptor T cell therapy for acute lymphoblastic leukemia. *Curr. Treat. Options Oncol.* **2020**, *21*, 16. [CrossRef]
109. Locke, F.L.; Go, W.Y.; Neelapu, S.S. Development and use of the anti-CD19 chimeric antigen receptor T-cell therapy axicabtagene ciloleucel in large B-cell lymphoma: A review. *JAMA Oncol.* **2019**, *6*, 281–290. [CrossRef]
110. Braendstrup, P.; Levine, B.L.; Ruella, M. The long road to the first FDA-approved gene therapy: Chimeric antigen receptor T cells targeting CD19. *Cytotherapy* **2020**, *22*, 57–69. [CrossRef]
111. van der Stegen, S.J.; Hamieh, M.; Sadelain, M. The pharmacology of second-generation chimeric antigen receptors. *Nat. Rev. Drug Discov.* **2015**, *14*, 499–509. [CrossRef]
112. Neelapu, S.S.; Locke, F.L.; Bartlett, N.L.; Lekakis, L.J.; Miklos, D.B.; Jacobson, C.A.; Braunschweig, I.; Oluwole, O.O.; Siddiqi, T.; Lin, Y.; et al. Axicabtagene ciloleucel CAR T-cell therapy in refractory large B-cell lymphoma. *N. Engl. J. Med.* **2017**, *377*, 2531–2544. [CrossRef]

113. Locke, F.L.; Ghobadi, A.; Jacobson, C.A.; Miklos, D.B.; Lekakis, L.J.; Oluwole, O.O.; Lin, Y.; Braunschweig, I.; Hill, B.T.; Timmerman, J.M.; et al. Long-term safety and activity of axicabtagene ciloleucel in refractory large B-cell lymphoma (ZUMA-1): A single-arm, multicentre, phase 1-2 trial. *Lancet Oncol.* **2019**, *20*, 31–42. [CrossRef]

114. Schuster, S.J.; Bishop, M.R.; Tam, C.S.; Waller, E.K.; Borchmann, P.; McGuirk, J.P.; Jäger, U.; Jaglowski, S.; Andreadis, C.; Westin, J.R.; et al. Tisagenlecleucel in adult relapsed or refractory diffuse large B-cell lymphoma. *N. Engl. J. Med.* **2019**, *380*, 45–56. [CrossRef] [PubMed]

115. Abramson, J.S.; Gordon, L.I.; Palomba, M.L.; Lunning, M.A.; Arnason, J.E.; Forero-Torres, A.; Wang, M.; Maloney, D.G.; Sehgal, A.; Andreadis, C.; et al. Updated safety and long term clinical outcomes in TRANSCEND NHL 001, pivotal trial of lisocabtagene maraleucel (JCAR017) in R/R aggressive NHL. *J. Clin. Oncol.* **2018**, *36*, 7505. [CrossRef]

116. Muranski, P.; Boni, A.; Wrzesinski, C.; Citrin, D.E.; Rosenberg, S.A.; Childs, R.; Restifo, N.P. Increased intensity lymphodepletion and adoptive immunotherapy–how far can we go? *Nat. Clin. Pract. Oncol.* **2006**, *3*, 668–681. [CrossRef]

117. Dudley, M.E.; Wunderlich, J.R.; Robbins, P.F.; Yang, J.C.; Hwu, P.; Schwartzentruber, D.J.; Topalian, S.L.; Sherry, R.; Restifo, N.P.; Hubicki, A.M.; et al. Cancer regression and autoimmunity in patients after clonal repopulation with antitumor lymphocytes. *Science* **2002**, *298*, 850–854. [CrossRef]

118. Hughes, M.S.; Yu, Y.Y.; Dudley, M.E.; Zheng, Z.; Robbins, P.F.; Li, Y.; Wunderlich, J.; Hawley, R.G.; Moayeri, M.; Rosenberg, S.A.; et al. Transfer of a TCR gene derived from a patient with a marked antitumor response conveys highly active T-cell effector functions. *Hum. Gene Ther.* **2005**, *16*, 457–472. [CrossRef]

119. Hirayama, A.V.; Gauthier, J.; Hay, K.A.; Voutsinas, J.M.; Wu, Q.; Gooley, T.; Li, D.; Cherian, S.; Chen, X.; Pender, B.S.; et al. The response to lymphodepletion impacts PFS in patients with aggressive non-Hodgkin lymphoma treated with CD19 CAR T cells. *Blood* **2019**, *133*, 1876–1887. [CrossRef]

120. Gattinoni, L.; Finkelstein, S.E.; Klebanoff, C.A.; Antony, P.A.; Palmer, D.C.; Spiess, P.J.; Hwang, L.N.; Yu, Z.; Wrzesinski, C.; Heimann, D.M.; et al. Removal of homeostatic cytokine sinks by lymphodepletion enhances the efficacy of adoptively transferred tumor-specific CD8+ T cells. *J. Exp. Med.* **2005**, *202*, 907–912. [CrossRef]

121. Ninomiya, S.; Narala, N.; Huye, L.; Yagyu, S.; Savoldo, B.; Dotti, G.; Heslop, H.E.; Brenner, M.K.; Rooney, C.M.; Ramos, C.A. Tumor indoleamine 2,3-dioxygenase (IDO) inhibits CD19-CAR T cells and is downregulated by lymphodepleting drugs. *Blood* **2015**, *125*, 3905–3916. [CrossRef]

122. Mateo, G.; Montalban, M.A.; Vidriales, M.B.; Lahuerta, J.J.; Mateos, M.V.; Gutierrez, N.; Rosinol, L.; Montejano, L.; Blade, J.; Martinez, R.; et al. Prognostic value of immunophenotyping in multiple myeloma: A study by the PETHEMA/GEM cooperative study groups on patients uniformly treated with high-dose therapy. *J. Clin. Oncol.* **2008**, *26*, 2737–2744. [CrossRef]

123. Cannizzo, E.; Carulli, G.; Del Vecchio, L.; Ottaviano, V.; Bellio, E.; Zenari, E.; Azzara, A.; Petrini, M.; Preffer, F. The role of CD19 and CD27 in the diagnosis of multiple myeloma by flow cytometry: A new statistical model. *Am. J. Clin. Pathol.* **2012**, *137*, 377–386. [CrossRef] [PubMed]

124. Zandecki, M.; Facon, T.; Bernardi, F.; Izydorczyk, V.; Dupond, L.; Francois, M.; Reade, R.; Iaru, T.; Bauters, F.; Cosson, A. CD19 and immunophenotype of bone marrow plasma cells in monoclonal gammopathy of undetermined significance. *J. Clin. Pathol.* **1995**, *48*, 548–552. [CrossRef] [PubMed]

125. Feinberg, D.; Paul, B.; Kang, Y. The promise of chimeric antigen receptor (CAR) T cell therapy in multiple myeloma. *Cell. Immunol.* **2019**, *345*, 103964. [CrossRef] [PubMed]

126. Garfall, A.L.; Stadtmauer, E.A.; Hwang, W.T.; Lacey, S.F.; Melenhorst, J.J.; Krevvata, M.; Carroll, M.P.; Matsui, W.H.; Wang, Q.; Dhodapkar, M.V.; et al. Anti-CD19 CAR T cells with high-dose melphalan and autologous stem cell transplantation for refractory multiple myeloma. *JCI Insight* **2018**, *3*, e120505. [CrossRef]

127. Hosen, N. Chimeric antigen receptor T-cell therapy for multiple myeloma. *Int. J. Hematol.* **2020**, *111*, 530–534. [CrossRef]

128. Huang, H.; Wu, H.W.; Hu, Y.X. Current advances in chimeric antigen receptor T-cell therapy for refractory/relapsed multiple myeloma. *J. Zhejiang Univ. Sci. B* **2020**, *21*, 29–41. [CrossRef]

129. Brudno, J.N.; Maric, I.; Hartman, S.D.; Rose, J.J.; Wang, M.; Lam, N.; Stetler-Stevenson, M.; Salem, D.; Yuan, C.; Pavletic, S.; et al. T cells genetically modified to express an anti-B-cell maturation antigen chimeric antigen receptor cause remissions of poor-prognosis relapsed multiple myeloma. *J. Clin. Oncol.* **2018**, *36*, 2267–2280. [CrossRef]

130. Raje, N.; Berdeja, J.; Lin, Y.; Siegel, D.; Jagannath, S.; Madduri, D.; Liedtke, M.; Rosenblatt, J.; Maus, M.V.; Turka, A.; et al. Anti-BCMA CAR T-cell therapy bb2121 in relapsed or refractory multiple myeloma. *N. Engl. J. Med.* **2019**, *380*, 1726–1737. [CrossRef]

131. Munshi, N.C.; Anderson, J.L.D.; Shah, N.; Jagannath, S.; Berdeja, J.G.; Lonial, S.; Raje, N.S.; DiCapua Siegel, D.S.; Lin, Y.; Oriol, A.; et al. Idecabtagene vicleucel (ide-cel; bb2121), a BCMA-targeted CAR T-cell therapy, in patients with relapsed and refractory multiple myeloma (RRMM): Initial KarMMa results. *J. Clin. Oncol.* **2020**, *38*, 8503. [CrossRef]

132. Press Release (Brisol Myers Squibb, 6 December 2019). Available online: https://news.bms.com/press-release/corporatefinancial-news/bristol-myers-squibb-and-bluebird-bio-announce-positive-top-li (accessed on 12 June 2020).

133. Berdeja, J.G.; Alsina, M.; Shah, N.D.; Siegel, D.S.; Jagannath, S.; Madduri, D.; Kaufman, J.L.; Munshi, N.C.; Rosenblatt, J.; Jasielec, J.K.; et al. Updated results from an ongoing phase 1 clinical study of bb21217 anti-Bcma CAR T cell therapy. *Blood* **2019**, *134*, 927. [CrossRef]

134. Xu, J.; Chen, L.J.; Yang, S.S.; Sun, Y.; Wu, W.; Liu, Y.F.; Xu, J.; Zhuang, Y.; Zhang, W.; Weng, X.Q.; et al. Exploratory trial of a biepitopic CAR T-targeting B cell maturation antigen in relapsed/refractory multiple myeloma. *Proc. Natl. Acad. Sci. USA* **2019**, *116*, 9543–9551. [CrossRef] [PubMed]

135. Zhao, W.H.; Liu, J.; Wang, B.Y.; Chen, Y.X.; Cao, X.M.; Yang, Y.; Zhang, Y.L.; Wang, F.X.; Zhang, P.Y.; Lei, B.; et al. A phase 1, open-label study of LCAR-B38M, a chimeric antigen receptor T cell therapy directed against B cell maturation antigen, in patients with relapsed or refractory multiple myeloma. *J. Hematol. Oncol.* **2018**, *11*, 141. [CrossRef] [PubMed]

136. Zhao, W.H.; Liu, J.; Wang, B.Y.; Chen, Y.X.; Cao, X.M.; Yang, Y.; Zhang, Y.L.; Wang, F.X.; Zhang, P.Y.; Lei, B.; et al. Updated analysis of a phase 1, open-label study of LCAR-B38M, a chimeric antigen receptor T cell therapy directed against B-cell maturation antigen, in patients with relapsed/refractory multiple myeloma. *Blood* **2018**, *132*, 955. [CrossRef]

137. Madduri, D.; Usmani, S.Z.; Jagannath, S.; Singh, I.; Zudaire, E.; Yeh, T.M.; Allred, A.J.; Banerjee, A.; Goldberg, J.D.; Schecter, J.M.; et al. Results from CARTITUDE-1: A phase 1b/2 study of JNJ-4528, a CAR-T cell therapy directed against B-cell maturation antigen (BCMA), in patients with relapsed and/or refractory multiple myeloma (R/R MM). *Blood* **2019**, *134*, 577. [CrossRef]

138. Gregory, T.; Cohen, A.D.; Costello, C.L.; Ali, S.A.; Berdeja, J.G.; Ostertag, E.M.; Martin, C.; Shedlock, D.J.; Resler, M.L.; Spear, M.A.; et al. Efficacy and safety of P-Bcma-101 CAR-T cells in patients with relapsed/refractory (r/r) multiple myeloma (MM). *Blood* **2018**, *132*, 1012. [CrossRef]

139. Costello, C.L.; Gregory, T.K.; Ali, S.A.; Berdeja, J.G.; Patel, K.K.; Shah, N.D.; Ostertag, E.; Martin, C.; Ghoddusi, M.; Shedlock, D.J.; et al. Phase 2 study of the response and safety of P-Bcma-101 CAR-T cells in patients with relapsed/refractory (r/r) multiple myeloma (MM) (PRIME). *Blood* **2019**, *134*, 3184. [CrossRef]

140. Mailankody, S.; Ghosh, A.; Staehr, M.; Purdon, T.J.; Roshal, M.; Halton, E.; Diamonte, C.; Pineda, J.; Anant, P.; Bernal, Y.; et al. Clinical responses and pharmacokinetics of MCARH171, a human-derived BCMA targeted CAR T cell therapy in relapsed/refractory multiple myeloma: Final results of a phase I clinical trial. *Blood* **2018**, *132*, 959. [CrossRef]

141. Green, D.J.; Pont, M.; Sather, B.D.; Cowan, A.J.; Turtle, C.J.; Till, B.G.; Nagengast, A.M.; Libby, I.E.N.; Becker, P.S.; Coffey, D.G.; et al. Fully human Bcma targeted chimeric antigen receptor T cells administered in a defined composition demonstrate potency at low doses in advanced stage high risk multiple myeloma. *Blood* **2018**, *132*, 1011. [CrossRef]

142. Mailankody, S.; Htut, M.; Lee, K.P.; Bensinger, W.; Devries, T.; Piasecki, J.; Ziyad, S.; Blake, M.; Byon, J.; Jakubowiak, A. JCARH125, anti-BCMA CAR T-cell therapy for relapsed/refractory multiple myeloma: Initial proof of concept results from a phase 1/2 multicenter study (EVOLVE). *Blood* **2018**, *132*, 957. [CrossRef]

143. Jiang, S.; Jin, J.; Hao, S.; Yang, M.; Chen, L.; Ruan, H.; Xiao, J.; Wang, W.; Li, Z.; Yu, K. Low dose of human scFv-derived BCMA-targeted CAR-T cells achieved fast response and high complete remission in patients with relapsed/refractory multiple myeloma. *Blood* **2018**, *132*, 960. [CrossRef]

144. Lin, L.; Xing, L.; Cho, S.-F.; Wen, K.; Hsieh, P.; Kurtoglu, M.; Zhang, Y.; Stewart, C.A.; Anderson, K.C.; Tai, Y.-T. Preclinical evaluation of CD8+ anti-BCMA mRNA CAR T-cells for control of multiple myeloma. *Clin. Lymphoma Myeloma Leuk.* **2019**, *19*, e169. [CrossRef]

145. Cohen, A.D.; Garfall, A.L.; Stadtmauer, E.A.; Melenhorst, J.J.; Lacey, S.F.; Lancaster, E.; Vogl, D.T.; Weiss, B.M.; Dengel, K.; Nelson, A.; et al. B cell maturation antigen-specific CAR T cells are clinically active in multiple myeloma. *J. Clin. Investig.* **2019**, *129*, 2210–2221. [CrossRef] [PubMed]

146. Bu, D.X.; Singh, R.; Choi, E.E.; Ruella, M.; Nunez-Cruz, S.; Mansfield, K.G.; Bennett, P.; Barton, N.; Wu, Q.; Zhang, J.; et al. Pre-clinical validation of B cell maturation antigen (BCMA) as a target for T cell immunotherapy of multiple myeloma. *Oncotarget* **2018**, *9*, 25764–25780. [CrossRef]

147. Cohen, A.D.; Garfall, A.L.; Stadtmauer, E.A.; Lacey, S.F.; Lancaster, E.; Vogl, D.T.; Dengel, K.; Ambrose, D.E.; Chen, F.; Plesa, G.; et al. B-cell maturation antigen (BCMA)-specific chimeric antigen receptor T cells (CART-BCMA) for multiple myeloma (MM): Initial safety and efficacy from a phase I study. *Blood* **2016**, *128*, 1147. [CrossRef]

148. Shi, X.; Yan, L.; Shang, J.; Qu, S.; Kang, L.; Zhou, J.; Jin, S.; Yao, W.; Yao, Y.; Yan, S.; et al. Tandom autologous transplantation and combined infusion of CD19 and BCMA-specific chimeric antigen receptor T cells for high risk MM: Initial safety and efficacy report from a clinical pilot study. *Blood* **2018**, *132*, 1009. [CrossRef]

149. Yan, L.; Shang, J.; Kang, L.; Shi, X.; Zhou, J.; Jin, S.; Yao, W.; Yao, Y.; Chen, G.; Zhu, Z.; et al. Combined infusion of CD19 and BCMA-specific chimeric antigen receptor T cells for RRMM: Initial safety and efficacy report from a clinical pilot study. *Blood* **2017**, *130*, 506.

150. Timmers, M.; Roex, G.; Wang, Y.; Campillo-Davo, D.; Van Tendeloo, V.F.I.; Chu, Y.; Berneman, Z.N.; Luo, F.; Van Acker, H.H.; Anguille, S. Chimeric antigen receptor-modified T cell therapy in multiple myeloma: Beyond B cell maturation antigen. *Front. Immunol.* **2019**, *10*, 1613. [CrossRef]

151. Mikkilineni, L.; Manasanch, E.E.; Lam, N.; Vanasse, D.; Brudno, J.N.; Maric, I.; Rose, J.J.; Stetler-Stevenson, M.; Wang, H.W.; Yuan, C.M.; et al. T cells expressing an anti-B-cell maturation antigen (BCMA) chimeric antigen receptor with a fully-human heavy-chain-only antigen recognition domain induce remissions in patients with relapsed multiple myeloma. *Blood* **2019**, *134*, 3230. [CrossRef]

152. Sachdeva, M.; Busser, B.W.; Temburni, S.; Jahangiri, B.; Gautron, A.S.; Marechal, A.; Juillerat, A.; Williams, A.; Depil, S.; Duchateau, P.; et al. Repurposing endogenous immune pathways to tailor and control chimeric antigen receptor T cell functionality. *Nat. Commun.* **2019**, *10*, 5100. [CrossRef]

153. Gautron, A.S.; Juillerat, A.; Guyot, V.; Filhol, J.M.; Dessez, E.; Duclert, A.; Duchateau, P.; Poirot, L. Fine and predictable tuning of TALEN gene editing targeting for improved T cell adoptive immunotherapy. *Mol. Ther. Nucleic Acids* **2017**, *9*, 312–321. [CrossRef]

154. Li, C.; Zhou, X.; Wang, J.; Hu, G.; Yang, Y.; Meng, L.; Hong, Z.; Chen, L.; Zhou, J. Clinical responses and pharmacokinetics of fully human BCMA targeting CAR T cell therapy in relapsed/refractory multiple myeloma. In Proceedings of the 17th International Myeloma Workshop, Boston, MA, USA, 12–15 September 2019. OAB-033.

155. Jurica, M.S.; Monnat, R.J., Jr.; Stoddard, B.L. DNA recognition and cleavage by the LAGLIDADG homing endonuclease I-CreI. *Mol. Cell* **1998**, *2*, 469–476. [CrossRef]

156. Lin, Q.; Zhao, J.; Song, Y.; Liu, D. Recent updates on CAR T clinical trials for multiple myeloma. *Mol. Cancer* **2019**, *18*, 154. [CrossRef] [PubMed]

157. Friedman, K.M.; Garrett, T.E.; Evans, J.W.; Horton, H.M.; Latimer, H.J.; Seidel, S.L.; Horvath, C.J.; Morgan, R.A. Effective targeting of multiple B-cell maturation antigen-expressing hematological malignancies by anti-B-cell maturation antigen chimeric antigen receptor T Cells. *Hum. Gene Ther.* **2018**, *29*, 585–601. [CrossRef] [PubMed]

158. Press Release (Bristol Myers Squibb, 31 March 2020). Available online: https://news.bms.com/press-release/celltherapy/bristol-myers-squibb-and-bluebird-bio-announce-submission-biologics-licens (accessed on 12 June 2020).

159. Zheng, W.; O'Hear, C.E.; Alli, R.; Basham, J.H.; Abdelsamed, H.A.; Palmer, L.E.; Jones, L.L.; Youngblood, B.; Geiger, T.L. PI3K orchestration of the in vivo persistence of chimeric antigen receptor-modified T cells. *Leukemia* **2018**, *32*, 1157–1167. [CrossRef]

160. Goldberg, S.D.; Cardoso, R.M.; Lin, T.; Spinka-Doms, T.; Klein, D.; Jacobs, S.A.; Dudkin, V.; Gilliland, G.; O'Neil, K.T. Engineering a targeted delivery platform using Centyrins. *Protein Eng. Des. Sel.* **2016**, *29*, 563–572. [CrossRef]

161. Gattinoni, L.; Speiser, D.E.; Lichterfeld, M.; Bonini, C. T memory stem cells in health and disease. *Nat. Med.* **2017**, *23*, 18–27. [CrossRef]

162. Sidana, S.; Shah, N. CAR T-cell therapy: Is it prime time in myeloma? *Blood Adv.* **2019**, *3*, 3473–3480. [CrossRef]
163. Wang, X.; Chang, W.C.; Wong, C.W.; Colcher, D.; Sherman, M.; Ostberg, J.R.; Forman, S.J.; Riddell, S.R.; Jensen, M.C. A transgene-encoded cell surface polypeptide for selection, in vivo tracking, and ablation of engineered cells. *Blood* **2011**, *118*, 1255–1263. [CrossRef]
164. Press Release (CARsgen Therapeutics Co. Ltd. 28 October 2019). Available online: https://www.prnewswire.com/news-releases/carsgen-announces-investigational-car-t-therapy-ct053-granted-rmat-designation-by-the-us-fda-for-rr-multiple-myeloma-300945966.html (accessed on 18 June 2020).
165. Li, C.; Wang, J.; Wang, D.; Hu, G.; Yang, Y.; Zhou, X.; Meng, L.; Hong, Z.; Chen, L.; Mao, X.; et al. Efficacy and safety of fully human BCMA targeting CAR T cell therapy in relapsed/refractory multiple myeloma. *Blood* **2019**, *134*, 929. [CrossRef]
166. Lam, N.; Alabanza, L.; Trinklein, N.; Buelow, B.; Kochenderfer, J.N. T cells expressing anti-B-cell maturation antigen (BCMA) chimeric antigen receptors with antigen recognition domains made up of only single human heavy chain variable domains specifically recognize BCMA and eradicate tumors in mice. *Blood* **2017**, *130*, 504.
167. Sommer, C.; Bentley, T.; Sutton, J.; Heyen, J.; Valton, J.; Ni, Y.J.; Justewicz, D.; Van Blarcom, T.; Smith, J.; Leonard, M.; et al. Off-the-shelf AlloCAR T (TM) cells targeting BCMA for the treatment of multiple myeloma. *Clin. Lymphoma Myeloma Leuk.* **2019**, *19*, E24. [CrossRef]
168. Valton, J.; Guyot, V.; Boldajipour, B.; Sommer, C.; Pertel, T.; Juillerat, A.; Duclert, A.; Sasu, B.J.; Duchateau, P.; Poirot, L. A versatile safeguard for chimeric antigen receptor T-cell immunotherapies. *Sci. Rep.* **2018**, *8*, 8972. [CrossRef] [PubMed]
169. Prieto, J.; Redondo, P.; Lopez-Mendez, B.; D'Abramo, M.; Merino, N.; Blanco, F.J.; Duchateau, P.; Montoya, G.; Molina, R. Understanding the indirect DNA read-out specificity of I-CreI meganuclease. *Sci. Rep.* **2018**, *8*, 10286. [CrossRef] [PubMed]
170. Maroto-Martin, E.; Encinas, J.; Garcia-Ortiz, A.; Ugalde, L.; Alonso, R.; Leivas, A.; Mari, L.P.; Garrido, V.; Martin-Antonio, B.; Sune, G.; et al. Generation of two new immunotherapeutic products with genetically modified NK cells. Comparison of clinically relevant CARS in multiple myeloma. *Haematologica* **2019**, *104*, 97.
171. Martin, E.M.; Encinas, J.; Garcia-Ortiz, A.; Ugalde, L.; Fernandez, R.A.; Leivas, A.; Paciello, M.L.; Garrido, V.; Martin-Antonio, B.; Sune, G.; et al. Exploring NKG2D and BCMA-CAR NK-92 for adoptive cellular therapy to multiple myeloma. *Clin. Lymphoma Myeloma Leuk.* **2019**, *19*, E24–E25. [CrossRef]

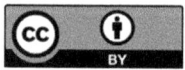

© 2020 by the author. Licensee MDPI, Basel, Switzerland. This article is an open access article distributed under the terms and conditions of the Creative Commons Attribution (CC BY) license (http://creativecommons.org/licenses/by/4.0/).

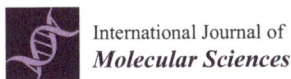
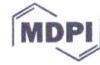

Review

CD38 and Anti-CD38 Monoclonal Antibodies in AL Amyloidosis: Targeting Plasma Cells and beyond

Dario Roccatello [1,*,†], Roberta Fenoglio [1,†], Savino Sciascia [1], Carla Naretto [1], Daniela Rossi [1], Michela Ferro [1], Antonella Barreca [2], Fabio Malavasi [3] and Simone Baldovino [1]

1. Nephrology and Dialysis Unit & CMID (Center of Research of Immunopathology and Rare Diseases), Coordinating Center of the Network for Rare Diseases of Piedmont and Aosta Valley, San Giovanni Bosco Hub Hospital of Turin, and Department of Clinical and Biological Sciences, University of Turin, 10154 Turin, Italy; roberta.fenoglio@unito.it (R.F.); savino.sciascia@unito.it (S.S.); carla.naretto@alscittaditorino.it (C.N.); daniela.rossi@unito.it (D.R.); michela.ferro@alscittaditorino.it (M.F.); simone.baldovino@unito.it (S.B.)
2. Pathology Division, Department of Oncology, University of Turin, 10154 Turin, Italy; antonella.barreca@unito.it
3. Department of Medical Science, University of Turin, and Fondazione Ricerca Molinette, 10154 Turin, Italy; fabio.malavasi@unito.it
* Correspondence: dario.roccatello@unito.it
† These authors contributed equally to this work.

Received: 21 May 2020; Accepted: 5 June 2020; Published: 10 June 2020

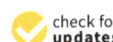

Abstract: Immunoglobulin light chain amyloidosis (AL amyloidosis) is a rare systemic disease characterized by monoclonal light chains (LCs) depositing in tissue as insoluble fibrils, causing irreversible tissue damage. The mechanisms involved in aggregation and deposition of LCs are not fully understood, but CD138/38 plasma cells (PCs) are undoubtedly involved in monoclonal LC production. CD38 is a pleiotropic molecule detectable on the surface of PCs and maintained during the neoplastic transformation in multiple myeloma (MM). CD38 is expressed on T, B and NK cell populations as well, though at a lower cell surface density. CD38 is an ideal target in the management of PC dyscrasia, including AL amyloidosis, and indeed anti-CD38 monoclonal antibodies (MoAbs) have promising therapeutic potential. Anti-CD38 MoAbs act both as PC-depleting agents and as modulators of the balance of the immune cells. These aspects, together with their interaction with Fc receptors (FcRs) and neonatal FcRs, are specifically addressed in this paper. Moreover, the initiallyavailable experiences with the anti-CD38 MoAb DARA in AL amyloidosis are reviewed.

Keywords: AL amyloidosis; CD38; anti-CD38 MoAb; Daratumumab; Isatuximab

1. Introduction

Systemic amyloidosis is characterized by abnormal production and deposition in the extracellular space of misfolded proteins, resulting in a heterogeneous spectrum of clinical conditions [1]. The most prevalent type, namely immunoglobulin light chain amyloidosis (AL amyloidosis), is associated with deposition in the targeted organs of the light chains (LCs) of the immunoglobulins [2]. AL amyloidosis is a rare disease with an incidence of about 1 person/million/year. Due to its rarity and non-specific presentation, diagnosis is often late and frequently occurs after one year from initial symptom presentations. AL amyloidosis can be detected in 30% of patients newly diagnosed as having MM, but it mostly complicates monoclonal gammopathies of undetermined significance [1], which have a 10-foldlower relative risk of developing AL amyloidosis. The clinical manifestations of AL amyloidosis depend on organ involvement. However, the diagnosis can be challenging as symptoms might mimic other more frequent conditions. The deposition of monoclonal light-chain proteins in AL amyloidosis can induce toxic damages in several organs, with the heart and kidney being most frequently affected [3].

AL amyloidosis is often associated with a poor prognosis, with patients having a mean survival ranging from six months to three years, according to the characteristics of the investigated cohort [4,5]. The degree of cardiac involvement represents a major determinant of the outcome in patients with AL amyloidosis, with up to a third of patients with severe cardiac damage having a fatal outcome within 12 months from diagnosis [1,6].

Renal involvement, as identified by the detection of decreased estimated glomerular filtration rate (eGFR) or the presence of proteinuria, is found in approximately 70% of patients [7–13]. The risk of dialysis at two years is 11%–25% in patients with eitherdecreased eGFR orproteinuria, and up to 60%–75% in patients with both decreased eGFR and proteinuria [14,15].

The goals of therapy should be to suppress the production of the pathologic LC precursor and lessen organ impairment. The latter is hard to achieve since the process of amyloid deposition is often irreversible [16]. Therefore, an effective treatment should be applied as soon as possible, before irreversible damage occurs. Only half of the patients treated with conventional regimens show normalization of LCs levels in serum (i.e., complete hematologic response) [17]. The absence of a complete hematologic response results in further deposition of amyloid and reduces the chances of the improvement of affected organs. Therefore, the standard escalation treatment in the attempt to control the hematological disorder (which is a milestone of conventional treatment) should not be applied to patients with rapid disease progression, such as those with renal involvement. Indeed, it could result in a delay in the effective management of the disease and in the consequent accumulation of irreversible lesions. These patients should be treated aggressively ab initio, and the availability of an effective target therapy is desirable.

The involvement of the CD138+ 38+ monoclonal PCs in LCs production is well established, and CD38 could be considered a suitable target of PCs.

The emerging therapeutic potential of anti-CD38 MoAbs in PC dyscrasias is addressed in this paper, and the initiallyavailable experiences with anti-CD38 MoAbs in AL amyloidosis are reviewed.

2. Evidence Supporting CD38 as an Ideal Target for Treating AL Amyloidosisand thePossible Therapeutic Role of Anti-CD38 Antibodies

Most of the available information about the therapeutic effects of targeting CD38 derives from studies on MM. AL amyloidosis and MM are both PC dyscrasias and share some genetic aberrations and therapeutic approaches; however, AL amyloidosis has a distinct phenotype and different prognostic features. The experience with anti-CD38 compounds in MM is critical for the development of novel strategies of management of AL amyloidosis. Indeed, the high expression of CD38 on the clonal PC surface represents the basis for target therapy.

Multiple roles have been described for CD38, as a receptor, adhesion molecule and ectoenzyme [18]. Due to these characteristics, CD38 could represent an effective molecule to be targeted by therapeutic antibodies in the management of AL amyloidosis, a pathologic condition characterized by high expression of this molecule at the cell surface level [19]. CD38 is not expressed by early stem cell progenitors [20]. Instead, B cells, activated T cells and NK express CD38 on their surface, making those cells a potential target for the anti-CD38 MoAbs [21–31].

Daratumumab (DARA), a fully human monoclonal antibody targeting CD38, is the first therapeutic anti-CD38 moAb clinically approved by the Food and Drug Administration for the management of relapsing MM. Its use has been approved in monotherapy as well as in association with lenalidomide or bortezomib. After DARA was approved, more anti-CD38 MoAbs have been reported, such as isatuximab (ISA) and MOR202 [32].

In order to speculate on the potential effect of anti-CD38 antibodies in AL amyloidosis, the mechanisms through which DARA (the most analyzed anti-CD38 agent) exerts its cytotoxic role on effector cells in MM (that is mainly mediated by anFcR-dependent mechanism) should be mentioned.

The principal effects of DARA include antibody-dependent cellular cytotoxicity (ADCC), antibody-dependent cellular phagocytosis (ADCP), complement-dependent cytotoxicity (CDC), and direct apoptosis after secondary cross-linking [20].

ADCC is induced by the release of cytotoxic cytokines and cellular mediators (to include perforins and granzymes) by NK cells. Immunomodulatory imide drugs (IMiDs) have a synergic effect when combined with anti-CD38 moAb by implementing the activity and the number of NK cells [31,32]. However, after treatment with anti-CD38 moAb, a paradoxical reduction of NK cells can be found, possibly due to cytotoxic crosstalk between NK cells and DARA [33]. Whether this mechanism reduces the synergic effect of ADCC in the context of MM is still under debate [34].

ADCP is a further potent mechanism through which DARA can exert its effect by inducing a trigger effect on monocytes and macrophages targeting antibody-opsonized MM cells. It has been speculated that the proportion of monocytes and MM cells can play a role in DARA-mediated antibody-dependent cellular phagocytosis. In this context, the mechanisms supporting the contribution of the CD47 pathway in the modulation of phagocytosis by monocytes has been investigated, showing that an anti-CD47 antibody might potentiate the ADCP effect induced by DARA [35].

CDC follows the ligation of DARA on CD38 on MM cells [29]. DARA is reportedly the most efficient among anti-CD38 MoAbs in triggering the classical complement pathway [29,36–38].

Moreover, CD38 has an ectoenzyme activity, associated with the release of extracellular adenosine (ADO) [39]. Several biological functions have been described for ADO, to include the ability of the nucleoside to exert an inhibitory effect on the immune system through modulation of the activity of several cells populations (e.g., NK cells, monocytes, dendritic cells, T and B lymphocytes, and macrophages) [39]. The potential additional therapeutic effect of targeting ADO in order to obtain an inhibition of the immune system is still under investigation.

Furthermore, DARA is able to reduce the expression of CD38 on the cell surface by trogocytosis. This effect is based on a switch of the CD38-antiCD38 MoAb complex between the abnormal PCs, monocytes, and neutrophils. Again, the process results in an inhibition of ADO levels, with a consequent effect on the tolerogenic microenvironment [40].

DARA also induces polarization and redistribution of CD38 on the myeloma cell membrane surface, resulting in the release of microvesicles expressing the CD38-antiCD38 complex. The role of these changes is not elucidated yet [20].

DARA also exerts a direct immunomodulatory activity on immune cells [13–41] and is able to deplete CD38+ suppressor cells, namely Breg, Treg and myeloid-derived suppressor cells. Remarkably, along with the known effect on Treg and myeloid-derived suppressor cells, emerging evidence is supporting the theory that the MM microenvironment supports the survival of Breg, leading to an overall immunosuppression effect [42].

Another recently launched anti-CD38 MoAb is ISA. This MoAb recognized a specific epitope on human CD38. Its molecular target is represented by a completely different amino acid sequence when compared to DARA [36,37]. ISA has been shown to exert both a potent pro-apoptotic effect, regardless of the presence of cross-linking agents, and robust ADCC (the most prevalent effector mechanism for the elimination of tumor plasma), CDC and ADCP against CD38+ malignant subpopulations [8].

Interestingly, a direct association between the level of CD38+ expression and mechanisms activated by ISA has been found in preclinical models [43,44].

ISA has also been shown to exert its immunomodulatory activity by reducing CD38+ Treg and, at the same time, by potentiating NK cells and T lymphocytes-mediated immune response [43,45,46]. Moreover, ISA has inhibitory effects on immune-checkpoint molecules, such as PD-L1 on osteoclasts [41–45].

MOR202 is a fully human anti-CD38 antibody that is currently under investigation in phase I/IIa clinical trials in MM. The ability of MOR202 of inducing both ADCC and ADCP effects in MM cells makes this molecule a promising candidate for new therapeutic regimens in the management of patients with MM [47]. As for the other anti-CD38 moAbs, the cytotoxic effect of MOR202 on MM cells is augmented by IMiD compounds, such as lenalidomide and pomalidomide. These compounds, apart from being involved in the activation of effector cells and direct cytotoxicity, are able to upregulate CD38. These mechanisms represent an indication for combining MOR202 with IMiD compounds.

Each of these three anti-CD38 MoAbs provided a strong case for being used in AL amyloidosis. However, the effects of ISA are strongly related to CD38 expression (which could be a drawback in the AL amyloidosis setting as this condition is characterized by a small burden of abnormal PCs) and both ISA and MOR202 seem to require IMiD co-operation to achieve an optimal effect. This might restrict their use in very co-morbid patients, such as subjects with AL amyloidosis. Moreover, insights of efficacy and safety in AL amyloidosis are presently limited to DARA.

3. From Basic Research to Clinical Application in AL Amyloidosis: Available Experiences

As previously emphasized, the relatively small percentage of clonally restricted plasma cells in AL amyloidosis expresses CD38, suggesting anti-CD38 MoAbs to be putatively effective in this disease [28].

DARA is the only anti-CD38 MoAb that has been formally examined over the last few years for the treatment of AL amyloidosis [46,48–52]. Nevertheless, information about organ improvement, especially the kidney, suffers from imprecise criteria of the definition of organ involvement.

Sanchorawala et al. showed high hematologic response rates (>80%) in 21 patients with relapsed AL amyloidosis [46]. No data were available on renal response.

Roussel et al. examined 84 AL amyloidosis patients who were given DARA either in combination with dexamethasone or other plasma-cell-directed therapies. Eighty-four percent of the patients had a hematologic response, in the majority of cases within one month. Several patients had cardiac involvement, and half of them showed a cardiac response within two months. Only 26 of the 53 patients with renal impairment or urinary abnormalities were evaluable. They showed some renal response within six months [50]. Unfortunately, none of the patients in this series were reported as having biopsy-proven renal involvement. As far as renal implications are concerned, the identification of amyloid deposits represents the only proof of kidney involvement. Moreover, the entity and distribution of renal amyloid deposition might also be important when comparing the outcome of these patients [51].

In a multicenter phase II study on DARA monotherapy [50], 40 patients from 15 centers, including 26 patients with presumptive renal involvement, who were previously treated with other agents, had been examined. This is another example of misinterpretation and confounding data, occurring when nephrologists are not involved in data evaluation. Indeed, no renal biopsies had been carried out and definitions of renal involvement were not provided. Twenty-one of these patients had <60 mL/min/1.73 m^2 eGFR. This figure, considering patients' mean age (69 years), is close to normal. Seven patients were defined as having had a renal response because of a 30% decrease in proteinuria without a 25% percent increase in eGFR.

With regard to renal response, these results are difficult to interpret.

We attempted DARA monotherapy in four severe cases of AL with multiorgan and biopsy-proven renal involvement. Two males and two females (mean age 64 years, ranging from 52 to 69) were treated with DARA following antibody testing and extended RBC antigen phenotyping. The treatment protocol included 16mg/kg DARA administered intravenously weekly for eight consecutive weeks, then every two weeks for another eight administrations, and lastly, monthly until the 52nd week. One patient was refractory to conventional schedules, one was treated for relapsing disease, one was intolerant and one was treated front-line. Administration of DARA resulted in the disappearance of serum M-component and Bence–Jones proteinuria, and normalization or improvement of the free light chain ratio with a decrease in N-terminal pro-peptide levels and a dramatic drop in urinary protein loss. Cytofluorimetric profiles showed complete disappearance of peripheral PCs with a decrease in both NK and B cell CD19+ve and a slight increase in T helper cells.

4. Expanding the Role of CD38: Future Perspectives

CD38 is identifiable on several non-pathological cell subpopulations, including NK cells, B lymphocytes and activated T cells. Therefore, anti CD38 MoAbs could also potentially exert an effect on non-pathological cells [20]. On the other hand, several investigations showed that anti-CD38 MoAbs can trigger a depletion of CD38+ immunosuppressive cells, including Treg, Breg and myeloid-derived suppressor elements cells [1,42]. These observations further support the rationale of an anti-CD38 MoAb-based regimen as a therapeutic tool for PC dyscrasias.

Further considerations are worth mentioning when considering expanding the potential indication for anti-CD38 MoAbs.

As NK cells mediate ADCC, these cells have a main role in enhancing the activity of anti-CD38 MoAbs [53–57]. DARA increases NK-cell cytotoxicity against cells expressing high, but not low, CD38 [50]. This could be used as a platform for a new therapeutic target for CD38+ cells beyond PC. Besides, in a syngeneic in vivo tumor model neoplasia study, the therapeutic effect of DARA was shown to trigger programmed cell death of myeloma cells via a cross-linking mechanism [20,53–57]. Intriguingly, the crosstalk between DARA and FcRs seems to play a pivotal role in triggering the activity of the MoAbs (Figure 1). The decreased levels of NK cells found in subjects treated with DARA could be due to an antibody-mediated fratricide between NK cells. However, NK cells reduction does not significantly affect DARA efficacy [58]. Moreover, this effect can be balanced by agonistic agents. For instance, IMiDs can have a synergic effect with MoAbs directly targeting CD38 (not limited to DARA) by bursting the activity of NK cells, with a consequent increase in the ADCC [59,60]. Similarly, ADCP is a further mechanism through which anti-CD38 mAbs exert their action on monocytes and macrophages by antibody-opsonized cells [61]. The proportions of monocytes and abnormal PCs could impact on DARA-mediated ADCP [61]. Moreover, the CD47 pathway has been shown to regulate monocyte-driven phagocytosis, and anti-CD47 antibody has been found to increase the ADCP activity triggered by DARA [62].

With regard to other potential agents upcoming as alternative options of anti-CD38 target therapy, ISA exerts both robust pro-apoptotic activity and strong ADCC-associated anti-neoplastic effects, ADCP and CDC. Several additional mechanisms have been described, including (a) homotypic aggregation-associated cell death (as observed in MM cells) that is influenced by the expression of CD38 on the cell surface and is related to the actin cytoskeleton and membrane lipid rafts [39]; (b) up-modulation of reactive oxygen species; (c) lysosome-mediated cell death via alteration of the lysosomes structure and upregulation of the lysosomal membrane permeability; (d) caspase 3 and 7-mediated apoptosis induced in cells highly expressing CD38 (typically MM PCs).

Research aimed at examining in depth the effects of the antibody binding to CD38 is crucial. It has been observed that the process of interaction between CD38 and anti-CD38 MoAbs can influence either internalization or externalization of the target/antibody complex, with a consequent effect on the release of microvesicles [53–57]. For instance, DARA creates a polarization and redistribution of CD38 on the MM cell surface and the development and shedding of microvesicles rich in CD38 bind to DARA in biological fluids. These microvesicles differ when compared to those spontaneously released. Indeed, they present antibody on their surface, express ectoenzymes able to metabolize adenosine triphosphate and nicotinamide adenine dinucleotide to produce adenosine. Besides, they have the potential to merge with neighboring cells and eventually escape the myeloma niche, reaching the blood.

Albeit the process has still to be fully elucidated, microvesicles can also undergo a process of uptake into the cytoplasm of myeloid-derived suppressor cells, NK and monocytes. Pilot in vitro data have shown that microvesicles derived from MM cells exposed to DARA might be able to modulate gene expression at the level of the immune response in purified NK cells.

The effects of microvesicles on dendritic cells for possible vaccinal effects are currently under evaluation.

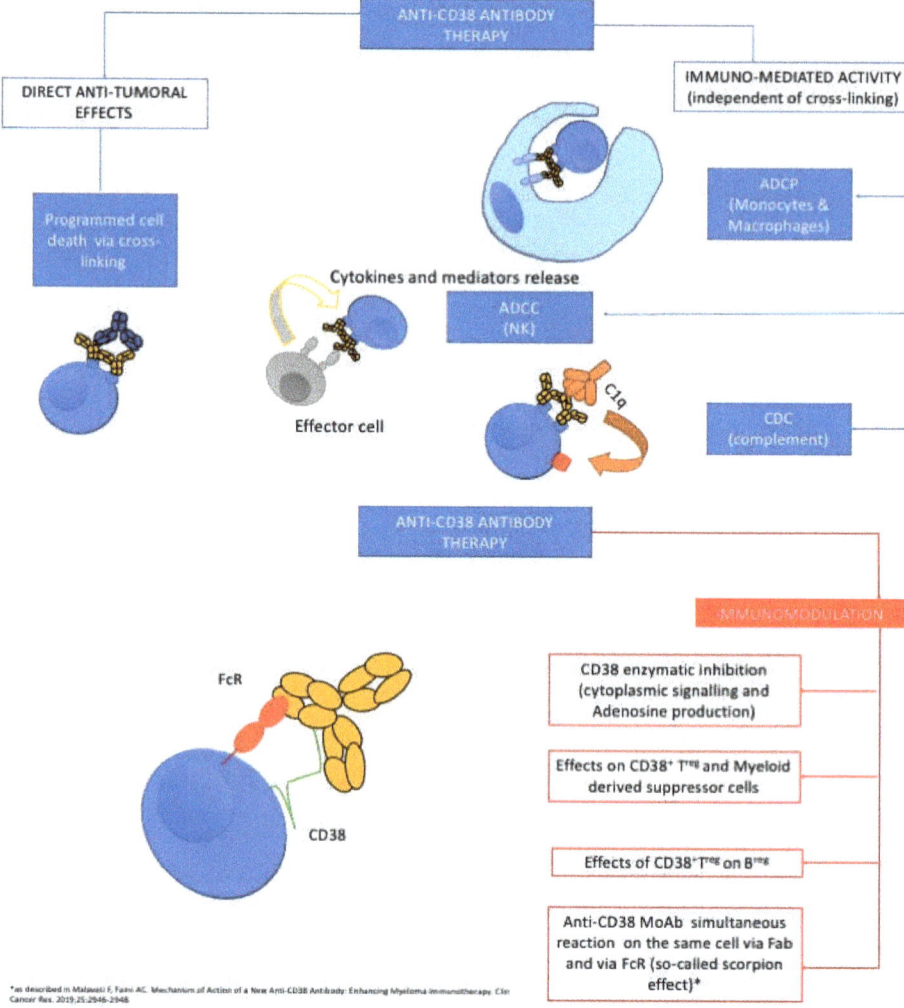

Figure 1. (UPPER PANEL) The left side of the figure illustrates the key effects of the anti-CD38 antibodies on the tumor target and on the main functional effector cells. On the right, a diagram of a hypothetical extension of the immunomodulatory effects mediated by anti-CD38 antibodies. The most intriguing hypothesis is based on the functional synergic interactions between the antibodies and their IgG Fc receptors expressed at various levels by myeloid and lymphoid effectors. The diagram (LOWER PANEL) also shows that the anti-CD38 antibodies may react simultaneously on the same cell via Fab and via FcR, through the so-called scorpion effect [54].

Another point to be considered as relevant for anti-CD38 MoAbs efficacy is the activation of CDC [63,64]. Among anti-CD38 moAbs, DARA has been proved to be the stronger activator of the classical complement cascade, whilst MOR202 shows a moderate CDC activity [63]. Instead, the greater direct pro-apoptotic effect has been associated with ISA, regardless of the cross-linking, and seems to be exerted through the activation of caspases 3 and 7 [65]. The latest effect was not reported for DARA and MOR202 and it might depend on the different epitope recognition in the target CD38 molecule by the different MoAbs [32,66]. When referring to the putative immunomodulatory effects following direct targeting of immune cells, DARA is able to deplete CD38+ immune-suppressor cells such as Treg and myeloid-derived suppressor cells [67]. Incidentally, emerging evidence shows that the MM microenvironment supports the survival of Breg which, in turn, exerts an immunosuppressive effect [41]. ISA is also capable of immunomodulatory effects. It decreases CD38+ Treg and increases NK cell activity proportionately [43]. ISA has also been shown to have an inhibitory effect on numerous immune-checkpoint molecules.

How the majority of these effects can enhance the efficacy of anti-CD38 compounds in AL amyloidosis is currently only speculative.

5. Conclusions

The understanding of the pathogenesis of tissue damage in AL amyloidosis has remarkably improved in recent years. Nevertheless, this condition, especially when heart and kidneys are involved, continues to have an unacceptably poor prognosis. Amyloid deposition is often a permanent process for which putatively effective treatments should be used in a timely manner, before irreversible damage has been established. Autologous stem cell transplantation is thought to be the most definite PC-directed therapy in AL amyloidosis [1]. However, due to the delay in diagnosis and the extent of cardiac involvement, only a minority of patients are eligible for transplantation. Consonant with this observation are our data from fifty-two AL amyloidosis subjects followed at our Center between 2007 and 2018. As many as thirty-one were ineligible for bone marrow transplantation. Therefore, alternative therapies with a high degree of safety due to the burden of co-morbidities of these patients are urgently needed. A better understating of the mechanisms underlying the regulation of PC survival in PC dyscrasia and of the crosstalk with the immune microenvironment have promoted the description of new target therapies.

CD38 target therapy should both deplete and modulate immune cells. While the majority of in vitro and in vivo observations have been done in MM, initial experiences might be a launching pad for expanding research on the use of anti-CD38 target therapy in AL amyloidosis. Different anti-CD38 MoAbs have been designed to target abnormal PCs via the Fc-dependent immune effector mechanism. Among the most widely used anti-CD38 compounds in an MM setting DARA is a full human MoAb while ISA is chimeric. It is rational to suppose that the dissimilarities in structure between DARA and ISA explain the diverse interactions with the FcRs and the different molecular mechanisms involved in their interaction with the target molecule. Available data on the use of anti-CD38 MoAbs, especially in AL amyloidosis, are pivotal, but pave the way to studies aimed at characterizing novel therapeutic protocols.

AL amyloidosis is characterized to a limited extent by abnormal PCs producing a huge amount of light chains susceptible to aggregation in insoluble form and deposition in target organs. Causal therapy is mainly addressed to interrupt the synthesis of abnormal proteins. It should be remembered that the extent of PC dyscrasias widely differs between MM and AL amyloidosis. Combination therapies (i.e., anti-CD38 MoAbs plus IMiDs and/or proteasome inhibitors) are needed to lessen the tumor burden in MM, and the rate of relapses justifies an escalation approach to improve patient survival. As compared to MM, management of AL amyloidosis probably needs less intensive treatment, due to the limited dimension of the clone. However, treatment should be extremely timely, maybe in an upfront setting, in order to prevent definitive organ damage. Target therapy with anti-CD38 MoAbs in AL amyloidosis could be revealed to be the most appropriate strategy, even when given alone, to reduce the adverse effects in these fragile patients, maybe at a personalized dose, and perhaps for a more prolonged time.

Finally, the experience with novel protocols for AL amyloidosis could be transferred to other diseases. Apart from incorporating the approaches used in MM into future strategies able to reduce the mortality of AL amyloidosis patients, the challenge for the near future will be to design novel therapeutic protocols for each disorder attributable to a PC dyscrasia. These conditions include those with a small clone of PCs producing harmful light chains causing irreversible organ damage distally to the production site. Ideally, a number of rare diseases could benefit from therapeutic schemes validated in AL amyloidosis i.e., monoclonal immunoglobulin deposition disease, proliferative glomerulonephritis with monoclonal IgG-K deposits, type I cryoglobulinemia with clonally restricted IgG, light chain nephropathy and fibrillary glomerulonephritis with a monotypic light chain.

Author Contributions: Conceptualization, D.R. (Dario Roccatello), R.B. and S.B.; Methodology, D.R. (Daniela Rossi), S.S. and C.N.; Formal Analysis, S.B., D.R. (Dario Roccatello) and F.M.; Investigation, D.R. (Daniela Rossi), R.B., A.B., C.N. and M.F.; Data Curation, M.F., C.N., A.B. and S.B.; Writing—Original Draft Preparation, D.R. (Dario Roccatello) and R.F.; Writing—Review & Editing, S.S., S.B., C.N., Daniela Rossi, M.F., A.B. and F.M. All authors have read and agreed to the published version of the manuscript.

Funding: This research received no external funding.

Conflicts of Interest: The authors declare no conflicts of interest.

References

1. Palladini, G.; Merlini, G. What is new in diagnosis and management of light chain amyloidosis? *Blood* **2016**, *128*, 159–168. [CrossRef] [PubMed]
2. Blancas-Mejia, L.M.; Misra, P.; Dick, C.J.; Cooper, S.A.; Redhage, K.R.; Bergman, M.R.; Jordan, T.L.; Maar, K.; Ramirez-Alvarado, M. Immunoglobulin light chain amyloid aggregation. *Chem. Commun.* **2018**, *54*, 10664–10674. [CrossRef] [PubMed]
3. Sanchorawala, V. Light-chain (AL) amyloidosis: Diagnosis and treatment. *Clin. J. Am. Soc. Nephrol.* **2006**, *1*, 1331–1341. [CrossRef] [PubMed]
4. Weiss, B.M.; Lund, S.H.; Bjorkholm, M. Improved survival in AL amyloidosis: A population-based study on 1430 patients diagnosed in Sweden 1995–2013. *Blood* **2016**, *128*, 4448. [CrossRef]
5. Lousada, I.; Comenzo, R.L.; Landau, H.; Guthrie, S.; Merlini, G. Light Chain Amyloidosis: Patients experience survey from the Amyloidosis Research Consortium. *Adv. Ther.* **2015**, *32*, 920–928. [CrossRef] [PubMed]
6. Falk, R.H.; Dubrey, S.W. Amyloid heart disease. Progress in Cardiovascular Diseases. *Open J. Clin. Diagn.* **2014**, *4*, 347–361.
7. Dispenzieri, A. Renal risk and response in amyloidosis. *Blood* **2014**, *124*, 2315–2316. [CrossRef] [PubMed]
8. Kastritis, E.; Gavriatopoulou, M.; Roussou, M.; Migkou, M.; Fotiou, D.; Ziogas, D.C.; Kanellias, N.; Eleutherakis-Papaiakovou, E.; Panagiotidis, I.; Giannouli, S.; et al. Renal outcome in patients with AL amyloidosis: Prognostic factors. *Am. J. Hematol.* **2017**, *92*, 632–639. [CrossRef] [PubMed]
9. Fuah, K.W.; Lim, C.T.S. Renal-limited AL amyloidosis—A diagnostic and management dilemma. *BMC Nephrol.* **2018**, *19*, 307. [CrossRef] [PubMed]
10. Sasatomi, Y.; Kiyoshi, Y.; Uesugi, N.; Hisano, S.; Takebayashi, S. Prognosis of renal amyloidosis: A clinic-pathological study using cluster analysis. *Nephron* **2001**, *87*, 42–49. [CrossRef] [PubMed]
11. Nuvolone, M.; Milani, P.; Palladini, G.; Merlini, G. Management of the elderly patient with AL amyloidosis. *Eur. J. Intern. Med.* **2018**, *58*, 48–56. [CrossRef] [PubMed]
12. Kalle, A.; Gudipati, A.; Raju, S.B.; Kalidindi, K.; Guditi, S.; Taduri, G.; Uppin, M.S. Revisiting renal amyloidosis with clinicopathological characteristics, grading, and scoring: A single-institutional experience. *J. Lab. Physicians* **2018**, *10*, 226–231. [CrossRef] [PubMed]
13. Rezk, T.; Lachmann, H.J.; Fontana, M.; Sachchithanantham, S.; Mahmood, S.; Petrie, A.; Whelan, C.J.; Pinney, J.H.; Foard, D.; Lane, T.; et al. Prolonged renal survival in light chain amyloidosis: Speed and magnitude of light chain reduction is the crucial factor. *Kidney. Int.* **2017**, *92*, 1476–1483. [CrossRef] [PubMed]
14. Palladini, G.; Hegenbart, U.; Milani, P.; Kimmich, C.; Foli, A.; Ho, A.D.; Rosin, M.V.; Albertini, R.; Moratti, R.; Merlini, G.; et al. A staging system for renal outcome and early markers of renal response to chemotherapy in AL amyloidosis. *Blood* **2014**, *124*, 2325–2332. [CrossRef] [PubMed]
15. Kyle, R.A.; Greipp, P.R.; O'Fallon, W.M. Primary systemic amyloidosis: Multivariate analysis for prognostic factors in 168 cases. *Blood* **1986**, *68*, 220–224. [CrossRef] [PubMed]
16. Angel-Korman, A.; Jaberi, A.; Sanchorawala, V.; Havasi, A. The utility of repeat kidney biopsy in systemic immunoglobulin light chain amyloidosis. *Amyloid* **2019**, *27*, 17–24. [CrossRef]
17. Kumar, S.K.; Dispenzieri, A.; Lacy, M.Q.; Hayman, S.R.; Buadi, F.K.; Zeldenrust, S.R.; Tan, T.; Sinha, S.; Leung, N.; Kyle, R.A.; et al. Changes in serum-free light chain rather than intact monoclonal immunoglobulin levels predicts outcome following therapy in primary amyloidosis. *Am. J. Hematol.* **2011**, *86*, 251–255. [CrossRef]

18. Malavasi, F.; Deaglio, S.; Damle, R.; Funaro, A.E.; Horenstein, A.L.; Ortolan, E.; Vaisitti, T.; Aydin, S. Evolution and function of the ADP ribosyl cyclase/CD38 gene family in physiology and pathology. CD38 and chronic lymphocytic leukemia: A decade later. *Physiol. Rev.* **2008**, *88*, 841–886. [CrossRef] [PubMed]
19. Matsuda, M.; Gono, T.; Shimojima, Y.; Hoshii, Y.; Ikeda, S. Phenotypic analysis of plasma cells in bone marrow using flow cytometry in AL amyloidosis. *Amyloid* **2003**, *10*, 110–116. [CrossRef] [PubMed]
20. Morandi, F.; Horenstein, A.L.; Costa, F.; Giuliani, N.; Pistoia, V.; Malavasi, F. CD38: A Target for Immunotherapeutic Approaches in Multiple Myeloma. *Front. Immunol.* **2018**, *9*, 2722. [CrossRef]
21. Nijhof, I.S.; Groen, R.W.; Lokhorst, H.M.; van Kessel, B.; Bloem, A.C.; van Velzen, J.; de Jong-Korlaar, R.; Yuan, H.; Noort, W.A.; Klein, S.K.; et al. Upregulation of CD38 expression on multiple myeloma cells by all-trans retinoic acid improves the efficacy of daratumumab. *Leukemia* **2015**, *29*, 2039–2049. [CrossRef] [PubMed]
22. García-Guerrero, E.; Gogishvili, T.; Danhof, S.; Schreder, M.; Pallaud, C.; Pérez-Simón, J.A.; Einsele, H.; Hudecek, M. Panobinostat induces CD38 upregulation and augments the antimyeloma efficacy of daratumumab. *Blood* **2017**, *129*, 3386–3388. [CrossRef] [PubMed]
23. Costa, F.; Toscani, D.; Chillemi, A.; Quarona, V.; Bolzoni, M.; Marchica, V.; Vescovini, R.; Mancini, C.; Martella, E.; Campanini, N.; et al. Expression of CD38 in myeloma bone niche: A rational basis for the use of anti-CD38 immunotherapy to inhibit osteoclast formation. *Oncotarget* **2017**, *8*, 56598–56611. [CrossRef] [PubMed]
24. Chillemi, A.; Zaccarello, G.; Quarona, V.; Lazzaretti, M.; Martella, E.; Giuliani, N.; Ferracini, R.; Pistoia, V.; Horenstein, A.L.; Malavasi, F. CD38 and bone marrow microenvironment. *Front. Biosci.* **2014**, *19*, 152–162. [CrossRef] [PubMed]
25. An, G.; Acharya, C.; Feng, X.; Wen, K.; Zhong, M.; Zhang, L.; Munshi, N.C.; Qiu, L.; Tai, Y.-T.; Anderson, K.C. Osteoclasts promote immune suppressive microenvironment in multiple myeloma: Therapeutic implication. *Blood* **2016**, *128*, 1590–1603. [CrossRef] [PubMed]
26. Mansour, A.; Wakkach, A.; Blin-Wakkach, C. Emerging Roles of Osteoclasts in the Modulation of Bone Microenvironment and Immune Suppression in Multiple Myeloma. *Front. Immunol.* **2017**, *8*, 954. [CrossRef] [PubMed]
27. Krejcik, J.; Frerichs, K.A.; Nijhof, I.S.; van Kessel, B.; van Velzen, J.F.; Bloem, A.C.; Broekmans, M.E.C.; Zweegman, S.; van Meerloo, J.; Musters, R.; et al. Monocytes and Granulocytes Reduce CD38 Expression Levels on Myeloma Cells in Patients Treated with Daratumumab. *Clin. Cancer Res.* **2017**, *23*, 7498–7511. [CrossRef] [PubMed]
28. Takedachi, M.; Oohara, H.; Smith, B.J.; Iyama, M.; Kobashi, M.; Maeda, K.; Long, C.L.; Humphrey, M.B.; Stoecker, B.J.; Toyosawa, S.; et al. CD73-generated adenosine promotes osteoblast differentiation. *J. Cell Physiol.* **2012**, *227*, 2622–2631. [CrossRef]
29. Bolzoni, M.; Toscani, D.; Costa, F.; Vicario, E.; Aversa, F.; Giuliani, N. The link between bone microenvironment and immune cells in multiple myeloma: Emerging role of CD38. *Immunol. Lett.* **2019**, *205*, 65–70. [CrossRef]
30. Sidana, S.; Muchtar, E.; Sidiqi, M.H.; Jevremovic, D.; Dispenzieri, A.; Gonsalves, W.; Buadi, F.; Lacy, M.Q.; Hayman, S.R.; Kourelis, T.; et al. Impact of minimal residual negativity using next generation flow cytometry on outcomes in light chain amyloidosis. *Am. J. Hematol.* **2020**, *95*, 497–502. [CrossRef]
31. Zambello, R.; Barilà, G.; Manni, S.; Piazza, F.; Semenzato, G. NK cells and CD38: Implication for (Immuno)Therapy in Plasma Cell Dyscrasias. *Cells* **2020**, *9*, 768. [CrossRef] [PubMed]
32. Van de Donk, N.W.C.J.; Richardson, P.G.; Malavasi, F. CD38 antibodies in multiple myeloma: Back to the future. *Blood* **2018**, *131*, 13–29. [CrossRef] [PubMed]
33. D'Agostino, M.; Mina, R.; Gay, F. Anti-CD38 monoclonal antibodies in multiple myeloma: Another cook in the kitchen? *Lancet Haematol.* **2020**, *7*, e355–e357.
34. Plesner, T.; van de Donk, N.; Richardson, P.G. Controversy in the Use of CD38 Antibody for Treatment of Myeloma: Is High CD38 Expression Good or Bad? *Cells* **2020**, *9*, 378. [CrossRef] [PubMed]
35. Storti, P.; Vescovini, R.; Costa, F.; Marchica, V.; Toscani, D.; Dalla Palma, B.; Craviotto, L.; Malavasi, F.; Giuliani, N. CD14(+) CD16(+) monocytes are involved in daratumumab-mediated myeloma cells killing and in anti-CD47 therapeutic strategy. *Br. J. Haematol.* **2020**, *12*. [CrossRef] [PubMed]

36. Deckert, J.; Wetzel, M.C.; Bartle, L.M.; Skaletskaya, A.; Goldmacher, V.S.; Vallée, F.; Zhou-Liu, Q.; Ferrari, P.; Pouzieux, S.; Lahoute, C.; et al. SAR650984, a novel humanized CD38-targeting antibody, demonstrates potent antitumor activity in models of multiple myeloma and other CD38+ hematologic malignancies. *Clin. Cancer Res.* **2014**, *20*, 4574–4583. [CrossRef] [PubMed]
37. Martin, T.G.; Corzo, K.; Chiron, M.; Velde, H.V.; Abbadessa, G.; Campana, F.; Solanki, M.; Meng, R.; Lee, H.; Wiederschain, D.; et al. Therapeutic opportunities with pharmacological inhibition of CD38 with Isatuximab. *Cells* **2019**, *8*, 1522. [CrossRef] [PubMed]
38. Nijhof, I.S.; Casneuf, T.; van Velzen, J.; van Kessel, B.; Axel, A.E.; Syed, K.; Groen, R.W.; van Duin, W.; Sonneveld, P.; Minnema, M.C.; et al. CD38 expression and complementinhibitors affect response and resistance to daratumumab therapy in myeloma. *Blood J. Am. Soc. Hematol.* **2016**, *128*, 959–970.
39. Morandi, F.; Horenstein, A.L.; Rizzo, R.; Malavasi, F. The Role of Extracellular Adenosine Generation in the Development of Autoimmune Diseases. *Mediators Inflamm.* **2018**, 7019398.
40. Kastritis, E.; Kostopoulos, I.V.; Terpos, E.; Paiva, B.; Fotiou, D.; Gavriatopoulou, M.; Kanellias, N.; Ziogas, D.C.; Roussou, M.; Migkou, M.; et al. Evaluation of minimal residual disease using next-generation flow cytometry in patients with AL amyloidosis. *Blood Cancer J.* **2018**, *8*, 46. [CrossRef] [PubMed]
41. Zhang, L.; Tai, Y.-T.; Ho, M.; Xing, L.; Chauhan, D.; Gang, A.; Qiu, L.; Anderson, K.C. Regulatory B cell-myeloma cell interaction confers immunosuppression and promotes their survival in the bone marrow milieu. *Blood Cancer J.* **2017**, *7*, e547. [CrossRef] [PubMed]
42. Zuch de Zafra, C.L.; Fajardo, F.; Zhong, W.; Bernett, M.J.; Muchhal, U.S.; Moore, G.L.; Stevens, J.; Case, R.; Pearson, J.T.; Liu, S.; et al. Targeting Multiple Myeloma with AMG 424, a Novel Anti-CD38/CD3 Bispecific T-cell-recruiting Antibody Optimized for Cytotoxicity and Cytokine Release. *Clin. Cancer Res.* **2019**, *25*, 3921–3933. [CrossRef] [PubMed]
43. Feng, X.; Zhang, L.; Acharya, C.; An, G.; Wen, K.; Qiu, L.; Munshi, N.C.; Tai, Y.T.; Anderson, K.C. Targeting CD38 suppresses induction and function of T regulatory cells to mitigate immunosuppression in multiple myeloma. *Clin. Cancer Res.* **2017**, *23*, 4290–4300. [CrossRef] [PubMed]
44. Moreno, L.; Perez, C.; Zabaleta, A.; Manrique, I.; Alignani, D.; Ajona, D.; Blanco, L.; Lasa, M.; Maiso, P.; Rodriguez, I.; et al. The mechanism of action of the anti-CD38 monoclonal antibody isatuxima. *Clin. Cancer Res.* **2019**, *25*, 3176–3187. [CrossRef] [PubMed]
45. Morandi, F.; Airoldi, I.; Marimpietri, D.; Bracci, C.; Faini, A.C.; Gramignoli, R. CD38, a Receptor with Multifunctional Activities: From Modulatory Functions on Regulatory Cell Subsets and Extracellular Vesicles, to a Target for Therapeutic Strategies. *Cells* **2019**, *8*, 1527. [CrossRef]
46. Sanchorawala, V.; Sarosiek, S.D.; Sloan, J.M.; Brauneis, D.; Migre, M.E.; Mistark, M.; Santos, S.; Cruz, R.; Fennessey, S.; Shelton, A.C. Safety, Tolerability and Response Rates of Daratumumab in Patients with Relapsed Light Chain (AL) Amyloidosis: Results of a Phase II Study. *Blood* **2005**, *132* (Suppl. 1). [CrossRef]
47. Raab, M.S.; Engelhardt, M.; Blank, A.; Goldschmidt, H.; Agis, H.; Blau, I.W.; Einsele, H.; Ferstl, B.; Schub, N.; Röllig, C.; et al. MOR202, a novel anti-CD38 monoclonal antibody, in patients with relapsed or refractory multiple myeloma: A first-in-human, multicentre, phase 1–2a trial. *Lancet Haematol.* **2020**, *7*, e381–e394. [CrossRef]
48. Chung, S.; Kaufman, G.P.; Sidana, S.; Eckhert, E.; Schrier, S.L.; Lafayette, R.A.; Arai, S.; Witteles, R.M.; Liedtke, M. Organ responses with daratumumab therapy in previously treated AL amyloidosis. *Blood Adv.* **2020**, *4*, 458–466. [CrossRef] [PubMed]
49. Itabashi, M.; Takei, T.; Tsukada, M.; Sugiura, H.; Uchida, K.; Tsuchiya, K.; Honda, K.; Nitta, K. Association between clinical characteristics and AL amyloid deposition in the kidney. *Heart Vessel* **2010**, *25*, 543–548. [CrossRef] [PubMed]
50. Roussel, M.; Merlini, G.; Arnulf, B.; Chevret, S.; Stoppa, A.M.; Perrot, A.; Palladini, G.; Karlin, L.; Royer, B.; Huart, A.; et al. A prospective phase II of daratumumab in previously treated systemic light chain amyloidosis patients. *Blood* **2020**, *135*, 1531–1540. [CrossRef]
51. Cherkasova, E.; Espinoza, L.; Kotecha, R.; Reger, R.N.; Berg, M.; Aue, G.; Attar, R.M.; Sasser, A.K.; Carlsten, M.; Childs, R.W.; et al. Treatment of Ex Vivo expanded NK cells with Daratumumab F(ab')2 fragments protects adoptively transferred NK cells from Daratumumab-mediated killing and augments Daratumumab-induced Antibody Dependent Cellular Toxicity (ADCC) of myeloma. *Blood* **2015**, *126*, 4244. [CrossRef]
52. Van de Donk, N.W.C.J.; Usmani, S.Z. CD38 Antibodies in Multiple Myeloma: Mechanisms of Action and Modes of Resistance. *Front Immunol.* **2018**, *9*, 2134. [CrossRef] [PubMed]

53. Overdijk, M.B.; Jansen, J.H.; Nederend, M.; Lammerts van Bueren, J.J.; Groen, R.W.; Parren, P.W.; Leusen, J.H.; Boross, P. The Therapeutic CD38 Monoclonal Antibody Daratumumab Induces Programmed Cell Death via Fcγ Receptor-Mediated Cross-Linking. *J. Immunol.* **2016**, *197*, 807–813. [CrossRef] [PubMed]
54. Giuliani, N.; Malavasi, F. Immunotherapy in Multiple Myeloma. *Front. Immunol.* **2019**, *10*, 1945. [CrossRef] [PubMed]
55. Deaglio, S.; Zubiaur, M.; Gregorini, A.; Ausiello, C.M.; Dianzani, U.; Sancho, U.; Malavasi, F. Human CD38 and CD16 are functionally dependent and physically associated in natural killer cells. *Bood* **2002**, *99*, 2490–2498. [CrossRef] [PubMed]
56. Malavasi, F.; Chillemi, A.; Castella, B.; Schiavoni, I.; Incarnato, D.; Oliva, S.; Horenstein, A.L. CD38 and antibody therapy: What can basic science add. *Blood* **2016**, *128*, SCI-36. [CrossRef]
57. Malavasi, F.; Faini, A.C. Mechanism of action of a new anti-CD38 antibody: Enhancing myeloma immunotherapy. *Clin. Cancer Res.* **2019**, *25*, 2946–2948. [CrossRef] [PubMed]
58. Casneuf, T.; Xu, X.S.; Adams, H.C.; Axel, A.E.; Chiu, C.; Khan, I.; Ahmadi, T.; Yan, X.; Lonial, S.; Plesner, T.; et al. Effects of daratumumab on natural killer cells and impact on clinical outcomes in relapsed or refractory multiple myeloma. *Blood Adv.* **2017**, *1*, 2105–2114. [CrossRef] [PubMed]
59. Nijhof, I.S.; Groen, R.W.; Noort, W.A.; van Kessel, B.; de Jong-Korlaar, R.; Bakker, J.; van Bueren, J.J.L.; Parren, P.W.; Lokhorst, H.M.; van De Donk, N.W.; et al. Preclinical evidence for the therapeutic potential of CD38-targeted immuno-chemotherapy in multiple myeloma patients refractory to lenalidomide and bortezomib. *Clin. Cancer Res.* **2015**, *21*, 2802–2810. [CrossRef] [PubMed]
60. van der Veer, M.S.; de Weers, M.; van Kessel, B.; Bakker, J.M.; Wittebol, S.; Parren, P.W.; Lokhorst, H.M.; Mutis, T. Towards effective immunotherapy of myeloma: Enhanced elimination of myeloma cells by combination of lenalidomide with the human CD38 monoclonal antibody daratumumab. *Haematologica* **2011**, *96*, 284–290. [CrossRef] [PubMed]
61. Rigalou, A.; Ryan, A.; Natoni, A.; Chiu, C.; Sasser, K.; O'Dwyer, M.E. Potentiation of Anti-Myeloma Activity of Daratumumab with Combination of Cyclophosphamide, Lenalidomide or Bortezomib Via a Tumor Secretory Response That Greatly Augments Macrophage-Induced ADCP. *Blood* **2016**, *22*, 2101. [CrossRef]
62. Overdijk, M.B.; Verploegen, S.; Bogels, M.; van Egmond, M.; van Bueren, J.J.L.; Mutis, T.; Groen, R.W.J.; Breij, E.; Martens, A.C.M.; Bleeker, W.K.; et al. Antibody-mediated phagocytosis contributes to the anti-tumor activity of the therapeutic antibody daratumumab in lymphoma and multiple myeloma. *MAbs* **2015**, *7*, 311–321. [CrossRef] [PubMed]
63. Van de Donk, N. Immunomodulatory effects of CD38-targeting antibodies. *Immunol. Lett.* **2018**, *199*, 16–22. [CrossRef] [PubMed]
64. de Weers, M.; Tai, Y.-T.; van der Veer, M.S.; Bakker, J.M.; Vink, T.; Jacobs, D.C.H.; Oomen, L.A.; Peipp, M.; Valerius, T.; Slootstra, J.W.; et al. Daratumumab, a novel therapeutic human CD38 monoclonal antibody, induces killing of multiple myeloma and other hematological tumors. *J. Immunol.* **2011**, *186*, 1840–1848. [CrossRef] [PubMed]
65. Jiang, H.; Acharya, C.; An, G.; Zhong, M.; Feng, X.; Wang, L.; Dasilva, N.; Song, Z.; Yang, G.; Adrian, F.; et al. SAR650984 directly induces multiplemyeloma cell death via lysosomal-associated and apoptotic pathways, which is further enhanced by pomalidomide. *Leukemia* **2016**, *30*, 399–408. [CrossRef] [PubMed]
66. Richter, J.; Sanchez, L.; Thibaud, S. Therapeutic potential of isatuximab in thetreatment of multiple myeloma: Evidence to date. *Semin Oncol.* **2020**, *S0093-7754*, 30036-1.
67. Bride, K.L.; Vincent, T.L.; Im, S.-Y.; Aplenc, R.; Barrett, D.M.; Carroll, W.L.; Carson, R.; Dai, Y.; Devidas, M.; Dunsmore, K.P.; et al. Preclinical efficacy of daratumumab in T-cell acute lymphoblastic leukemia. *Blood J. Am. Soc. Hematol.* **2018**, *131*, 995–999. [CrossRef] [PubMed]

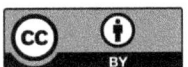

© 2020 by the authors. Licensee MDPI, Basel, Switzerland. This article is an open access article distributed under the terms and conditions of the Creative Commons Attribution (CC BY) license (http://creativecommons.org/licenses/by/4.0/).

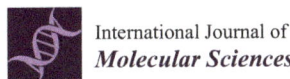 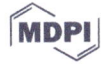

Article

An Affibody Molecule Is Actively Transported into the Cerebrospinal Fluid via Binding to the Transferrin Receptor

Sebastian W. Meister, Linnea C. Hjelm, Melanie Dannemeyer, Hanna Tegel, Hanna Lindberg, Stefan Ståhl and John Löfblom *

Department of Protein Science, School of Engineering Sciences in Chemistry, Biotechnology and Health, KTH Royal Institute of Technology, AlbaNova University Centre, SE-106 91 Stockholm, Sweden; smeister@kth.se (S.W.M.); lhjelm@kth.se (L.C.H.); melanied@kth.se (M.D.); hannat@biotech.kth.se (H.T.); hanli@kth.se (H.L.); ssta@kth.se (S.S.)
* Correspondence: lofblom@kth.se; Tel.: +46-8-790-9659

Received: 6 March 2020; Accepted: 22 April 2020; Published: 23 April 2020

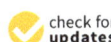

Abstract: The use of biotherapeutics for the treatment of diseases of the central nervous system (CNS) is typically impeded by insufficient transport across the blood–brain barrier. Here, we investigate a strategy to potentially increase the uptake into the CNS of an affibody molecule (Z_{SYM73}) via binding to the transferrin receptor (TfR). Z_{SYM73} binds monomeric amyloid beta, a peptide involved in Alzheimer's disease pathogenesis, with subnanomolar affinity. We generated a tri-specific fusion protein by genetically linking a single-chain variable fragment of the TfR-binding antibody 8D3 and an albumin-binding domain to the affibody molecule Z_{SYM73}. Simultaneous tri-specific target engagement was confirmed in a biosensor experiment and the affinity for murine TfR was determined to 5 nM. Blockable binding to TfR on endothelial cells was demonstrated using flow cytometry and in a preclinical study we observed increased uptake of the tri-specific fusion protein into the cerebrospinal fluid 24 h after injection.

Keywords: neurodegenerative disorders; affibody molecules; blood–brain barrier; receptor-mediated transcytosis; transferrin receptor

1. Introduction

The blood–brain barrier (BBB) is defined as the structural, physiological, and molecular mechanisms regulating the exchange of molecules between the systemic circulation and the brain [1]. Morphologically, the BBB consists of brain capillary endothelial cells (BCECs) within the microvasculature of the brain [2]. On the abluminal site the BCECs are joined by pericytes and the end-feet of astrocytes [3]. Paracellular passage through the BBB is limited by the presence of tight junction proteins between the individual endothelial cells [4]. Only small hydrophilic molecules can enter the brain via this route [5]. The entry of amphiphilic molecules into the brain is reduced due to expression of efflux transporters in BCECs [6]. While the presence of this tight barrier is essential for central nervous system (CNS) homeostasis, it presents an obstacle for the treatment of diseases of the CNS using biotherapeutics. Only around 0.1%–0.2% of peripherally administered antibodies are typically crossing into the brain [7–9]. Potential receptor-mediated transcytosis (RMT) mechanisms of endogenous ligands have been investigated with the aim to increase the brain uptake of biologics in a non-invasive manner. To this end, therapeutic macromolecules have been conjugated to antibodies against receptors or transporters expressed on the BBB. Examples of RMT target proteins include the insulin receptor, low-density lipoprotein receptor-related protein 1, glucose transporter 1, basignin,

CD98hc, and the transferrin receptor (TfR) [9]. TfR, which naturally transports iron to the brain [10], is the most widely used target protein for this purpose and has been used in several studies aiming to transport cargo proteins across the BBB [11]. Investigation of the trafficking mechanism using TfR has shed light on the relationship between TfR binding and TfR trafficking [12,13]. In order to achieve optimal brain exposure of the therapeutic cargo, the antibody needs to dissociate from the receptor during or after transcytosis. This can be achieved by utilizing an antibody with moderate to low affinity for TfR [14]. Yu and coworkers could also demonstrate that a high affinity TfR binding antibody is cleared faster from circulation compared to an antibody with lower affinity for TfR [14]. High-affinity TfR binding has been shown to promote degradation of the transferrin receptor in mice [13]. Monovalent binding to the heterodimeric TfR has been shown to induce a more favorable route of intracellular sorting compared to bivalent TfR binding [12,15].

Another possible route for drug delivery into the CNS is via passage over the blood-cerebrospinal fluid (CSF) barrier, which is formed by the epithelium of the choroid plexus [16]. The choroid plexus epithelium expresses TfR and is thought to be involved in iron transport into the brain [17]. CSF communicates freely with brain interstitial fluid through convective flow and diffusion [18]. Systemically administered drugs can reach the brain interstitial fluid by transfer across the BBB, or indirectly by passage over the choroid plexus followed by diffusion/convection transport [19].

In Alzheimer's disease (AD), the most common form of dementia, an important pathological feature is the deposition of extracellular senile plaques consisting of amyloid beta (Aß) in the brains of patients [20]. Soluble, monomeric Aß peptides self-aggregate into neurotoxic oligomers and insoluble ß-sheet-rich plaques. Aß, in different physical forms, has been the target of numerous active and passive immunotherapeutic campaigns [21]. While several anti-Aß antibodies have proven efficacious in preclinical models [22], most of these antibodies have failed to show sufficient clinical benefits in AD clinical trials [23]. Although antibodies that are specific for the monomeric form of Aß have not yet demonstrated better efficacy than agents targeting for example the amyloid plaques, it has been suggested that they might still have a higher potential. The motivation is mainly that potential future therapies probably need to start at the pre-symptomatic stage of the disease and thus should target Aß species that are found early in the disease progression [24]. We have recently reported on the generation of an affibody molecule that binds monomeric Aß with 60 pM affinity. Affibody molecules are alternative scaffold proteins that are engineered by directed evolution (e.g., phage display technology). We have previously developed an affibody-based Aβ-binder by phage display technology. In a subsequent affinity-maturation effort, we isolated a high-affinity variant (denoted Z_{SYM73}) from second-generation affibody libraries displayed on bacteria [25].

Z_{SYM73} has an unusual structure and forms a disulfide-stabilized heterodimer in complex with the Aß peptide. Upon binding, both the affibody and the Aß peptide fold, forming a beta-sheet with Aß in a beta-hairpin conformation [26]. When bound, the aggregation-prone parts of Aß are buried in a tunnel-like cavity and the affibody efficiently inhibits the aggregation. In an APP/PS1 double transgenic mouse study, treatment with Z_{SYM73} led to prevention of the amyloid burden build up in both cortex and hippocampus as well as prevention of decline in cognitive function [27].

Encouraged by these positive results, the aim here was to investigate strategies that might be employed in future therapeutic studies to increase brain exposure of Z_{SYM73}, which has the potential to also improve efficacy. It has previously been demonstrated that the CNS uptake of rat 8D3 mAb against mouse TfR is substantially higher than for non-TfR binding antibodies [28–30]. We genetically fused Z_{SYM73} to a single-chain variable fragment (scFv) of the 8D3 mAb and an engineered albumin-binding domain (ABD) [31], which was included also in the preclinical study with Z_{SYM73} [27]. The engineered ABD and its binding to serum albumin has been shown in a number of both preclinical and clinical studies to prolong the circulatory half-life of fusion proteins by decreasing renal filtration and indirect recycling via the neonatal Fc receptor [32–35]. The tri-specific fusion protein thus comprised (i) a monovalent TfR-binding scFv, (ii) the therapeutic candidate Z_{SYM73} with affinity for monomeric Aß, and (iii) the ABD for prolonged in vivo circulation, at less than a third of the molecular weight of a standard IgG mAb (44 kDa compared to 150 kDa).

2. Results

2.1. Design and Production of scFv8D3-Z_{SYM73}-ABD and Z_{SYM73}-ABD

Z_{SYM73} is a heterodimeric affibody with high and specific affinity for the monomeric amyloid beta peptide (Figure 1A,B). The two subunits are connected by a flexible glycine/serine linker. For extending the in vivo half-life, we fused the affibody to a small albumin-binding domain (ABD; 46 amino acids) that is originally derived from streptococcal protein G [36] (Figure 1A,B). The albumin-binding domain used in this study (ABD$_{035}$ [21]; denoted only ABD hereinafter) has been engineered to femtomolar affinity for human serum albumin by directed evolution [21]. It also binds to serum albumin from other species, including mouse, and has successfully been used to extend the circulatory half-life of affibody fusion proteins in both preclinical and clinical studies [37,38]. Z_{SYM73}-ABD was included in this study to compare CSF uptake in absence of TfR-binding (Figure 1A,B).

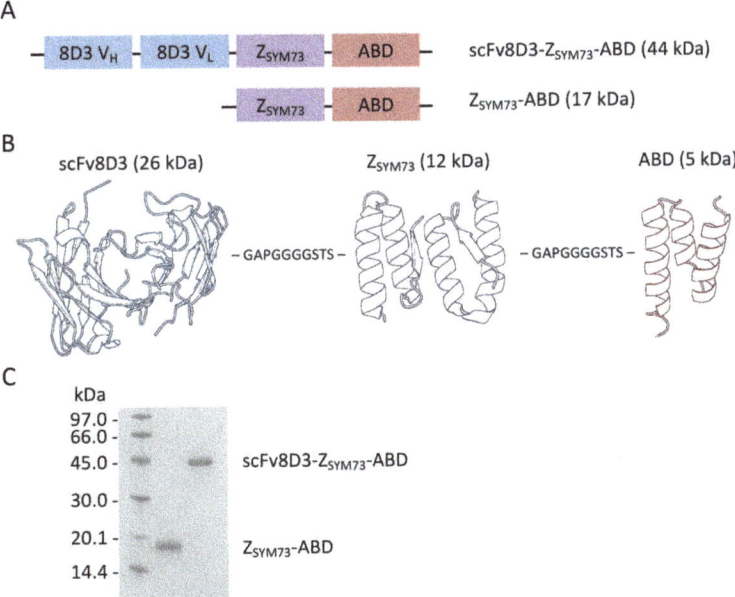

Figure 1. (**A**) Schematic representation of the tri-specific scFv8D3-Z_{SYM73}-ABD and the control protein Z_{SYM73}-ABD. Abbreviations scFv = single-chain variable fragment, Z = affibody, ABD = albumin-binding domain. (**B**) Schematic picture over the structure of scFv8D3-Z_{SYM73}-ABD with linkers between the subunits as amino acid sequences. The schematic structure is composed of following PDB IDs: scFv: 1KTR Zsym: 2OTK and ABD: 1GJT. (**C**) SDS-PAGE analysis of purified proteins. Purified scFv8D3-Z_{SYM73}-ABD and Z_{SYM73}-ABD appear as a single band of the correct size. The original and non-cropped gel is shown in Supplementary Figure S1.

To investigate the potential of transferrin-receptor (TfR) targeting for increasing the uptake of Z_{SYM73} in the central nervous system (CNS), we used the previously investigated TfR-specific antibody 8D3 [39]. The rat 8D3 mAb is specific for mouse TfR [40] and was reformatted into a synthetic scFv in the heavy (V_H) to light (V_L) chain orientation, separated by a 16 amino-acid flexible linker (^{N}GTTAASGSSGGSSSGA^C) [39]. The resulting scFv8D3 was then fused to the N-terminus of Z_{SYM73}-ABD [17] via a 10 amino-acid linker (^{N}GAPGGGGSTS^C).

ScFv8D3-Z_{SYM73}-ABD and Z_{SYM73}-ABD were produced in CHO cells and purified using affinity chromatography with human serum albumin (HSA) immobilized as ligand on a sepharose matrix, and followed by endotoxin removal by purification on EndoTrap columns. Both fusion proteins were observed as single bands of correct size after SDS-PAGE, demonstrating high sample purity (Figure 1C, the non-cropped gel is shown in Supplementary Figure S1). Quantification of the recovered proteins via amino acid analysis was carried out to determine protein concentrations. Production yields were approximately 35 mg of purified protein per liter cell culture medium for both proteins.

2.2. SPR Assays for Analysis of the Interaction between Recombinant Mouse TfR, MSA, and Aß$_{1-40}$ with the Trispecific Fusion Protein

First, we performed an in vitro binding analysis to evaluate the retained functionality of each of the domains (scFv8D3, Z_{SYM73}, and ABD) in the designed fusion protein using SPR-based biosensor assays. ScFv8D3-Z_{SYM73}-ABD or Z_{SYM73}-ABD were injected over a streptavidin surface on which biotinylated Aβ$_{1-40}$ was first indirectly immobilized. Mouse TfR and mouse serum albumin (MSA) were subsequently injected over the surface without regeneration. The results showed that scFv8D3-Z_{SYM73}-ABD is capable of simultaneously binding to Aß$_{1-40}$, TfR, and MSA (Figure 2A), demonstrating that both the N-terminus and C-terminus of Z_{SYM73} tolerate conjugation to fusion partners. As expected, no binding of Z_{SYM73}-ABD to TfR could be observed (Figure 2B).

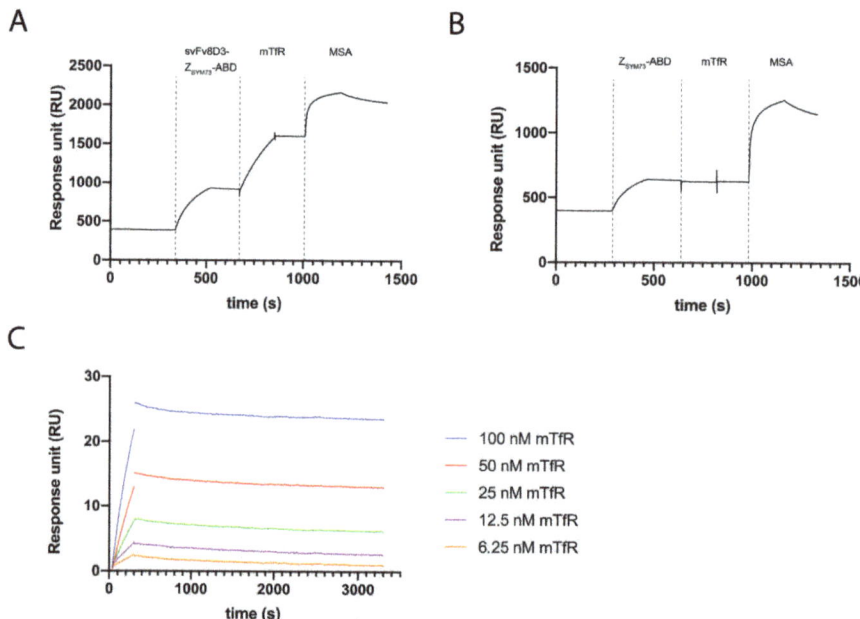

Figure 2. Surface plasmon resonance (SPR)-based biosensor assays. (**A**) Representative sensorgram showing the results from a triple co-inject assay. Aβ$_{1-40}$ is immobilized on the surface, and scFv8D3-Z_{SYM73}-ABD, mTfR, and mouse serum albumin (MSA) are injected subsequently. (**B**) Representative sensorgram showing the results from a triple co-inject assay. Aβ$_{1-40}$ is immobilized on the surface, and Z_{SYM73}-ABD, mTfR, and MSA are injected subsequently. Respective start points of injections are marked with a dashed line and the injected protein is stated over respective part of the sensorgram. (**C**) Representative sensorgram from the kinetic analysis of the interaction between mTfR and scFv8D3-Z_{SYM73}-ABD. All experiments were performed in duplicates. The gaps in the sensorgrams at the end of injection are from removal of spikes in signal by the Biacore evaluation software.

Next, the affinity of the interaction between scFv8D3-Z_{SYM73}-ABD and mouse TfR was investigated. In nature, TfR is a homodimeric receptor [41] and the two domains are covalently connected by two disulfide bonds between Cys 89 and Cys 98 in the respective domain, which can lead to avidity effects when interacting with surface-captured scFv8D3-Z_{SYM73}-ABD. The recombinant extracellular domain of TfR that was used in SPR starts at Cys 89 and is then most likely forming the two disulfide bonds and consequently has potential for dimerization. In order to assess the dimeric status of the receptor, we analyzed dithiothreitol (DTT)-treated TfR and non-treated TfR using SDS-PAGE. The results demonstrated that a relatively large proportion of the receptor is in a multimeric form (Supplementary Figure S2). Hence, to control for avidity effects in the kinetic analysis, we captured scFv8D3-Z_{SYM73}-ABD on HSA surfaces at three different immobilization levels. The mean equilibrium dissociation constant for the kinetic analysis was determined to be 5 nM. We only observed a small increase in off-rates for lower capture levels indicating small avidity effects (Table 1). Representative SPR measurement for the kinetic analysis of the interaction between mouse TfR and scFv8D3-Z_{SYM73}-ABD are shown in Figure 2C.

Table 1. Results from the kinetic analysis of the interaction between mTfR and scFv8D3-Z_{SYM73}-ABD using SPR. ScFv8D3-Z_{SYM73}-ABD was captured on human serum albumin (HSA) surfaces at three different levels and mTfR was injected over the surfaces. Mean values of two separate experiments and standard deviations are shown.

Immobilization Level	R_{max} (RU)	k_a (1/Ms)	k_d (1/s)	K_D (nM)
Surface 1: High (747 RU)	73.3 ± 9.8	1.4 ± 0.1 × 10^4	3.5 ± 0.1 × 10^{-5}	2.3 ± 0.02
Surface 2: Intermediate (487 RU)	61.3 ± 19.4	1.2 ± 0.3 × 10^4	7.6 ± 0.9 × 10^{-5}	6.6 ± 1.2
Surface 3: Low (229 RU)	21.9 ± 4.2	2.0 ± 0.3 × 10^4	9.9 ± 0.5 × 10^{-5}	5.2 ± 0.6

R_{max}, maximal capacity of the sensor chip surface; k_a, association rate constant; k_d, dissociation rate constant; K_D, equilibrium constant.

2.3. Flow Cytometry for Analysis of the Interaction between the Trispecific Fusion Protein and Mouse TfR-Expressing Endothelial Cells

Flow cytometry was used to assess whether scFv8D3-Z_{SYM73}-ABD could bind TfR in a cellular context. Mouse brain endothelial cells (bEnd.3) were treated with 37.5 nM, 75 nM, 150 nM, and 300 nM scFv8D3-Z_{SYM73}-ABD as well as PBS as control, and HSA labeled with Alexa Fluor 647 (HSA-AF647) was used as a secondary reagent. A concentration-dependent shift in fluorescence signal was observed for cells treated with scFv8D3-Z_{SYM73}-ABD compared to the PBS control, confirming binding to TfR in a cellular context (Figure 3A and Supplementary Figure S3B). Since fluorescently labeled HSA was used as secondary reagent, the results also confirmed simultaneous binding to albumin and TfR. Co-incubation of bEnd.3 cells with scFv8D3-Z_{SYM73}-ABD and a 6.6-fold molar excess of unlabeled parental monoclonal antibody 8D3 resulted in decrease in signal, indicating specific binding to TfR (Figure 3B). We did not observe binding of the control protein Z_{SYM73}-ABD to bEnd.3 cells or binding of scFv8D3-Z_{SYM73}-ABD to the human cell line SKOV-3 (murine TfR negative) (Figure 3C,D).

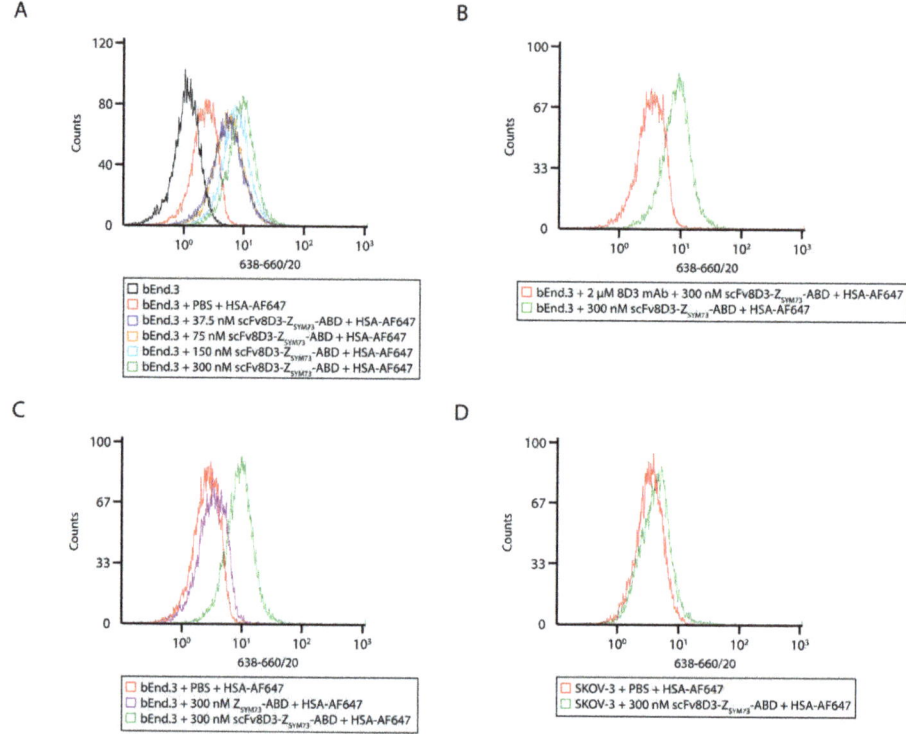

Figure 3. Flow-cytometric analysis of scFv8D3-Z_{SYM73}-ABD binding to cells. (**A**) Representative histograms showing results from the flow-cytometric analysis of bEnd.3 cells treated with 37.5 nM, 75 nM, 150 nM, and 300 nM scFv8D3-Z_{SYM73}-ABD. As a control, cells labeled only with HSA-AF647 and unlabeled cells were analyzed. (**B**) Representative histograms showing results from a blocking experiment using the parental mAb 8D3. (**C**) Representative histograms showing results from a control experiment using Z_{SYM73}-ABD. The MFI for cells treated with scFv8D3-Z_{SYM73}-ABD was 8.8 ± 0.2 and the MFI for cells treated with Z_{SYM73}-ABD was 3.7 ± 0.5. An unpaired t test demonstrated significant difference (p value = 0.0059). (**D**) Representative histograms showing results from the flow-cytometric analysis of SKOV-3 cells treated with 300 nM scFv8D3-Z_{SYM73}-ABD. As a control, cells labeled only with HSA-AF647 were analyzed. The wavelength of the excitation laser and bandwidth of the fluorescence detection filter is shown on the x-axis label in nm.

2.4. Bioavailability of the Affibody Fusion Proteins in Mouse CSF

The CSF bioavailability of scFv8D3-Z_{SYM73}-ABD and Z_{SYM73}-ABD was investigated in a mouse study. Male NMRI mice received a single 87.8 nmol/kg intravenous dose of either scFv8D3-Z_{SYM73}-ABD or Z_{SYM73}-ABD. One animal died directly after the injected dose, due to an air bubble in the syringe. CSF and serum samples were obtained from mice terminated after 3 h, 24 h, and 48 h. The specific concentrations of the two proteins in the biological samples were determined in an ELISA (Supplementary Table S1).

We first evaluated the pharmacokinetic profile of scFv8D3-Z_{SYM73}-ABD and Z_{SYM73}-ABD in serum over the time-course of 48 h (Figure 4A,B). By fitting the data using a one phase decay model, we estimated a serum half-life of around 26 h for Z_{SYM73}-ABD, which is in accordance with the 28.8 h serum half-life of MSA in mice [42]. We observed a faster serum clearance for scFv8D3-Z_{SYM73}-ABD, resulting in an estimated serum half-life of around 7 h.

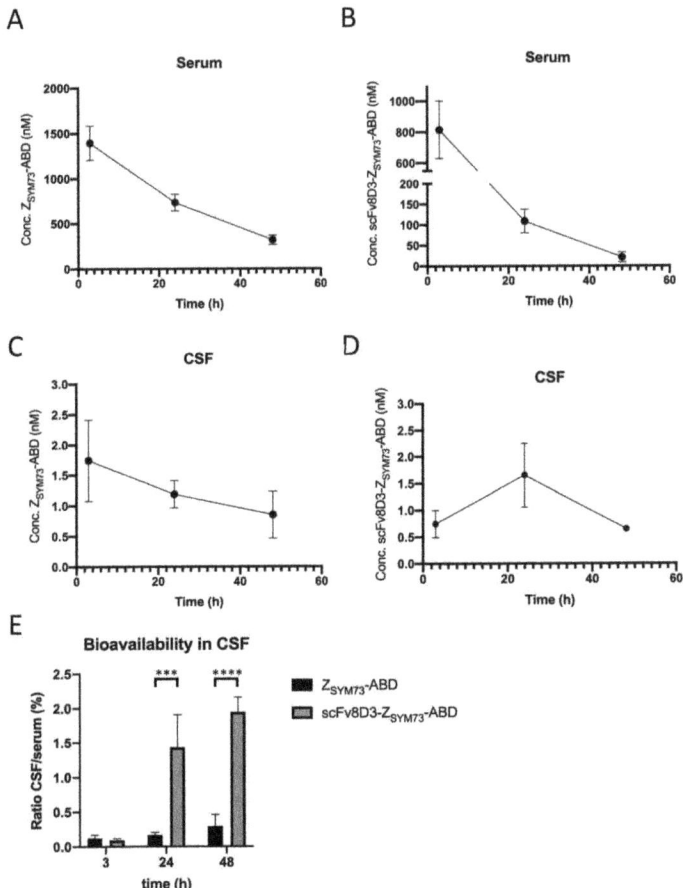

Figure 4. Concentrations of Z_{SYM73}-ABD and scFv8D3-Z_{SYM73}-ABD in NMRI mouse serum and CSF at 3 h, 24 h, and 48 h post administration. (**A**) Pharmacokinetic profile of Z_{SYM73}-ABD in mouse serum. (**B**) Pharmacokinetic profile of scFv8D3-Z_{SYM73}-ABD in mouse serum. (**C**) Pharmacokinetic profile of Z_{SYM73}-ABD in mouse cerebrospinal fluid (CSF). (**D**) Pharmacokinetic profile of scFv8D3-Z_{SYM73}-ABD in mouse CSF. (**E**) Bioavailability in CSF, expressed as CSF-to-serum ratio, of Z_{SYM73}-ABD and scFv8D3-Z_{SYM73}-ABD at 3 h, 24 h, and 48 h post administration. Unpaired t tests on data from 24 and 48 h demonstrated significant differences between CSF/serum ratios for Z_{SYM73}-ABD and scFv8D3-Z_{SYM73}-ABD (*** p value ≤ 0.001, **** p value ≤ 0.0001).

Next, we determined the absolute concentrations of the two proteins in CSF at 3 h, 24 h, and 48 h. Some of the CSF samples had to be excluded from the analysis due to contamination with blood or protein concentrations below the ELISA's sensitivity (Supplementary Table S1). The CSF concentrations of Z_{SYM73}-ABD steadily declined over the observed time course, with concentrations of 1.74 nM, 1.19 nM, and 0.85 nM at 3 h, 24 h, and 48 h, respectively (Figure 4C). The CSF concentration of scFv8D3-Z_{SYM73}-ABD doubled from 0.75 nM to 1.66 nM between 3 h and 24 h post injection (Figure 4D). We determined a mean concentration of 0.65 nM scFv8D3-Z_{SYM73}-ABD in the CSF samples after 48 h (Figure 4D).

Based on this data, we determined CSF bioavailability, expressed as CSF-to-serum ratios, of the two proteins over 48 h. We observed a steep increase in CSF bioavailability of scFv8D3-Z_{SYM73}-ABD between 3 h and 24 h, with CSF-to-serum ratios of 0.09% and 1.43%, respectively (Figure 4E). At 48 h post injection, the CSF-to-serum ratio of scFv8D3-Z_{SYM73}-ABD was 1.94%. The CSF bioavailability of the control protein Z_{SYM73}-ABD was 0.12%, 0.16%, and 0.29% at 3 h, 24 h, and 48 h, respectively (Figure 4E). The CSF bioavailability of Z_{SYM73}-ABD is in accordance with a recent study carried out in rats [27] and reflects values reported for passive protein uptake into the CNS [43]. The fusion of scFv8D3 to Z_{SYM73}-ABD led to an 9-fold increase in CSF bioavailability after 24 h indicating an active transport mechanism into CSF.

3. Discussion

In this present study we explored a strategy that could potentially increase the brain uptake of an affibody molecule via transferrin receptor-mediated transcytosis in the future. Engagement of the TfR has successfully been used in previous studies to transport cargo proteins across the BBB [14,28,44].

Here, we designed a tri-specific fusion protein consisting of a single-chain variable fragment (scFv) of the mouse TfR-specific antibody 8D3, the Aβ-specific affibody molecule Z_{SYM73}, and an engineered albumin-binding domain (ABD) (Figure 1A,B). There is a risk that fusion to ABD and scFv might affect the interaction with Aβ. In an SPR assay, we demonstrated that scFv8D3-Z_{SYM73}-ABD was able to simultaneously engage with Aβ$_{1-40}$, mouse TfR, and MSA, confirming the tri-specific nature of the fusion protein. We have also previously reported on the therapeutic effect of Z_{SYM73}-ABD in a murine AD model with promising results, and since ABD is cross reactive to MSA, this is further indication that albumin-binding has no dramatic negative effect on target binding. We report an affinity (K_D) of scFv8D3-Z_{SYM73}-ABD for mouse TfR of 5 nM (Figure 2C and Table 1). The observed affinity is about 3-fold stronger than previously reported monomeric 8D3 affinity, as determined by ELISA [28]. When investigating the relationship between TfR affinity and brain uptake of TfR antibodies, Yu et al. reported highest brain exposure for antibodies with an affinity for TfR of around 50 nM–100 nM [14]. More recently, apparent TfR affinities of 0.6 nM and 8 nM led to increased brain uptake of antibody variants [28,44]. Our engineered fusion protein engages with TfR in a monovalent binding mode, which has been shown to be important for transport across the BBB [12]. We next demonstrated blockable binding of scFv8D3-Z_{SYM73}-ABD to TfR on mouse brain endothelial cells (bEnd.3).

The CSF uptake and serum pharmacokinetics of scFv8D3-Z_{SYM73}-ABD and the control protein Z_{SYM73}-ABD were assessed in NMRI mice. It has recently been shown that Z_{SYM73}-ABD treatment leads to prevention of the amyloid burden build up in both cortex and hippocampus as well as prevention of cognitive function decline in APP/PS1 double transgenic mice. The brain bioavailability of Z_{SYM73}-ABD in mice is however unknown [27].

We decided to assess protein uptake into CSF as a surrogate for brain uptake. It has been reported that drug concentrations in CSF can be used for estimating the concentration in brain interstitial fluid [45,46]. We reasoned that affibody concentrations in CSF do not take into account proteins bound to TfR on the BBB and hence reflect active, free affibody concentrations in CSF. Wang and coworkers concluded that CSF-to-serum ratios are indicators of antibody CNS uptake after the antibody concentration in CSF reached a maximum [43].

In contrast to the results for Z_{SYM73}-ABD, we observed a steep increase in CSF concentration of the scFv8D3-Z_{SYM73}-ABD between 3 and 24 h post injection, indicating active receptor-mediated uptake (Figure 4D). It should be noted that the concentration of the trispecific protein in CSF was approximately 2-fold lower at 3 h p.i., and only moderately higher (1.4-fold) at 24 h p.i. compared to the control protein. Clearance from serum was drastically faster for scFv8D3-Z_{SYM73}-ABD compared to the control protein Z_{SYM73}-ABD, with estimated circulatory serum half-lives of 7 h and 26 h, respectively (Figure 4A,B). Fast serum clearance has been reported for TfR antibodies and is likely due to binding to TfR expressed in peripheral tissues such as liver and kidney [44]. The CSF bioavailability, expressed as the ratio of CSF-to-serum concentrations, for Z_{SYM73}-ABD was 0.12%, 0.16%, and 0.29% at 3 h, 24 h, and 48 h, respectively. We observed a significant increase in CSF bioavailability for scFv8D3-Z_{SYM73}-ABD, with ratios of 1.43% and 1.94% at 24 h and 48 h, respectively. Brain-to-serum concentration ratios between 0.91% to 2.11% at 24 h post injection have been reported by Yu and coworkers for monovalent TfR antibodies following injection of a similar dose (20 mg/kg or approximately 130 nmol/kg) [14], indicating that protein concentrations in CSF might be used as a surrogate for brain protein concentrations.

In this study, we investigated CSF bioavailability of affibody fusion proteins after administrating a therapeutically relevant dose of 87.8 nmol/kg. These doses are comparable to doses administered in a preclinical study of Z_{SYM73}-ABD and significantly larger than doses used in previous studies exploiting TfR brain uptake using the 8D3 antibody [27,28,44].

The increase in CSF bioavailability could be the result of either active transport over BBB, followed by diffusion transport from the brain interstitial fluid into CSF or by passage over the epithelium of the choroid plexus [16]. However, uptake at the choroid plexus has been demonstrated to inversely correlate with the molecular weight of compounds [47]. Since the bioavailability of the larger scFv8D3-Z_{SYM73}-ABD (44 kDa) is higher compared with the smaller Z_{SYM73}-ABD (17 kDa), this indicates that the uptake into CSF is not primarily driven by passive passage over the epithelium of the choroid plexus. Still, using CSF as a surrogate for estimating uptake into brain parenchyma is controversial and should be considered as indications [47]. Future studies on target engagement and therapeutic effect will hopefully contribute to the understanding of the mechanisms. Another option is to measure the concentration of the affibody fusion proteins using ELISA on brain homogenate. In such studies, it is important to note that measurements on brain homogenates typically do not distinguish between proteins that have passed over the endothelium layer into the brain parenchyma, and the fraction of proteins still associated with the endothelial cells, and more sophisticated methods (e.g., capillary depletion methods [48]) should hence be used to avoid overestimating the uptake [49].

Although the results indicate active uptake into CSF that is mediated by binding to TfR, the much faster blood clearance of the scFv8D3-Z_{SYM73}-ABD is far from optimal. In future studies, it would be interesting to investigate both the brain uptake and the pharmacokinetics of the scFv8D3-Z_{SYM73}-ABD at different doses. Due to the fast serum clearance of the protein, higher doses might be necessary to achieve a therapeutic relevant concentration in CSF, but this might impede the future clinical utility. Moreover, we would like to explore lower affinity binding domains for TfR and different valences of 8D3, which could influence both uptake into CNS as well as the blood clearance rate. Dissociation of the brain shuttle molecules from TfR expressed on the BBB might be slow, leading to lower active concentration in brain and consequently lower amounts of protein detectable in CSF. This could be achieved by mutating scFv8D3 and selection of lower affinity variants or by replacing the antibody fragment for an affibody molecule with moderate affinity towards TfR. It should also be noted that the 8D3 antibody is not cross-reactive to human TfR and was only used in this study to explore the potential of TfR-targeting for increasing uptake into CNS. If TfR-specific affibody molecules were to be developed in the future, achieving cross-reactivity between human TfR and corresponding TfRs in model animals should be a focus.

At 44 kDa, the scFv8D3-Z_{SYM73}-ABD presented in this study is significantly smaller than comparable therapeutic bispecific antibodies. It should be noted that the drug complex would be substantially larger in blood when associated with albumin, which will affect parameters such as diffusion and penetration in tissues. There is still a potential positive effect of small size in terms of possibilities for higher molar concentrations in formulations which could open up for alternative routes of administration (e.g., subcutaneous injections) in the future. Moreover, since albumin concentration is lower in the brain, the fraction of non-HSA associated drug might be higher in this compartment, which could have positive effects on brain biodistribution. Moreover, CSF is only an indication of increased uptake in the brain. Target engagement by measuring therapeutic effect is an important next step to obtain more experimental evidence on brain uptake and follow-up efforts will be focused on such studies.

4. Materials and Methods

4.1. Design and Molecular Cloning of Affibody Fusion Proteins

The rat 8D3 mAb against mouse TfR was reformatted into a synthetic scFv in the heavy (V_H) to light (V_L) chain orientation, separated by a 16 amino-acid flexible linker (^{N}GTTAASGSSGGSSSGA^C). The 8D3 scFv was fused to the N-terminus of Z_{SYM73}-ABD [27] via a 10 amino-acid linker (^{N}GAPGGGGSTS^C). The albumin-binding domain used in this study (ABD$_{035}$ [21]; denoted only ABD hereinafter) has been engineered to femtomolar affinity for human serum albumin by directed evolution [21]. The resulting fusion protein is hereafter denoted as scFv8D3-Z_{SYM73}-ABD. The gene encoding scFv8D3-Z_{SYM73}-ABD was ordered from Genewiz (GENEWIZ Germany GmbH, Leipzig, Germany). The genes encoding scFv8D3-Z_{SYM73}-ABD and Z_{SYM73}-ABD were inserted into pQMCF1 (Icosagen Cell Factory OU, Tartu, Estonia) [50]. The genes encoding scFv8D3-Z_{SYM73}-ABD and Z_{SYM73}-ABD were amplified by polymerase chain reaction (PCR) using Q5 high-fidelity polymerase (New England Biolabs, Ipswich, MA, USA). Specific primers were used to introduce a *Not*I sequence upstream-, and an *Asc*I sequence downstream of the respective gene. The pQMCF1 vector (Icosagen Cell Factory OU, Tartu, Estonia) and the two PCR products were digested using *Not*I-HF and *Asc*I restriction enzymes (NEB). The digested vector and inserts were purified using QIAquick Gel Extraction Kit (Qiagen GmbH, Hilden, Germany) and QIAquick PCR Purification Kit (Qiagen), respectively. The purified vector and inserts were subsequently ligated using T4 DNA Ligase (NEB). By utilizing the *Not*I and *Asc*I restriction sites the genes were ligated in fusion with a N-terminal CD33 secretion signal peptide present in the vector. The pQMCF1 plasmid moreover contains a CMV promoter [50]. The two plasmids (pQMCF1 scFv8D3-ZSYM73-ABD and pQMCF1 ZSYM73-ABD) were transformed into chemically competent TOP10 *Escherichia coli* cells by heat shock (Thermo Fisher Scientific, Waltham, MA, USA). Plasmids were prepared using QIAprep Spin Miniprep Kit (Qiagen GmbH, Hilden, Germany) and the sequences were verified by Sanger DNA sequencing (Microsynth AG, Balgach, Switzerland).

4.2. Protein Expression, Purification, and Quality Control

ScFv8D3-Z_{SYM73}-ABD and Z_{SYM73}-ABD were expressed in Chinese hamster ovary (CHO) EBNALT 85 cells using the Icosagen QMCF technology (an episomal protein expression system, which uses mammalian cells that are genetically modified and designed plasmids). After 12 days of cultivation, cell culture supernatants were spiked with 10× tris-buffered saline (TST) to a final concentration of 1× TST. ScFv8D3-Z_{SYM73}-ABD and Z_{SYM73}-ABD were recovered from the cell culture supernatant using affinity chromatography with human serum albumin (HSA) as a ligand immobilized to sepharose matrix, as described elsewhere [51]. The recovered proteins were buffer-exchanged to phosphate-buffered saline (PBS) using PD-10 desalting columns (GE Healthcare Life Sciences, Uppsala, Sweden). Endotoxin removal was carried out using EndoTrap® red columns (Lionex GmbH, Braunschweig, Germany) according to the manufacturer's instructions. The purity of the recovered proteins was evaluated by SDS-PAGE. Quantification of the proteins was carried out by amino acid analysis (Alphalyse A/S, Odense, Denmark). All proteins were stored in PBS at −80 °C.

4.3. Analysis of Binding to Recombinant Proteins Using SPR-Based Biosensor Assays

All surface plasmon resonance (SPR) experiments were performed on a Biacore T200 (GE Healthcare Life Sciences, Uppsala, Sweden) with PBS containing 0.5% Tween 20 as running buffer. Firstly, trispecific simultaneous binding of the affibody fusion proteins was analyzed. Biotinylated amyloid beta 1-40 (AnaSpec, Fremont, CA, USA) was captured on a streptavidin sensor chip (GE Healthcare Life Sciences, Uppsala, Sweden) according the manufacturer's recommendations to a capture level of 130 RU. Three hundred nanomoles of either scFv8D3-Z_{SYM73}-ABD or Z_{SYM73}-ABD was initially injected over the surface for 180 s at a flow rate of 30 µL/min. After a dissociation phase of approximately 150 s, 300 nM of recombinant his-tagged mouse TfR (Sino Biological Inc., Beijing, China) was injected over the surface for 180 s. Following another dissociation phase of approximately 150 s, 300 nM mouse serum albumin (Merck KGaA, Darmstadt, Germany) was injected for 180 s.

Kinetic data on the scFv8D3 interaction with mouse TfR was obtained by capturing scFv8D3-Z_{SYM73}-ABD on human serum albumin (HSA) immobilized on the surface, followed by injections of various concentrations of mouse TfR. To this end, albumin from human serum (Merck KGaA, Darmstadt, Germany) was immobilized on three different surfaces of a CM5 sensor chip (GE Healthcare Life Sciences, Uppsala, Sweden) according to the manufacturer's protocol. Immobilization levels of HSA reached 747 response units (RU), 487 RU, and 229 RU for the three different surfaces. The flow rate for all following injections was 30 µL/min. 80 nM scFv8D3-Z_{SYM73}-ABD was injected over all surfaces for 10 s, followed by 300 s injections of mouse TfR (Sino Biological Inc., Beijing, China) in concentrations of 100 nM, 50 nM, 25 nM, 12.5 nM, 6.25 nM, and 0 nM. Dissociation was monitored by injecting running buffer for 3000 s. The surfaces were regenerated by injecting 10 mM HCl for 30 s. All SPR experiments were carried out in duplicates.

4.4. Analysis of Binding to TfR on Mouse Brain Endothelial Cells Using Flow Cytometry

The monoclonal anti-mouse TfR antibody 8D3 was purchased from Novus Biologicals (Novus Biologicals LLC, Centennial, CO, USA). The bEnd.3 mouse brain endothelial cell line (ATCC) was cultured in Dulbecco's Modified Eagle's Medium (Merck KGaA) complemented with 10% fetal bovine serum. The SKOV-3 cell line (ATCC) was cultured according to the manufacturer's protocol. At approximately 80% confluency, cells were harvested using TrypLE™ Express (ThermoFisher Scientific, Waltham, MA, USA) according to the manufacturer's protocol. Around 100,000 cells were resuspended in the respective protein solution in PBS + 1% bovine serum albumin (BSA; PBSB) and incubated for 45 min at 4 °C under constant agitation. The supernatant was discarded by centrifugation at 1700 rpm and 4 °C for 4 min. Cells were subsequently resuspended in 100 nM HSA-Alexa Fluor 647 conjugate (produced in-house) in PBSB and incubated for 20 min at 4 °C under constant agitation. The supernatant was discarded as described above and the cells were resuspended in 400 uL ice-cold PBSB. The cells were analyzed using a Gallios™ flow cytometer (Beckman Coulter Inc., Indianapolis, IN, USA). Gates based on forward and side scatter intensities were used to analyze intact and single cells (Supplementary Figure S3A). All flow cytometry experiments were carried out in duplicates on separate biological samples.

4.5. Analysis of CNS Uptake in a Mouse Model

The animal study was carried out by Adlego Biomedical AB, Solna, Sweden. Ethics permit No. 4570-2019 approved by the regional animal experimental committee in Stockholm (North). 36 male NMRI mice were divided into two groups. Twenty-one mice received an 87.8 nmol/kg dose of Z_{SYM73}-ABD and 15 mice received an 87.8 nmol/kg dose of scFv8D3-Z_{SYM73}-ABD via intravenous injection in a lateral tail vein. Subgroups of 7 (Z_{SYM73}-ABD) or 5 (scFv8D3-Z_{SYM73}-ABD) mice were terminated at 3, 24, and 48 h after administration. Blood samples were collected from the orbital plexus and CSF samples were collected from the cisterna magna at termination. Serum was extracted from the blood samples and all sampled were stored at −20 °C within 1 h of collection. Samples were thawed on ice and measured in an ELISA including a freshly prepared calibration standard (reference material from identical batch). Briefly, a 96-well plate was coated with mouse monoclonal anti-affibody antibodies (Affibody AB, Solna, Sweden). Serum received from one untreated mouse was used to prepare a 1% (v/v) solution in Blocker™ Casein in PBS (ThermoFisher Scientific, Waltham, MA, USA). All serum samples and serum standards were diluted in the 1% (v/v) serum solution. For dilution of the CSF samples and CSF standards, a 1% (v/v) solution of CSF received from one untreated rat in Blocker™ Casein (ThermoFisher Scientific, Waltham, MA, USA) was prepared. The samples and calibration standards were diluted and added to the wells. Polyclonal rabbit anti-ABD antibodies (Affibody AB) were added, followed by horseradish peroxidase (HRP)-conjugated polyclonal donkey-anti-rabbit-IgG antibodies (Jackson Immunoresearch, West Grove, PA, USA). Detection was carried out by addition of

TMB substrate (ThermoFisher Scientific, Waltham, MA, USA) and the reaction was stopped using 2 M sulfuric acid. Independent experiments (*N*) were performed on individual animals. Parallel ELISA experiments (*n*) were performed in triplicate on separate biological samples and calibration standards in parallel on the same day.

Supplementary Materials: The following are available online at http://www.mdpi.com/1422-0067/21/8/2999/s1, Figure S1: Non-cropped SDS-PAGE analysis of purified proteins, Figure S2: SDS-PAGE analysis of reduced- and non-reduced recombinant proteins, Figure S3: Representative plot from flow-cytometric analysis with gating indicated, Table S1: Serum and CSF concentrations, and C_{CSF}/C_{serum} ratios of the two investigated proteins in individual mice.

Author Contributions: Conceptualization, S.W.M., S.S. and J.L.; methodology, S.W.M. and J.L.; investigation, S.W.M., L.C.H., M.D. and H.L.; data curation, S.W.M.; writing—original draft preparation, S.W.M.; writing—review and editing, S.W.M., L.C.H., M.D., H.T., H.L., S.S., J.L.; visualization, S.W.M. and J.L.; supervision, H.T., S.S. and J.L.; project administration, J.L.; funding acquisition, H.T., S.S. and J.L. All authors have read and agreed to the published version of the manuscript.

Funding: This research was funded by grants from the Swedish Brain foundation (grant FO2018-0094), the Wallenberg Center for Protein Research (KAW 2019.0341), the Tussilago foundation (FL-0002.025.551-7) and the Schörling Family foundation via the Swedish FTD Initiative.

Acknowledgments: The authors wish to thank Ingmarie Höidén-Guthenberg and Fredrik Y. Frejd at Affibody AB, Solna, Sweden for providing the protocol and reagents for the affibody pharmacokinetics ELISA.

Conflicts of Interest: The authors declare no conflict of interest. The funders had no role in the design of the study; in the collection, analyses, or interpretation of data; in the writing of the manuscript, or in the decision to publish the results.

References

1. Saunders, N.R.; Habgood, M.D.; Møllgård, K.; Dziegielewska, K.M. The biological significance of brain barrier mechanisms: Help or hindrance in drug delivery to the central nervous system? *F1000Research* **2016**, *5*, F1000 Faculty Rev-313. [CrossRef] [PubMed]
2. Thomsen, M.S.; Routhe, L.J.; Moos, T. The vascular basement membrane in the healthy and pathological brain. *J. Cereb. Blood Flow. Metab.* **2017**, *37*, 3300–3317. [CrossRef] [PubMed]
3. Abbott, N.J.; Rönnbäck, L.; Hansson, E. Astrocyte–endothelial interactions at the blood–brain barrier. *Nat. Rev. Neurosci.* **2006**, *7*, 41–53. [CrossRef] [PubMed]
4. Brightman, M.W.; Reese, T.S. Junctions between intimately apposed cell membranes in the vertebrate brain. *J. Cell Biol.* **1969**, *40*, 648–677. [CrossRef] [PubMed]
5. Hawkins, B.T.; Davis, T.P. The Blood-Brain Barrier/Neurovascular Unit in Health and Disease. *Pharmacol. Rev.* **2005**, *57*, 173–185. [CrossRef]
6. Abbott, N.J.; Patabendige, A.A.K.; Dolman, D.E.M.; Yusof, S.R.; Begley, D.J. Neurobiology of Disease Structure and function of the blood—brain barrier. *Neurobiol. Dis.* **2010**, *37*, 13–25. [CrossRef]
7. Poduslo, J.F.; Curran, G.L.; Berg, C.T. Macromolecular permeability across the blood-nerve and blood-brain barriers. *Proc. Natl. Acad. Sci. USA* **1994**, *91*, 5705–5709. [CrossRef]
8. Yu, Y.J.; Watts, R.J. Developing Therapeutic Antibodies for Neurodegenerative Disease. *Neurotherapeutics* **2013**, *10*, 459–472. [CrossRef]
9. Zuchero, Y.J.Y.; Chen, X.; Bien-Ly, N.; Bumbaca, D.; Tong, R.K.; Gao, X.; Zhang, S.; Hoyte, K.; Luk, W.; Huntley, M.A.; et al. Discovery of Novel Blood-Brain Barrier Targets to Enhance Brain Uptake of Therapeutic Antibodies Article Discovery of Novel Blood-Brain Barrier Targets to Enhance Brain Uptake of Therapeutic Antibodies. *Neuron* **2016**, *89*, 70–82. [CrossRef]
10. Duck, K.A.; Connor, J.R. Iron uptake and transport across physiological barriers. *Biometals* **2016**, *29*, 573–591. [CrossRef]
11. Pulgar, V.M. Transcytosis to Cross the Blood Brain Barrier, New Advancements and Challenges. *Front. Neurosci.* **2018**, *12*, 1019. [CrossRef] [PubMed]
12. Niewoehner, J.; Bohrmann, B.; Collin, L.; Urich, E.; Sade, H.; Maier, P.; Rueger, P.; Stracke, J.O.; Lau, W.; Tissot, A.C.; et al. Increased Brain Penetration and Potency of a Therapeutic Antibody Using a Monovalent Molecular Shuttle. *Neuron* **2014**, *81*, 49–60. [CrossRef] [PubMed]

13. Bien-Ly, N.; Yu, J.Y.; Bumbaca, D.; Elstrott, J.; Boswell, C.A.; Zhang, Y.; Luk, W.; Lu, Y.; Dennis, M.S.; Weimer, R.M.; et al. Transferrin receptor (TfR) trafficking determines brain uptake of TfR antibody affinity variants. *J. Exp. Med.* **2014**, *211*, 233–244. [CrossRef] [PubMed]
14. Yu, Y.J.; Zhang, Y.; Kenrick, M.; Hoyte, K.; Luk, W.; Lu, Y.; Atwal, J.; Elliott, J.M.; Prabhu, S.; Watts, R.J.; et al. Boosting brain uptake of a therapeutic antibody by reducing its affinity for a transcytosis target. *Sci. Transl. Med.* **2011**, *3*, 84ra44. [CrossRef] [PubMed]
15. Villasenor, R.; Schilling, M.; Sundaresan, J.; Lutz, Y.; Collin, L. Sorting Tubules Regulate Blood-Brain Barrier Transcytosis. *Cell Rep.* **2017**, *21*, 3256–3270. [CrossRef] [PubMed]
16. Gonzalez, A.M.; Leadbeater, W.E.; Burg, M.; Sims, K.; Terasaki, T.; Johanson, C.E.; Stopa, E.G.; Eliceiri, B.P.; Baird, A. Targeting choroid plexus epithelia and ventricular ependyma for drug delivery to the central nervous system. *BMC Neurosci.* **2011**, *12*, 4. [CrossRef]
17. Rouault, T.A.; Zhang, D.-L.; Jeong, S.Y. Brain iron homeostasis, the choroid plexus, and localization of iron transport proteins. *Metab. Brain Dis.* **2009**, *24*, 673–684. [CrossRef]
18. Abbott, N.J.; Pizzo, M.E.; Preston, J.E.; Janigro, D.; Thorne, R.G. The role of brain barriers in fluid movement in the CNS: Is there a 'glymphatic' system? *Acta Neuropathol.* **2018**, *135*, 387–407. [CrossRef]
19. Haqqani, A.S.; Caram-Salas, N.; Ding, W.; Brunette, E.; Delaney, C.E.; Baumann, E.; Boileau, E.; Stanimirovic, D. Multiplexed evaluation of serum and CSF pharmacokinetics of brain-targeting single-domain antibodies using a NanoLC-SRM-ILIS method. *Mol. Pharm.* **2013**, *10*, 1542–1556. [CrossRef]
20. Querfurth, H.W.; LaFerla, F.M. Alzheimer's disease. *N. Engl. J. Med.* **2010**, *362*, 329–344. [CrossRef]
21. Spencer, B.; Masliah, E. Immunotherapy for Alzheimer's disease: Past, present and future. *Front. Aging Neurosci.* **2014**, *6*, 114. [CrossRef] [PubMed]
22. Sevigny, J.; Chiao, P.; Bussière, T.; Weinreb, P.H.; Williams, L.; Maier, M.; Dunstan, R.; Salloway, S.; Chen, T.; Ling, Y.; et al. The antibody aducanumab reduces Aβ plaques in Alzheimer's disease. *Nat. Publ. Gr.* **2016**, *537*, 50–56. [CrossRef] [PubMed]
23. Panza, F.; Lozupone, M.; Logroscino, G.; Imbimbo, B.P. A critical appraisal of amyloid-β-targeting therapies for Alzheimer disease. *Nat. Rev. Neurol.* **2019**, *15*, 73–88. [CrossRef] [PubMed]
24. Selkoe, D.J.; Hardy, J. The amyloid hypothesis of Alzheimer's disease at 25 years. *EMBO Mol. Med.* **2016**, *8*, 1–14. [CrossRef]
25. Lindberg, H.; Hard, T.; Lofblom, J.; Stahl, S. A truncated and dimeric format of an Affibody library on bacteria enables FACS-mediated isolation of amyloid-beta aggregation inhibitors with subnanomolar affinity. *Biotechnol. J.* **2015**, *10*, 1707–1718. [CrossRef]
26. Hoyer, W.; Grönwall, C.; Jonsson, A.; Ståhl, S.; Härd, T. Stabilization of a β-hairpin in monomeric Alzheimer's amyloid-β peptide inhibits amyloid formation. *Proc. Natl. Acad. Sci. USA* **2008**, *105*, 5099–5104. [CrossRef]
27. Boutajangout, A.; Lindberg, H.; Awwad, A.; Paul, A.; Baitalmal, R.; Almokyad, I.; Höidén-Guthenberg, I.; Gunneriusson, E.; Frejd, F.Y.; Härd, T.; et al. Affibody-Mediated Sequestration of Amyloid β Demonstrates Preventive Efficacy in a Transgenic Alzheimer's Disease Mouse Model. *Front. Aging Neurosci.* **2019**, *11*, 64. [CrossRef]
28. Hultqvist, G.; Syvanen, S.; Fang, X.T.; Lannfelt, L.; Sehlin, D. Bivalent Brain Shuttle Increases Antibody Uptake by Monovalent Binding to the Transferrin Receptor. *Theranostics* **2017**, *7*, 308–318. [CrossRef]
29. Lee, H.J.; Engelhardt, B.; Lesley, J.; Bickel, U.; Pardridge, W.M. Targeting Rat Anti-Mouse Transferrin Receptor Monoclonal Antibodies through Blood-Brain Barrier in Mouse. *J. Pharmacol. Exp. Ther.* **2000**, *292*, 1048–1052.
30. Cabezón, I.; Manich, G.; Martín-Venegas, R.; Camins, A.; Pelegrí, C.; Vilaplana, J. Trafficking of Gold Nanoparticles Coated with the 8D3 Anti-Transferrin Receptor Antibody at the Mouse Blood–Brain Barrier. *Mol. Pharm.* **2015**, *12*, 4137–4145. [CrossRef]
31. Jonsson, A.; Dogan, J.; Herne, N.; Abrahmsén, L.; Nygren, P.-Å. Engineering of a femtomolar affinity binding protein to human serum albumin. *Protein Eng. Des. Sel.* **2008**, *21*, 515–527. [CrossRef] [PubMed]
32. Zorzi, A.; Linciano, S.; Angelini, A. Non-covalent albumin-binding ligands for extending the circulating half-life of small biotherapeutics. *MedChemComm* **2019**, *10*, 1068–1081. [CrossRef] [PubMed]
33. Kim, D.; Jeon, H.; Ahn, S.; Choi, W.I.; Kim, S.; Jon, S. An approach for half-life extension and activity preservation of an anti-diabetic peptide drug based on genetic fusion with an albumin-binding aptide. *J. Control Release* **2017**, *256*, 114–120. [CrossRef] [PubMed]
34. Tan, H.; Su, W.; Zhang, W.; Wang, P.; Sattler, M.; Zou, P. Recent Advances in Half-life Extension Strategies for Therapeutic Peptides and Proteins. *Curr. Pharm. Des.* **2018**, *24*, 4932–4946. [CrossRef]

35. Sleep, D.; Cameron, J.; Evans, L.R. Albumin as a versatile platform for drug half-life extension. *Biochim. Biophys. Acta* **2013**, *1830*, 5526–5534. [CrossRef]
36. Johansson, M.U.; Frick, I.M.; Nilsson, H.; Kraulis, P.J.; Hober, S.; Jonasson, P.; Linhult, M.; Nygren, P.-Å.; Uhlén, M.; Björck, L.; et al. Structure, specificity, and mode of interaction for bacterial albumin-binding modules. *J. Biol. Chem.* **2002**, *277*, 8114–8120. [CrossRef]
37. Ståhl, S.; Gräslund, T.; Eriksson Karlström, A.; Frejd, F.Y.; Nygren, P.Å.; Löfblom, J. Affibody Molecules in Biotechnological and Medical Applications. *Trends Biotechnol.* **2017**, *35*, 691–712. [CrossRef]
38. Affibody. ClinicalTrials.gov Identifier: NCT03591887, A Study to Evaluate ABY-035 in Subjects With Moderate-to-severe Plaque Psoriasis (AFFIRM-35); 2018 Jul 19 (cited 2020 Feb 19). Available online: https://clinicaltrials.gov/ct2/show/NCT03591887 (accessed on 19 July 2018).
39. Luz, D.; Chen, G.; Maranhão, A.Q.; Rocha, L.B.; Sidhu, S.; Piazza, R.M. Development and Characterization of Recombinant Antibody Fragments That Recognize and Neutralize In Vitro Stx2 Toxin from Shiga Toxin-Producing Escherichia coli. *PLoS ONE* **2015**, *10*, e0120481. [CrossRef]
40. Boado, R.J.; Zhang, Y.; Wang, Y.; Pardridge, W.M. Engineering and expression of a chimeric transferrin receptor monoclonal antibody for blood–brain barrier delivery in the mouse. *Biotechnol. Bioeng.* **2009**, *102*, 1251–1258. [CrossRef]
41. Giannetti, A.M.; Snow, P.M.; Zak, O.; Björkman, P.J. Mechanism for Multiple Ligand Recognition by the Human Transferrin Receptor. *PLoS Biol.* **2003**, *1*, e51. [CrossRef]
42. Yang, B.; Kim, J.C.; Seong, J.; Tae, G.; Kwon, I. Comparative studies of the serum half-life extension of a protein via site-specific conjugation to a species-matched or -mismatched albumin. *Biomater. Sci.* **2018**, *6*, 2092–2100. [CrossRef] [PubMed]
43. Wang, Q.; Delva, L.; Weinreb, P.H.; Pepinsky, R.B.; Graham, D.; Veizaj, E.; Cheung, A.E.; Chen, W.; Nestorov, I.; Rohde, E.; et al. Monoclonal antibody exposure in rat and cynomolgus monkey cerebrospinal fluid following systemic administration. *Fluids Barriers CNS* **2018**, *15*, 10. [CrossRef] [PubMed]
44. Stocki, P.; Szary, J.M.; Jacobsen, C.L.; Demydchuk, M.; Northall, L.; Moos, T.; Walsh, F.S.; Rutkowski, J.L. High efficiency blood-brain barrier transport using a VNAR targeting the Transferrin Receptor 1 (TfR1). *bioRxiv* **2019**, 816900. [CrossRef]
45. Liu, X.; Van Natta, K.; Yeo, H.; Vilenski, O.; Weller, P.E.; Worboys, P.D.; Monshouwer, M. Unbound Drug Concentration in Brain Homogenate and Cerebral Spinal Fluid at Steady State as a Surrogate for Unbound Concentration in Brain Interstitial Fluid. *Drug Metab. Dispos.* **2007**, *37*, 787–793. [CrossRef]
46. Shen, D.D.; Artru, A.A.; Adkison, K.K. Principles and applicability of CSF sampling for the assessment of CNS drug delivery and pharmacodynamics. *Adv. Drug Deliv. Rev.* **2004**, *56*, 1825–1857. [CrossRef]
47. Pardridge, W.M. Blood-Brain Barrier and Delivery of Protein and Gene Therapeutics to Brain. *Front. Aging Neurosci.* **2020**, *11*, 373. [CrossRef]
48. Triguero, D.; Buciak, J.; Pardridge, W.M. Capillary depletion method for quantification of blood-brain barrier transport of circulating peptides and plasma proteins. *J. Neurochem.* **1990**, *54*, 1882–1888. [CrossRef]
49. Bickel, U. How to measure drug transport across the blood-brain barrier. *NeuroRx* **2005**, *2*, 15–26. [CrossRef]
50. Jennbacken, K.; Wågberg, F.; Karlsson, U.; Eriksson, J.; Magnusson, L.; Chimienti, M.; Ricchiuto, P.; Bernström, J.; Ding, M.; Ross-Thriepland, D.; et al. Phenotypic Screen with the Human Secretome Identifies FGF16 as Inducing Proliferation of iPSC-Derived Cardiac Progenitor Cells. *Int. J. Mol. Sci.* **2019**, *20*, 6037. [CrossRef]
51. Altai, M.; Leitao, C.D.; Rinne, S.S.; Vorobyeva, A.; Atterby, C.; Ståhl, S.; Tolmachev, V.; Löfblom, J.; Orlova, A. Influence of Molecular Design on the Targeting Properties of ABD-Fused Mono- and Bi-Valent Anti-HER3 Affibody Therapeutic Constructs. *Cells* **2018**, *7*, 164. [CrossRef]

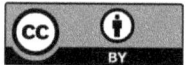

© 2020 by the authors. Licensee MDPI, Basel, Switzerland. This article is an open access article distributed under the terms and conditions of the Creative Commons Attribution (CC BY) license (http://creativecommons.org/licenses/by/4.0/).

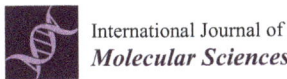

Article

Identification of a Novel Linear B-Cell Epitope on the Nucleocapsid Protein of Porcine Deltacoronavirus

Jiayu Fu [1,†], Rui Chen [1,†], Jingfei Hu [1], Huan Qu [1], Yujia Zhao [1], Sanjie Cao [1,2,3], Xintian Wen [1], Yiping Wen [1], Rui Wu [1], Qin Zhao [1], Xiaoping Ma [2] and Xiaobo Huang [1,2,3,*]

1. Research Center of Swine Disease, College of Veterinary Medicine, Sichuan Agricultural University, Chengdu 611130, China
2. Sichuan Science-observation Experimental station of Veterinary Drugs and Veterinary Diagnostic Technology, Ministry of Agriculture, Chengdu 611130, China
3. National Teaching and Experiment Center of Animal, Sichuan Agricultural University, Chengdu 611130, China
* Correspondence: huangxiaobo@sicau.edu.cn; Tel.: +86-180-4845-1618
† These authors contributed equally to this work.

Received: 3 December 2019; Accepted: 13 January 2020; Published: 19 January 2020

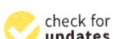

Abstract: Porcine deltacoronavirus (PDCoV), first identified in 2012, is a swine enteropathogen now found in many countries. The nucleocapsid (N) protein, a core component of PDCoV, is essential for virus replication and is a significant candidate in the development of diagnostics for PDCoV. In this study, monoclonal antibodies (mAbs) were generated and tested for reactivity with three truncations of the full protein (N1, N2, N3) that contained partial overlaps; of the five monoclonals chosen tested, each reacted with only the N3 truncation. The antibody designated 4E88 had highest binding affinity with the N protein and was chosen for in-depth examination. The 4E88 epitope was located to amino acids 308-AKPKQQKKPKK-318 by testing the 4E88 monoclonal for reactivity with a series of N3 truncations, then the minimal epitope, 309-KPKQQKKPK-317 (designated EP-4E88), was pinpointed by testing the 4E88 monoclonal for reactivity with a series of synthetic peptides of this region. Homology analysis showed that the EP-4E88 sequence is highly conserved among PDCoV strains, and also shares high similarity with sparrow coronavirus (HKU17), Asian leopard cat coronavirus (ALCCoV), quail coronavirus (UAE-HKU30), and sparrow deltacoronavirus (SpDCoV). Of note, the PDCoV EP-4E88 sequence shared very low similarity (<22.2%) with other porcine coronaviruses (PEDV, TGEV, PRCV, SADS-CoV, PHEV), demonstrating that it is an epitope that can be used for distinguishing PDCoV and other porcine coronavirus. 3D structural analysis revealed that amino acids of EP-4E88 were in close proximity and may be exposed on the surface of the N protein.

Keywords: porcine deltacoronavirus; nucleocapsid; monoclonal antibodies

1. Introduction

The genus *Deltacoronavirus* is a relatively new member of the Coronavirus subfamily, that consists of avian and mammalian CoVs [1]. Among these is porcine deltacoronavirus (PDCoV), originally discovered from fecal samples of pigs in Hong Kong in 2012 [2]. Since then, PDCoV has been reported in multiple states of the United States and Canada [3–6], South Korea [7], mainland China [8,9] and Thailand [10] causing economic losses to each country's swine industry. Clinically, Porcine deltacoronavirus (PDCoV) is indistinguishable from porcine epidemic diarrhea virus (PEDV) and transmissible gastroenteritis virus (TGEV), both Alphacoronaviruses, it is characterized by severe diarrhea, vomiting, and dehydration in piglets, and histopathological lesions typical of atrophic enteritis [11]. The clinical and epidemiological similarities between PDCoV and other porcine intestinal pathogenic coronaviruses make diagnosis and treatment of these viruses a challenge, highlighting the need for discriminating diagnostic methods [12].

PDCoV is an enveloped, single-stranded, positive-sense RNA virus with a 25 kb genome [13]. In the genome opening reading frames(ORFs), ORF1a and ORF1b account for two-thirds of its genome, which encode two polymerase proteins, pp1a and pp1ab [14]. The last one-third of the genome encodes four structural proteins: spike (S protein), envelope (E protein), membrane (M protein), nucleocapsid (N protein), and three accessory proteins (NS6 and NS7/NS7a) [15,16]. NS7 ORF is included into N gene sequence. Moreover, NS7a is contained into NS7 ORF [16]. The N protein is a phosphoprotein and binds to RNA genome, which supplies a structural basis to the helical nucleocapsid [17,18]. The common characteristics for all CoVs N proteins are high expression levels early in the infection and high anti-N antibody levels. N protein also owns multiple functions in pathogenesis, viral replication, and immune system interference [17]. These characteristics make the N protein an ideal target for development of serological methods based on purified protein [19] or antigenic epitopes [20].

PDCoV N protein is highly conserved among PDCoV strains but had low sequence identity with other porcine coronavirus, such as PEDV, TGEV, and PRCV [21]. Although CoV N proteins have low sequence identity, all share the same domain and structure organization [18,22]. For diagnosis of PDCoV, serological assays based on N protein, such as indirect ELISA and fluorescent microsphere immunoassay, have proven to be highly sensitive [23]. Monoclonal antibodies of PDCoV N protein have also proven useful in fluorescent antibody and immunohistochemistry staining methods for identification of PDCoV-infected cells or intestinal tissues [23]. However, the cross-reactivity between porcine coronaviruses in these assays makes accurate diagnoses difficult [24–26], thus development of discriminate diagnostic assays for PDCoV is essential.

In this study, the N protein of PDCoV was expressed in E. coli, purified, then used to produce mouse monoclonal antibodies. The epitope (EP-4E88/309-KPKQQKKPK-317) of the antibody with the highest N protein binding affinity was extensively investigated. Sequence alignment analysis revealed that the sequence of EP-4E88 is highly conserved among porcine deltacoronavirus strains, but has very low sequence similarity to other porcine coronavirus (PEDV, TGEV, PRCV, SADS-CoV, PHEV). Among them, TGEV, PRCV N protein are identical, because PRCV is a S gene deletion of TGEV [27]. Besides, SADS-CoV also known as swine enteric alphacoronavirus (SeACoV) [28] and porcine enteric alphacoronavirus (PEAV) [29]. The results of I-TASSER server for 3D structure prediction showed that amino acids of EP-4E88 was in close proximity and may be exposed on the surface of the N protein. Our findings on this PDCoV N protein epitope added insight for developing epitope-associated diagnostics and vaccines.

2. Results

2.1. Expression, Purification, and Characterization of Full-Length Porcine Deltacoronavirus (PDCoV) Recombinant N Protein (rNP)

As seen in the SDS-PAGE results (Figure 1A), the expressed PDCoV-rNP was soluble and found predominantly in the supernatant post sonication (lane 4), and lanes 6 show the Ni-NTA purified rNP at the expected size, 44 kDa. The Western blot (Figure 1B), demonstrates that the recombinant N protein was specifically recognized by the pig anti-PDCoV hyperimmune serum at a 1:200 dilutions.

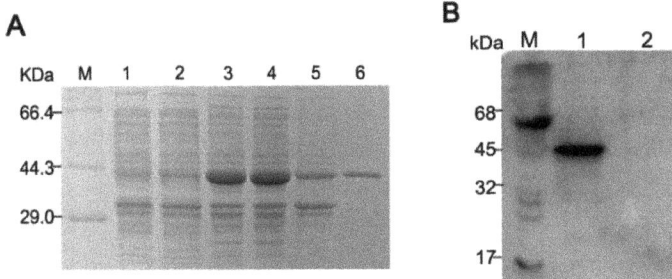

Figure 1. Expression and purification of His-tagged Porcine deltacoronavirus (PDCoV) N-protein. (**A**) SDS-PAGE of pET28a-N transfected BL21 (DE3) cells. M, protein molecular weight marker; lane 1: *E. coli* BL21 with empty vector pET-28a (+); lane 2: Uninduced *E.coli* BL21 with pET-28a-N; lane 3, IPTG-induced pET28a-N transfected cells prior to sonication, lane 4, supernatant of pET28a-N transfected cells post sonication; lane 5: the precipitates of bacterium solution; lane 6: Ni-NTA purified rNP from supernatant; (**B**) Western blot of *E. coli* expressed pET28a-N (lane 1) and empty vector pET-28a (lane 2), probed with hyperimmune pig anti-PDCoV.

2.2. Production and Screening of PDCoV rNP mAbs

Purified PDCoV rNP was used to immunize BALB/c mice; the mouse with the highest antibody titer was sacrificed for hybridoma production. Hybridomas were screened four times by indirect ELISA, and ultimately five hybridomas (11E, 7D2, 4E88, 6A5, and 3B5) were chosen for further testing. The hybridomas were identified as IgG1 k light chain isotype using a mouse monoclonal antibody isotyping ELISA kit (Proteintech Group, Inc.). As can be seen from the representative indirect immunoinfluscent assay (IFA) images (Figure 2A) the monoclonal 4E88 showed the greatest reactivity with the N protein in infected cells. The reactivity of infected cells detected by each monoclonal was quantitated by Imagine Pro plus 6.0 and the results are shown in the bar graph in Figure 2B. ELISA results (Figure 2C) also demonstrated that monoclonal 4E88 had greater reactivity with the N-protein than did the other mAbs. PDCoV NS6 was used as a negative control. To determine if the binding of the mAbs to the N protein required its conformational integrity, native and denatured N was dotted onto PVDF membrane and reacted with each mAb. The results (Figure 2D) show that 4E88, 3B5, 11E, and 7D2 react well with denatured N protein, indicating they recognize linear epitopes. Monoclonal 6A5 did not react with denatured N protein, indicating that it may recognize a conformational epitope.

Next, IEDB Analysis Resource online analysis software was used to predict the B-cell epitope of N protein. Based on the analysis results, we divided the N protein into three parts: N1 (1-124aa), N2 (113-240aa), N3 (221-342aa). The ELISA results (Figure 2E), showed that all the five mAbs recognized the N3 fragment but did not react with N1 and N2.

2.3. Epitope Mapping of PDCoV NP

To locate the epitope on N3 recognized by mAb 4E88, three truncations of N3 were constructed: N3-1 (221-267 aa), N3-2 (261-307 aa), and N3-3 (301-342 aa) (Figure 3A). ELISA (Figure 3D) and dot blot (Figure 3E) results showed that mAb 4E88 reacted only with the N3-3 fragment. From here, four truncations of the N3-3 fragment were constructed: N3-3-1 (301-330 aa), N3-3-2 (308-342aa), N3-3-3 (221-328 aa), and N3-3-4 (221-318 aa). N3-3-1 was not expressed successfully, and although mAb 4E88 did react with N3-3-2 the signal was weak. Both N3-3-3 and N3-3-4, which contain most of the N3-3-1 region, reacted with mAb 4E88, but the N3-3-3 region reacted strongly while N3-3-4 reacted somewhat weakly. These results demonstrated that the amino acids 308-318 are at a minimum necessary for the 4E88 interaction. Peptides spanning these amino acids were synthesized (Sangon Biotech, China) (Figure 4A,B) for subsequent experiments.

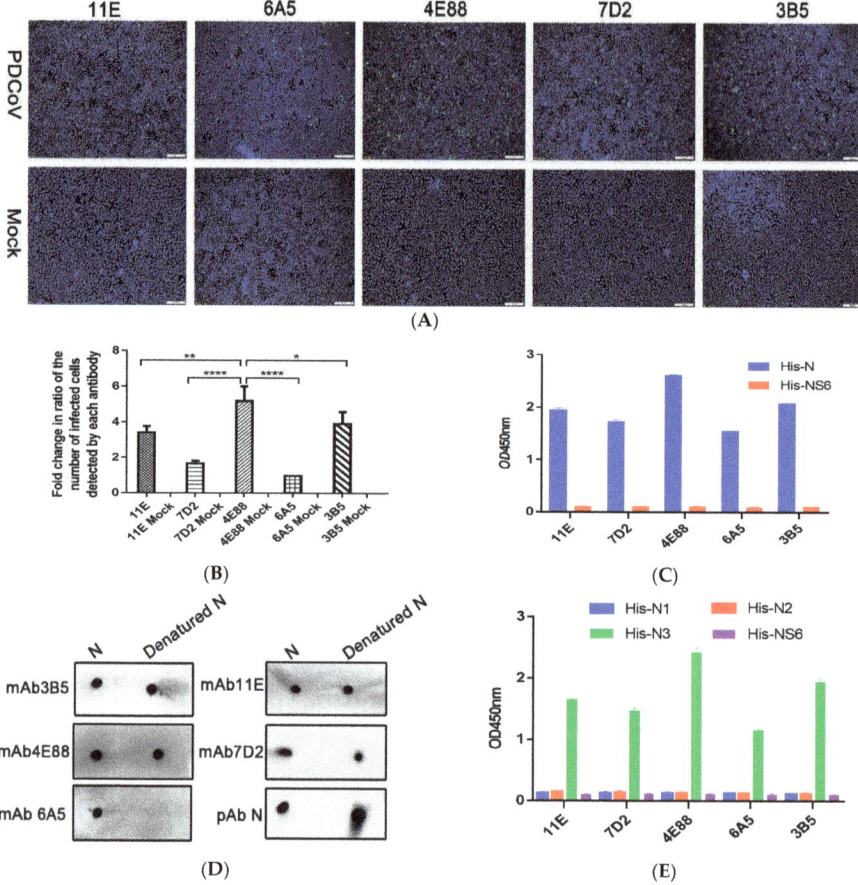

Figure 2. Activity of anti-PDCoV rNP mAbs. (**A**) Immunoinfluscent assay (IFA) of the five mAbs in PDCoV infected cells. Magnification = 10×; (**B**) Quantification of the virus-infected cells detected by each monoclonal shown in panel A. * $p = 0.0483$, ** $p = 0.0049$, **** $p < 0.0001$ for 4E88 compared to 3B5, 11E, 7D2, 6A5, respectively; (**C**) Activity of the antibodies with His-N and His-NS6 by ELISA; (**D**) Linear epitope identification of five monoclonals by dot blot with denatured and native N protein; (**E**) ELISA assay of the reactivity of each monoclonal with the N1,N2, and N3 protein. The experiments were repeated three times.

2.4. Identification of the Minimal Epitope

The synthesized peptides were used as antigens in ELISA (Figure 4C) and dot blot assays (Figure 4D), the results showed that mAb 4E88 reacted most strongly with P1, reacted about half as well with P2, P3, and P6, and did not react with P4 or P5, demonstrating that the 4E88 minimal epitope is amino acids 309-317.

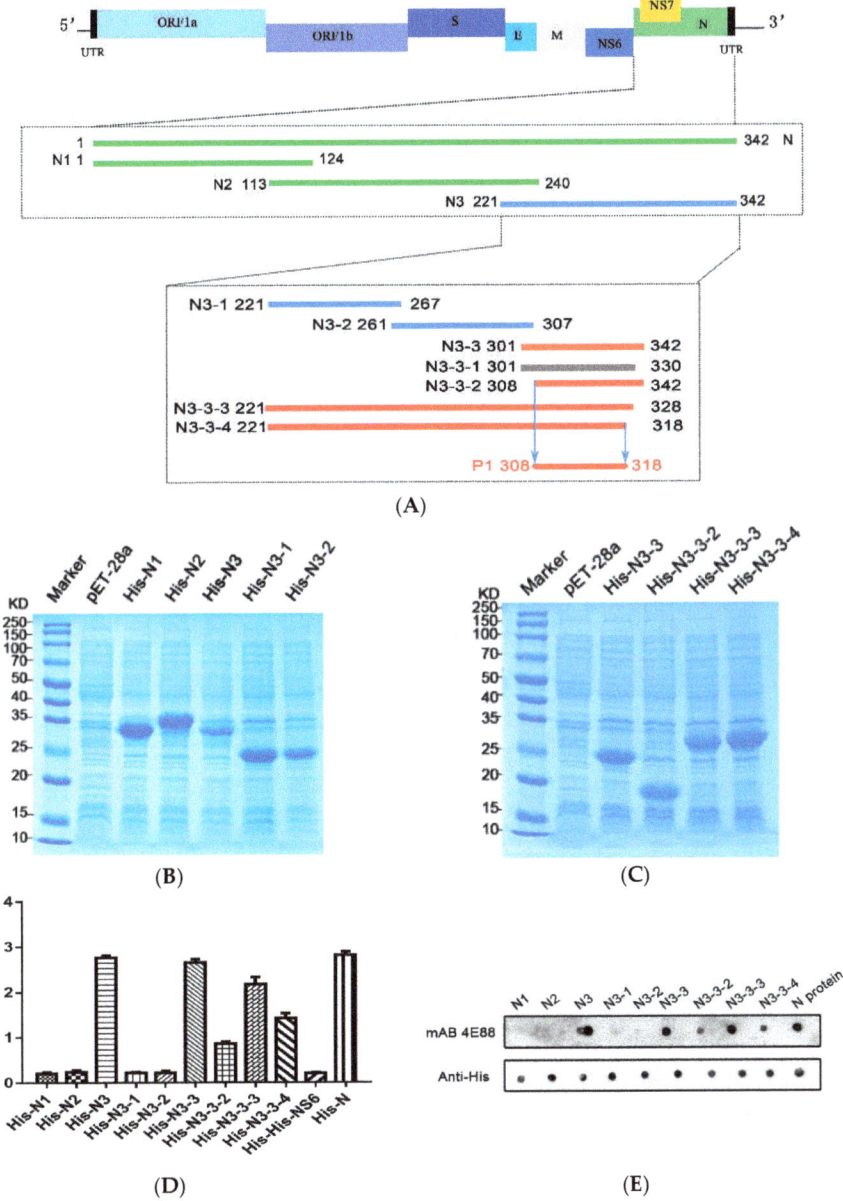

Figure 3. PDCoV N-protein epitope mapping. (**A**) Schematic of PDCoV genome organization and N-protein epitope mapping. The segments recognized by monoclonal 4E88 are represented by red lines, the segments unrecognized by 4E88 are represented by green and blue lines, and the segment that was unsuccessfully expressed is represented by gray; (**B**,**C**) SDS-PAGE of the N-protein truncations expressed in *E. coli*; (**D**,**E**) ELISA and dot blot assays of the reactivity of monoclonal 4E88 with the N-protein truncations. The experiments were performed in triplicate.

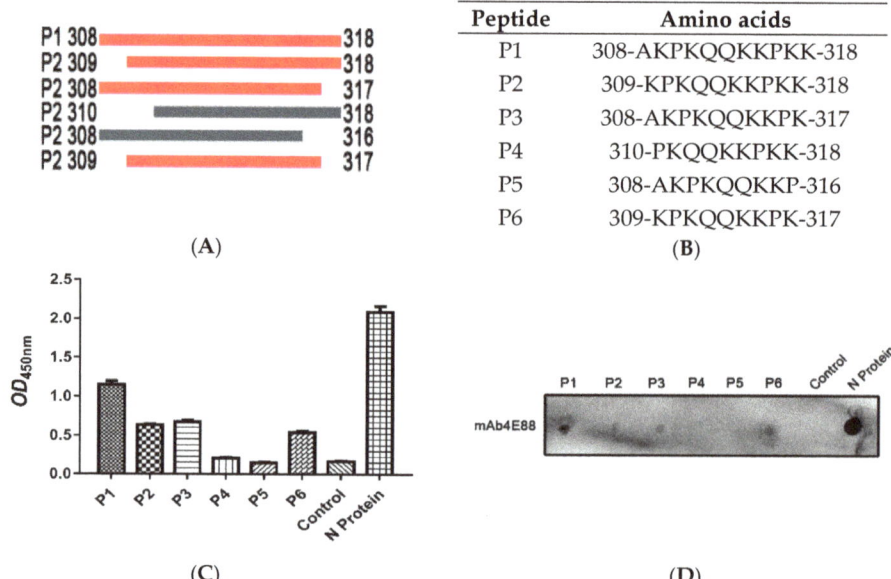

Figure 4. Identification of the minimal 4E88 epitope. Six peptides (P1, P2, P3, P4, P5, P6) were synthesized to detect the minimal epitope (**A,B**) and tested for reactivity with 4E88 by ELISA (**C**) and dot blot assays (**D**). The experiments were repeated three times.

2.5. Cross-Reactivity Analysis

IFA was performed to investigate whether PDCoV cross-reacts with PEDV and TGEV on the epitope of EP-4E88 (aa 309-KPKQQKKPK-317). The mAb 4E88 was used as primary antibody. Figure 5 shows that no fluorescent signals were observed in TGEV infected ST cells and PEDV-infected Vero cells. This result shows that PDCoV EP-4E88 does not cross-react with TGEV and PEDV.

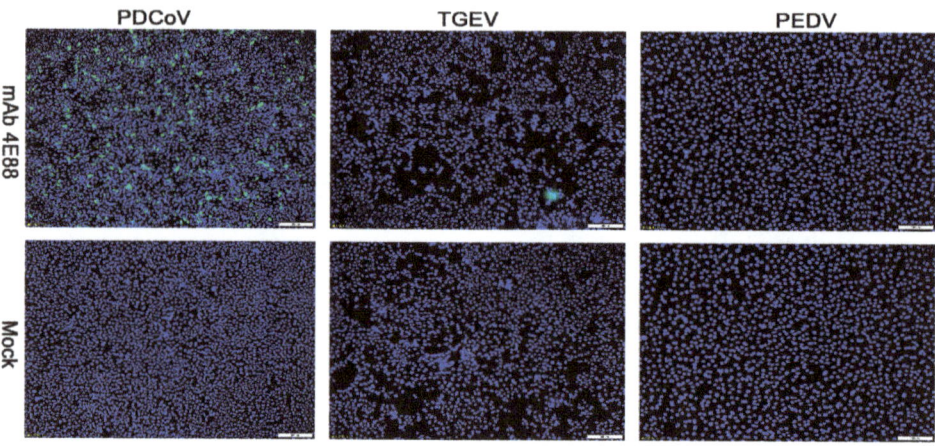

Figure 5. Reactivity of mAb 4E88 with PDCoV, TGEV, and PEDV-infected cells determined by IFA. Binding was visualized with FITC labeled goat anti-mouse antibody, while DAPI was used to visualize the cell nuclei. The strain used for cell infection is shown at the top, and the antibody used for the assay are indicated on the left. Magnification = 10×.

2.6. Homology Analysis

To explore the level of conservation of the 4E88 epitope, 25 PDCoV strains from GenBank were selected for sequence alignment (Figure 6A), which was done using DNA Star. The results show that the EP-4E88 (aa 309-KPKQQKKPK-317) is highly conserved among the PDCoV strains analyzed, with shared sequence similarity of 100% (Figure 6A). Sixteen strains in the genus *Deltacoronavirus* were chosen for further sequence alignment. The results revealed that PDCoV, sparrow coronavirus (HKU17) and Asian leopard cat coronavirus (ALCCoV) share 100% sequence similarity in the position of epitope 4E88 (Figure 6B). The newly discovered Quail deltacoronavirus (UAE-HKU30) and Sparrow deltacoronavirus (SpDCoV) share 90% sequence similarity with PDCoV in epitope 4E88, having one amino acid deletion at lys^{314}. The other deltacoronavirus have 30–60% sequence similarity with PDCoV in epitope 4E88.

PDCoV is the only porcine deltacoronavirus; sequence alignment of the 4E88 epitope with other porcine coronaviruses was performed to determine conservation among coronavirus genera. The results showed very low sequence similarity, the highest being 22.2% (Figure 6C).

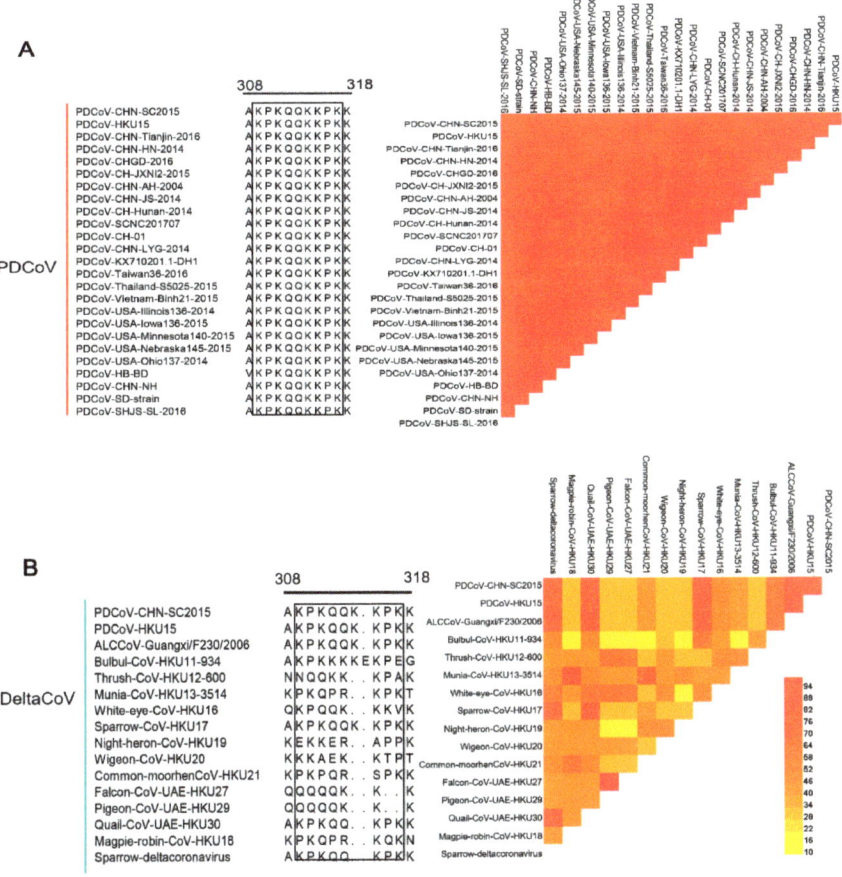

Figure 6. *Cont.*

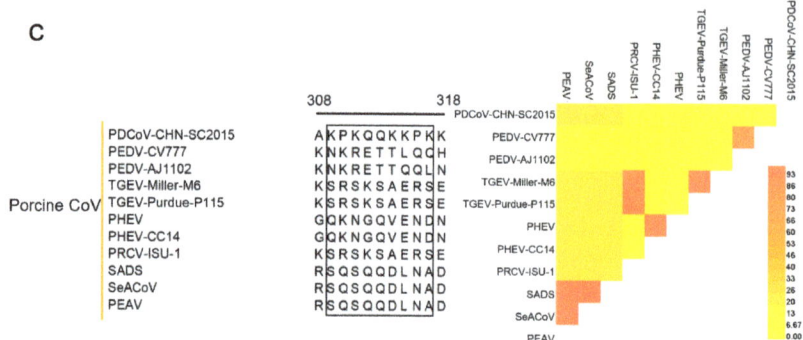

Figure 6. Comparison of the 4E88 epitope amino acid sequence among different virus strains. (**A**) EP-4E88 sequences from strains of PDCoV. Heat map of homology comparison between PDCoV CHN-SC2015 strain and other 24 PDCoV reference strains in GenBank. The sequences of EP-4E88 for all strains are surrounded by black frames; (**B**) EP-4E88 sequences from strains of other 15 deltacoronaviruses. Heat map of homology comparison between PDCoV CHN-SC2015 strain and 15 deltacoronavirus strains in GenBank; (**C**) EP-4E88 sequences from strains of other 11 porcine coronavirus. Heat map of homology comparison between PDCoV CHN-SC2015 strain and 11 porcine coronavirus reference strains in GenBank. The level of homology were analyzed by MAFFT v7.037 and analyzed by DNASTAR.

2.7. Distructure of EP-4E88

A 3-dimensional model of the PDCoV N-protein was constructed based on seven templates in the I-TASSER server website(Figure 7). Top five final models predicted by I-TASSER and its C-score. In I-TASSER, C-score has the function of estimating the quality of predicted models. Our models had C-scores in the range of [−4.26, −3.58], which is nomal for predicted models. The amino acids of EP-4E88 are located in close proximity to one another and are predicted to be exposed on the surface of the N protein, suggesting that EP-4E88 is highly likely to be a linear epitope.

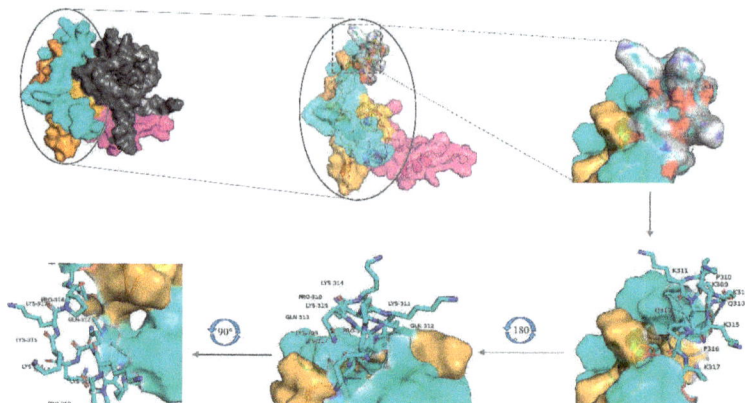

Figure 7. Model of the I-TASSER predicted 3D structure of the N-protein, visualized using the PyMOL molecular graphics and modeling system. The overall structure is shown on the upper left, the yellow areas represent aa231-291, blue areas represent aa292-342, grey areas represent aa1-171, and pink areas represent aa172-230. The EP-4E88 residues (aa 309-KPKQQKKPK-317) are shown as a stick figure and are displayed at different angles of rotation.

3. Discussion

PDCoV, a novel swine enteropathogen, has spread quickly since first discovered in 2012 in Hong Kong. Its distribution is now nearly worldwide and is causing increasing economic losses to commercial pig industries. Co-infections of PDCoV and other enteric viruses complicates diagnosis and leads to increased morbidity and mortality [12,30]. A discriminate diagnostic tool would be invaluable for efforts in the control of PDCoV and similar viruses.

Coronavirus nucleocapsid protein is one of the most abundant viral proteins and is the major antigen recognized by convalescent antisera [31]. Compared with other coronavirus proteins, the N protein is a preferred candidate for serological diagnostics because it is abundant and highly conserved among coronavirus species [26]. Leung et al. found [32] that in patients with SARS, IgG most frequently dominated the antibody response and predominantly targeted the viral nucleocapsid. With respect to PDCoV, the S and N proteins have frequently been the focus for the development of diagnostics [15]. The CoV spike protein however, varies due to mutation to a much greater extent that does the N protein, the result of this variation is a lack of diagnostic accuracy [33].

In this study, monoclonal antibodies were produced against purified recombinant N-protein and their epitopes investigated. The five antibodies we tested, all recognized the 122 C-terminal amino acids of the N-protein (aa 221-341), indicating that this section contains the main antigenic epitope of N protein. IEDB (Immune Epitope Database and Analysis Resource) prediction analysis software (http://www.iedb.org/) also proved our point, the results indicated that three epitopes located at the C-terminal of the N-protein sequence, and the largest of 10 predicted epitopes is in amino acids 221-342, this fragment we termed N3. B-cell epitopes are classified as linear or conformational, though it has been reported that 90% of B cell-recognizing epitopes are conformational epitopes, this is due to most of the B-cells epitopes can form conformation in the three dimensional structure, the antigen internalizing process and antigen recognizing ability [34–36]. To determine whether our monoclonals recognized conformational epitopes, the N protein was denatured and then tested for reactivity with the mAbs by dot-blot. One mAb (6A5) did not react with the denatured N protein, so we speculated that it recognizes a conformational epitope, the remaining mAbs did react with the denatured N protein so we speculated that these recognize linear epitopes. One mAb (4E88) from our panel was selected for further study of the antigenic epitope of N protein; we chose this antibody because it had the highest reactivity with N-protein in ELISA and dot blot, as well as in PDCoV-infected cells. Moreover, the dominant epitope of the N protein has a greater potential use for early diagnostics than the others.

Identification of PDCoV B-cell epitopes is fundamental for the development of epitope-based diagnostic tools, vaccines, and therapeutic antibodies. Approaches for epitope identification are structural and functional. Structural methods include X-ray crystallography, which can precisely locate the epitope position but it is limited to small soluble proteins, the method is also time consuming and costly, together these impede its widespread use [37]. Functional methods are used to detect the binding activity of antibody with antigen fragments, synthetic peptides or recombinant antigens, and have the advantage of being simpler to conduct [37]. Here, the epitope region recognized by 4E88 (308-AKPKQQKKPKK-318 aa) was determined by serially truncating the N3 portion of the N-protein. From there a series of peptides were synthesized and used as antigen in ELISA and dot blot assays, thus we determined that 309-KPKQQKKPK-317 was the minimal epitope.

Woo et al. [1] found that avian and mammalian deltacoronaviruses share similar genome characteristics and structure, and that avian coronaviruses are the gene source of gamma- and deltacoronaviruses. In our study alignment analysis revealed that the sequence of epitope 4E88 is highly conserved among PDCoV strains; the sequence similarity was also extremely high with Sparrow coronavirus (HKU17), Asian leopard cat coronavirus (ALCCoV), Quail coronavirus (UAE-HKU30), and Sparrow deltacoronavirus (SpDCoV). PDCoV may come from a host jumps event between mammals and birds [38], also supporting this view is genome analysis showing that PDCoV shares a close relationship with HKU17 (96.8% of sequence identity in N), HKU30 (90.9% of sequence identity in N), and SpDCoV (95.3% of sequence identity in N) [1,39]. The shared sequence at position

309-317aa (epitope 4E88) among PDCoV, HKU17, ALCCoV, HKU30, and SpDCoV may contribute to the understanding of the evolutionary relationship between birds and mammals. Similar phenomenon was also found in other virus. Li et al. [40] found a shared epitope, EXE/DPPFG, among six flaviviruses and verified the cross-reactivity by positive sera detection. Chen et al. [41] found that PDCoV N gene-based PCR cross-reacts with SpDCoV because of their relatively conserved regions. The relationship between PDCoV and other animal-originated deltacoronavirus needs further exploration and whether PDCoV EP-4E88 cross-reacts with HKU17, ALCCoV, HKU30, or SpDCoV should be analyzed using two-way serum cross-reactivity.

To date, six porcine coronavirus diseases (PEDV, TGEV, PRCV, SADS-CoV, PHEV, PDCoV) have been reported [42,43]. Because they present with similar clinical symptoms, diagnosis is a challenge, a sensitive and discriminate serologic method is clearly needed. The PDCoV epitope, 4E88 (aa 309-KPKQQKKPK-317), found in this study shares very low sequence similarity (<22.2%) with other swine coronavirus (Figure 6C), such as PEDV (aa 309-NKRETTLQQ-317) and TGEV (aa 309-SRSKSAERS-317), PHEV (aa 309-QKNGQVEND-317), PRCV (aa 309-SRSKSAERS-317), SADS-CoV (aa 309-SQSQDLNA-317) indicating the EP-4E88 is unique to PDCoV and could be used to distinguish PDCoV and from other swine coronaviruses. Cross-reactivity among swine coronaviruses has been reported and is usually associated with the epitope of N protein [24,26,44]. Lin et al. [24] observed that one-way cross-reaction between TGEV Miller hyperimmune pig antisera and various PEDV strains with the TGEV Miller N protein mAb (14G9.3C) was based on an N protein epitope. Xie et al. [26] found two N-terminal epitopes (58-RWRMRRGERIE-68 and 78-LGTGPHAD-85) of the PEDV N protein contribute to the cross-reaction between PEDV and TGEV. Ma et al. [44] found that N protein is responsible for two-way cross-reactivity between PEDV and PDCoV; four regions (47-GYW-49, 67-FYYTGTGPRGNLKY-82, 194-PKG-197, and 329-EWD-332) are highly conserved and likely account for the cross-reaction [44].

To our knowledge, this is the first report to identify the PDCoV N-protein antigenic epitope EP-4E88 (aa 309-NKRETTLQQ-317). It is a linear B-cell epitope and highly conserved among PDCoV strains and other porcine coronaviruses, EP-4E88 also shares high sequence identity with four non-swine deltacoronavirus. Our findings provide valuable insight into the evolutionary and serological relationship among PDCoV and non-swine deltacoronavirus, and for the development of PDCoV epitope-associated diagnostics and vaccine design.

4. Materials and Methods

4.1. Ethics Statement

All animal experiments were approved by the Institutional Animal Care and Use Committee of Sichuan Agricultural University (IACUC#RW2016-090, approval date: 8 September 2016), and were performed in strict accordance with the Care and Use of Laboratory Animals guidelines and regulations of the Ministry of Science and Technology of the People's Republic of China.

4.2. Virus and Cells

ST cells (ATCC CRL-1746), Sp2/0-Ag14 (ATCC CRL-1581) cells and Vero cells (ATCC CCL-81) were maintained at 37 °C in a humidified 5% CO_2 atmosphere in Dulbecco's modified Eagle medium (DMEM; Gibco, Carlsbad, CA, USA) supplemented with 10% heat-inactivated fetal bovine serum (PAN-Biotech, Aigenbach, Germany) and 1% antibiotic-antimycotic (Solarbio, Beijing, China). The PDCoV strain CHN-SC2015 (GenBank accession No.MK355396), PEDV-CV777 strain (GenBank accession No. AF353511.1), TGEV-H strain was preserved by the Laboratory of Research Center of Swine Disease in Sichuan Agricultural University. For PDCoV propagation, ST cells at 90% confluence were washed three times with DMEM supplemented with 5 µg/mL trypsin-EDTA (maintenance medium) and then inoculated with 1 mL of PDCoV. The virus was removed and 6 mL of maintenance medium was added. When CPE was observed, generally at 2 days post-infection, the cells were harvested then stored at −80 °C until further use. The titers of CHN-SC2015 obtained were up to $10^{6.64}$ TCID50/mL. For PEDV propagation, Vero cells at 90% confluence were washed three times with DMEM supplemented with 10 μg/mL trypsin-EDTA (maintenance medium) and then inoculated with 1 mL of PEDV. When CPE was observed, generally at 3 days post-infection, the cells were harvested then stored at −80 °C until further use. For TGEV propagation, ST cells at 90% confluence were washed three times with DMEM supplemented with 5 μg/mL trypsin-EDTA (maintenance medium) and then inoculated with 1 mL of TGEV. When CPE was observed, generally at 2 days post-infection, the cells were harvested then stored at −80 °C until further use.

4.3. Construction of Full-Length and Truncated Recombinant N-Protein

PDCoV CHN-SC2015 genomic RNA was extracted using TRIzol Reagent (Sangon Biotech, Shanghai, China) according to the manufacturer's instructions. The N gene was amplified by RT-PCR with primers (Table 1) designed with Primer 5.0. The N gene amplicon (1029 bp) was inserted into the pET-28a (+) expression vector (Novagen, Madison, WI, USA) between the EcoR I and Xho I sites. The integrity of the resulting construct (pET28-N) was verified by restriction enzyme digestion, PCR, and DNA sequencing. pET28-N was transformed into Transetta (DE3) *Escherichia coli*. Protein expression was induced with 0.8 mM isopropyl-β-galactopyranoside (IPTG) for 3 h at 30 °C. Bacteria were collected by centrifugation and lysed by ultrasonication, then centrifuged again; the recombinant N protein (rNP) was purified from the supernatant post sonication by Ni-NTA His-Bind Resin (Bio-Rad, Hercules, CA, USA) according to the instructions. The concentration of the purified rNP was analyzed by SDS-PAGE. Using the same methodology, a series of truncated N-proteins were produced: His-N1, His-N2, His-N3, His-N3-1, His-N3-2, His-N3-3, His-N3-3-1, His-N3-3-2, His-N3-3-3, His-N3-3-4 (Figure 3A).

Table 1. Sequence of the oligonucleotides used for PCR.

Segment		Sequences (5'-3')	Positions (Amino Acids)
N1	N1-F	CGGGATCC ATGGCCGCACCAGTAGTC	1-124
	N1-R	*CCCTCGAG* TAGCAGCTGATGTTTAGGATT	
N2	N2-F	CGGGATCC TCGGGAGCTGACACTTCTATTA	113-240
	N2-R	*CCCTCGAG* TGCCCCTGCCTGAAAGTTG	
N3	N3-F	CGGGATCC AAGACGGGTATGGCTGATCC	221-342
	N3-R	*CCCTCGAG* CTACGCTGCTGATTCCTGCT	
N3-1	N3-1-F	CGGGATCC TCTCGTACTGGTGCCAATGTCG	221-267
	N3-1-R	*CCCTCGAG* GAGCGCATCCTTAAGTCTCTCATAG	
N3-2	N3-2-F	CGGGATCC TTCTCTTACTCAATCACAGTCAAGG	261-307
	N3-2-R	*CCCTCGAG* GACTGGTCTTGTTTGTCAGGCTT	
N3-3	N3-3-F	CGGGATCC CCTGACAAACAAGACCAGTCTG	301-342
	N3-3-R	*CCCTCGAG* CGCTGCTGATTCCTGCTTTA	
N3-3-1	N3-3-1-F	CGGGATCC CCTGACAAACAAGACCAGTCTGCTA	301-330
	N3-3-1-R	*CCCTCGAG* CCACTCCCAATCCTGTTTGTCTG	
N3-3-2	N3-3-2-F	CGGGATCC GCTAAACCCAAACAGCAGAAGAAAC	308-342
	N3-3-2-R	*CCCTCGAG* CGCTGCTGATTCCTGCTTTAT	
N3-3-3	N3-3-3-F	CGGGATCC AAGACGGGTATGGCTGATCC	221-328
	N3-3-3-R	*CCCTCGAG* CCAATCCTGTTTGTCTGCTG	
N3-3-4	N3-3-4-F	CGGGATCC AAGACGGGTATGGCTGATCC	221-318
	N3-3-4-R	*CCCTCGAG* CTTTTTAGGTTTCTTCTGCTGTTTG	

Restriction endonuclease sites: BamHI (underlined) and XhoI (italic).

4.4. Western Blotting

Western blotting was used to test the reactivity of hyperimmune pig anti-serum against the recombinant N protein. Purified N protein and pET-28a (+) empty vector were subjected to SDS-PAGE then transferred to a PVDF membrane. The membrane was blocked with 5% skim milk in PBST (PBS/0.05% Tween-20) for 1.5 h then incubated with anti-PDCoV pig hyperimmune serum (1:200) overnight at 4 °C overnight. The membrane was washed three times with PBST then incubated with HRP-goat anti-pig IgG (1:5000) for 1 h at 37 °C. The membrane was washed four times with PBST and the proteins were visualized using enhanced chemiluminescence reagents (ECL; Bio-Rad, Hercules, CA, USA).

4.5. Production of Anti-rNP mAbs

Six-week-old female BALB/c mice purchased from Chengdu Dossy Experimental Animal Co, Ltd., were inoculated via subcutaneous injection with purified rN protein (100 µg/mouse) mixed with an equal volume of Montanide Gel 01 PR adjuvant (Montanide, SEPPIC, Puteaux, France). Mice were boosted twice, at 2-week intervals, with the same immunogen and adjuvant. Pre-immune serum samples were taken from all mice and tested for reactivity against purified rNP by indirect ELISA. Two weeks after the final boost, mice were sacrificed and spleens removed. Spleen cells were fused with Sp2/0 Ag14 cells, and hybridomas were selected in HAT and HT medium. Culture supernatants from individual hybridoma clones were screened for reactivity with rNP by indirect ELISA. Reactive hybridomas were subcloning three times by limiting dilution, stable hybridomas were injected into the abdominal cavity of sensitized mice to produce ascites. Antibodies were purified twice, first using the octylic acid ammonium sulfate method (CA-AS), then by HPLC through a diethylaminoethyl column. The identification of isotype in prepared mAbs by mouse monoclonal antibody isotyping ELISA kit (Proteintech Group, Inc., Wuhan, China).

4.6. Denatured Protein

To identify mAbs that recognize conformational or linear epitopes, the N3 proteins were denatured as previously described [34]. Briefly, the purified rN proteins were mixed with 6× protein-loading buffer with DTT (TransGen Biotech, Beijing, China) then heated for 8 min at 95 °C; this procedure fully denatures secondary structure. The denatured proteins were tested with the mAbs using a dot-blot assay.

4.7. IFA

ST cells were grown in 12-well plates until 80% confluent. Half the wells were infected with PDCoV (MOI = 0.1) and half were mock infected. After 36 h post-infection, cells were then washed twice with PBS, fixed with 4% formaldehyde in PBS for 30 min, then permeabilized with 0.5% Triton-X-100 for 30 min at room temperature. Cells were washed again and blocked with 2% BSA in PBS for 1.5 h then incubated with each of the five anti-N mAb for 1 h in PBS with 1% BSA. Cells were washed three times and incubated with FITC labeled goat anti-rabbit IgG (1:500 in PBST). Nuclei were stained with DAPI (Solarbio, Beijing, China). The Image-Pro Plus 6.0 was used to analyze number of immunfluoresnce from six different stained images. The FITC-positive cells of mAb 6A5 was set to one-fold.

4.8. ELISA

Indirect ELISA was performed as described in Guo et al. 2006 [45]. Briefly, the wells of a 96-well ELISA plate were coated with 1 µg/well of protein overnight at 4 °C. The wells were rinsed, then blocked with 5% non-fat dry milk in TBST for 1 h at room temperature. Wells were rinsed three times with TBST then incubated with mAb (1:500) for 1 h at 37 °C. Wells were rinsed again and incubated with HRP-conjugated goat anti-mouse IgG, (1:5000) for 1 h at 37 °C. After final rinsing wells were incubated with tetramethylbenzidine (TMB) for 15 min, color development was stopped with 3M H$_2$SO$_4$. The OD_{450} was read by ELISA plate reader (Bio-Rad, Hercules, CA, USA).

4.9. Dot-Blot Analysis

Dot-blot hybridization for identification of linear epitopes was based on the method described by Chen et al. 2017 [46]. Briefly, PVDF membranes were soaked in dimethyl sulfoxide then in methanol. Total of 1 µL (0.5 µg) of protein was spotted onto the treated membrane, then air-dried for 10 min. The membrane was blocked with 2% BSA in TBST for 30 min at room temperature, then incubated with mAb (1:200) in 2% BSA/TBST for 1 h at 37 °C. The membrane was rinsed then incubated with goat anti-mouse IgG (1:5000) for 1 h at 37 °C. The signal was developed using enhanced chemiluminescence reagents (ECL; Bio-Rad, Hercules, CA, USA).

4.10. Identification of the Minimal 4E88 Epitope

To determine the minimal B-cell epitope recognized by mAb 4E88, five peptides spanning various lengths of aa308-318 were commercially synthesized (Sangon Biotech, Shanghai, China). The amino acid sequence of these peptides (P1–P6) are shown in Figure 3A,B. The reactivity of 4E88 with the peptides was tested by dot-blotting and ELISA as previous described [47]. Specially, peptides were dissolved in DMSO (Solarbio) to a concentration of 10 mg/mL, for dot-blotting 1 µL (10 µg) was spotted onto PVDF membrane, and for ELISA, 100 µL (1 mg) were aliquoted into wells and incubated at 4 °C for 15 h.

4.11. Sequence Homology

To determine whether the epitope recognized by mAb 4E88 was conserved among PDCoV strains, the amino acid sequences of 25 PDCoV strains in GenBank (Table 2) were aligned with the sequence in EP-4E88 using MAFFT v7.037 and analyzed by DNASTAR. The EP-4E88 sequence was also aligned with other deltacoronavirus and porcine coronavirus (Tables 3 and 4) as described. The results were rendered in figure form with ESPript 3.

Table 2. PDCoV strains used to align the sequences of EP-4E88.

Strains	Country	Collection Date	Accession Number	Lengths of N-Protein (Amino Acid)
PDCoV-CHN-SC2015	China	2015	QDH76192.1	342
PDCoV-CHN-JXJGS01-2016	China	2016	ASK86338.1	342
PDCoV-CHN-Tianjin-2016	China	2016	APG38202.1	342
PDCoV-CHN-HN-2014	China	2014	ALS54090.1	342
PDCoV-CHGD-2016	China	2016	AYU65238.1	342
PDCoV-CH-JXNI2-2015	China	2015	ALA13749.1	342
PDCoV-CHN-AH-2004	China	2004	AKC54432.1	342
PDCoV-CHN-JS-2014	China	2014	AKC54446.1	342
PDCoV-CH-Hunan-2014	China	2014	AUG59160.1	342
PDCoV-SCNC201707	China	2017	AZL30771.1	342
PDCoV-CH-01	China	2016	AQS99157.1	342
PDCoV-CHN-LYG-2014	China	2014	AML83920.1	342
PDCoV-KX710201.1-DH1	China	2016	ASW22235.1	342
PDCoV-Taiwan36-2016	China	2016	KY586149.1	342
PDCoV-Thailand-S5025-2015	Thailand	2015	KU051656.1	342
PDCoV-Vietnam-Binh21-2015	Vietnam	2015	APZ76702.1	342
PDCoV-USA-Illinois136-2014	USA	2014	AIB07804.1	342
PDCoV-USA-Iowa136-2015	USA	2015	ANI85829.1	342
PDCoV-USA-Minnesota140-2015	USA	2015	ANI85836.1	342
PDCoV-USA-Nebraska145-2015	USA	2015	ANI85850.1	342
PDCoV-USA-Ohio137-2014	USA	2014	KJ601780.1	342
PDCoV-HB-BD	China	2017	ATJ00133.1	342
PDCoV-CHN-NH	China	2015	ANA78447.1	342
PDCoV-SD-strain	China	2014	ASR75150.1	342
PDCoV-SHJS-SL-2016	China	2016	AUH28254.1	342

Table 3. Deltacoronavirus strains used for EP-4E88 sequence alignment.

Strains	Country	Collection Date	Accession Number	Lengths of N-Protein (Amino Acid)
PDCoV-HKU15	China	2009	YP_005352835.1	342
Asian leopard cat coronavirus (ALCCoV) Guangxi/F230/2006	China	2006	ABQ39962.1	342
Bulbul-CoV-HKU11-934	China	2007	ACJ12039.1	349
Thrush-CoV-HKU12-600	China	2007	ACJ12057.1	343
Munia-CoV-HKU13-3514	China	2007	ACJ12066.1	352
White-eye-CoV-HKU16	China	2007	YP-005352842.1	347
Sparrow-CoV-HKU17	China	2007	YP-005352850.1	342
Night-heron-CoV-HKU19	China	2007	YP-005352867.1	342
Wigeon-CoV-HKU20	China	2008	YP-005352875.1	350
Common-moorhen CoV-HKU21	China	2007	YP-005352885.1	351
Falcon-CoV-UAE-HKU27	China	2013	BBC54826.1	344
Pigeon-CoV-UAE-HKU29	China	2017	BBC54846.1	344
Quail-CoV-UAE-HKU30	China	2017	BBC54865.1	341
Magpie-robin-CoV-HKU18	China	2007	YP-005352858.1	346
Sparrow-deltacoronavirus	USA	2017	AWV67111.1	341

Table 4. Porcine coronavirus strains used for EP-4E88 sequence alignment.

Strains	Country	Collection Date	Accession Number	Lengths of N-Protein (Amino Acid)
PEDV-CV777	Belgium	1977	AF353511	441
PEDV-AJ1102	China	2011	JX188454	441
TGEV-Purdue P115	USA	2006	DQ811788	382
TGEV-Miller M6	USA	2006	DQ811785	382
PRCV-ISU-1	USA	2006	DQ811787	382
PHEV-VW572	Belgium	2005	DQ011855	449
PHEV-CC14	China	2014	MF083115	449
SADS-CoV/CN/GDWT/2017	China	2017	MG557844	375
PEAV-GDS04	China	2017	MH697599	375
SeACoV-p10	China	2018	MK977618	375

4.12. Three-Dimensional Structure Prediction

I-TASSER (https://zhanglab.ccmb.med.umich.edu/I-TASSER/) was used to predict the three-dimensional structure of the full-length PDCoV N-protein as described [48–50]. Seven threading templates in Protein Data Bank (PDB) were selected for construction by this program (2gecB, 5gaoE, 1sskA, 4n16A, 4j3kA, 1ssk, 2gecA). Figures were generated using the PyMOL molecular visualization system.

4.13. Statistical Analysis

The experiments were repeated three times. All statistical data were analyzed by GraphPad Prism version 7.0 and expressed as mean ± SD. The differences among the five monoclonals were analyzed using the one-way ANOVA. Statistical changes marked by * p value < 0.05, ** p value < 0.01, *** p value < 0.001, **** p value < 0.0001.

5. Conclusions

In this study, five monoclonals of PDCoV N protein were produced. Of the five monoclonals, mAB 4E88 had highest binding affinity with the N protein and was chosen for identifying epitope. EP-4E88 (aa309-KPKQQKKPK-317) was the minimal epitope which recognized by mAb 4E88. Homology analysis showed that the EP-4E88 sequence is highly conserved among PDCoV strains and several deltacoronavirus but shared very low similarity with other porcine coronaviruses. Therefore, EP-4E88 lays a good foundation for applied research associated with PDCoV diagnosis.

Author Contributions: J.F., R.C. made major contributions to this work; X.H. and S.C. designed the study and revised the manuscript; J.H., Y.Z., H.Q. Performed the virus isolation and identification; Y.W., R.W., Q.Z., X.W., analyzed some experimental data. X.M. commented on the manuscript and provided valuable feedback. All authors have read and agreed to the published version of the manuscript.

Funding: This study was supported by the National Key Research and Development Program of China (award 2016YFD0500700).

Acknowledgments: We would like to thank Rui Chen and Xiaobo Huang at the Sichuan agricultural University for critical reading and revising this manuscript.

Conflicts of Interest: The authors declare no conflict of interest.

References

1. Woo, P.C.Y.; Lau, S.K.P.; Lam, C.S.F.; Lau, C.C.Y.; Tsang, A.K.L.; Lau, J.H.N.; Bai, R.; Teng, J.L.L.; Tsang, C.C.C.; Wang, M.; et al. Discovery of seven novel Mammalian and avian coronaviruses in the genus deltacoronavirus supports bat coronaviruses as the gene source of alphacoronavirus and betacoronavirus and avian coronaviruses as the gene source of gammacoronavirus and deltacoronavirus. *J. Virol.* **2012**, *86*, 3995–4008. [CrossRef] [PubMed]
2. Woo, P.C.; Lau, S.K.; Tsang, C.-C.; Lau, C.C.; Wong, P.-C.; Chow, F.W.; Fong, J.Y.; Yuen, K.-Y. Coronavirus HKU15 in respiratory tract of pigs and first discovery of coronavirus quasispecies in 5′-untranslated region. *Emerg. Microbes Infect.* **2017**, *6*, e53. [CrossRef] [PubMed]
3. Li, G.; Chen, Q.; Harmon, K.M.; Yoon, K.-J.; Schwartz, K.J.; Hoogland, M.J.; Gauger, P.C.; Main, R.G.; Zhang, J. Full-Length Genome Sequence of Porcine Deltacoronavirus Strain USA/IA/2014/8734. *Genome Announc.* **2014**, *2*, e00278-14. [CrossRef] [PubMed]
4. Marthaler, D.; Jiang, Y.; Collins, J.; Rossow, K. Complete Genome Sequence of Strain SDCV/USA/Illinois121/2014, a Porcine Deltacoronavirus from the United States. *Genome Announc.* **2014**, *2*, 00218-14. [CrossRef] [PubMed]
5. Wang, L.; Byrum, B.; Zhang, Y. Detection and genetic characterization of deltacoronavirus in pigs, Ohio, USA, 2014. *Emerg. Infect. Dis.* **2014**, *20*, 1227–1230. [CrossRef]
6. Wang, L.; Byrum, B.; Zhang, Y. Porcine coronavirus HKU15 detected in 9 US states, 2014. *Emerg. Infect. Dis.* **2014**, *20*, 1594–1595. [CrossRef]
7. Lee, S.; Lee, C. Complete Genome Characterization of Korean Porcine Deltacoronavirus Strain KOR/KNU14-04/2014. *Genome Announc.* **2014**, *2*, e01191-14. [CrossRef]
8. Song, D.; Zhou, X.; Peng, Q.; Chen, Y.; Zhang, F.; Huang, T.; Zhang, T.; Li, A.; Huang, D.; Wu, Q.; et al. Newly Emerged Porcine Deltacoronavirus Associated With Diarrhoea in Swine in China: Identification, Prevalence and Full-Length Genome Sequence Analysis. *Transbound. Emerg. Dis.* **2015**, *62*, 575–580. [CrossRef]
9. Wang, Y.-W.; Yue, H.; Fang, W.; Huang, Y.-W. Complete Genome Sequence of Porcine Deltacoronavirus Strain CH/Sichuan/S27/2012 from Mainland China. *Genome Announc.* **2015**, *3*, e00945-15. [CrossRef]
10. Janetanakit, T.; Lumyai, M.; Bunpapong, N.; Boonyapisitsopa, S.; Chaiyawong, S.; Nonthabenjawan, N.; Kesdaengsakonwut, S.; Amonsin, A. Porcine Deltacoronavirus, Thailand, 2015. *Emerg. Infect. Dis.* **2016**, *22*, 757–759. [CrossRef]
11. Wang, L.; Hayes, J.; Sarver, C.; Byrum, B.; Zhang, Y. Porcine deltacoronavirus: Histological lesions and genetic characterization. *Arch. Virol.* **2016**, *161*, 171–175. [CrossRef] [PubMed]
12. Jung, K.; Hu, H.; Saif, L.J. Porcine deltacoronavirus infection: Etiology, cell culture for virus isolation and propagation, molecular epidemiology and pathogenesis. *Virus Res.* **2016**, *226*, 50–59. [CrossRef] [PubMed]
13. Zhang, J. Porcine deltacoronavirus: Overview of infection dynamics, diagnostic methods, prevalence and genetic evolution. *Virus Res.* **2016**, *226*, 71–84. [CrossRef] [PubMed]
14. Zhao, Y.; Qu, H.; Hu, J.; Fu, J.; Chen, R.; Li, C.; Cao, S.; Wen, Y.; Wu, R.; Zhao, Q.; et al. Characterization and Pathogenicity of the Porcine Deltacoronavirus Isolated in Southwest China. *Viruses* **2019**, *11*, 1074. [CrossRef]
15. Fang, P.; Fang, L.; Hong, Y.; Liu, X.; Dong, N.; Ma, P.; Bi, J.; Wang, D.; Xiao, S. Discovery of a novel accessory protein NS7a encoded by porcine deltacoronavirus. *J. Gen. Virol.* **2017**, *98*, 173–178. [CrossRef]
16. Chen, R.; Fu, J.; Hu, J.; Li, C.; Zhao, Y.; Qu, H.; Wen, X.; Cao, S.; Wen, Y.; Wu, R.; et al. Identification of the immunodominant neutralizing regions in the spike glycoprotein of porcine deltacoronavirus. *Virus Res.* **2020**, *276*, 197834. [CrossRef]

17. Hsin, W.-C.; Chang, C.-H.; Chang, C.-Y.; Peng, W.-H.; Chien, C.-L.; Chang, M.-F.; Chang, S.C. Nucleocapsid protein-dependent assembly of the RNA packaging signal of Middle East respiratory syndrome coronavirus. *J. Biomed. Sci.* **2018**, *25*, 47. [CrossRef]
18. Chang, C.-K.; Sue, S.-C.; Yu, T.-H.; Hsieh, C.-M.; Tsai, C.-K.; Chiang, Y.-C.; Lee, S.-J.; Hsiao, H.-H.; Wu, W.-J.; Chang, W.-L.; et al. Modular organization of SARS coronavirus nucleocapsid protein. *J. Biomed. Sci.* **2006**, *13*, 59–72. [CrossRef]
19. Hou, X.-L.; Yu, L.-Y.; Liu, J. Development and evaluation of enzyme-linked immunosorbent assay based on recombinant nucleocapsid protein for detection of porcine epidemic diarrhea (PEDV) antibodies. *Vet. Microbiol.* **2007**, *123*, 86–92. [CrossRef]
20. Wang, K.; Xie, C.; Zhang, J.; Zhang, W.; Yang, D.; Yu, L.; Jiang, Y.; Yang, S.; Gao, F.; Yang, Z.; et al. The Identification and Characterization of Two Novel Epitopes on the Nucleocapsid Protein of the Porcine Epidemic Diarrhea Virus. *Sci. Rep.* **2016**, *6*, 39010. [CrossRef]
21. Su, M.; Li, C.; Guo, D.; Wei, S.; Wang, X.; Geng, Y.; Yao, S.; Gao, J.; Wang, E.; Zhao, X.; et al. A recombinant nucleocapsid protein-based indirect enzyme-linked immunosorbent assay to detect antibodies against porcine deltacoronavirus. *J. Vet. Med. Sci.* **2016**, *78*, 601–606. [CrossRef] [PubMed]
22. Zúñiga, S.; Sola, I.; Moreno, J.L.; Sabella, P.; Plana-Durán, J.; Enjuanes, L. Coronavirus nucleocapsid protein is an RNA chaperone. *Virology* **2007**, *357*, 215–227. [CrossRef] [PubMed]
23. Okda, F.; Lawson, S.; Liu, X.; Singrey, A.; Clement, T.; Hain, K.; Nelson, J.; Christopher-Hennings, J.; Nelson, E.A. Development of monoclonal antibodies and serological assays including indirect ELISA and fluorescent microsphere immunoassays for diagnosis of porcine deltacoronavirus. *BMC Vet. Res.* **2016**, *12*, 95. [CrossRef] [PubMed]
24. Lin, C.-M.; Gao, X.; Oka, T.; Vlasova, A.N.; Esseili, M.A.; Wang, Q.; Saif, L.J. Antigenic relationships among porcine epidemic diarrhea virus and transmissible gastroenteritis virus strains. *J. Virol.* **2015**, *89*, 3332–3342. [CrossRef] [PubMed]
25. Gimenez-Lirola, L.G.; Zhang, J.; Carrillo-Avila, J.A.; Chen, Q.; Magtoto, R.; Poonsuk, K.; Baum, D.H.; Piñeyro, P.; Zimmerman, J. Reactivity of Porcine Epidemic Diarrhea Virus Structural Proteins to Antibodies against Porcine Enteric Coronaviruses: Diagnostic Implications. *J. Clin. Microbiol.* **2017**, *55*, 1426–1436. [CrossRef] [PubMed]
26. Xie, W.; Ao, C.; Yang, Y.; Liu, Y.; Liang, R.; Zeng, Z.; Ye, G.; Xiao, S.; Fu, Z.F.; Dong, W.; et al. Two critical N-terminal epitopes of the nucleocapsid protein contribute to the cross-reactivity between porcine epidemic diarrhea virus and porcine transmissible gastroenteritis virus. *J. Gen. Virol.* **2019**, *100*, 206–216. [CrossRef]
27. Bernard, S.; Bottreau, E.; Aynaud, J.M.; Have, P.; Szymansky, J. Natural infection with the porcine respiratory coronavirus induces protective lactogenic immunity against transmissible gastroenteritis. *Vet. Microbiol.* **1989**, *21*, 1–8. [CrossRef]
28. Pan, Y.; Tian, X.; Qin, P.; Wang, B.; Zhao, P.; Yang, Y.-L.; Wang, L.; Wang, D.; Song, Y.; Zhang, X.; et al. Discovery of a novel swine enteric alphacoronavirus (SeACoV) in southern China. *Vet. Microbiol.* **2017**, *211*, 15–21. [CrossRef]
29. Wang, X.; Fang, L.; Liu, S.; Ke, W.; Wang, D.; Peng, G.; Xiao, S. Susceptibility of porcine IPI-2I intestinal epithelial cells to infection with swine enteric coronaviruses. *Vet. Microbiol.* **2019**, *233*, 21–27. [CrossRef]
30. Marthaler, D.; Raymond, L.; Jiang, Y.; Collins, J.; Rossow, K.; Rovira, A. Rapid detection, complete genome sequencing, and phylogenetic analysis of porcine deltacoronavirus. *Emerg. Infect. Dis.* **2014**, *20*, 1347–1350. [CrossRef]
31. Cong, Y.; Ulasli, M.; Schepers, H.; Mauthe, M.; V'Kovski, P.; Kriegenburg, F.; Thiel, V.; de Haan, C.A.M.; Reggiori, F. Nucleocapsid protein recruitment to replication-transcription complexes plays a crucial role in coronaviral life cycle. *J. Virol.* **2019**, *JVI*, 01925-19. [CrossRef] [PubMed]
32. Leung, D.T.M.; Tam, F.C.H.; Ma, C.H.; Chan, P.K.S.; Cheung, J.L.K.; Niu, H.; Tam, J.S.L.; Lim, P.L. Antibody response of patients with severe acute respiratory syndrome (SARS) targets the viral nucleocapsid. *J. Infect. Dis.* **2004**, *190*, 379–386. [CrossRef] [PubMed]
33. Yang, W.; Chen, W.; Huang, J.; Jin, L.; Zhou, Y.; Chen, J.; Zhang, N.; Wu, D.; Sun, E.; Liu, G. Generation, identification, and functional analysis of monoclonal antibodies against porcine epidemic diarrhea virus nucleocapsid. *Appl. Microbiol. Biotechnol.* **2019**, *103*, 3705–3714. [CrossRef] [PubMed]

34. Chang, C.-Y.; Cheng, I.-C.; Chang, Y.-C.; Tsai, P.-S.; Lai, S.-Y.; Huang, Y.-L.; Jeng, C.-R.; Pang, V.F.; Chang, H.-W. Identification of Neutralizing Monoclonal Antibodies Targeting Novel Conformational Epitopes of the Porcine Epidemic Diarrhoea Virus Spike Protein. *Sci. Rep.* **2019**, *9*, 2529. [CrossRef] [PubMed]
35. Van Regenmortel, M.H.V. Mapping Epitope Structure and Activity: From One-Dimensional Prediction to Four-Dimensional Description of Antigenic Specificity. *Methods* **1996**, *9*, 465–472. [CrossRef] [PubMed]
36. Barlow, D.J.; Edwards, M.S.; Thornton, J.M. Continuous and discontinuous protein antigenic determinants. *Nature* **1986**, *322*, 747–748. [CrossRef]
37. Potocnakova, L.; Bhide, M.; Pulzova, L.B. An Introduction to B-Cell Epitope Mapping and In Silico Epitope Prediction. *J. Immunol. Res.* **2016**, *2016*, 6760830. [CrossRef]
38. Li, W.; Hulswit, R.J.G.; Kenney, S.P.; Widjaja, I.; Jung, K.; Alhamo, M.A.; van Dieren, B.; van Kuppeveld, F.J.M.; Saif, L.J.; Bosch, B.-J. Broad receptor engagement of an emerging global coronavirus may potentiate its diverse cross-species transmissibility. *Proc. Natl. Acad. Sci. USA* **2018**, *115*, E5135–E5143. [CrossRef]
39. Lau, S.K.P.; Wong, E.Y.M.; Tsang, C.-C.; Ahmed, S.S.; Au-Yeung, R.K.H.; Yuen, K.-Y.; Wernery, U.; Woo, P.C.Y. Discovery and Sequence Analysis of Four Deltacoronaviruses from Birds in the Middle East Reveal Interspecies Jumping with Recombination as a Potential Mechanism for Avian-to-Avian and Avian-to-Mammalian Transmission. *J. Virol.* **2018**, *92*, e00265-18. [CrossRef]
40. Li, C.; Bai, X.; Meng, R.; Shaozhou, W.; Zhang, Q.; Hua, R.; Liu, J.-H.; Liu, M.; Zhang, Y. Identification of a New Broadly Cross-reactive Epitope within Domain III of the Duck Tembusu Virus E Protein. *Sci. Rep.* **2016**, *6*, 36288. [CrossRef]
41. Chen, Q.; Wang, L.; Yang, C.; Zheng, Y.; Gauger, P.C.; Anderson, T.; Harmon, K.M.; Zhang, J.; Yoon, K.-J.; Main, R.G.; et al. The emergence of novel sparrow deltacoronaviruses in the United States more closely related to porcine deltacoronaviruses than sparrow deltacoronavirus HKU17. *Emerg. Microbes Infect.* **2018**, *7*, 105. [CrossRef] [PubMed]
42. Zhou, P.; Fan, H.; Lan, T.; Yang, X.-L.; Shi, W.-F.; Zhang, W.; Zhu, Y.; Zhang, Y.-W.; Xie, Q.-M.; Mani, S.; et al. Fatal swine acute diarrhoea syndrome caused by an HKU2-related coronavirus of bat origin. *Nature* **2018**, *556*, 255–258. [CrossRef] [PubMed]
43. Li, K.; Li, H.; Bi, Z.; Song, D.; Zhang, F.; Lei, D.; Luo, S.; Li, Z.; Gong, W.; Huang, D.; et al. Significant inhibition of re-emerged and emerging swine enteric coronavirus in vitro using the multiple shRNA expression vector. *Antivir. Res.* **2019**, *166*, 11–18. [CrossRef] [PubMed]
44. Ma, Y.; Zhang, Y.; Liang, X.; Oglesbee, M.; Krakowka, S.; Niehaus, A.; Wang, G.; Jia, A.; Song, H.; Li, J. Two-way antigenic cross-reactivity between porcine epidemic diarrhea virus and porcine deltacoronavirus. *Vet. Microbiol.* **2016**, *186*, 90–96. [CrossRef] [PubMed]
45. Guo, H.; Zhou, E.M.; Sun, Z.F.; Meng, X.J.; Halbur, P.G. Identification of B-cell epitopes in the capsid protein of avian hepatitis E virus (avian HEV) that are common to human and swine HEVs or unique to avian HEV. *J. Gen. Virol.* **2006**, *87*, 217–223. [CrossRef] [PubMed]
46. Chen, C.-W.; Chang, C.-Y. Peptide Scanning-assisted Identification of a Monoclonal Antibody-recognized Linear B-cell Epitope. *J. Vis. Exp. JoVE* **2017**, *121*, e55417. [CrossRef]
47. Chen, C.-W.; Wu, M.-S.; Huang, Y.-J.; Cheng, C.-A.; Chang, C.-Y. Recognition of Linear B-Cell Epitope of Betanodavirus Coat Protein by RG-M18 Neutralizing mAB Inhibits Giant Grouper Nervous Necrosis Virus (GGNNV) Infection. *PLoS ONE* **2015**, *10*, e0126121. [CrossRef]
48. Yang, J.; Yan, R.; Roy, A.; Xu, D.; Poisson, J.; Zhang, Y. The I-TASSER Suite: Protein structure and function prediction. *Nat. Methods* **2015**, *12*, 7–8. [CrossRef]
49. Roy, A.; Kucukural, A.; Zhang, Y. I-TASSER: A unified platform for automated protein structure and function prediction. *Nat. Protoc.* **2010**, *5*, 725–738. [CrossRef]
50. Zhang, Y. I-TASSER server for protein 3D structure prediction. *BMC Bioinform.* **2008**, *9*, 40. [CrossRef]

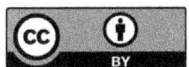

© 2020 by the authors. Licensee MDPI, Basel, Switzerland. This article is an open access article distributed under the terms and conditions of the Creative Commons Attribution (CC BY) license (http://creativecommons.org/licenses/by/4.0/).

MDPI
St. Alban-Anlage 66
4052 Basel
Switzerland
Tel. +41 61 683 77 34
Fax +41 61 302 89 18
www.mdpi.com

International Journal of Molecular Sciences Editorial Office
E-mail: ijms@mdpi.com
www.mdpi.com/journal/ijms

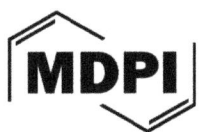

www.ingramcontent.com/pod-product-compliance
Lightning Source LLC
LaVergne TN
LVHW070137100526
838202LV00015B/1838